Comparative Effectiveness Review
Number 143

Imaging Techniques for the Diagnosis and Staging of Hepatocellular Carcinoma

Prepared for:
Agency for Healthcare Research and Quality
U.S. Department of Health and Human Services
540 Gaither Road
Rockville, MD 20850
www.ahrq.gov

Contract No. 290-2012-00014-I

Prepared by:
Pacific Northwest Evidence-based Practice Center
Portland, OR

Investigators:
Roger Chou, M.D., FACP
Carlos Cuevas, M.D.
Rongwei Fu, Ph.D.
Beth Devine, Ph.D., Pharm.D., M.B.A.
Ngoc Wasson, M.P.H.
Alexander Ginsburg, M.A., M.C.R.P.
Bernadette Zakher, M.B.B.S.
Miranda Pappas, M.A.
Elaine Graham, M.L.S.
Sean Sullivan, Ph.D.

AHRQ Publication No. 14(15)-EHC048-EF
October 2014

This report is based on research conducted by the Pacific Northwest Evidence-based Practice Center (EPC) under contract to the Agency for Healthcare Research and Quality (AHRQ), Rockville, MD (Contract No. 290-2012-00014-I). The findings and conclusions in this document are those of the authors, who are responsible for its contents; the findings and conclusions do not necessarily represent the views of AHRQ. Therefore, no statement in this report should be construed as an official position of AHRQ or of the U.S. Department of Health and Human Services.

The information in this report is intended to help health care decisionmakers—patients and clinicians, health system leaders, and policymakers, among others—make well informed decisions and thereby improve the quality of health care services. This report is not intended to be a substitute for the application of clinical judgment. Anyone who makes decisions concerning the provision of clinical care should consider this report in the same way as any medical reference and in conjunction with all other pertinent information, i.e., in the context of available resources and circumstances presented by individual patients.

This report may be used, in whole or in part, as the basis for development of clinical practice guidelines and other quality enhancement tools, or as a basis for reimbursement and coverage policies. AHRQ or U.S. Department of Health and Human Services endorsement of such derivative products may not be stated or implied.

This report may periodically be assessed for the urgency to update. If an assessment is done, the resulting surveillance report describing the methodology and findings will be found on the Effective Health Care Program Web site at www.effectivehealthcare.ahrq.gov. Search on the title of the report.

This document is in the public domain and may be used and reprinted without permission except those copyrighted materials that are clearly noted in the document. Further reproduction of those copyrighted materials is prohibited without the specific permission of the copyright holder.

Persons using assistive technology may not be able to fully access information in this report. For assistance contact EffectiveHealthCare@ahrq.hhs.gov.

None of the investigators have any affiliations or financial involvement that conflicts with the material presented in this report.

Suggested citation: Chou R, Cuevas C, Fu R, Devine B, Wasson N, Ginsburg A, Zakher B, Pappas M, Graham E, Sullivan S. Imaging Techniques for the Diagnosis and Staging of Hepatocellular Carcinoma. Comparative Effectiveness Review No. 143. (Prepared by the Pacific Northwest Evidence-based Practice Center under Contract No. 290-2012-00014-I.) AHRQ Publication No. 14(15)-EHC048-EF. Rockville, MD: Agency for Healthcare Research and Quality; October 2014. www.effectivehealthcare.ahrq.gov/reports/final.cfm.

Preface

The Agency for Healthcare Research and Quality (AHRQ), through its Evidence-based Practice Centers (EPCs), sponsors the development of systematic reviews to assist public- and private-sector organizations in their efforts to improve the quality of health care in the United States. These reviews provide comprehensive, science-based information on common, costly medical conditions, and new health care technologies and strategies.

Systematic reviews are the building blocks underlying evidence-based practice; they focus attention on the strength and limits of evidence from research studies about the effectiveness and safety of a clinical intervention. In the context of developing recommendations for practice, systematic reviews can help clarify whether assertions about the value of the intervention are based on strong evidence from clinical studies. For more information about AHRQ EPC systematic reviews, see www.effectivehealthcare.ahrq.gov/reference/purpose.cfm.

AHRQ expects that these systematic reviews will be helpful to health plans, providers, purchasers, government programs, and the health care system as a whole. Transparency and stakeholder input are essential to the Effective Health Care Program. Please visit the Web site (www.effectivehealthcare.ahrq.gov) to see draft research questions and reports or to join an email list to learn about new program products and opportunities for input.

We welcome comments on this systematic review. They may be sent by mail to the Task Order Officer named below at: Agency for Healthcare Research and Quality, 540 Gaither Road, Rockville, MD 20850, or by email to epc@ahrq.hhs.gov.

Richard G. Kronick, Ph.D.
Director
Agency for Healthcare Research and Quality

Yen-pin Chiang, Ph.D.
Acting Deputy Director
Center for Evidence and Practice
 Improvement
Agency for Healthcare Research and Quality

Stephanie Chang, M.D., M.P.H.
Director, EPC Program
Center for Evidence and Practice
 Improvement
Agency for Healthcare Research and Quality

Nahed El-Kassar, M.D., Ph.D.
Task Order Officer
Center for Evidence and Practice
 Improvement
Agency for Healthcare Research and Quality

Acknowledgments

The authors gratefully acknowledge the following individuals for their contributions to this project: Tracy Dana, M.L.S., for assistance with literature search strategy development; Leah Williams, B.S., for editorial support; our Task Order Officer, Nahed El-Kassar, M.D., Ph.D., for her support and guidance in developing this report; and our Associate Editor, Issa Dahabreh, M.D., M.S., for his review of the report and helpful comments.

Key Informants

In designing the study questions, the EPC consulted several Key Informants who represent the end-users of research. The EPC sought the Key Informant input on the priority areas for research and synthesis. Key Informants are not involved in the analysis of the evidence or the writing of the report. Therefore, in the end, study questions, design, methodological approaches, and/or conclusions do not necessarily represent the views of individual Key Informants.

Key Informants must disclose any financial conflicts of interest greater than $10,000 and any other relevant business or professional conflicts of interest. Because of their role as end-users, individuals with potential conflicts may be retained. The TOO and the EPC work to balance, manage, or mitigate any conflicts of interest.

The list of Key Informants who participated in developing this report follows:

James Adamson, M.D.
Arkansas Blue Cross and Blue Shield
Little Rock, AR

Jeffrey W. Clark, M.D.
Dana-Farber/Harvard Cancer Center
Massachusetts General Hospital
Boston, MA

Adrian Di Bisceglie, M.D., FACP
American Association for the Study of Liver Diseases
Saint Louis University School of Medicine
St. Louis, MO

Darla McCloskey, R.N., B.S.N., P.H.N.
Indian Health Service
Winnebago, NE

Morris Sherman, M.B., B.Ch., Ph.D.
University of Toronto
Toronto, Ontario, Canada

Jeffrey C. Weinreb, M.D., FACR, FISMRM, FSCBT/MR
American College of Radiology
Yale School of Medicine
New Haven, CT

A patient representative and a patient advocate (family member) also served as Key Informants.

Technical Expert Panel

In designing the study questions and methodology at the outset of this report, the EPC consulted several technical and content experts. Broad expertise and perspectives were sought. Divergent and conflicted opinions are common and perceived as healthy scientific discourse that results in a thoughtful, relevant systematic review. Therefore, in the end, study questions, design, methodologic approaches, and/or conclusions do not necessarily represent the views of individual technical and content experts.

Technical Experts must disclose any financial conflicts of interest greater than $10,000 and any other relevant business or professional conflicts of interest. Because of their unique clinical or content expertise, individuals with potential conflicts may be retained. The TOO and the EPC work to balance, manage, or mitigate any potential conflicts of interest identified.

The list of Technical Experts who participated in developing this report follows:

Mark Ghany, M.D.
National Institute of Diabetes and Digestive
 and Kidney Diseases
Bethesda, MD

Devan Kansagara, M.D.
Portland Veterans Affairs Evidence-based
 Synthesis Program
Portland, OR

Tom Oliver, B.A., C.R.A.
American Society of Clinical Oncology
Alexandria, VA

Morris Sherman, M.B., B.Ch., Ph.D.
University of Toronto
Toronto, Ontario, Canada

Claude Sirlin, M.D.
American College of Radiology
University of California, San Diego
La Jolla, CA

Christoph Wald, M.D., Ph.D.
Tufts University Medical School
Boston, MA

Peer Reviewers

Prior to publication of the final evidence report, EPCs sought input from independent Peer Reviewers without financial conflicts of interest. However, the conclusions and synthesis of the scientific literature presented in this report do not necessarily represent the views of individual reviewers.

Peer Reviewers must disclose any financial conflicts of interest greater than $10,000 and any other relevant business or professional conflicts of interest. Because of their unique clinical or content expertise, individuals with potential nonfinancial conflicts may be retained. The TOO and the EPC work to balance, manage, or mitigate any potential nonfinancial conflicts of interest identified.

The list of Peer Reviewers follows:

Mark Ghany, M.D.
National Institute of Diabetes and Digestive
 and Kidney Diseases
Bethesda, MD

Devan Kansagara, M.D.
Portland Veterans Affairs Evidence-based
Synthesis Program
Portland, OR

Tom Oliver, B.A., C.R.A.
American Society of Clinical Oncology
Alexandria, VA

Mark Russo, M.D., M.P.H.
Carolinas Medical Center and HealthCare
 System
Charlotte, NC

Morris Sherman, M.B., B.Ch., Ph.D.
University of Toronto
Toronto, Ontario, Canada

Mark Somerfield, Ph.D.
American Society of Clinical Oncology
Alexandria, VA

Christoph Wald, M.D., Ph.D.
Tufts University Medical School
Boston, MA

Stephanie Wilson, M.D., FRCPC
University of Calgary
Calgary, Alberta, Canada

Imaging Techniques for the Diagnosis and Staging of Hepatocellular Carcinoma

Structured Abstract

Objectives. Hepatocellular carcinoma (HCC) is the most common primary malignant neoplasm of the liver, and accurate diagnosis and staging of HCC are important for guiding treatment and other clinical decisions. A number of imaging modalities are available for detection of HCC in surveillance and nonsurveillance settings, evaluation of focal liver lesions to identify HCC, and staging of HCC. The purpose of this review is to compare the effectiveness of imaging techniques for HCC on test performance, clinical decisionmaking, clinical outcomes, and harms.

Data sources. Articles were identified from searches (from 1998 to 2013) of electronic databases, including Ovid MEDLINE®, Scopus, and the Cochrane Libraries. The searches were supplemented by reviewing reference lists and searching clinical trials registries.

Review methods. We used predefined criteria to determine study eligibility. We selected studies of ultrasound (US), computed tomography (CT), magnetic resonance imaging (MRI), and positron emission tomography (PET) that evaluated test performance for detection of HCC lesions, evaluation of focal liver lesions, or staging of HCC. We also included randomized trials and comparative observational studies on effects of imaging on clinical decisionmaking, clinical outcomes, and harms. The risk of bias (quality) of included studies was assessed, data were extracted, and results were summarized quantitatively (through meta-analysis) and qualitatively. Analyses were stratified by imaging type and unit of analysis (patient or HCC lesion). Additional analyses were conducted to evaluate the effects of the reference standard used and study, patient, tumor, and technical characteristics on estimates of test performance.

Results. Of the 4,846 citations identified at the title and abstract level, we screened and reviewed 851 full-length articles. A total of 281 studies were included, 274 of which evaluated test performance. No body of evidence was rated high strength of evidence due to methodological shortcomings, imprecision, and/or inconsistency. Moderate strength-of-evidence ratings were primarily limited to estimates of diagnostic accuracy for CT and MRI and to some direct comparisons involving US versus CT or MRI. Few studies evaluated diagnostic accuracy in surveillance settings, and the only two studies that directly compared imaging modalities found US without contrast associated with lower sensitivity and specificity than CT for detection of patients with HCC (low strength of evidence). For detection of HCC in nonsurveillance settings, based on studies that directly compared imaging modalities and using HCC lesions as the unit of analysis, sensitivity was lower for US without contrast than for CT or MRI (difference in sensitivity based on within-study comparisons of 0.11 to 0.22) (moderate strength of evidence) and sensitivity was higher for MRI than CT (pooled difference 0.09; 95% confidence interval [CI], 0.07 to 12) (moderate strength of evidence). For evaluation of detected focal liver lesions, we found no clear differences in sensitivity for identifying HCC between US with contrast, CT, and MRI (moderate strength of evidence). Across imaging modalities and indications for imaging, specificity was generally 0.85 or higher, but specificity was not reported in a number of studies. Sensitivity of ^{18}F-fluorodeoxyglucose (FDG) PET for identification of metastatic HCC lesions was 0.82 (95% CI, 0.72 to 0.90) (low strength of evidence), but sensitivity of FDG PET for intrahepatic lesions was poor (moderate strength of evidence). Evidence suggests that imaging strategies involving more than one imaging modality, in which a positive test is defined as typical imaging findings on one or more imaging modalities, is associated with higher sensitivity than a single test, with little effect on specificity (moderate strength of evidence).

Across imaging modalities, factors associated with lower estimates of sensitivity included use of explanted liver as the reference standard, use of HCC lesions as the unit of analysis, smaller HCC lesion size, and more well-differentiated HCC lesions. For MRI, hepatic-specific contrast agents were associated with slightly higher sensitivity than nonspecific contrast agents. For PET, evidence suggested higher sensitivity with use of PET/CT than with PET alone and with ^{11}C-acetate than with FDG.

Evidence on the comparative effects of imaging for HCC on clinical decisionmaking was extremely limited. The proportion of patients correctly assessed with CT for transplant eligibility based on Milan criteria ranged from 40 to 96 percent (moderate strength of evidence). Evidence on the effects of surveillance with imaging versus no surveillance on clinical outcomes was limited to a single randomized trial (low strength of evidence). Although it found an association between surveillance with US and alpha-fetoprotein (AFP) and decreased liver-specific mortality, the trial was conducted in China, potentially limiting applicability to screening in the United States, and there were important methodological shortcomings. Evidence on comparative harms associated with imaging was also extremely limited but indicates low rates of serious direct harms.

Conclusions. Several imaging modalities have relatively high sensitivity and specificity for diagnosis or staging of HCC, although test performance is suboptimal for small or well-differentiated HCC. Although there are some potential differences in test performance between different imaging modalities and techniques, more research is needed to understand the effects of such differences on clinical decisionmaking and clinical outcomes.

Contents

Executive Summary ES-1
Background and Objectives 1
Methods 10
   Topic Refinement and Review Protocol 10
   Searching for the Evidence 10
      Populations and Conditions of Interest 10
      Study Selection 10
      Data Abstraction and Data Management 12
   Assessment of Methodological Risk of Bias of Individual Studies 13
   Data Synthesis 14
      Approaches to Data Analysis 14
   Grading the Strength of Evidence for Individual Comparisons and Outcomes 15
   Assessing Applicability 16
   Peer Review and Public Commentary 16
Results 21
   Introduction 21
   Results of Literature Searches 21
   Key Question 1. What is the comparative effectiveness of available imaging-based strategies, used singly or in sequence, for detection of hepatocellular carcinoma among individuals in surveillance and nonsurveillance settings? 23
      Description of Included Studies 23
      Key Points 23
      Detailed Synthesis 29
   Key Question 2. What is the comparative effectiveness of imaging techniques, used singly, in combination, or in sequence, in diagnosing HCC among individuals in whom a focal liver lesion has been detected? 50
      Description of Included Studies 50
      Key Points 50
      Detailed Synthesis 53
   Key Question 3. What is the comparative effectiveness of imaging techniques, used singly, in combination, or in sequence, in staging hepatocellular carcinoma among patients diagnosed with hepatocellular carcinoma? 64
      Description of Included Studies 64
      Key Points 64
      Detailed Synthesis 66
Discussion 109
   Key Findings and Strength of Evidence 109
   Findings in Relationship to What Is Already Known 124
   Applicability 124
   Implications for Clinical and Policy Decisionmaking 125
   Limitations of the Review Process 127
   Limitations of the Evidence Base 128
   Research Gaps 129

Conclusions 130
References 131
Abbreviations and Acronyms 154

Tables
Table A. Summary of evidence for Key Question 1.a (detection): test performance ES-12
Table B. Summary of evidence for Key Question 1.a.i (detection): effects of reference standard on test performance (based on HCC lesions as the unit of analysis) ES-15
Table C. Summary of evidence for Key Question 1.a.ii (detection): effects of patient, tumor, technical, and other factors on test performance ES-15
Table D. Summary of evidence for Key Question 1.b (detection): clinical decisionmaking ES-17
Table E. Summary of evidence for Key Question 1.c (detection): clinical and patient-centered outcomes ES-17
Table F. Summary of evidence for Key Question 1.d (detection): harms ES-18
Table G. Summary of evidence for Key Question 2.a (evaluation of focal liver lesions): test performance ES-18
Table H. Summary of evidence for Key Question 2.a.i (evaluation of focal liver lesions): effects of reference standard on test performance (based on HCC lesions as the unit of analysis) ES-21
Table I. Summary of evidence for Key Question 2.a.ii (evaluation of focal liver lesions): effects of patient, tumor, technical, and other factors on test performance ES-21
Table J. Summary of evidence for Key Question 2.b (evaluation of focal liver lesions): clinical decisionmaking ES-22
Table K. Summary of evidence for Key Question 2.c (evaluation of focal liver lesions): clinical and patient-centered outcomes ES-22
Table L. Summary of evidence for Key Question 2.d (evaluation of focal liver lesions): harms ES-22
Table M. Summary of evidence for Key Question 3.a (staging): test performance ES-22
Table N. Summary of evidence for Key Question 3.a.i (staging): effects of reference standard on test performance ES-23
Table O. Summary of evidence for Key Question 3.a.ii (staging): effects of patient, tumor, and technical factors on test performance ES-23
Table P. Summary of evidence for Key Question 3.b (staging): clinical decisionmaking ES-23
Table Q. Summary of evidence for Key Question 3.c (staging): clinical and patient-centered outcomes ES-24
Table R. Summary of evidence for Key Question 3.d (staging): harms ES-24
Table 1. Imaging techniques used in the surveillance, diagnosis, and staging of hepatocellular carcinoma 7
Table 2. Recommended minimum technical specifications for dynamic contrast-enhanced computed tomography (CT) of the liver 8
Table 3. Recommended minimum technical specifications for dynamic contrast-enhanced MR imaging of the liver 9
Table 4. Search strategy—Ovid MEDLINE® (1998–2013) 17
Table 5. Inclusion and exclusion criteria by Key Question 18
Table 6. Test performance of ultrasound imaging for identification and diagnosis of hepatocellular carcinoma 73

Table 7. Test performance of computed tomography imaging for identification of intrahepatic and extrahepatic hepatocellular carcinoma 77
Table 8. Test performance of magnetic resonance imaging for identification of intrahepatic and extrahepatic hepatocellular carcinoma 81
Table 9. Test performance of positron emission tomography for identification of intrahepatic and extrahepatic hepatocellular carcinoma 84
Table 10. Pooled direct (within-study) comparisons of test performance of imaging modalities for identification and diagnosis of hepatocellular carcinoma 87
Table 11. Comparisons of test performance for hepatocellular carcinoma of single compared with multiple modality imaging 91
Table 12. Pooled direct (within-study) comparisons of ultrasound for identification and diagnosis of hepatocellular carcinoma 93
Table 13. Direct comparisons of diagnostic accuracy according to lesion size <10, 10-20, and >20 mm 94
Table 14. Pooled direct (within-study) comparisons of computed tomography for identification and diagnosis of hepatocellular carcinoma 95
Table 15. Pooled direct (within-study) comparisons of magnetic resonance imaging for identification and diagnosis of hepatocellular carcinoma 96
Table 16. Pooled direct (within-study) comparisons of positron emission tomography for identification and diagnosis of hepatocellular carcinoma 98
Table 17. Test performance of ^{18}F-fluorodeoxyglucose positron emission tomography for hepatocellular carcinoma, stratified by lesion size 100
Table 18. Test performance of ^{18}F-fluorodeoxyglucose positron emission tomography for hepatocellular carcinoma, stratified by degree of tumor differentiation 100
Table 19. Studies on accuracy of imaging for differentiating hepatocellular carcinoma from other hepatic lesions 101
Table 20. Pooled direct (within-study) comparisons of test performance of one imaging modality versus another imaging modality for identification and diagnosis of hepatocellular carcinoma 104
Table 21. Accuracy of imaging for staging of hepatocellular carcinoma 107
Table 22. Test performance of ^{18}F-fluorodeoxyglucose positron emission tomography for metastatic hepatocellular carcinoma, stratified by location of metastasis 108
Table 23. Summary of evidence for Key Question 1.a (detection): test performance 112
Table 24. Summary of evidence for Key Question 1.a.i (detection): effects of reference standard on test performance (based on HCC lesions as the unit of analysis) 115
Table 25. Summary of evidence for Key Question 1.a.ii (detection): effects of patient, tumor, technical, and other factors on test performance 115
Table 26. Summary of evidence for Key Question 1.b (detection): clinical decisionmaking 117
Table 27. Summary of evidence for Key Question 1.c (detection): clinical and patient-centered outcomes 117
Table 28. Summary of evidence for Key Question 1.d (detection): harms 118
Table 29. Summary of evidence for Key Question 2.a (evaluation of focal liver lesions): test performance 119
Table 30. Summary of evidence for Key Question 2.a.i (evaluation of focal liver lesions): effects of reference standard on test performance (based on HCC lesions as the

unit of analysis) 121
Table 31. Summary of evidence for Key Question 2.a.ii (evaluation of focal liver lesions): effects of patient, tumor, technical, and other factors on test performance 121
Table 32. Summary of evidence for Key Question 2.b (evaluation of focal liver lesions): clinical decisionmaking 122
Table 33. Summary of evidence for Key Question 2.c (evaluation of focal liver lesions): clinical and patient-centered outcomes 122
Table 34. Summary of evidence for Key Question 2.d (evaluation of focal liver lesions): harms 122
Table 35. Summary of evidence for Key Question 3.a (staging): test performance 122
Table 36. Summary of evidence for Key Question 3.a.i (staging): effects of reference standard on test performance 123
Table 37. Summary of evidence for Key Question 3.a.ii (staging): effects of patient, tumor, and technical factors on test performance 123
Table 38. Summary of evidence for Key Question 3.b (staging): clinical decisionmaking 123
Table 39. Summary of evidence for Key Question 3.c (staging): clinical and patient-centered outcomes 124
Table 40. Summary of evidence for Key Question 3.d (staging): harms 124
Table 41. Post-test probability of HCC with different imaging modalities in detection of HCC or for evaluation of focal liver lesions 126

Figures
Figure A. Analytic framework—detection (Key Question 1) ES-3
Figure B. Analytic framework—evaluation of focal liver lesions (Key Question 2) ES-4
Figure C. Analytic framework—staging (Key Question 3) ES-5
Figure 1. Analytic framework—detection (Key Question 1) 5
Figure 2. Analytic framework—evaluation of focal liver lesions (Key Question 2) 5
Figure 3. Analytic framework—staging (Key Question 3) 6
Figure 4. Study flow diagram 22
Figure 5. Test performance of ultrasound without contrast for detection of patients with hepatocellular carcinoma in surveillance settings 30
Figure 6. Test performance of ultrasound without contrast for detection of patients with hepatocellular carcinoma in nonsurveillance settings 31
Figure 7. Sensitivity of ultrasound without contrast for detection of hepatocellular carcinoma lesions in nonsurveillance settings 32
Figure 8. Sensitivity of ultrasound with contrast for detection of hepatocellular carcinoma lesions in nonsurveillance settings 33
Figure 9. Test performance of CT for detection of patients with hepatocellular carcinoma in nonsurveillance settings 35
Figure 10. Test performance of CT for detection of hepatocellular carcinoma lesions in nonsurveillance settings 36
Figure 11. Test performance of MRI for detection of patients with hepatocellular carcinoma in nonsurveillance settings 37
Figure 12. Test performance of MRI for detection of hepatocellular carcinoma lesions in nonsurveillance settings 38
Figure 13. Test performance of FDG PET for detection of patients with hepatocellular carcinoma in nonsurveillance settings 40

Figure 14. Test performance of FDG PET for detection of hepatocellular carcinoma lesions in nonsurveillance settings 41
Figure 15. Sensitivity of ^{11}C-acetate PET for detection of patients with hepatocellular carcinoma in nonsurveillance settings 42
Figure 16. Sensitivity of ^{11}C-acetate PET for detection of hepatocellular carcinoma lesions in nonsurveillance settings 42
Figure 17. Test performance of ultrasound with contrast in evaluation of focal liver lesions for identification of patients with hepatocellular carcinoma 54
Figure 18. Test performance of ultrasound with contrast for evaluation of focal liver lesions for identification of hepatocellular carcinoma lesions 55
Figure 19. Test performance of CT in evaluation of focal liver lesions for identification of patients with hepatocellular carcinoma 57
Figure 20. Test performance of CT in evaluation of focal liver lesions for hepatocellular carcinoma lesions 58
Figure 21. Test performance of MRI in evaluation of focal liver lesions for patients with hepatocellular carcinoma 60
Figure 22. Test performance of MRI in evaluation of focal liver lesions for hepatocellular carcinoma lesions 61
Figure 23. Test performance of FDG PET for detection of patients with metastatic hepatocellular carcinoma 68
Figure 24. Test performance of FDG PET for detection of metastatic hepatocellular carcinoma lesions 69

Appendixes
Appendix A. Included Studies
Appendix B. Excluded Studies
Appendix C. Risk of Bias
Appendix D. Evidence Table: Diagnostic Accuracy Studies of Ultrasound Imaging
Appendix E. Evidence Table: Diagnostic Accuracy Studies of Computed Tomography Imaging
Appendix F. Evidence Table: Diagnostic Accuracy Studies of Magnetic Resonance Imaging
Appendix G. Evidence Table: Diagnostic Accuracy Studies of Positron Emission Tomography Imaging
Appendix H. Evidence Table: Patient Outcomes for Staging (Randomized Controlled Trials)
Appendix I. Evidence Table: Comparative Effectiveness of Imaging Strategies on Clinical Decisionmaking and Patient Outcomes (Cohort Studies)
Appendix J. Strength of Evidence
Appendix K. Appendix References

Executive Summary

Background and Objectives

Hepatocellular carcinoma (HCC) is the most common primary malignant neoplasm of the liver, usually developing in individuals with chronic liver disease or cirrhosis. Worldwide, it is the fifth most common cancer and the third most common cause of cancer death.[1] There were 156,940 deaths attributed to liver and intrahepatic bile duct cancer in the United States in 2011, with 221,130 new cases diagnosed.[2] The lifetime risk of developing liver and intrahepatic bile duct cancer in the United States is about 1 in 132, with an age-adjusted incidence rate of 7.3 per 100,000 people per year.[3]

The American Association for the Study of Liver Diseases (AASLD) recommends surveillance for the following groups at high risk for developing HCC: Asian male hepatitis B virus (HBV) carriers age 40 and older, Asian female HBV carriers age 50 and older, HBV carriers with a family history of HCC, African/North American Black HBV carriers, HBV or hepatitis C virus carriers with cirrhosis, all individuals with other causes for cirrhosis (including alcoholic cirrhosis), and patients with stage 4 primary biliary cirrhosis.[4]

The natural history of HCC is variable, but it is often an aggressive tumor associated with poor survival without treatment.[5] When diagnosed early, HCC may be amenable to potentially curative therapy. The three phases of pretherapy evaluation of HCC are detection, further evaluation of focal liver lesions, and staging.[4] Detection often occurs in the setting of surveillance or in the use of periodic testing in people without HCC to identify lesions in the liver that are clinically suspicious for HCC.[4] The evaluation phase involves the use of additional tests (radiological and/or histopathological) to confirm that a focal liver lesion is indeed HCC. Staging determines the extent and severity of a person's cancer to inform prognosis and treatment decisions. A number of staging systems are available, including the widely used TNM (tumor, node, metastasis) staging system and the more recent Barcelona Clinic Liver Cancer (BCLC) staging system,[6] which has become the de facto staging reference standard;[4] the Milan criteria have been used to identify patients likely to experience better post-transplantation outcomes, although other methods have been proposed.[7]

A number of imaging techniques are available to detect the presence of lesions, evaluate focal liver lesions, and determine the stage of the disease. They include ultrasound (US), computed tomography (CT), magnetic resonance imaging (MRI), and positron emission tomography (PET). Understanding the diagnostic accuracy of imaging methods and how they affect clinical decisionmaking, and ultimately patient outcomes, is a challenge. Imaging techniques may be used alone, in various combinations or algorithms, and/or with liver-specific biomarkers, resulting in many potential comparisons. Technical aspects of imaging methods are complex, and they are continuously evolving.

Diagnostic accuracy studies use different reference standards, such as explanted liver specimens from patients undergoing transplantation, percutaneous or surgical biopsy, imaging, clinical followup, or combinations of these methods. Use of these different reference standards introduces heterogeneity that may limit comparisons of techniques. Reference standards also are susceptible to misclassification due to sampling error, inadequate specimens, insufficient followup, or other factors. Other considerations may impact the diagnostic accuracy or clinical utility of imaging strategies; they include risk factors for HCC and lesion characteristics, such as tumor size or degree of differentiation, severity of hepatic fibrosis, and etiology of liver disease.

Accurate diagnosis and staging of HCC are critical for providing optimal patient care. However, clinical uncertainty remains regarding optimal imaging strategies due to the factors described above. The purpose of this report is to comprehensively review the comparative effectiveness and diagnostic performance of different imaging modalities and strategies for detection of HCC, evaluation of focal liver lesions to identify HCC, and staging of HCC.

Scope and Key Questions

The Key Questions and corresponding analytic frameworks used to guide this report are shown below. Separate analytic frameworks address detection (Figure A), diagnosis (Figure B), and staging (Figure C). The analytic frameworks show the target populations, interventions (imaging tests), and outcomes (diagnostic accuracy, clinical decisionmaking, clinical outcomes, and harms) that we examined.

Key Question 1. What is the comparative effectiveness of available imaging-based strategies, used singly or in sequence, for detection of hepatocellular carcinoma among individuals in surveillance and nonsurveillance settings?

   a. What is the comparative test performance of imaging-based strategies for detecting HCC?
      i. How is a particular technique's test performance modified by use of various reference standards (e.g., explanted liver samples, histological diagnosis, or clinical and imaging followup)?
      ii. How is the comparative effectiveness modified by patient (e.g., severity of liver disease, underlying cause of liver disease, body mass index, age, sex, race), tumor (e.g., tumor diameter, degree of differentiation, location), technical, or other factors (e.g., results of biomarker tests, setting)?
   b. What is the comparative effectiveness of imaging-based strategies on intermediate outcomes related to clinical decisionmaking (e.g., use of subsequent diagnostic tests and treatments)?
   c. What is the comparative effectiveness of imaging-based strategies on clinical and patient-centered outcomes?
   d. What are the adverse effects or harms associated with imaging-based surveillance strategies?

Key Question 2. What is the comparative effectiveness of imaging techniques, used singly, in combination, or in sequence, in diagnosing hepatocellular carcinoma among individuals in whom a focal liver lesion has been detected?

   a. What is the comparative test performance of imaging techniques for diagnosing HCC in patients with a focal liver lesion?
      i. How is a particular technique's test performance modified by use of various reference standards (e.g., explanted liver samples, histological diagnosis, or clinical imaging and followup)?
      ii. How is the comparative effectiveness modified by patient, tumor, technical, or other factors?
   b. What is the comparative effectiveness of the various imaging techniques on intermediate outcomes related to clinical decisionmaking?

c. What is the comparative effectiveness of the various imaging techniques on clinical and patient-centered outcomes?
d. What are the adverse effects or harms associated with imaging-based diagnostic strategies?

Key Question 3. What is the comparative effectiveness of imaging techniques, used singly, in combination, or in sequence, in staging hepatocellular carcinoma among patients diagnosed with hepatocellular carcinoma?

a. What is the comparative test performance of imaging techniques to predict HCC tumor stage?
   i. How is a particular technique's test performance modified by use of various reference standards (e.g., explanted liver samples, histological diagnosis, or clinical and imaging followup)?
   ii. How is the comparative effectiveness modified by patient, tumor, technical, or other factors?
b. What is the comparative test performance effectiveness of imaging techniques on intermediate outcomes related to clinical decisionmaking?
c. What is the comparative effectiveness of imaging techniques on clinical and patient-centered outcomes?
d. What are the adverse effects or harms associated with imaging-based staging strategies?

Figure A. Analytic framework—detection (Key Question 1)

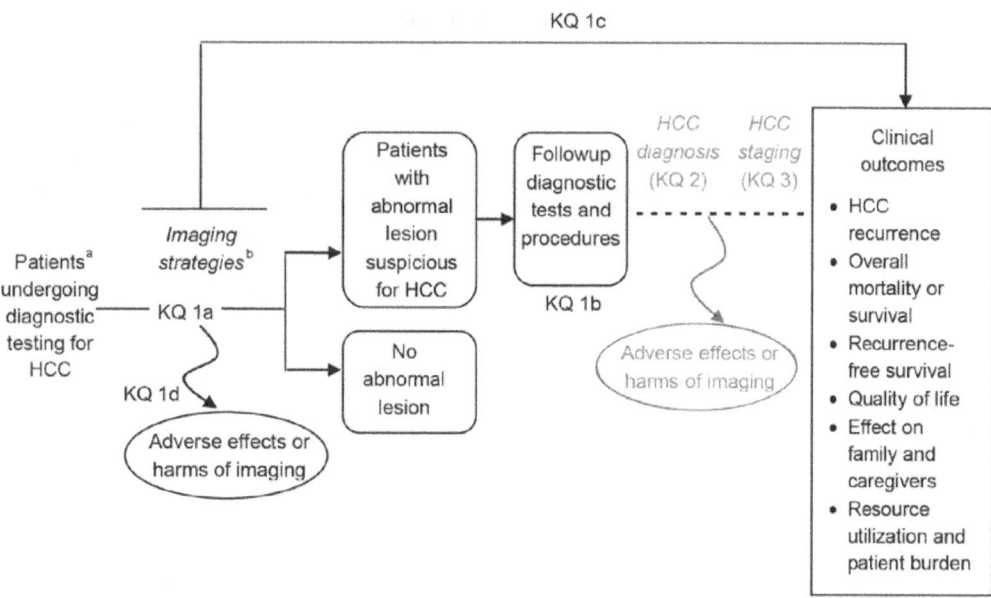

HCC = hepatocellular carcinoma; KQ = Key Question.
[a] Potential modifiers of test performance include patient (e.g., severity of liver disease, underlying cause of liver disease, body mass index, age, sex, race), tumor (e.g., tumor diameter, degree of differentiation, location), technical, and other factors (e.g., biomarker levels, setting).
[b] Imaging techniques are used singly, in combination, or in sequence with or without biomarkers used as modifiers.
Note: Shaded figure elements illustrate the relationship of KQ 1 to KQ 2 and KQ 3.

Figure B. Analytic framework—evaluation of focal liver lesions (Key Question 2)

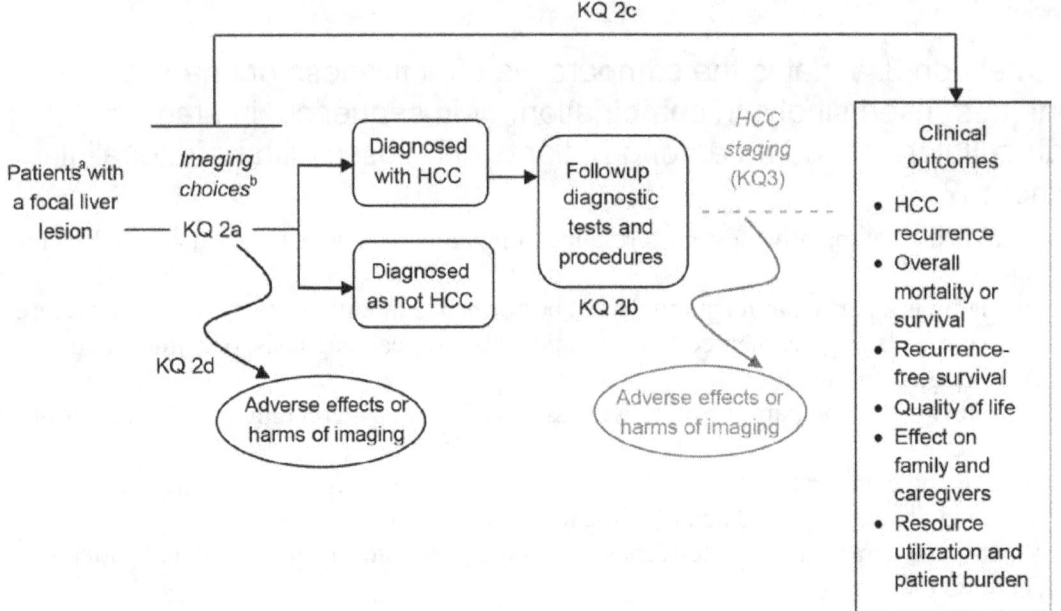

HCC = hepatocellular carcinoma; KQ = Key Question.
Note: Shaded elements show the relationship of KQ 2 to KQ 3.

[a] Potential modifiers of test performance include patient (e.g., severity of liver disease, underlying cause of liver disease, body mass index, age, sex, race), tumor (e.g., tumor diameter, degree of differentiation, location), technical, and other factors (e.g., biomarker levels, setting).
[b] Imaging techniques are used singly, in combination, or in sequence with or without biomarkers used as modifiers.

Figure C. Analytic framework—staging (Key Question 3)

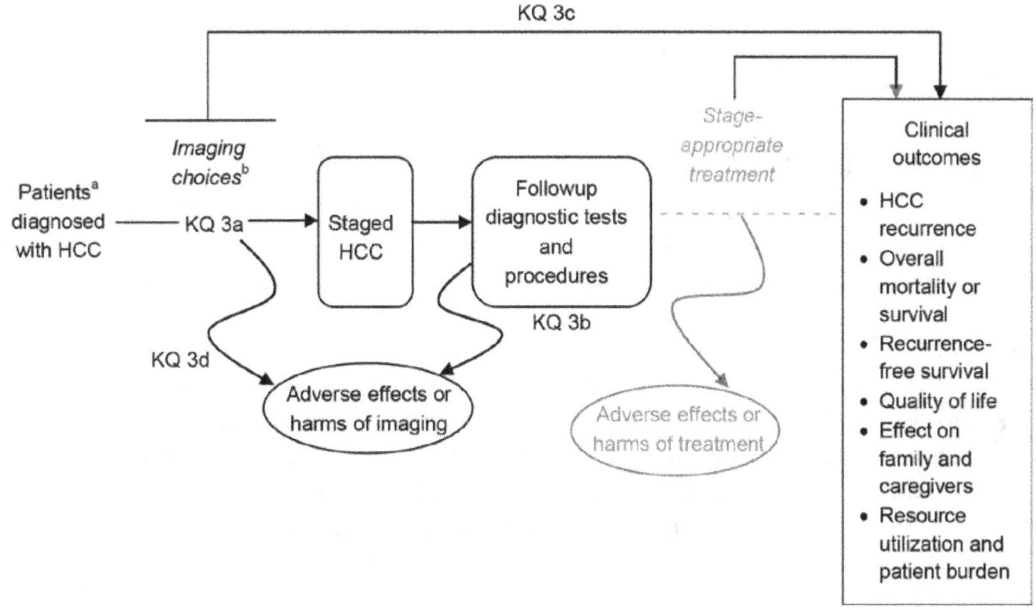

```
                                    KQ 3c
         ┌──────────────────────────────────────────────────────┐
         │                                                      ▼
                        Imaging          Stage-         ┌──────────────┐
                        choices ᵇ      appropriate      │   Clinical   │
  Patientsᵃ                             treatment       │   outcomes   │
  diagnosed ──── KQ 3a ──► Staged ──► Followup  ─ ─ ─ ─►│ • HCC        │
  with HCC                  HCC      diagnostic tests   │   recurrence │
                                     and procedures    │ • Overall    │
                    KQ 3d              KQ 3b            │   mortality or│
                      ╲                  ╲              │   survival   │
                       ▼                  ▼             │ • Recurrence-│
                 ╭──────────────╮   ╭──────────────╮    │   free survival│
                 │ Adverse effects│   │ Adverse effects│ │ • Quality of life│
                 │ or harms of  │   │ or harms of  │    │ • Effect on  │
                 │ imaging      │   │ treatment    │    │   family and │
                 ╰──────────────╯   ╰──────────────╯    │   caregivers │
                                                        │ • Resource   │
                                                        │   utilization and│
                                                        │   patient burden│
                                                        └──────────────┘
```

ᵃ Potential modifiers of test performance include patient (e.g., severity of liver disease, underlying cause of liver disease, body mass index, age, sex, race), tumor (e.g., tumor diameter, degree of differentiation, location), technical, and other factors (e.g., biomarker levels, setting).
ᵇ Imaging techniques are used singly, in combination, or in sequence with or without biomarkers used as modifiers.
Note: Shaded elements show subsequent treatment that may follow detection (KQ 1), diagnosis (KQ 2), and staging (KQ 3).
HCC = hepatocellular carcinoma; KQ = Key Question.

Methods

The methods for this systematic review follow the methods suggested in the AHRQ Effective Health Care Program methods guides.[8,9]

Searching for the Evidence

For the primary literature, we searched Ovid MEDLINE®, Scopus, Evidence-Based Medicine Reviews (Ovid), the Cochrane Central Register of Controlled Trials, the Cochrane Database of Systematic Reviews, the Database of Abstracts of Reviews of Effects, and the Health Technology Assessment Database from 1998 to December 2013. We searched for unpublished studies in clinical trial registries (ClinicalTrials.gov, Current Controlled Trials, ClinicalStudyResults.org, and the World Health Organization International Clinical Trials Registry Platform), regulatory documents (U.S. Food and Drug Administration Medical Devices Registration and Listing), and individual product Web sites. Scientific information packets (SIPs) were solicited through the *Federal Register*.[10] We also searched the reference lists of relevant studies and previous systematic reviews for additional studies.

Study Selection

We developed criteria for inclusion and exclusion of studies based on the Key Questions and the populations, interventions, comparators, outcomes, timing, and setting (PICOTS) of interest. Titles and abstracts from all searches were reviewed for inclusion. Full-text articles were obtained for all articles identified as potentially meeting inclusion criteria. Papers were selected for inclusion in our review if they were about imaging for HCC with US (with or without contrast), CT with contrast, or MRI with contrast; were relevant to one or more Key Questions; met the predefined inclusion criteria; and reported original data.

We excluded studies that reported diagnostic accuracy of imaging for non-HCC malignant lesions; studies of nonspiral CT and MRI using machines ≤1.0 T, as these are considered outdated techniques;[11] studies that evaluated MRI with agents that are no longer produced commercially and are unavailable for clinical use; studies of CT arterial portography and CT hepatic angiography; studies published prior to 1998; studies in which imaging commenced prior to 1995, unless those studies reported use of imaging meeting minimum technical criteria; and studies of intraoperative US. We also excluded studies published only as conference abstracts, non–English-language articles, and studies of nonhuman subjects.

For studies of test performance (e.g., sensitivity, specificity, and likelihood ratios), we included studies that evaluated one or more imaging methods against a reference standard. Reference standards were histopathology (based on explanted liver or nonexplant histological specimen from surgery or percutaneous biopsy), imaging plus clinical followup (e.g., lesion growth), or some combination of these standards. We excluded studies in which the reference standard involved one of the imaging tests under evaluation and that did not perform clinical followup and studies that had no reference standard (i.e., reported the number of lesions identified with an imaging technique but did not evaluate accuracy against another reference technique).

To assess comparative effects of imaging on clinical outcomes (e.g., mortality, HCC recurrence, quality of life, and harms), we included randomized controlled trials that compared different imaging modalities or strategies. A systematic review funded by the Department of Veterans Affairs Evidence Synthesis Program on effects of screening for HCC on clinical outcomes is forthcoming and will include comparative observational studies.[12]

To assess comparative effects of imaging on intermediate outcomes related to clinical decisionmaking (e.g., subsequent diagnostic testing, treatments, or resource utilization), we included randomized trials and cohort studies that compared different imaging modalities or strategies.

Data Abstraction and Data Management

We extracted the following data from included studies into evidence tables using Excel spreadsheets: study design, year, setting, country, sample size, method of data collection (retrospective or prospective), eligibility criteria, population and clinical characteristics (including age, sex, race, underlying cause of liver disease, proportion of patients in sample with HCC, HCC lesion size, and proportion with cirrhosis), the number of imaging readers, criteria used for a positive test, and the reference standard used. We abstracted results for diagnostic accuracy, intermediate outcomes, and clinical outcomes, including results stratified according to patient, lesion, and imaging characteristics. Technical information for different imaging tests was abstracted.[11]

Assessment of Methodological Risk of Bias of Individual Studies

We assessed risk of bias (quality) for each study based on predefined criteria. Randomized trials and cohort studies were evaluated using criteria and methods developed by the U.S. Preventive Services Task Force.[13] These criteria were applied in conjunction with the approach recommended in the Agency for Healthcare Research and Quality (AHRQ) "Methods Guide for Effectiveness and Comparative Effectiveness Reviews."[8] Studies of diagnostic test performance were assessed using the approach recommended in the AHRQ "Methods Guide for Medical Test Reviews,"[9] which is based on methods developed by the Quality Assessment of Diagnostic Accuracy Studies (QUADAS) group.[14] Individual studies were rated as having "low," "moderate," or "high" risk of bias.

Data Synthesis

We performed meta-analyses on measures of test performance in order to help summarize data and obtain more precise estimates.[15] All quantitative analyses were conducted using SAS® 9.3 (SAS Institute Inc., Cary, NC). We pooled only studies that were clinically comparable and could provide a meaningful combined estimate (based on the variability among studies in design, patient population, imaging methods, and outcomes) and magnitude of effect size. We conducted separate analyses for each imaging modality, stratified according to the unit of analysis used (patients with HCC, HCC lesions, or liver segments with HCC) and analyzed studies of US with contrast separately from studies of US without contrast. For studies that used multiple readers, we averaged results across readers using the binomial specification of Proc NLMIXED on SAS.

We evaluated a number of potential sources of heterogeneity and modifiers of diagnostic accuracy. We performed analyses stratified according to the reference standard used and on domains related to risk of bias, aspects of study design (retrospective or prospective, use of a confidence rating scale), setting (based on country in which imaging was performed), and technical factors (such as scanner types, type of contrast or tracer used, use of recommended imaging phases, timing of delayed phase imaging, and section thickness). We also evaluated diagnostic accuracy in subgroups stratified according to HCC lesion size, degree of tumor differentiation, and tumor location, as well as patient characteristics such as severity of underlying liver disease, underlying cause of liver disease, and body mass index. Because of the effects of lesion size on estimates of diagnostic accuracy, subgroup analyses for each imaging modality were performed on the subgroup of studies that were not restricted to small (<2–3 cm) HCC lesions.

We performed separate analyses on the subset of studies that directly compared two or more imaging modalities or techniques in the same population against a common reference standard. Research indicates that results based on such direct comparisons differ from results based on noncomparative studies and may be better suited for evaluating comparative diagnostic test performance.[16]

We did not perform meta-analysis on staging accuracy and intermediate or clinical outcomes due to the small number of studies. Rather, we synthesized these studies qualitatively, using the methods described below for assessing the strength of evidence.

Grading the Strength of Evidence for Individual Comparisons and Outcomes

The strength of evidence for each Key Question was assessed by one researcher for each outcome described in the PICOTS using the approach described in the AHRQ "Methods Guide for Effectiveness and Comparative Effectiveness Reviews."[8] The strength of evidence pertains to the overall quality of each body of evidence and is based on the risk of bias (graded low, moderate, or high); the consistency of results between studies (graded consistent, inconsistent, or unknown/not applicable when only one study was available); the directness of the evidence linking the intervention and health outcomes (graded direct or indirect); and the precision of the estimate of effect, based on the number and size of studies and confidence intervals for the estimates (graded precise or imprecise). We did not assess studies of diagnostic test performance for publication bias using graphical or statistical methods because research indicates that such methods can be misleading. Rather, we searched for unpublished studies through searches of clinical trials registries and regulatory documents and by soliciting SIPs.

Assessing Applicability

We recorded factors important for understanding the applicability of studies, such as whether the publication adequately described the study population, the country in which the study was conducted, the prevalence of HCC in the patients who underwent imaging, the magnitude of differences in measures of diagnostic accuracy and clinical outcomes, and whether the imaging techniques were reasonably representative of standard practice.[17] We also recorded the funding source and role of the sponsor.

Results

The bulk of the available evidence addresses diagnostic accuracy of different imaging techniques for hepatocellular carcinoma. Few studies compared effects of different imaging modalities or strategies on clinical decisionmaking and clinical outcomes, and almost no studies reported harms.

Results of Literature Searches

We reviewed titles and abstracts of the 4,846 citations identified by literature searches. Of these, 851 articles appeared to meet inclusion criteria and were selected for further full-text review. Following review at the full-text level, a total of 281 studies met inclusion criteria.

We identified 274 studies that evaluated diagnostic accuracy of imaging tests. Of these, 70 evaluated US imaging, 134 evaluated CT, 129 evaluated MRI, and 32 evaluated PET; 28 studies evaluated more than one imaging modality. We rated 3 studies low risk of bias, 189 moderate risk of bias, and 89 high risk of bias. Almost all studies reported sensitivity, but only 130 reported specificity or provided data to calculate specificity. We found that 119 studies avoided use of a case-control design, 151 used blinded ascertainment, and 75 used a prospective design. More studies were conducted in Asia (182 studies) than in Australia, Canada, the United States, or Europe combined (92 studies). In 155 studies, imaging was conducted starting in or after 2003.

Data for outcomes other than measures of test performance were sparse. Seven studies reported comparative effects on clinical decisionmaking, three studies reported comparative clinical and patient-centered outcomes, and three studies reported harms associated with imaging for HCC.

Key Question 1. What is the comparative effectiveness of available imaging-based strategies, used singly or in sequence, for detection of HCC among individuals in surveillance and nonsurveillance settings?

Six studies evaluated diagnostic accuracy of imaging techniques for surveillance, and 182 studies reported diagnostic accuracy in nonsurveillance settings (e.g., imaging performed to assess detection rates in a series of patients undergoing treatment for HCC or patients with otherwise known prevalence of HCC prior to imaging). Four studies of PET evaluated accuracy specifically for identification of recurrent HCC. One randomized trial (rated high risk of bias) evaluated clinical outcomes associated with imaging-based surveillance versus no screening, and two trials evaluated clinical outcomes associated with different US surveillance intervals. No study compared effects of different imaging surveillance strategies on diagnostic thinking or clinical decisionmaking. Two studies reported harms associated with imaging for HCC. Tables A–F summarize the key findings and strength of evidence for these studies.

Key Question 2. What is the comparative effectiveness of imaging techniques, used singly, in combination, or in sequence, in diagnosing HCC among individuals in whom a focal liver lesion has been detected?

Fifty-four studies evaluated diagnostic accuracy of imaging tests in diagnosing HCC among individuals in whom an abnormal lesion has been detected, and 19 studies evaluated the accuracy of imaging tests for distinguishing HCC from another specific type of liver lesion. No study compared effects of different imaging modalities or strategies on diagnostic thinking or on clinical or patient-centered outcomes. One study reported harms. Tables G–L summarize the key findings and strength of evidence for these studies.

Key Question 3. What is the comparative effectiveness of imaging techniques, used singly, in combination, or in sequence, in staging HCC among patients diagnosed with HCC?

Six studies reported test performance of various imaging techniques for staging of patients with HCC based on TNM criteria. Ten studies reported test performance of PET for detection of metastatic disease. Seven studies reported effects of imaging on transplant decisions, and one study reported comparative effects of imaging on clinical and patient-centered outcomes. No study reported harms associated with imaging for HCC staging. Tables M–R summarize the key findings and strength of evidence for these studies.

Discussion

Key Findings and Strength of Evidence

The key findings of this review, including strength-of-evidence grades, are summarized in Tables A–R. The preponderance of evidence on imaging for HCC was in the area of diagnostic test performance. However, few studies evaluated test performance of imaging for HCC in true surveillance settings of patients at high risk for HCC, but without a prior diagnosis of HCC, undergoing periodic imaging. Among the limited evidence available in this setting, there was no clear difference between US without contrast and CT, based on across-study comparisons of sensitivity using either HCC lesions or patients with HCC as a unit of analysis. The strength of evidence is low for sensitivity. However, two studies that directly compared sensitivity of US without contrast and CT reported lower sensitivity with US for detection of patients with HCC.[18,19] The strength of evidence was also rated as low.

Many more studies evaluated test performance of imaging for HCC in populations of patients undergoing treatment such as liver transplantation, hepatic resection, or ablation therapy, or in series of patients previously diagnosed with HCC or with HCC and other liver conditions. Such studies were considered as part of Key Question 1 with studies of surveillance because they were not designed to further characterize previously identified HCC lesions (the focus of Key Question 2). Rather, their purpose was to evaluate test performance for lesion identification, therefore providing information that could potentially be extrapolated to surveillance. We analyzed these studies separately from studies conducted in true surveillance settings, given the differences in the reason for imaging and the populations evaluated, including a generally much higher prevalence of HCC, with some studies enrolling only patients with HCC. In these studies, sensitivity was lower for US without contrast than for CT or MRI, with a difference based on within-study (direct) comparisons that ranged from 0.11 to 0.22, using HCC lesions as the unit of analysis. This conclusion is graded moderate strength of evidence. MRI and CT performed similarly when patients with HCC were the unit of analysis, but sensitivity was higher for MRI than for CT when HCC lesions were the unit of analysis (pooled difference 0.09; 95% confidence interval, 0.07 to 12; moderate strength of evidence).

US with contrast did not perform better than US without contrast for identification of HCC[20,21] (low strength of evidence). This is probably related to the short duration in which microbubble contrast is present within the liver, so that it is not possible to perform a comprehensive contrast-enhanced examination of the liver.[22] Rather, the main use of US with contrast appears to be for evaluation of previously identified focal liver lesions.

For characterization of previously identified lesions, we found no clear differences in sensitivity between US with contrast, CT, and MRI (moderate strength of evidence). Although some evidence was available on the accuracy of imaging modalities for distinguishing between HCC and other (non-HCC) liver lesions, it was not possible to draw strong conclusions due to variability in the types of non-HCC lesions evaluated (regenerative nodules, dysplastic nodules, hypervascular pseudolesions, hemangiomas, etc.), small numbers of studies, and some inconsistency in findings.

Studies of patients with HCC were generally associated with somewhat higher sensitivity than studies that used HCC lesions as the unit of analysis. Studies that used explanted livers as the reference standard reported lower sensitivity than studies that used a nonexplant reference standard (moderate strength of evidence). Use of multiple reference standards poses a challenge to assessment of diagnostic accuracy.[23] Across imaging modalities, sensitivity was markedly lower for HCC lesions <2 cm versus those ≥2 cm (differences in sensitivity ranged from 0.30 to

0.39), and further declined for lesions <10 mm in diameter (moderate strength of evidence). Evidence also consistently indicated substantially lower sensitivity for well-differentiated lesions than moderately or poorly differentiated lesions (low strength of evidence).

Evidence on the effects of other patient, tumor, and technical factors on test performance was more limited (low strength of evidence). For US, there was no clear effect of use of Doppler, lesion depth, or body mass index on test performance. For CT, some evidence indicated higher sensitivity for studies that used a contrast rate of ≥3 ml/s than those with a contrast rate <3 ml/s, and higher sensitivity for studies that used delayed phase imaging. For MRI, hepatic-specific contrast agents were associated with slightly higher sensitivity than nonspecific contrast agents, but there were no clear effects of magnetic field strength (3.0 vs. 1.5 T), use of delayed phase imaging, timing of delayed phase imaging (≥120 seconds after administration of contrast or <120 s), section thickness (≤5 mm vs. >5 mm), or use of diffusion-weighted imaging. For identification of intrahepatic HCC lesions, limited evidence found PET with ^{11}C-acetate and other alternative tracers such as ^{18}F-fluorocholine and ^{18}F-fluorothymidine associated with substantially higher sensitivity than ^{18}F-fluorodeoxyglucose (FDG) PET. Sensitivity of FDG PET was lower than sensitivity of FDG PET/CT.

The limited available evidence suggests that using multiple imaging tests and defining a positive test as typical imaging findings on at least one imaging modality increases sensitivity without substantively reducing specificity (moderate strength of evidence).

Conclusions were generally robust on sensitivity and stratified analyses based on study factors such as setting (Asia vs. United States or Europe), prospective collection of data, interpretation of imaging findings blinded to results of the reference standard, avoidance of case-control design, and overall risk of bias.

Across analyses, specificity was generally high, with most pooled estimates around 0.85 or higher and few clear differences between imaging modalities. However, many studies did not report specificity and pooled estimates of specificity were frequently imprecise, precluding strong conclusions regarding comparative test performance. Since likelihood ratios are sensitive to small changes in estimates when the specificity is high, it was also difficult to draw strong conclusions regarding comparative diagnostic test performance based on differences in positive or negative likelihood ratios. Most likelihood ratio estimates fell into or near the "moderately useful" range (positive likelihood ratio of 5–10 and negative likelihood ratio of 0.1–0.2), with the exception of FDG PET for identification of intrahepatic HCC lesions, which was associated with a negative likelihood ratio of 0.50.

Evidence regarding the accuracy of imaging modalities for staging was primarily limited to CT. Most studies addressed accuracy of CT, with 28 to 58 percent correctly staged based on TNM criteria and somewhat more understaging (25% to 52%) than overstaging (2% to 27%) (moderate strength of evidence). Studies on the accuracy of imaging for identifying metastatic HCC disease were primarily limited to FDG PET or PET/CT, with a pooled sensitivity of 0.82 to 0.85 (low strength of evidence).

Evidence on the comparative effectiveness of imaging for HCC on diagnostic thinking, use of subsequent procedures, or resource utilization was extremely limited. In studies that compared the accuracy of transplant decisions based on CT against primarily explanted livers as the reference standard, the proportion correctly assessed for transplant eligibility based on Milan criteria ranged from 40 to 96 percent (moderate strength of evidence). Evidence on the effects of surveillance with imaging versus no surveillance on clinical outcomes was limited to a single randomized trial[24] (low strength of evidence).

Evidence on comparative harms associated with imaging was also extremely limited, with no study measuring downstream harms related to false-positive tests or subsequent workup, or potential harms related to labeling or psychological effects. A handful of studies reported low rates of serious direct harms (e.g., allergic reactions) associated with imaging. However, evidence on administration of contrast for radiological procedures in general also suggests a low rate of serious adverse events. No study on US with contrast reported harms. Although PET and CT are associated with risk of radiation exposure, no study of imaging for HCC was designed to evaluate potential long-term clinical outcomes associated with radiation exposure.

Table A. Summary of evidence for Key Question 1.a (detection): Test performance

Subquestion	Imaging Modality or Comparison	Strength of Evidence	Summary
Surveillance settings *Unit of analysis: patients with HCC*	US without contrast	Sensitivity: Low Specificity: Low	Sensitivity was 0.78 (95% CI, 0.60 to 0.89; 4 studies) and specificity 0.89 (95% CI, 0.80 to 0.94; 3 studies), for an LR+ of 6.8 (95% CI, 4.2 to 11) and LR- of 0.25 (95% CI, 0.13 to -0.46).
Surveillance settings *Unit of analysis: patients with HCC*	CT	Sensitivity: Low Specificity: Low	Sensitivity was 0.84 (95% CI, 0.59 to 0.95; 2 studies) and specificity 0.999 (95% CI, 0.86 to 0.99; 2 studies), for an LR+ of 60 (95% CI, 5.9 to 622) and LR- of 0.16 (95% CI, 0.06 to 0.47).
Surveillance settings *Unit of analysis: patients with HCC*	MRI or PET	Insufficient	No evidence
Surveillance settings *Unit of analysis: HCC lesions*	US without contrast	Sensitivity: Low Specificity: Insufficient	Sensitivity was 0.60 (95% CI, 0.24 to 0.87; 1 study); specificity was not reported.
Surveillance settings *Unit of analysis: HCC lesions*	CT	Sensitivity: Low Specificity: Insufficient	Sensitivity was 0.62 (95% CI, 0.46 to 0.76; 1 study).
Surveillance settings *Unit of analysis: HCC lesions*	MRI or PET	Insufficient	No evidence
Nonsurveillance settings *Unit of analysis: patients with HCC*	US without contrast	Sensitivity: Low Specificity: Low	Sensitivity was 0.73 (95% CI, 0.46 to 0.90; 8 studies) and specificity 0.93 (95% CI, 0.85 to 0.97; 6 studies), for an LR+ of 11 (95% CI, 5.4 to 21) and LR- of 0.29 (95% CI, 0.13 to 0.65).
Nonsurveillance settings *Unit of analysis: patients with HCC*	CT	Sensitivity: Moderate Specificity: Moderate	Sensitivity was 0.83 (95% CI, 0.75 to 0.89; 16 studies) and specificity 0.92 (95% CI, 0.86 to 0.96; 11 studies), for an LR+ of 11 (95% CI, 5.6 to 20) and LR- of 0.19 (95% CI, 0.12 to 0.28).
Nonsurveillance settings *Unit of analysis: patients with HCC*	MRI	Sensitivity: Moderate Specificity: Moderate	Sensitivity was 0.85 (95% CI, 0.76 to 0.91; 10 studies) and specificity 0.90 (95% CI, 0.81 to 0.94; 8 studies), for an LR+ of 8.1 (95% CI, 4.3 to 15) and LR- of 0.17 (95% CI, 0.10 to 0.28).

Table A. Summary of evidence for Key Question 1.a (detection): Test performance (continued)

Subquestion	Imaging Modality or Comparison	Strength of Evidence	Summary
Nonsurveillance settings *Unit of analysis: patients with HCC*	PET	Sensitivity: Moderate Specificity: Low	For FDG PET, sensitivity was 0.52 (95% CI, 0.39 to 0.66; 15 studies) and specificity was 0.95 (95% CI, 0.82 to 0.99; 5 studies), for an LR+ of 11 (95% CI, 2.6 to 49) and LR- of 0.50 (95% CI, 0.37 to 0.68). For ^{11}C-acetate PET or PET/CT, sensitivity was 0.85 (95% CI, 0.67 to 0.94; 4 studies); specificity was not reported.
Nonsurveillance settings *Unit of analysis: HCC lesions*	US without contrast	Sensitivity: Moderate Specificity: Low	Sensitivity was 0.59 (95% CI, 0.42 to 0.74; 11 studies). Only 2 studies reported specificity, with inconsistent results (0.63; 95% CI, 0.53 to 0.73, and 0.95; 95% CI, 0.85 to 0.99).
Nonsurveillance settings *Unit of analysis: HCC lesions*	US with contrast	Sensitivity: Low Specificity: Insufficient	Sensitivity was 0.73 (95% CI, 0.52 to 0.87; 8 studies). No study evaluated specificity.
Nonsurveillance settings *Unit of analysis: HCC lesions*	CT	Sensitivity: Moderate Specificity: Moderate	Sensitivity was 0.77 (95% CI, 0.72 to 0.80; 79 studies) and specificity 0.89 (95% CI, 0.84 to 0.93; 21 studies), for an LR+ of 7.1 (95% CI, 4.7 to 11) and LR- of 0.26 (95% CI, 0.22 to 0.31).
Nonsurveillance settings *Unit of analysis: HCC lesions*	MRI	Sensitivity: Moderate Specificity: Moderate	Sensitivity was 0.82 (95% CI, 0.79 to 0.85; 75 studies) and specificity 0.87 (95% CI, 0.77 to -0.93; 16 studies), for an LR+ of 6.4 (95% CI, 3.5 to 12) and LR- of 0.20 (95% CI, 0.16 to 0.25).
Nonsurveillance settings *Unit of analysis: HCC lesions*	PET	Sensitivity: Moderate Specificity: Low	For FDG PET, sensitivity was 0.53 (95% CI, 0.41 to 0.65; 5 studies) and specificity 0.91 (95% CI, 0.76 to 0.98; 1 study). For ^{11}C-acetate PET, sensitivity was 0.78 (95% CI, 0.61 to 0.89; 4 studies); specificity was not reported.
Direct (within-study) comparisons of imaging modalities *Unit of analysis: patients with HCC*	US without contrast vs. CT	Sensitivity: Moderate Specificity: Moderate	Sensitivity was 0.68 (95% CI, 0.54 to 0.80) vs. 0.80 (95% CI, 0.68 to 0.88), for a difference of -0.12 (95% CI, -0.20 to -0.03), based on 6 studies. Two studies were performed in surveillance settings. (Low strength of evidence for sensitivity and specificity.)
Direct (within-study) comparisons of imaging modalities *Unit of analysis: patients with HCC*	US without contrast vs. MRI	Sensitivity: Moderate Specificity: Moderate	Sensitivity was 0.61 (95% CI, 0.48 to 0.74) vs. 0.81 (95% CI, 0.69 to 0.89), for a difference of -0.19 (95% CI, -0.30 to -0.08), based on 3 studies, none of which were performed in surveillance settings.
Direct (within-study) comparisons of imaging modalities *Unit of analysis: patients with HCC*	MRI vs. CT	Sensitivity: Moderate Specificity: Moderate	Sensitivity was 0.88 (95% CI, 0.53 to 0.98) vs. 0.82 (95% CI, 0.41 to 0.97), for a difference of 0.06 (95% CI, -0.05 to 0.17), based on 4 studies, none of which were performed in surveillance settings.
Direct (within-study) comparisons of imaging modalities *Unit of analysis: HCC lesions*	US without contrast vs. CT	Sensitivity: Moderate Specificity: Moderate	Sensitivity was 0.55 (95% CI, 0.43 to 0.66) vs. 0.66 (95% CI, 0.54 to 0.76), for a difference of -0.11 (95% CI, -0.18 to -0.04), based on 3 studies, none of which were performed in surveillance settings.

Table A. Summary of evidence for Key Question 1.a (detection): Test performance (continued)

Subquestion	Imaging Modality or Comparison	Strength of Evidence	Summary
Direct (within-study) comparisons of imaging modalities *Unit of analysis: HCC lesions*	US without contrast vs. MRI	Sensitivity: Moderate Specificity: Moderate	Sensitivity was 0.57 (95% CI, 0.42 to 0.71) vs. 0.79 (95% CI, 0.67 to 0.88), for a difference of -0.22 (95% CI, -0.31 to 0.14), based on 3 studies, none of which were performed in surveillance settings.
Direct (within-study) comparisons of imaging modalities *Unit of analysis: HCC lesions*	US with contrast vs. CT	Sensitivity: Moderate Specificity: Insufficient	Sensitivity was 0.51 (95% CI, 0.29 to 0.74) vs. 0.61 (95% CI, 0.38 to 0.81), for a difference of -0.10 (95% CI, -0.20 to -0.00), based on 4 studies, none of which were performed in surveillance settings.
Direct (within-study) comparisons of imaging modalities *Unit of analysis: HCC lesions*	US with contrast vs. MRI	Sensitivity: Moderate Specificity: Insufficient	Sensitivity was 0.65 (95% CI, 0.41 to 0.84) vs. 0.73 (95% CI, 0.50 to 0.88), for a difference of -0.08 (95% CI, -0.19 to 0.02), based on 3 studies, none of which were performed in surveillance settings.
Direct (within-study) comparisons of imaging modalities *Unit of analysis: HCC lesions*	MRI vs. CT	Sensitivity: Moderate Specificity: Moderate	Sensitivity was 0.81 (95% CI, 0.76 to 0.84) vs. 0.71 (95% CI, 0.66 to 0.76), for a difference of 0.09 (95% CI, 0.07 to 0.12), based on 31 studies, none of which were performed in surveillance settings. Findings were similar when studies were stratified according to use of nonhepatic-specific or hepatic-specific contrast and when the analysis was restricted to HCC lesions <2–3 cm. For HCC lesions <2–3 cm, the difference in sensitivity was greater for studies of hepatic-specific MRI contrast (0.23; 95% CI, 0.17 to 0.29; 12 studies) than for studies of nonhepatic-specific MRI contrast (0.06; 95% CI, -0.01 to 0.13; 6 studies).
Multiple imaging modalities	Various combinations	Sensitivity: Insufficient Specificity: Insufficient	One study found sensitivity of imaging with various combinations of 2 imaging modalities was similar or lower than with single-modality imaging, based on concordant positive findings on 2 imaging modalities. The other study reported higher sensitivity with multiple imaging modalities than with single-modality imaging, but criteria for positive results based on multiple imaging modalities were unclear.

CI = confidence interval; CT = computed tomography; FDG = ^{18}F-fluorodeoxyglucose; HCC = hepatocellular carcinoma; LR+ = positive likelihood ratio; LR- = negative likelihood ratio; MRI = magnetic resonance imaging; PET = positron emission tomography; US = ultrasound.

Table B. Summary of evidence for Key Question 1.a.i (detection): Effects of reference standard on test performance (based on HCC lesions as the unit of analysis)

Imaging Modality or Comparison	Strength of Evidence	Summary
US without contrast	Sensitivity: Moderate Specificity: Insufficient	Using HCC lesions as the unit of analysis, sensitivity was 0.34 (95% CI, 0.22 to 0.47) in 5 studies that used explanted liver as the reference standard and ranged from 0.72 to 0.75 in studies that used other reference standards.
US with contrast	Sensitivity: Low Specificity: Insufficient	No study using HCC lesions as the unit of analysis used an explanted liver reference standard. Sensitivity was 0.58 (95% CI, 0.39 to 0.75) using a nonexplant histopathological reference standard and 0.98 (95% CI, 0.88 to 0.997) using a mixed reference standard.
CT	Sensitivity: Moderate Specificity: Moderate	Using HCC lesions as the unit of analysis, sensitivity was 0.67 (95% CI, 0.59 to 0.75) in 23 studies that used explanted liver as the reference standard and ranged from 0.65 to 0.86 in studies that used other reference standards.
MRI	Sensitivity: Moderate Specificity: Moderate	Using HCC lesions as the unit of analysis, sensitivity was 0.69 (95% CI, 0.59 to 0.77) in 15 studies that used explanted liver as the reference standard and ranged from 0.85 to 0.88 in studies that used a nonexplant histopathological reference standard or mixed reference standard; only 3 studies evaluated an imaging/clinical reference standard (sensitivity, 0.65; 95% CI, 0.43 to 0.83).
PET	Sensitivity: Low Specificity: Insufficient	No study of FDG PET used an explanted liver reference standard. Four of the 5 studies that used HCC lesions as the unit of analysis used a nonexplant histological reference standard (sensitivity, 0.49; 95% CI, 0.37 to 0.61).

CI = confidence interval; CT = computed tomography; FDG = ^{18}F-fluorodeoxyglucose; HCC = hepatocellular carcinoma; MRI = magnetic resonance imaging; PET = positron emission tomography; US = ultrasound.

Table C. Summary of evidence for Key Question 1.a.ii (detection): Effects of patient, tumor, technical, and other factors on test performance

Subquestion	Imaging Modality or Comparison	Strength of Evidence	Summary
Lesion size	US without contrast	Sensitivity: Moderate Specificity: Low	Sensitivity was 0.82 (95% CI, 0.68 to 0.91) for lesions ≥2 cm and 0.34 (95% CI, 0.19 to 0.53) for lesions <2 cm, for a difference of 0.48 (95% CI, 0.39 to 0.57). Sensitivity was 0.09 (95% CI, 0.02 to 0.29; 4 studies) for lesions <10 mm, to 0.50 (95% CI, 0.23 to 0.78; 4 studies) for lesions 10–20 mm and 0.88 (95% CI, 0.66 to 0.96; 4 studies) for lesions >20 mm, for a difference of 0.37 (95% CI, 0.18 to 0.57) for lesions >20 mm vs. 10–20 mm and 0.41 (95% CI, 0.19 to 0.63) for lesions 10–20 mm vs. <10 mm.
Lesion size	US with contrast	Sensitivity: Low Specificity: Low	Sensitivity was 0.94 (95% CI, 0.83 to 0.98) for lesions ≥>2 cm and 0.77 (95% CI, 0.53 to 0.91) for lesions <2 cm, for a difference of 0.17 (95% CI, 0.03 to 0.32), based on 5 studies. Three studies found sensitivity of 0.64 (95% CI, 0.33 to 0.87) for lesions 10–20 mm and 0.91 (95% CI, 0.71 to 0.98) for lesions >20 mm, for a difference of 0.26 (95% CI, 0.04 to 0.48).
Lesion size	CT	Sensitivity: Moderate Specificity: Low	Sensitivity was 0.94 (95% CI, 0.92 to 0.95) for lesions ≥2 cm and 0.63 (95% CI, 0.57 to 0.69) for lesions <2 cm, for an absolute difference in sensitivity of 0.31 (95% CI, 0.26 to 0.36), based on 34 studies. Sensitivity was 0.32 (95% CI, 0.25 to 0.41; 21 studies) for lesions <10 mm, 0.74 (95% CI, 0.67 to 0.80; 23 studies) for lesions 10–20 mm, and 0.95 (95% CI, 0.92 to 0.97; 20 studies), for a difference of 0.21 (95% CI, 0.15 to 0.26) for lesions >20 vs. 10–20 mm and 0.42 (95% CI, 0.36 to 0.48) for lesions 10–20 vs. <10 mm.

Table C. Summary of evidence for Key Question 1.a.ii (detection): Effects of patient, tumor, technical, and other factors on test performance (continued)

Subquestion	Imaging Modality or Comparison	Strength of Evidence	Summary
Lesion size	MRI	Sensitivity: Moderate Specificity: Moderate	Sensitivity was 0.96 (95% CI, 0.93 to 0.97) for lesions ≥2 cm and 0.66 (95% CI, 0.58 to 0.74) for lesions <2 cm, for an absolute difference in sensitivity of 0.29 (95% CI, 0.23 to 0.36), based on 29 studies. Sensitivity was 0.45 (95% CI, 0.34 to 0.56; 20 studies) for lesions <10 mm, 0.78 (95% CI, 0.69 to 0.85; 21 studies) for lesions 10–20 mm, and 0.97 (95% CI, 0.94 to 0.98, 14 studies) for lesions >20 mm (95% CI, 0.94 to 0.98; 18 studies), for a difference of 0.19 (95% CI, 0.12 to 0.26) for >20 vs. 10–20 mm and 0.33 (95% CI, 0.26 to 0.40) for 10–20 vs. <10 mm.
Lesion size	PET	Sensitivity: Low Specificity: Insufficient	For FDG PET, sensitivity was consistently higher for larger lesions, based on 5 studies. Data were not pooled due to differences in the tumor size categories evaluated. Two studies of ^{11}C-acetate PET found inconsistent effects of lesion size on sensitivity.
Degree of tumor differentiation	US with contrast	Sensitivity: Low Specificity: Insufficient	Sensitivity was 0.83 (95% CI, 0.55 to 0.95) for moderately or poorly differentiated HCC lesions and 0.43 (95% CI, 0.15 to 0.76) for well differentiated lesions, for an absolute difference in sensitivity of 0.40 (95% CI, 0.17 to 0.64), based on 3 studies.
Degree of tumor differentiation	CT	Sensitivity: Low Specificity: Insufficient	Sensitivity was 0.82 (95% CI, 0.66 to 0.91) for moderately or poorly differentiated HCC lesions and 0.50 (95% CI, 0.29 to 0.70) for well differentiated lesions, for an absolute difference in sensitivity of 0.32 (95% CI, 0.19 to 0.45), based on 5 studies.
Degree of tumor differentiation	MRI	Sensitivity: Low Specificity: Insufficient	Sensitivity was 0.68 (95% CI, 0.44 to 0.86) for moderately or poorly differentiated HCC lesions and 0.37 (95% CI, 0.17 to 0.62) for well differentiated lesions, for an absolute difference in sensitivity of 0.31 (95% CI, 0.13 to 0.49), based on 3 studies.
Degree of tumor differentiation	PET	Sensitivity: Low Specificity: Insufficient	For FDG PET, sensitivity was 0.72 (95% CI, 0.59 to 0.83) for moderately or poorly differentiated HCC lesions and 0.39 (95% CI, 0.26 to 0.55) for well differentiated lesions, for an absolute difference in sensitivity of 0.33 (95% CI, 0.20 to 0.46), based on 6 studies. In 3 studies of ^{11}C-acetate PET and 1 study of ^{18}F-fluorochorine PET, sensitivity for more well differentiated lesions was not lower than for more poorly differentiated lesions.
Other factors	US	Low	In 2 studies that directly compared US with vs. without contrast, there was no clear difference in sensitivity (-0.04; 95% CI, -0.11 to 0.04). One study that directly compared use of Doppler vs. no Doppler showed no clear effect on estimates of sensitivity. Lesion depth and body mass index had no effect on estimates of sensitivity.
Other factors	CT	Low	Using patients with HCC as the unit of analysis, studies with a contrast rate ≥3 ml/s reported a higher sensitivity (0.87; 95% CI, 0.77 to 0.93; 8 studies) than studies with a contrast rate <3 ml/s (0.71; 95% CI, 0.50 to -0.85; 4 studies). Studies with delayed phase imaging reported somewhat higher sensitivity (0.89; 95% CI, 0.81 to 0.94; 7 studies) than studies without delayed phase imaging (0.74; 95% CI, 0.66 to 0.87; 7 studies). However, neither of these technical parameters had clear effects in studies that used HCC lesions as the unit of analysis.

Table C. Summary of evidence for Key Question 1.a.ii (detection): Effects of patient, tumor, technical, and other factors on test performance (continued)

Subquestion	Imaging Modality or Comparison	Strength of Evidence	Summary
Other factors	MRI	Low	There were no clear differences in estimates of diagnostic accuracy when studies were stratified according to MRI scanner type (1.5 vs. 3.0 T), imaging phases evaluated (with or without delayed phase imaging), timing of delayed phase imaging (≥120 seconds vs. <120 seconds), section thickness (≤5 mm for enhanced images vs. >5 mm), or use of diffusion-weighted imaging. In studies that directly compared diagnostic accuracy with different types of contrast, hepatic-specific contrast agents were associated with slightly higher sensitivity than nonhepatic-specific contrast agents (0.83; 95% CI, 0.75 to 0.90, vs. 0.74; 95% CI, 0.62 to 0.83; difference 0.10; 95% CI, 0.04 to 0.15; 6 studies).
Other factors	PET	Low	FDG PET was associated with lower sensitivity that ^{11}C-acetate PET when either patients (0.58 vs. 0.81, for a difference of -0.23; 95% CI, -0.34 to -0.13; 3 studies) or HCC lesions (0.52 vs. 0.79, for a difference of -0.27; 95% CI, -0.36 to -0.17; 3 studies) were the unit of analysis. FDG PET was also associated with lower sensitivity that dual tracer PET with FDG and ^{11}C-acetate or ^{18}F-choline PET, but evidence was limited to 1 or 2 studies for each of these comparisons. Using patients as the unit of analysis, sensitivity of FDG PET (0.39; 95% CI, 0.24 to 0.56; 8 studies) was lower than sensitivity of FDG PET/CT (0.65; 95% CI, 0.50 to 0.78; 7 studies).

CI = confidence interval; CT = computed tomography; FDG = ^{18}F-fluorodeoxyglucose; HCC = hepatocellular carcinoma; MRI = magnetic resonance imaging; PET = positron emission tomography; US = ultrasound.

Table D. Summary of evidence for Key Question 1.b (detection): Clinical decisionmaking

Imaging Modality or Comparison	Strength of Evidence	Summary
Effects of different imaging modalities or strategies on clinical decisionmaking	Low	One randomized controlled trial (n = 163) found no clear differences between surveillance with US without contrast vs. CT in HCC detection rates, subsequent imaging, or cost per HCC detected.

CT = computed tomography; HCC = hepatocellular carcinoma; US = ultrasound.

Table E. Summary of evidence for Key Question 1.c (detection): Clinical and patient-centered outcomes

Imaging Modality or Comparison	Strength of Evidence	Summary
US plus serum AFP	Low	One cluster randomized controlled trial (n = 18,816) conducted in China found screening every 6 months with noncontrast US plus serum AFP vs. no screening in persons 35 to 79 years of age (mean, 42 years) with HBV infection or chronic hepatitis without HBV infection to be associated with lower risk of HCC-related mortality (32 vs. 54 deaths; rate ratio, 0.63; 95% CI, 0.41 to 0.98) at 5-year followup, but was rated high risk of bias due to multiple methodological shortcomings.
US screening at different intervals, mortality	Moderate	Two trials (n = 2,022) found no clear differences in mortality with US screening at 4- vs. 12-month intervals, or at 3- vs. 6-month intervals. One trial (n = 163) found no difference in HCC mortality between surveillance with US without contrast vs. CT, but was underpowered to detect differences.

AFP = alpha-fetoprotein; CI = confidence interval; CT = computed tomography; HBV = hepatitis B virus; HCC = hepatocellular carcinoma; US = ultrasound.

Table F. Summary of evidence for Key Question 1.d (detection): Harms

Imaging Modality or Comparison	Strength of Evidence	Summary
MRI, CT, US	Insufficient	One study reported no serious adverse events associated with administration of gadoxetic acid for MRI, and 1 study reported no clear differences in adverse events between CT with contrast at 3 ml/s vs. 5 ml/s. No study reported rates of adverse events associated with use of microbubble contrast agents in US, and harms were not reported in randomized trials of screening with imaging.

CT = computed tomography; MRI = magnetic resonance imaging; US = ultrasound.

Table G. Summary of evidence for Key Question 2.a (evaluation of focal liver lesions): Test performance

Subquestion	Imaging Modality or Comparison	Strength of Evidence	Summary
Evaluation of focal liver lesion *Unit of analysis: patients with HCC*	US with contrast	Sensitivity: Moderate Specificity: Moderate	Sensitivity was 0.87 (95% CI, 0.79 to 0.92; 12 studies) and specificity 0.91 (95% CI, 0.83 to 0.95; 8 studies), for an LR+ of 9.6 (95% CI, 5.1 to 18) and LR- of 0.14 (95% CI, 0.09 to 0.23).
Evaluation of focal liver lesion *Unit of analysis: patients with HCC*	US without contrast	Sensitivity: Low Specificity: Insufficient	Sensitivity was 0.78 (95% CI, 0.69 to 0.86) in 1 study; specificity was not reported.
Evaluation of focal liver lesion *Unit of analysis: patients with HCC*	CT	Sensitivity: Moderate Specificity: Low	Sensitivity was 0.86 (95% CI, 0.75 to 0.92; 8 studies) and specificity 0.88 (95% CI, 0.76 to 0.95; 5 studies), for an LR+ of 7.4 (95% CI, 3.3 to 17) and LR- of 0.16 (95% CI, 0.09 to 0.30).

Table G. Summary of evidence for Key Question 2.a (evaluation of focal liver lesions): Test performance (continued)

Subquestion	Imaging Modality or Comparison	Strength of Evidence	Summary
Evaluation of focal liver lesion *Unit of analysis: patients with HCC*	MRI	Sensitivity: Low Specificity: Low	Sensitivity was 0.77 (95% CI, 0.66 to 0.84; 4 studies) and specificity was 0.81 (95% CI, 0.52 to 0.94; 4 studies), for an LR+ of 4.0 (95% CI, 1.4 to 12) and LR- of 0.29 (95% CI, 0.21 to 0.39).
Evaluation of focal liver lesion *Unit of analysis: HCC lesions*	US with contrast	Sensitivity: Moderate Specificity: Moderate	Sensitivity was 0.87 (95% CI, 0.80 to 0.92; 21 studies) and specificity 0.91 (95% CI, 0.85 to 0.95; 10 studies) for an LR+ of 9.8 (95% CI, 5.7 to 17) and LR- of 0.14 (95% CI, 0.09 to 0.23).
Evaluation of focal liver lesion *Unit of analysis: HCC lesions*	CT	Sensitivity: Moderate Specificity: Moderate	Sensitivity was 0.79 (95% CI, 0.67 to 0.87; 13 studies) and specificity 0.90 (95% CI, 0.37 to 0.99; 6 studies), for an LR+ of 7.7 (95% CI, 0.71 to 84) and LR- of 0.24 (95% CI, 0.15 to 0.38).
Evaluation of focal liver lesion *Unit of analysis: HCC lesions*	MRI	Sensitivity: Moderate Specificity: Moderate	Sensitivity was 0.81 (95% CI, 0.72 to 0.87; 14 studies) and specificity 0.93 (95% CI, 0.80 to 0.98; 11 studies), for an LR+ of 12 (95% CI, 3.8 to 39) and LR- of 0.21 (95% CI, 0.15 to 0.30).
Evaluation of focal liver lesion *Unit of analysis: HCC lesions*	PET	Sensitivity: Low Specificity: Low	Sensitivity was 0.56 to 0.57 and specificity 1.0 in 2 studies of FDG PET.
For distinguishing HCC lesions from non-HCC hepatic lesions	US with contrast	Sensitivity: Low Specificity: Low	One study found US with sulfur hexafluoride contrast associated with a sensitivity of 0.94 (62/66) and a specificity of 0.68 (23/34) for distinguishing hypervascular HCC from focal nodular hyperplasia using quantitative methods, and 1 study found US with perflubutane contrast associated with a sensitivity of 0.59 (32/54) and specificity of 1.0 (13/13) for distinguishing small (<3 cm) well differentiated HCC lesions from regenerative nodules.
For distinguishing HCC lesions from non-HCC hepatic lesions	CT	Sensitivity: Low Specificity: Low	Five studies evaluated accuracy of CT for distinguishing HCC from non-HCC lesions, but the non-HCC lesions varied in the studies, precluding strong conclusions.
For distinguishing HCC lesions from non-HCC hepatic lesions	MRI	Sensitivity: Moderate Specificity: Moderate	Four studies reported inconsistent results for distinguishing small (<2 to 3 cm) hypervascular HCC lesions from hypervascular pseudolesions, with sensitivity 0.47 and 0.52 in 2 studies, and 0.91 and 0.92 in the other 2. Specificity was 0.93 or higher in all 4 studies. Eight other studies evaluated accuracy of MRI for distinguishing HCC from non-HCC lesions, but the non-HCC hepatic lesions varied in the studies.

Table G. Summary of evidence for Key Question 2.a (evaluation of focal liver lesions): Test performance (continued)

Subquestion	Imaging Modality or Comparison	Strength of Evidence	Summary
Direct (within-study) comparisons of imaging modalities *Unit of analysis: patients with HCC*	US without contrast vs. CT	Sensitivity: Low Specificity: Insufficient	Sensitivity was 0.78 (95% CI, 0.70 to 0.85) vs. 0.89 (95% CI, 0.84 to 0.95), for a difference of -0.12 (95% CI, -0.21 to -0.02), based on 1 study.
Direct (within-study) comparisons of imaging modalities *Unit of analysis: patients with HCC*	US with contrast vs. CT	Sensitivity: Moderate Specificity: Low	Sensitivity was 0.91 (95% CI, 0.85 to 0.94) vs. 0.88 (95% CI, 0.81 to 0.92), for a difference of 0.03 (95% CI, -0.02 to 0.08), based on 5 studies.
Direct (within-study) comparisons of imaging modalities *Unit of analysis: patients with HCC*	MRI vs. CT	Sensitivity: Low Specificity: Low	Sensitivity was 0.81 (95% CI, 0.70 to 0.92) vs. 0.74 (95% CI, 0.62 to 0.87), for a difference of 0.06 (-0.10 to 0.23), based on 1 study.
Direct (within-study) comparisons of imaging modalities *Unit of analysis: HCC lesions*	US with contrast vs. CT	Sensitivity: Moderate Specificity: Insufficient	Sensitivity was 0.92 (95% CI, 0.88 to 0.96) vs. 0.89 (95% CI, 0.83 to 0.93), for a difference of 0.04 (95% CI, -0.02 to 0.09), based on 4 studies.
Direct (within-study) comparisons of imaging modalities *Unit of analysis: HCC lesions*	US with contrast vs. MRI	Sensitivity: Low Specificity: Low	Sensitivity was 0.79 (95% CI, 0.65 to 0.94) vs. 0.83 (95% CI, 0.69 to 0.97), for a difference of -0.03 (95% CI, -0.24 to 0.17), based on 1 study.
Direct (within-study) comparisons of imaging modalities *Unit of analysis: HCC lesions*	MRI vs. CT	Sensitivity: Low Specificity: Low	One study found MRI associated with higher sensitivity (0.84; 95% CI, 0.76 to 0.92 vs. 0.62; 95% CI, 0.52 to 0.72, for a difference of 0.22; 95% CI, 0.09 to 0.35) but lower specificity (0.36; 95% CI, 0.20 to 0.52 vs. 0.72; 95% CI, 0.58 to 0.87, for a difference of -0.36; 95% CI, -0.58 to -0.15) than CT.

Table G. Summary of evidence for Key Question 2.a (evaluation of focal liver lesions): Test performance (continued)

Subquestion	Imaging Modality or Comparison	Strength of Evidence	Summary
Multiple imaging modalities	Various combinations	Moderate	In 4 studies in which positive results with multiple modality imaging were defined as concordant typical findings for HCC on 2 imaging modalities, sensitivity was lower than with a single modality (difference in sensitivity ranged from 0.09 to 0.27), with no clear difference in specificity. In 3 studies in which positive results with multiple modality imaging were defined as typical findings for HCC on at least 1 of the imaging techniques, sensitivity was higher than with a single modality (increase in sensitivity ranged from 0.09 to 0.25), with no clear difference in specificity. One study found that a sequential imaging strategy in which a second imaging test was performed only for indeterminate results on initial CT increased sensitivity for HCC from 0.53 to 0.74 to 0.79.

CI = confidence interval; CT = computed tomography; FDG = ^{18}F-fluorodeoxyglucose; HCC = hepatocellular carcinoma; LR+ = positive likelihood ratio; LR- = negative likelihood ratio; MRI = magnetic resonance imaging; PET = positron emission tomography; US = ultrasound.

Table H. Summary of evidence for Key Question 2.a.i (evaluation of focal liver lesions): effects of reference standard on test performance (based on HCC lesions as the unit of analysis)

Imaging Modality or Comparison	Strength of Evidence	Summary
All	Sensitivity: Moderate Specificity: Moderate	No study used explanted liver as the reference standard. There were no clear differences across imaging modalities in estimates of diagnostic accuracy in analyses stratified by use of different nonexplant reference standards.

HCC = hepatocellular carcinoma.

Table I. Summary of evidence for Key Question 2.a.ii (evaluation of focal liver lesions): effects of patient, tumor, technical, and other factors on test performance

Subquestion	Imaging Modality or Comparison	Strength of Evidence	Summary
Other factors	US	Low	In 2 studies that directly compared US with vs. without contrast, US with contrast was associated with sensitivity of 0.89 (95% CI, 0.83 to 0.93) and US without contrast with a sensitivity of 0.39 (95% CI, 0.32 to 0.47), for a difference in sensitivity of 0.50 (95% CI, 0.41 to 0.58). Based on across-study comparisons, there were no clear differences in sensitivity between different US contrast agents; no study directly compared different contrast agents. There were no differences in sensitivity of US based on lesion depth (3 studies) or body mass index (2 studies).
Other factors	CT	Low	Evidence on effects of technical parameters (type of CT scanner, use of delayed phase imaging, section thickness) was limited by small numbers of studies with wide CIs and methodological limitations, precluding reliable conclusions. Two studies found no clear difference in sensitivity of CT for HCC in patients with vs. without cirrhosis.
Other factors	MRI	Low	There were no clear differences in estimates of sensitivity based on the type of MRI machine (3.0 T vs. 1.5 T), type of contrast, use of delayed phase imaging, timing of delayed phase imaging, and section thickness. Estimates were similar when studies that used diffusion-weighted imaging were excluded.

CI = confidence interval; CT = computed tomography; HCC = hepatocellular carcinoma; MRI = magnetic resonance imaging; US = ultrasound.

Table J. Summary of evidence for Key Question 2.b (evaluation of focal liver lesions): clinical decisionmaking

Imaging Modality or Comparison	Strength of Evidence	Summary
All	Insufficient	No evidence

Table K. Summary of evidence for Key Question 2.c (evaluation of focal liver lesions): clinical and patient-centered outcomes

Imaging Modality or Comparison	Strength of Evidence	Summary
All	Insufficient	No evidence

Table L. Summary of evidence for Key Question 2.d (evaluation of focal liver lesions): harms

Imaging Modality or Comparison	Strength of Evidence	Summary
US and CT	Insufficient	One study of US (with and without contrast) and CT reported harms, but did not stratify results by imaging technique. The overall rate of adverse drug-related events was 10%, with all events classified as mild.

CT = computed tomography; US = ultrasound.

Table M. Summary of evidence for Key Question 3.a (staging): test performance

Subquestion	Imaging Modality or Comparison	Strength of Evidence	Summary
Staging accuracy, using TNM criteria	CT	Moderate	The proportion correctly staged using TNM or BCLC criteria ranged from 28% to 58%, the proportion overstaged from 2% to 27%, and the proportion understaged from 25% to 52%, based on 6 studies.
Staging accuracy, using TNM criteria	MRI	Low	The proportion correctly staged ranged from 40% to 75%, the proportion overstaged from 3.1% to 31%, and the proportion understaged from 19% to 31%, based on 3 studies.
Staging accuracy, using TNM criteria	PET	Low	One study found 26% of patients were correctly staged with FDG PET and 91% with ^{11}C-choline PET.
Staging accuracy, using TNM criteria	MRI vs. CT	Low	Two studies reported similar staging accuracy.
Identification of metastatic disease *Unit of analysis: patients with metastatic HCC*	PET	Sensitivity: Low Specificity: Low	Sensitivity of FDG PET was 0.85 (95% CI, 0.71 to 0.93; 6 studies) and specificity 0.93 (95% CI, 0.89 to 0.95; 5 studies), for an LR+ of 11 (95% CI, 7.8 to 17) and LR- of 0.16 (95% CI, 0.08 to 0.33). One study that directly compared sensitivity of FDG PET vs. ^{11}C-acetate PET reported comparable sensitivity (0.79 vs. 0.71), although sensitivity was higher when both tracers were used (0.98).
Identification of metastatic disease *Unit of analysis: patients with metastatic HCC*	PET/CT vs. CT	Low	Three studies found no difference in sensitivity (0.82; 95% CI, 0.61 to 0.93 vs. 0.85; 95% CI, 0.66 to 0.95).
Identification of metastatic disease *Unit of analysis: metastatic HCC lesions*	PET	Sensivity: Low Specificity: Insufficient	Sensitivity of FDG PET was 0.82 (95% CI, 0.72 to 0.90; 5 studies). One study that directly compared sensitivity of FDG vs. ^{11}C-acetate PET reported comparable sensitivity (0.86 vs. 0.77).

BCLC = Barcelona Clinic Liver Cancer; CI = confidence interval; CT = computed tomography; FDG = ^{18}F-fluorodeoxyglucose; HCC = hepatocellular carcinoma; LR+ = positive likelihood ratio; LR- = negative likelihood ratio; MRI = magnetic resonance imaging; PET = positron emission tomography; TNM = tumor, node, metastasis staging.

Table N. Summary of evidence for Key Question 3.a.i (staging): effects of reference standard on test performance

Imaging Modality or Comparison	Strength of Evidence	Summary
CT, MRI, PET	Sensitivity: Insufficient Specificity: Insufficient	Evidence was insufficient to determine effects of different reference standards on accuracy of staging using TNM criteria or accuracy of PET for identifying metastatic HCC because few studies evaluated alternative reference standards.

CT = computed tomography; HCC = hepatocellular carcinoma; MRI = magnetic resonance imaging; PET = positron emission tomography; TNM = tumor, node, metastasis staging.

Table O. Summary of evidence for Key Question 3.a.ii (staging): effects of patient, tumor, and technical factors on test performance

Imaging Modality or Comparison	Strength of Evidence	Summary
CT, MRI, PET	Insufficient	For accuracy of staging using TNM criteria, no study evaluated effects of patient-level characteristics or other factors on accuracy of imaging techniques for staging.
PET	Low	In 1 study that directly compared sensitivity of PET vs. PET/CT for identifying metastatic HCC lesions, there was no clear difference in sensitivity. Four studies of FDG PET found sensitivity increased as lesion size increased, but the number of lesions <1 cm was small (total of 20). Eight studies generally found sensitivity of FDG PET higher for lymph and bone metastasis than for lung metastasis, but samples were small, precluding strong conclusions.

CT = computed tomography; FDG = ^{18}F-fluorodeoxyglucose; HCC = hepatocellular carcinoma; MRI = magnetic resonance imaging; PET = positron emission tomography; TNM = tumor, node, metastasis staging.

Table P. Summary of evidence for Key Question 3.b (staging): clinical decisionmaking

Subquestion	Imaging Modality or Comparison	Strength of Evidence	Summary
Transplant eligibility, using Milan criteria	CT	Moderate	The proportion correctly assessed for transplant eligibility ranged from 40% to 96%. The proportion of patients who met transplant criteria based on CT but exceeded criteria based on the reference standard was 3.5% to 7.8%, based on 3 studies. Two studies found that 2.3% and 16% of patients who underwent transplantation based on Milan criteria had no HCC lesions on examination of explanted livers.
Transplant eligibility, using Milan criteria	CT vs. MRI	Low	One study reported similar accuracy.
Transplant eligibility, using Milan criteria	PET vs. CT	Low	One study found ^{11}C-choline PET more accurate than CT (95% vs. 40%).
Use of resection and ablative therapies	MRI vs. CT	Low	One study reported that the proportion of decisions to perform resection or ablative therapies that were classified as correct were similar for MRI (90% and 90%, respectively) and CT (80% and 77%, respectively).

CT = computed tomography; HCC = hepatocellular carcinoma; MRI = magnetic resonance imaging; PET = positron emission tomography.

Table Q. Summary of evidence for Key Question 3.c (staging): clinical and patient-centered outcomes

Imaging Modality or Comparison	Strength of Evidence	Summary
US with contrast vs. US without contrast plus CT	Low	One cohort study found that contrast-enhanced US identified more small (≤2 cm) HCC lesions than noncontrast US plus CT (36 vs. 31) and was associated with a higher complete necrosis rate following ablation (92%, or 106/115, vs. 83%, or 93/112 lesions; p = 0.036) but was rated high risk of bias. Another study that appeared to be performed in the same series of patients found US with contrast prior to radiofrequency ablation associated with lower local tumor progression rate (7.2% vs. 18%; rate ratio, 0.40; 95% CI, 0.16 to 0.87) and longer tumor-free survival (38 vs. 26 months), but was also rated high risk of bias.

CI = confidence interval; CT = computed tomography; HCC = hepatocellular carcinoma; US = ultrasound.

Table R. Summary of evidence for Key Question 3.d (staging): harms

Imaging Modality or Comparison	Strength of Evidence	Summary
All	Insufficient	No evidence

Findings in Relationship to What Is Already Known

Unlike our review, several previously published reviews on detection of HCC and evaluation of focal liver lesions found no clear differences in test performance between US, CT, and MRI for HCC.[25-28] Several factors may explain these discrepancies: we included more studies than any prior review, separately analyzed studies based on the reason for imaging, stratified studies according to the unit of analysis, and focused on within-study (direct) comparisons of two or more imaging modalities against a common reference standard instead of relying primarily or solely on across-study (indirect) estimates of test performance. Our review's findings are consistent with those of previous reviews regarding lower sensitivity of imaging for detection of small and well-differentiated HCC lesions.

Our findings regarding test performance of PET for detection of metastatic HCC are consistent with those from a recently published systematic review and meta-analysis.[29] Like our review, a recent systematic review found insufficient evidence to determine effects of surveillance with imaging on clinical outcomes.[30] A systematic review on screening for HCC in chronic liver disease funded by the U.S. Department of Veterans Affairs was conducted at the same time as our review.[12]

Applicability

A number of potential issues could impact the applicability of our findings. Over half of the studies were conducted in Asia, where the prevalence, underlying causes, course, evaluation, and management of chronic liver disease may be different than in the United States. To mitigate potential effects of study country on applicability, we excluded invasive imaging techniques not typically used in the United States, such as CT arterial portography and CT hepatic arteriography, as well as imaging techniques considered inadequate in the United States (such as C-arm CT). We also performed stratified analyses focusing on studies performed in the United States and Europe to evaluate effects on estimates of diagnostic accuracy and found no clear effects on estimates.

Imaging techniques are rapidly evolving, which is another factor that could affect applicability. To mitigate effects of outdated techniques on applicability, we excluded imaging technologies considered outdated, such as MRI with magnetic field strength <1.5 T and nonspiral

CT, and included only studies published since 1998. We also performed additional analyses on technical factors such as contrast rate, imaging phases evaluated, timing of imaging phases, section thickness, use of hepatobiliary contrast (for MRI), use of diffusion-weighted imaging, and newer technologies (e.g., dual-source or spectral CT). We included studies of US with microbubble contrast even though no agent is currently approved for abdominal imaging in the United States, because efforts to obtain U.S. Food and Drug Administration approval are ongoing and this technique is commonly used in other areas of the world, including Canada and Europe.

As noted above, few studies were performed in true surveillance settings (i.e., in patients at high risk for HCC but not previously diagnosed with this condition). Rather, most studies of test performance that were not performed specifically to evaluate or characterize previously identified lesions were conducted in patients undergoing imaging for other reasons, including series of patients undergoing liver transplantation, surgical resection, or other treatments for HCC. Although such studies are likely to provide some useful findings regarding diagnostic accuracy, results may not be directly applicable to patients undergoing surveillance. In particular, the high prevalence of HCC (many studies enrolled only patients with HCC) could overestimate test performance in true surveillance settings, in which the prevalence of HCC would be much lower.[31]

Implications for Clinical and Policy Decisionmaking

Our review has important potential implications for clinical and policy decisionmaking. Due to the lack of direct evidence regarding clinical benefits and downstream harms associated with different imaging tests for surveillance, diagnosis, and staging of HCC, most decisions regarding use of imaging tests must necessarily be made primarily on the basis of diagnostic test performance. Despite limited evidence in true surveillance settings, current guidelines from the AASLD recommend US without contrast for surveillance of HCC in at-risk individuals. Evidence from true surveillance settings to evaluate the comparative test performance of different imaging modalities was limited. Based primarily on studies conducted in nonsurveillance settings, our study suggests that US without contrast is less sensitive than MRI or CT for detecting HCC.[4] Although sensitivity for identifying HCC was higher for CT and MRI than for US in studies conducted in nonsurveillance settings, findings may not be directly applicable to clinical and policy decisions related to surveillance, as the spectrum of patients evaluated in these studies could have affected estimates.

In patients found to have an HCC lesion on surveillance, our review supports use of CT and MRI to further characterize lesions >1 cm in size, as in the AASLD guideline, based on high sensitivity and specificity. Evidence is limited but appears consistent with the sequential diagnostic imaging algorithm as outlined in the AASLD guideline, in which typical findings for HCC on sequentially performed CT or MRI are considered sufficient to make a diagnosis.

Our findings also support minimal technical specifications for MRI and CT for HCC imaging, as suggested in recent guidance, such as those regarding minimum contrast rates and use of delayed phase imaging.[11] Evidence suggesting superior test performance of MRI with hepatic-specific versus nonhepatic-specific contrast appears promising, although differences were relatively small. Therefore, clinical and policy decisions around use of nonhepatic-specific contrast may be impacted by additional factors other than test performance, such as cost, harms, or convenience.

US with contrast was associated with test performance similar to that of MRI and CT for evaluation of lesions, although no microbubble contrast agents are currently approved for use in the United States. Although the role of PET is likely to remain focused on identification of metastatic HCC and staging, additional research could help clarify the role of PET with alternative tracers for identification and evaluation of intrahepatic HCC.

Research Gaps

Significant research gaps limit the full understanding of the comparative effectiveness of imaging for surveillance, diagnosis, and staging of HCC. The only randomized trial of effects of surveillance for HCC with imaging on clinical outcomes had important methodological shortcomings and was performed in China, potentially limiting applicability to screening in the United States.[24] Although conducting a randomized trial of surveillance versus no screening in the United States could be difficult because screening is recommended in clinical practice guidelines and routinely performed in high-risk patients, randomized trials that compare screening using different imaging modalities or combinations of modalities would be helpful for understanding optimal approaches.

In lieu of such studies, evidence on effects of alternative imaging strategies on intermediate outcomes such as clinical decisionmaking, subsequent procedures, and resource utilization could also be informative. Such studies could potentially enroll smaller samples than randomized trials to compare screening using different imaging modalities and would probably not require the extended followup needed to assess clinical outcomes.

Although many studies are available on test performance of alternative imaging modalities and strategies, important research gaps remain. Notably, few studies evaluated imaging in true surveillance settings, and evidence on accuracy of imaging for identifying HCC lesions from nonsurveillance settings may not be directly applicable to surveillance due to spectrum effects. More studies are also needed to clarify the role of promising alternative techniques, such as US with contrast, MRI with hepatic-specific contrast, and PET with alternative tracers, on estimates of accuracy. Research should focus on improving methods for identifying small or well-differentiated HCC lesions, for which imaging remains suboptimal.

Conclusions

Based on estimates of test performance, several imaging modalities appear to be reasonable options for detection of HCC, evaluation of focal liver lesions for HCC, or staging of HCC. Although there are some potential differences in test performance between different imaging modalities and techniques, more research is needed to understand the effects of such differences on clinical decisionmaking and clinical outcomes.

References

1. Parkin DM. Global cancer statistics in the year 2000. Lancet Oncol. 2001 Sep;2(9):533-43. PMID: 11905707.

2. National Cancer Institute. Liver Cancer. www.cancer.gov/cancertopics/types/liver. Accessed September 21, 2011.

3. Howlader N, Noone AM, Krapcho M, et al., eds. SEER Cancer Statistics Review, 1975-2010. National Cancer Institute: Bethesda, MD; 2013. http://seer.cancer.gov/csr/1975_2010/.

4. Bruix J, Sherman M. Management of hepatocellular carcinoma: an update. Hepatology. 2011 Mar;53(3):1020-2. PMID: 21374666.

5. Cabibbo G, Enea M, Attanasio M, et al. A meta-analysis of survival rates of untreated patients in randomized clinical trials of hepatocellular carcinoma. Hepatology. 2010 Apr;51(4):1274-83. PMID: 20112254.

6. Forner A, Reig ME, de Lope CR, et al. Current strategy for staging and treatment: the BCLC update and future prospects. Semin Liver Dis. 2010 Feb;30(1):61-74. PMID: 20175034.

7. Mazzaferro V, Bhoori S, Sposito C, et al. Milan criteria in liver transplantation for hepatocellular carcinoma: an evidence-based analysis of 15 years of experience. Liver Transpl. 2011;17(S2):S44-S57. PMID: 21695773.

8. Methods Guide for Effectiveness and Comparative Effectiveness Reviews. AHRQ Publication No. 10(14)-EHC063-EF. Rockville, MD: Agency for Healthcare Research and Quality; January 2014. Chapters available at www.effectivehealthcare.ahrq.gov.

9. Methods Guide for Medical Test Reviews. AHRQ Publication No. 12-EHC017. Rockville, MD: Agency for Healthcare Research and Quality; June 2012. www.effectivehealthcare.ahrq.gov/reports/final.cfm.

10. Submit Scientific Information Packets. Rockville, MD: Agency for Healthcare Research and Quality; 2013. www.effectivehealthcare.ahrq.gov/index.cfm/submit-scientific-information-packets/. Accessed November 12, 2013.

11. Wald C, Russo MW, Heimbach JK, et al. New OPTN/UNOS policy for liver transplant allocation: standardization of liver imaging, diagnosis, classification, and reporting of hepatocellular carcinoma. Radiology. 2013 Feb;266(2):376-82. PMID: 23362092.

12. Kansagara D, Papak J, Pasha A, et al. Screening for Hepatocellular Cancer in Chronic Liver Disease: A Systematic Review. Washington: Department of Veterans Affairs; January 2014. www.ncbi.nlm.nih.gov/books/NBK2221841.

13. Harris RP, Helfand M, Woolf SH, et al. Current methods of the U.S. Preventive Services Task Force: a review of the process. Am J Prev Med. 2001 Apr;20(3 Suppl):21-35. PMID: 11306229.

14. Whiting PF, Rutjes AW, Westwood ME, et al. QUADAS-2: a revised tool for the quality assessment of diagnostic accuracy studies. Ann Intern Med. 2011 Oct 18;155(8):529-36. PMID: 22007046.

15. Fu R, Gartlehner G, Grant M, et al. Conducting quantitative synthesis when comparing medical interventions: AHRQ and the Effective Health Care Program. In: Methods Guide for Effectiveness and Comparative Effectiveness Reviews. AHRQ Publication No. 10(14)-EHC063-EF. Chapters available at www.effectivehealthcare.ahrq.gov/.

16. Takwoingi Y, Leeflang MM, Deeks JJ. Empirical evidence of the importance of comparative studies of diagnostic test accuracy. Ann Intern Med. 2013 Apr 2;158(7):544-54. PMID: 23546566.

17. Atkins D, Chang SM, Gartlehner G, et al. Assessing applicability when comparing medical interventions: AHRQ and the Effective Health Care Program. J Clin Epidemiol. 2011 Nov;64(11):1198-207. PMID: 21463926.

18. Chalasani N, Horlander JC Sr, Said A, et al. Screening for hepatocellular carcinoma in patients with advanced cirrhosis. Am J Gastroenterol. 1999 Oct;94(10):2988-93. PMID: 10520857.

19. Van Thiel DH, Yong S, Li SD, et al. The development of de novo hepatocellular carcinoma in patients on a liver transplant list: frequency, size, and assessment of current screening methods. Liver Transpl. 2004 May;10(5):631-7. PMID: 15108254.

20. Goto E, Masuzaki R, Tateishi R, et al. Value of post-vascular phase (Kupffer imaging) by contrast-enhanced ultrasonography using Sonazoid in the detection of hepatocellular carcinoma. J Gastroenterol. 2012;47(4):477-85. PMID: 22200940.

21. Kunishi Y, Numata K, Morimoto M, et al. Efficacy of fusion imaging combining sonography and hepatobiliary phase MRI with Gd-EOB-DTPA to detect small hepatocellular carcinoma. AJR Am J Roentgenol. 2012 Jan;198(1):106-14. PMID: 22194485.

22. Lencioni R, Piscaglia F, Bolondi L. Contrast-enhanced ultrasound in the diagnosis of hepatocellular carcinoma. J Hepatol. 2008 May;48(5):848-57. PMID: 18328590.

23. Naaktgeboren CA, de Groot JA, van Smeden M, et al. Evaluating diagnostic accuracy in the face of multiple reference standards. Ann Intern Med. 2013 Aug 6;159(3):195-202. PMID: 23922065.

24. Zhang BH, Yang BH, Tang ZY. Randomized controlled trial of screening for hepatocellular carcinoma. J Cancer Res Clin Oncol. 2004 Jul;130(7):417-22. PMID: 15042359.

25. Colli A, Fraquelli M, Casazza G, et al. Accuracy of ultrasonography, spiral CT, magnetic resonance, and alpha-fetoprotein in diagnosing hepatocellular carcinoma: a systematic review. Am J Gastroenterol. 2006 Mar;101(3):513-23. PMID: 16542288.

26. Westwood M, Joore M, Grutters J, et al. Contrast-enhanced ultrasound using SonoVue(R) (sulphur hexafluoride microbubbles) compared with contrast-enhanced computed tomography and contrast-enhanced magnetic resonance imaging for the characterisation of focal liver lesions and detection of liver metastases: a systematic review and cost-effectiveness analysis. Health Technol Assess. 2013 Apr;17(16):1-243. PMID: 23611316.

27. Guang Y, Xie L, Ding H, et al. Diagnosis value of focal liver lesions with SonoVue-enhanced ultrasound compared with contrast-enhanced computed tomography and contrast-enhanced MRI: a meta-analysis. J Cancer Res Clin Oncol. 2011 Nov;137(11):1595-605. PMID: 21850382.

28. Xie L, Guang Y, Ding H, et al. Diagnostic value of contrast-enhanced ultrasound, computed tomography and magnetic resonance imaging for focal liver lesions: a meta-analysis. Ultrasound Med Biol. 2011 Jun;37(6):854-61. PMID: 21531500.

29. Lin C-Y, Chen J-H, Liang J-A, et al. 18F-FDG PET or PET/CT for detecting extrahepatic metastases or recurrent hepatocellular carcinoma: a systematic review and meta-analysis. Eur J Radiol. 2012 Sep;81(9):2417-22. PMID: 21899970.

30. Aghoram R, Cai P, Dickinson JA. Alpha-foetoprotein and/or liver ultrasonography for screening of hepatocellular carcinoma in patients with chronic hepatitis B. Cochrane Database Syst Rev. 2012;(9):CD002799. PMID: 22972059.

31. Lachs MS, Nachamkin I, Edelstein PH, et al. Spectrum bias in the evaluation of diagnostic tests: lessons from the rapid dipstick test for urinary tract infection. Ann Intern Med. 1992 Jul 15;117(2):135-40. PMID: 1605428.

Background and Objectives

Hepatocellular carcinoma (HCC) is the most common primary malignant neoplasm of the liver, usually developing in individuals with chronic liver disease or cirrhosis. Worldwide, it is the fifth most common cause of cancer and the third most common cause of cancer death.[1] There were 156,940 deaths attributed to liver and intrahepatic bile duct cancer in the United States in 2011, with 221,130 new cases diagnosed.[2] The lifetime risk of developing liver and intrahepatic bile duct cancer in the United States is about 1 in 132, with an age-adjusted incidence rate of 7.3 per 100,000 people per year.[3] The highest incidence rates in the United States are found in Asian/Pacific Islanders (22.1 per 100,000 men and 8.4 per 100,000 women). The age-adjusted death rate is estimated at 5.2 per 100,000 people per year in the United States, with the highest rates among men occurring in Asian/Pacific Islanders (14.7 per 100,000) and among women in American Indian/Alaskan Natives (6.6 per 100,000). The overall 5-year relative survival rate with HCC is 14.4 percent.

Deaths from liver cancer significantly increased from 1998 to 2007 in both men and women.[4] The increase was mostly attributable to cirrhosis due to hepatitis B virus (HBV) infection, hepatitis C virus (HCV) infection, or long-term alcohol abuse, with HCV infection accounting for at least half of the observed increase[5,6] In the United States, HCV infection is the most frequently identified cause of HCC, and is present in about half of all cases, although 15 to 50 percent of patients have no identifiable etiology.[6] Worldwide, HBV infection is responsible for the majority of HCC cases, particularly in developing countries,[7] although the incidence of HBV infection and associated complications has declined following to the widespread implementation of universal vaccination programs.[8] The American Association for the Study of Liver Diseases (AASLD) recommends surveillance for the following groups at high risk for developing HCC: Asian male HBV carriers age 40 and older, Asian female HBV carriers age 50 and older, HBV carriers with a family history of HCC, African/North American black HBV carriers, HBV or HCV carriers with cirrhosis, all individuals with other causes for cirrhosis (including alcoholic cirrhosis), and patients with stage 4 primary biliary cirrhosis.[9]

The natural history of HCC is variable, but it is often an aggressive tumor associated with poor survival without treatment.[10] When diagnosed early, HCC may be amenable to potentially curative therapy. The three phases of pretherapy evaluation of HCC are detection, further evaluation of focal liver lesions, and staging.[9] Detection often occurs in the setting of surveillance, or in the use of periodic testing in persons without HCC to identify lesions in the liver that are clinically suspicious for HCC.[9] The evaluation phase involves the use of additional tests (radiological and/or histopathological) to confirm that a focal liver lesion is indeed HCC. Once the lesion is confirmed as HCC, staging is important for informing prognosis and treatment decisions. A number of staging systems are available, including the traditional TNM (tumor, node, metastasis) classification, based on the size, number, and location of primary lesions, the presence of invasion into vascular and biliary structures, and the presence of regional nodal and distant metastases.[11] More recently, the Barcelona Clinic Liver Cancer (BCLC) staging system,[12] which incorporates additional factors associated with prognosis such as liver functional status, physical status, cancer related symptoms, and impact of treatment, has become the de facto staging reference standard.[9] To select patients who are suitable for liver transplantation, the Milan criteria (one lesion <5 cm or up to 3 lesions <3 cm, with no extrahepatic manifestations or vascular invasion) have been used to identify patients likely to experience better post-transplantation outcomes, although other methods have been proposed.[13]

A number of imaging techniques are available to detect the presence of lesions, evaluate focal liver lesions, and determine the stage of the disease (Table 1). These include ultrasound (US), computed tomography (CT), magnetic resonance imaging (MRI), and positron emission tomography (PET). The typical use of each of these imaging modalities varies. For example, PET scan is typically used for staging and identification of metastatic disease, but not for initial detection or lesion characterization. US without contrast is the most frequently used modality for surveillance and recommended by the AASLD for this purpose.[9] Because HCC is typically a hypervascular lesion, arterial enhancing contrast agents are frequently used to increase the sensitivity and specificity of imaging techniques such as CT or MRI. Similarly, microbubble-enhanced US is performed to evaluate liver lesions in regions of the world such as Europe and Asia, although agents are not yet approved by the U.S. Food and Drug Administration (FDA) for this purpose.[14] Because the microbubbles are present for only a limited period of time in the liver, a comprehensive contrast-enhanced ultrasonographic evaluation of the entire liver is not possible. Therefore contrast-enhanced US is typically performed for the targeted evaluation and characterization of focal liver lesions previously identified on US without contrast or other imaging studies, rather than for initial evaluation of the entire liver.

Understanding the diagnostic accuracy of imaging methods and how they affect clinical decisionmaking and, ultimately, patient outcomes is a challenge. Imaging techniques may be used alone, in various combinations or algorithms, and/or with liver-specific biomarkers, resulting in many potential comparisons. In addition, detection and evaluation strategies vary. For example, some centers use periodic US alone for surveillance, while others use US alternatively with either CT or MRI every 6 months, with or without use of biomarkers such as alpha-fetoprotein. Technical aspects of imaging methods are complex and continuously evolving. Published standards for CT and MRI are available, providing guidance regarding minimum recommended technical specifications with regard to scanner types, section thickness, imaging phases, timing of imaging phases, and other factors (Tables 2 and 3).[15] Other technical variations have also been introduced, including MRI with liver-specific contrast agents[16] such as gadobenate or gadoxetic acid disodium (rather than standard nonspecific contrast agents such as gadodiamide or gadopentetate),[17] CT utilizing dual energy source or spectral techniques,[18,19] US with use of contrast enhancement,[20] and PET with use of tracers such as ^{18}F-fluorothymidine (FLT) or ^{11}C-choline,[21] rather than the standard ^{18}F-fluorodeoxyglucose (FDG). The use of different reference standards—such as explanted liver specimens from patients undergoing transplantation, percutaneous or surgical biopsy, imaging, clinical followup, or combinations of these methods—could introduce heterogeneity. Reference standards are also susceptible to misclassification due to sampling errors, inadequate specimens, insufficient followup, or other factors. Finally, other considerations may impact the diagnostic accuracy or clinical utility of imaging strategies; they include risk factors for HCC and lesion characteristics, such as tumor size or degree of differentiation, severity of hepatic fibrosis, and etiology of liver disease..

In addition to imaging studies, serological biomarkers for HCC can be used to aid in diagnosis. Alpha-fetoprotein is the most widely used serological marker for HCC surveillance, but recommended only as an adjunct to imaging due to limited sensitivity and specificity.[9] A newer biomarker is des-gamma-carboxy prothrombin, although its role in the surveillance and early diagnosis of HCC has not yet been defined.[22] Other biomarkers, such as glypican 3, heat shock protein 70, and glutamine synthetase, have not been validated in the clinical setting and are not currently recommended for use in screening.[9,23]

Accurate diagnosis and staging of HCC are critical for providing optimal patient care. However, clinical uncertainty remains regarding optimal imaging strategies, due to the factors described above. The purpose of this report is to comprehensively review the comparative effectiveness and diagnostic performance of different imaging modalities and strategies for detection of HCC, evaluation of focal liver lesions to identify HCC, and staging of HCC.

Scope and Key Questions

The Key Questions and corresponding analytic frameworks used to guide this report are shown below. Separate analytic frameworks address surveillance (Key Question 1, Figure 1), diagnosis (Key Question 2, Figure 2), and staging (Key Question 3, Figure 3). The analytic frameworks show the target populations, interventions (imaging tests), and outcomes (diagnostic accuracy, clinical decisionmaking, clinical outcomes, and harms) that we examined.

Key Question 1. What is the comparative effectiveness of available imaging-based strategies, used singly or in sequence, for detection of hepatocellular carcinoma among individuals in surveillance and nonsurveillance settings?

  a. What is the comparative test performance of imaging-based strategies for detecting HCC?
     i. How is a particular technique's test performance modified by use of various reference standards (e.g., explanted liver samples, histological diagnosis, or clinical and imaging followup)?
     ii. How is the comparative effectiveness modified by patient (e.g., severity of liver disease, underlying cause of liver disease, body mass index, age, sex, race), tumor (e.g., tumor diameter, degree of differentiation, location), technical, or other factors (e.g., results of biomarker tests, setting)?
  b. What is the comparative effectiveness of imaging-based strategies on intermediate outcomes related to clinical decisionmaking (e.g., use of subsequent diagnostic tests and treatments)?
  c. What is the comparative effectiveness of imaging-based strategies on clinical and patient-centered outcomes?
  d. What are the adverse effects or harms associated with imaging-based strategies?

Key Question 2. What is the comparative effectiveness of imaging techniques, used singly, in combination, or in sequence, in diagnosing hepatocellular carcinoma among individuals in whom a focal liver lesion has been detected?

  a. What is the comparative test performance of imaging techniques for diagnosing HCC in patients with a focal liver lesion?
     i. How is a particular technique's test performance modified by use of various reference standards (e.g., explanted liver samples, histological diagnosis, or clinical imaging and followup?

ii. How is the comparative effectiveness modified by patient, tumor, technical, or other factors?
  b. What is the comparative effectiveness of the various imaging techniques on intermediate outcomes related to clinical decisionmaking?
  c. What is the comparative effectiveness of the various imaging techniques on clinical and patient-centered outcomes?
  d. What are the adverse effects or harms associated with imaging-based diagnostic strategies?

Key Question 3. What is the comparative effectiveness of imaging techniques, used singly, in combination, or in sequence, in staging hepatocellular carcinoma among patients diagnosed with hepatocellular carcinoma?

  a. What is the comparative test performance of imaging techniques to predict HCC tumor stage?
     i. How is a particular technique's test performance modified by use of various reference standards (e.g., explanted liver samples, histological diagnosis, or clinical and imaging followup)?
     ii. How is the comparative effectiveness modified by patient, tumor, technical, or other factors?
  b. What is the comparative effectiveness of imaging techniques on intermediate outcomes related to clinical decisionmaking?
  c. What is the comparative effectiveness of imaging techniques on clinical and patient-centered outcomes?
  d. What are the adverse effects or harms associated with imaging-based staging strategies?

Figure 1. Analytic framework—detection (Key Question 1)

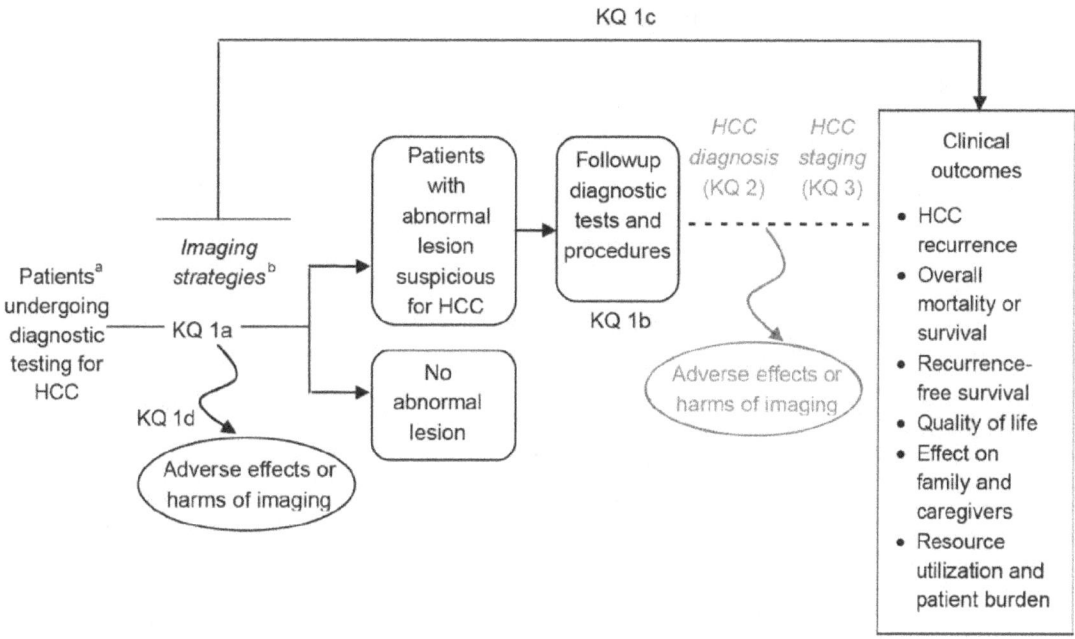

HCC = hepatocellular carcinoma; KQ = Key Question. Shaded elements show the relationship of KQ1 to KQ2 and KQ3.
[a] Potential modifiers of test performance include patient (e.g., severity of liver disease, underlying cause of liver disease, body mass index, age, sex, race), tumor (e.g., tumor diameter, degree of differentiation, location), technical, and other factors (e.g., biomarker levels, setting).
[b] Imaging techniques are used singly, in combination, or in sequence with or without biomarkers used as modifiers.

Figure 2. Analytic framework—evaluation of focal liver lesions (Key Question 2)

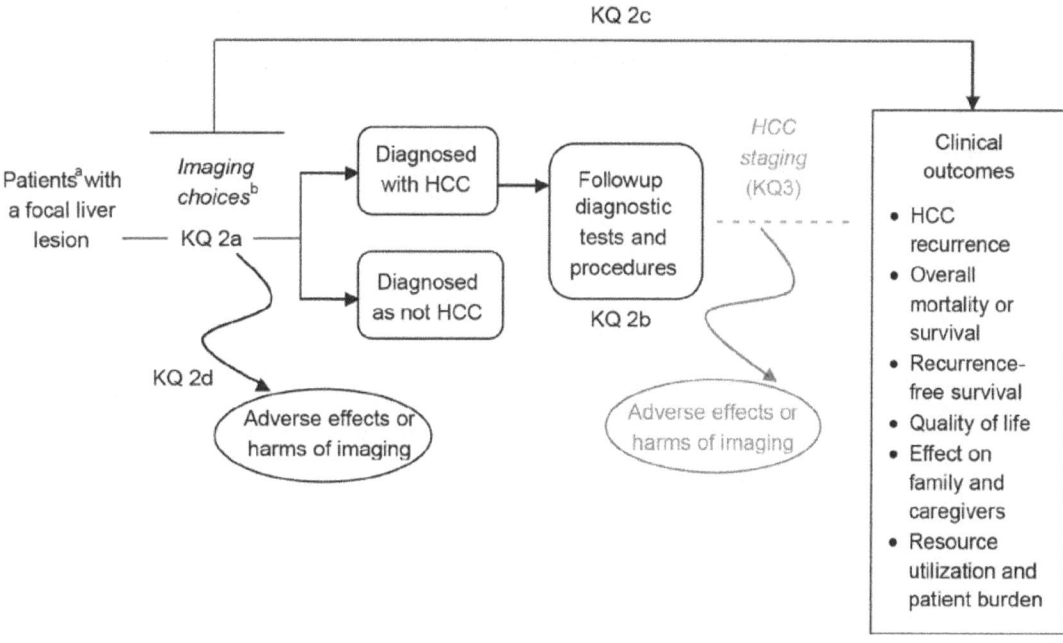

HCC = hepatocellular carcinoma; KQ = Key Question. Shaded elements show the relationship of KQ2 to KQ3.

[a] Potential modifiers of test performance include patient (e.g., severity of liver disease, underlying cause of liver disease, body mass index, age, sex, race), tumor (e.g., tumor diameter, degree of differentiation, location), technical, and other factors (e.g., biomarker levels, setting).
[b] Imaging techniques are used singly, in combination, or in sequence with or without biomarkers used as modifiers.

Figure 3. Analytic framework—staging (Key Question 3)

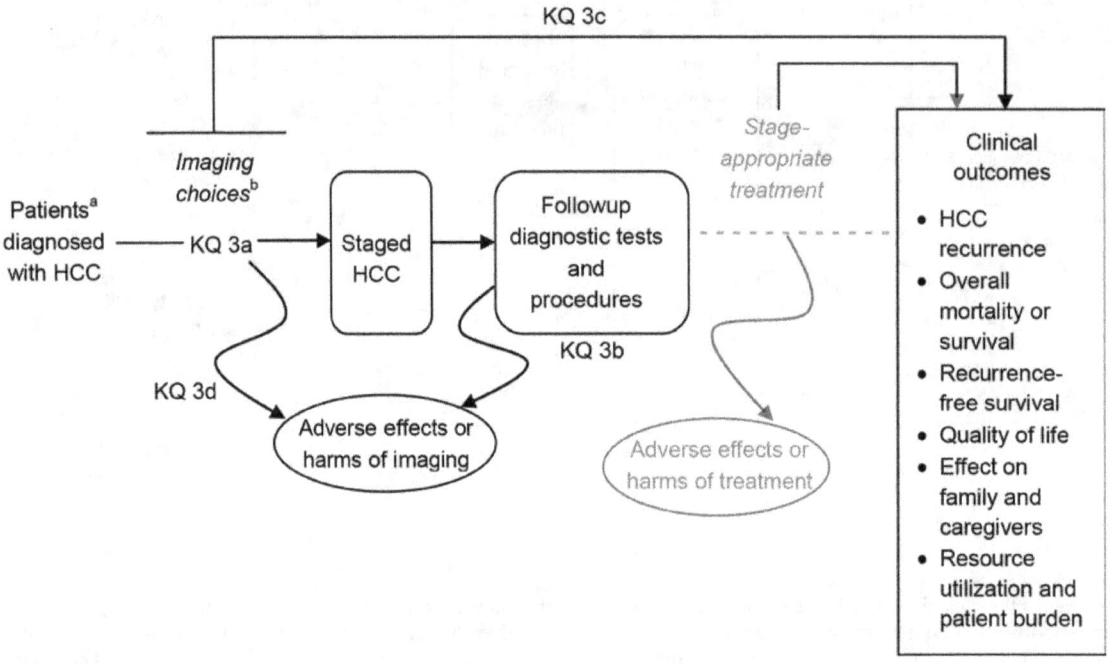

HCC = hepatocellular carcinoma; KQ = Key Question.
Note: Shaded elements show subsequent treatment that may follow detection (KQ1), diagnosis (KQ2), and staging (KQ3) [a] Potential modifiers of test performance include patient (e.g., severity of liver disease, underlying cause of liver disease, body mass index, age, sex, race), tumor (e.g., tumor diameter, degree of differentiation, location), technical, and other factors (e.g., biomarker levels, setting).
[b] Imaging techniques are used singly, in combination, or in sequence with or without biomarkers used as modifiers.

Table 1. Imaging techniques used in the surveillance, diagnosis, and staging of hepatocellular carcinoma

Imaging Modality	Key Characteristics	Surveillance	Diagnosis	Staging
Transabdominal ultrasound (US)	This modality uses ultrasound waves and their reflection from tissue interfaces to generate images of the underlying anatomy. Conventional (noncontrast) ultrasound is limited in its ability characterize hepatic lesions. Use of intravenous (IV) microbubble contrast agents has been proposed as a method for improving the characterization of liver masses. Most studies of contrast-enhanced US have focused on targeted evaluation of lesions identified on nonenhanced US or other imaging studies, due to the limited duration that contrast is present in the liver.	●	● (IV contrast only)	
Computed tomography (CT)	This imaging modality is based on x-ray exposure and acquisition of data through a set of detectors arrayed in a linear fashion. Contrast-enhanced CT images are obtained after injecting iodinated IV contrast media. Multiple passes are performed at specific times following contrast administration (multiphase contrast study). **Spiral CT** performs continuous scans, acquiring information to generate images in multiple planes. **Multidetector CT** scanners are based on the same imaging principles as spiral CT but utilize a two-dimensional array of detectors. MDCT permits faster scanning, resulting in fewer motion artifacts and improved image quality. **Dual energy CT** is a newer technique that uses x-rays of varying energy (70–140 kVp) to increase tissue contrast and detect different elements (e.g., iodine, calcium) within the liver. **Spectral CT** is a related technique that can separate and utilize information from the whole x-ray spectrum.	●	●	●
Magnetic resonance imaging (MRI)	This imaging technique uses a strong magnetic field and radiofrequency pulses to obtain anatomic images of the body. MRI scanning is slower than CT scanning and requires that the patient remain still during image acquisition. Like CT, multiphase MRI images are obtained in multiple passes following the IV administration of gadolinium-based contrast agents. MRI imaging acquisition techniques can preferentially assess tissues for fat content, diffusion characteristics, and edema. Different gadolinium contrast media are available, including nonspecific arterially enhancing agents such as gadopentetate and gadodiamide, and newer hepatic-specific agents like gadoxetic acid disodium or gadobenate that are preferentially taken up by functioning hepatocytes and excreted in the biliary system.	●	●	●
Positron emission tomography (PET)	This functional imaging technique uses radioisotope-tagged tracers to examine the level and type of biochemical activity in lesions suspected to be cancerous throughout the body (making it useful to study metastases). The most commonly used tracer is ^{18}F-fluorodeoxyglucose (FDG), which detects cells exhibiting increased glucose transport and metabolism (cancer cells typically exhibit such metabolic activity). Alternative tracers have also been investigated.			●

CT = computed tomography; FDG = ^{18}F-fluorodeoxyglucose; IV = intravenous; MRI = magnetic resonance imaging; PET = positron emission tomography; US = ultrasound

Table 2. Recommended minimum technical specifications for dynamic contrast-enhanced computed tomography (CT) of the liver[a]

Feature	Specification	Comment
Scanner type	Multidetector row scanner	...
Detector type	Minimum of 8 detector rows	Need to be able to image entire liver during brief late arterial phase time window
Reconstructed section thickness	Minimum of 5-mm reconstructed section thickness	Thinner sections are preferable, especially if multiplanar reconstructions are obtained
Injector	Power injector, preferably dual-chamber injector with saline flush	Bolus tracking recommended
Contrast agent injection rate	Minimum, 3 mL/sec; better, 4–6 mL/sec with minimum of 300 mg iodine per milliliter or higher, for dose of 1.5 mL/kg of body weight	...
Mandatory dynamic phases during contrast-enhanced CT*	Late arterial phase, portal venous phase, and delayed phase	Artery fully enhanced, beginning contrast enhancement of portal vein; portal vein enhanced, peak liver parenchymal enhancement, beginning contrast enhancement of hepatic veins; variable appearance, >120 sec after initial injection of contrast agent
Dynamic phases (timing)	Bolus tracking or timing bolus recommended for accurate timing	...

CT = computed tomography

*Comments describe typical hallmark image features

[a]Adapted with permission of the copyright holder, Radiological Society of North America (RSNA), from Wald C, Russo MW, Heimbach JK, et al. New OPTN/UNOS policy for liver transplant allocation: standardization of liver imaging, diagnosis, classification, and reporting of hepatocellular carcinoma. Radiology. 2013 Feb;266(2):376-82.[15]

Table 3. Recommended minimum technical specifications for dynamic contrast-enhanced MR imaging of the liver[a]

Feature	Specification	Comment
MR unit type	1.5-T or greater main magnetic field strength	Low-field-strength magnets not suitable
Coil type	Phased-array multichannel torso coil	Unless patient-related factors preclude use (e.g., body habitus)
Minimum sequences	Nonenhanced and dynamic gadolinium-enhanced T1-weighted GRE sequence (3D preferable), T2-weighted (with and without fat saturation), T1-weighted in- and opposed-phase imaging	...
Injector	Dual-chamber power injector	Bolus tracking recommended
Contrast agent injection rate	For extracellular gadolinium chelate that does not have dominant biliary excretion, 2–3 mL/sec	Preferably resulting in vendor-recommended total dose
Mandatory dynamic phases at contrast-enhanced MR imaging*	Nonenhanced T1 weighted, late arterial phase, portal venous phase, delayed phase	For nonenhanced T1 weighted, do not change imaging parameters for contrast-enhanced imaging; for late arterial phase, artery fully enhanced, beginning contrast enhancement of portal vein; for portal veinous phase, portal vein enhanced, peak liver parenchymal enhancement, beginning contrast enhancement of hepatic veins; for delayed phase, variable appearance, >120 sec after initial injection of contrast agent
Dynamic phases, timing	Use of a bolus-tracking method for timing contrast agent arrival for late aterial phase imaging is preferable; portal venous phase (35–55 sec after initiation of late arterial phase imaging); delayed phase (120–180 sec after initial contrast agent injection)	...
Section thickness	For dynamic series, 5 mm or less; for other imaging, 8 mm or less	...
Breath holding	Maximum length of series requiring breath hold should be about 20 sec, with a minimum matrix of 128 x 256	Compliance with breath-held instructions is very important; technologists need to understand the importance of patient instruction before and during imaging

GRE = gradient echo; MR = magnetic resonance; 3D = three-dimensional.

*Comments describe typical hallmark image features.

[a]Adapted with permission of the copyright holder, Radiological Society of North America (RSNA), from Wald C, Russo MW, Heimbach JK, et al. New OPTN/UNOS policy for liver transplant allocation: standardization of liver imaging, diagnosis, classification, and reporting of hepatocellular carcinoma. Radiology. 2013 Feb;266(2):376-82.[15]

Methods

The methods for this systematic review follow the methods suggested in the Agency for Healthcare Research and Quality (AHRQ) Effective Health Care Program methods guides.[24,25]

Topic Refinement and Review Protocol

This topic was selected for review based on a nomination from the Tufts Evidence-Based Practice Center (EPC) topic identification project, which included a set of draft proposed Key Questions. The Key Questions and scope were further developed with input from a Technical Expert Panel (TEP). The TEP provided high-level content and methodological guidance to the review process through involvement of clinicians and researchers with expertise in the diagnosis and management of liver diseases and cancers, radiologists, hepatologists, clinical outcomes researchers, and patient and payer representatives. TEP members disclosed all financial and other conflicts of interest prior to participation. The AHRQ Task Order Officer and the investigators reviewed the disclosures and determined that the panel members had no conflicts of interest that precluded participation.

The protocol for this comparative effectiveness review (CER) was posted on the Agency for Healthcare Research and Quality (AHRQ) Web site on July 25, 2013.[26] The protocol was also registered in the PROSPERO international database of prospectively registered systematic reviews.[27]

Searching for the Evidence

For the primary literature, we searched Ovid MEDLINE®, Scopus, Evidence-Based Medicine Reviews (Ovid), the Cochrane Central Register of Controlled Trials, the Cochrane Database of Systematic Reviews, the Database of Abstracts of Reviews of Effects, and the Health Technology Assessment Database from 1998 to December 2013 (see Table 4 for search strategy). We searched for unpublished studies in clinical trial registries (ClinicalTrials.gov, Current Controlled Trials, ClinicalStudyResults.org, and the World Health Organization International Clinical Trials Registry Platform), regulatory documents (U.S. Food and Drug Administration Medical Devices Registration and Listing), and individual product Web sites. Scientific information packets (SIPs) were solicited via a notice published in the *Federal Register* that invited interested parties to submit relevant published and unpublished studies using the publicly accessible AHRQ Effective Health Care online SIP portal.[28] One SIP response was received, but it yielded no additional relevant studies. We also hand-searched the reference lists of relevant studies and previous systematic reviews for additional studies.

Populations and Conditions of Interest

The populations and conditions of interest for each key question are described in Table 5.

Study Selection

We developed criteria for inclusion and exclusion of studies based on the Key Questions and the populations, interventions, comparators, outcomes, timing, and setting (PICOTS) approach (Table 5). Papers were selected for full review if they were about imaging for HCC, were relevant to one or more Key Questions, and met the predefined inclusion criteria. We excluded studies published only as conference abstracts, restricted inclusion to English language articles, and excluded studies of nonhuman subjects. Studies had to report original data to be included.

Each abstract was reviewed for inclusion. Full-text articles were obtained for all studies that investigators identified as potentially meeting inclusion criteria. Two investigators independently reviewed all full-text articles for final inclusion or exclusion. Discrepancies were resolved through discussion and consensus.

We selected studies of adults without HCC undergoing surveillance (Key Question 1), imaging for further evaluation of a focal liver lesion or to distinguish HCC from another type of hepatic lesion (Key Question 2), and staging of HCC (Key Question 3). For Key Question 1, we also included studies on diagnostic accuracy of imaging for detection of HCC in nonsurveillance settings. These included series of patients undergoing treatments for HCC (e.g., liver transplantation, hepatic resection, or ablative therapy) or patients with a known prevalence of HCC who were undergoing imaging for purposes other than surveillance. These studies were reviewed under Key Question 1 because they provide information about the test performance of imaging modalities for detecting HCC lesions, rather than to further characterize or assess a previously identified lesion (Key Question 2). We excluded studies that reported diagnostic accuracy of imaging for non-HCC malignant lesions, including metastatic lesions to the liver. We included studies that reported diagnostic accuracy for HCC and cholangiocarcinoma together if the proportion of patients with cholangiocarcinoma was <10 percent.

We selected studies of US (with or without contrast enhancement), contrast-enhanced CT (nonmultidetector or multidetector spiral CT, and dual energy or spectral CT), contrast-enhanced MRI, and PET or PET/CT using various tracers. We excluded studies of nonspiral CT and MRI using machines ≤1.0 T, as these are considered outdated techniques.[15] We excluded studies published prior to 1998 and also excluded studies in which imaging commenced prior to 1995, unless those studies reported use of imaging meeting minimum technical criteria (defined as nonmultidetector or multidetector spiral CT and MRI with a 1.5 or 3.0 T machine). We excluded studies that evaluated MRI with contrast agents that are no longer produced commercially and are unavailable for clinical use—for example, superparamagnetic iron oxide (ferumoxides or ferucarbotran) or mangafodipir contrast—unless results based on gadolinium-enhanced imaging phases were reported separately. Although US microbubble contrast agents are not approved by the U.S. Food and Drug Administration (FDA) for evaluation of liver lesions, we included such studies because these agents are available commercially outside the United States, US with contrast is commonly performed in other countries, and efforts to obtain FDA approval are ongoing.[29-31] We excluded studies of CT arterial portography and CT hepatic angiography, which are invasive techniques not typically utilized in the United States for diagnosis and staging of HCC. We also excluded studies of intraoperative US.

For studies of test performance (e.g., sensitivity, specificity, and likelihood ratios), we included studies that evaluated one or more imaging methods against a reference standard. Reference standards were histopathology (based on explanted liver or nonexplant histological specimen from surgery or percutaneous biopsy), imaging plus clinical followup (e.g., lesion growth), or some combination of these standards. We excluded studies in which the reference standard involved one of the imaging tests under evaluation and that did not perform clinical followup, and we also excluded studies that had no reference standard (i.e., reported the number of lesions identified with an imaging technique, but did not evaluate accuracy against another reference technique).

To assess comparative effects of imaging on clinical outcomes (e.g., mortality, HCC recurrence, quality of life, and harms), we included randomized controlled trials that compared different imaging modalities or strategies. A systematic review funded by the Department of Veterans Affairs Evidence Synthesis program on effects of screening for HCC on clinical outcomes is forthcoming and will include comparative observational studies.[32]

To assess comparative effects of imaging on intermediate outcomes related to clinical decisionmaking (e.g., subsequent diagnostic testing, treatments, or resource utilization), we included randomized trials and cohort studies that compared different imaging modalities or strategies.

Data Abstraction and Data Management

We extracted the following data from included studies into evidence tables using Excel spreadsheets: study design, year, setting, country, sample size, method of data collection (retrospective or prospective), eligibility criteria, population and clinical characteristics (including age, sex, race, underlying cause of liver disease, proportion of patients in sample with HCC, HCC lesion size, and proportion with cirrhosis), the number of imaging readers, criteria used for a positive test, and the reference standard used. We abstracted results for diagnostic accuracy, intermediate outcomes, and clinical outcomes, including results stratified according to patient, lesion, and imaging characteristics. Technical information for different imaging tests was abstracted as follows:[15]

- Ultrasound
  - Use of contrast
  - Type of contrast
  - Ultrasound operator (technician, physician, or other)
  - Transducer frequency
  - Use of Doppler

- Computed tomography
  - Use of multidetector scanner and the number of rows
  - Imaging sequences with timing
  - Contrast rate
  - Section thickness for contrast-enhanced images
  - Use of dual energy or spectral CT techniques

- Magnetic resonance imaging
  - MRI unit type (number of Teslas)
  - Imaging sequences with timing
  - Type of contrast
  - Section thickness
  - Use of diffusion-weighted imaging sequences
  - Spatial resolution

- Positron emission tomography
  - Scanner type (PET versus PET/CT)
  - Tracer type

Data abstraction for each study was completed by two investigators: the first abstracted the data, and the second reviewed the abstracted data for accuracy and completeness against the original articles. A team member with expertise in abdominal imaging reviewed data abstractions related to technical specifications.

Assessment of Methodological Risk of Bias of Individual Studies

We assessed risk of bias (quality) for each study based on predefined criteria. Randomized trials and cohort studies were evaluated using criteria and methods developed by the U.S. Preventive Services Task Force.[33] These criteria were applied in conjunction with the approach recommended in the Agency for Health Care Research and Quality (AHRQ) "Methods Guide for Effectiveness and Comparative Effectiveness Reviews."[24] Studies of diagnostic test performance were assessed using the approach recommended in the AHRQ "Methods Guide for Medical Test Reviews,"[25] which is based on methods developed by the Quality Assessment of Diagnostic Accuracy Studies (QUADAS) group.[34]

Individual studies were rated as having "low," "moderate," or "high" risk of bias. Studies rated "low" risk of bias are generally considered valid. Randomized trials and cohort studies assessed as having low risk of bias have a valid method for allocating patients to treatment (for randomized trials); clear reporting of dropouts with low dropout rates; blinding of patients, clinicians, and/or outcome assessors to the interventions received; appropriate measurement of and analysis of confounders (for cohort studies); and appropriate measurement of outcomes. Studies of diagnostic test performance that are assessed as having low risk of bias enroll consecutive or randomly sampled patients, avoid use of a case-control design, use a credible reference standard, apply the same reference standard to all patients, use blinded interpretation of the diagnostic test as well as the reference standard, use preset criteria to define a positive test, avoid long delays between the imaging test and the reference standard, and have limited (defined for this report as <10%) loss to followup.[7,12] We considered studies in which all patients had HCC as utilizing a case-control design, even if some patients also had other (non-HCC) lesions. We considered studies that utilized a histopathological reference standard or a reference standard consistent with European Association for the Study of the Liver (EASL) or AASLD criteria to be adequate, provided that the imaging test used as the reference standard was not the same as the test being evaluated. The AASLD criteria is based on tumor size, with lesions <1 cm undergoing serial imaging followup.[9] Based on AASLD criteria, for lesions >1 cm, presence of a typical enhancement pattern on CT or MRI is considered diagnostic for HCC; for lesions without typical enhancement on one of these imaging tests, biopsy is required.

Studies rated as having "moderate" risk have some methodological shortcomings, but no flaw or combination of flaws judged likely to cause major bias. In some cases, the study may be missing information, making it difficult to assess its methods or potential limitations. The moderate risk of bias category is broad, and studies with this rating will vary in their strengths and weaknesses; the results of some studies assessed to have moderate risk of bias are likely to be valid, while others may be only possibly valid.

Studies rated as having "high" risk of bias have significant flaws that may invalidate the results. They have a serious or "fatal" flaw in design, analysis, or reporting; large amounts of missing information; or serious discrepancies in reporting. The results of these studies are at least as likely to reflect flaws in the study design as the differences between the compared interventions. We did not exclude studies rated as having high risk of bias a priori, but they were considered the least reliable when synthesizing the evidence, particularly when discrepancies between studies were present.

Data Synthesis

We performed meta-analyses on measures of test performance in order to help summarize data and obtain more precise estimates.[35] All quantitative analyses were conducted using SAS® 9.3 (SAS Institute Inc., Cary, NC). We only pooled studies that were clinically comparable and could provide a meaningful combined estimate (based on the variability among studies in design, patient population, imaging methods, and outcomes) and magnitude of effect size. We conducted separate analyses for each imaging modality, stratified according to the unit of analysis used (patients with HCC, HCC lesions, or liver segments with HCC), and analyzed studies of US with contrast separately from studies of US without contrast. For studies that used multiple readers, we averaged results across readers using the binomial specification of Proc NLMIXED on SAS. For Key Question 1, we also stratified analyses according to whether imaging was performed for surveillance or if imaging was performed in a series of patients for some other reason. For Key Question 2, we separately analyzed studies that evaluated further imaging of a focal liver lesion identified on previous imaging and studies evaluating the ability of imaging tests to distinguish between HCC and another specific non-HCC lesion. For Key Question 3, we separately analyzed studies on test performance of imaging for identifying metastatic HCC and accuracy of imaging for staging based on tumor, node, metastasis staging (TNM), Barcelona Liver Cancer Clinic (BLCC), and other criteria.

We evaluated a number of potential sources of heterogeneity (see below) and modifiers of diagnostic accuracy. We performed analyses stratified according to the reference standard used and on domains related to risk of bias, aspects of study design (retrospective or prospective, use of a confidence rating scale), setting (based on country in which imaging was performed), and technical factors (such as scanner types, type of contrast or tracer used, use of recommended imaging phases, timing of delayed phase imaging, and section thickness). We also evaluated diagnostic accuracy in subgroups stratified according to HCC lesion size, degree of tumor differentiation, and tumor location, as well as patient characteristics such as severity of underlying liver disease, underlying cause of liver disease, and body mass index. For analyzing effects of tumor size and degree of differentiation on estimates of accuracy, we analyzed studies on surveillance and diagnosis together. Because of the effects of lesion size on estimates of diagnostic accuracy, subgroup analyses for each imaging modality were performed on the subgroup of studies that were not restricted to small (<2-3 cm) HCC lesions.

We performed separate analyses on the subset of studies that directly compared two or more imaging modalities or techniques in the same population against a common reference standard. Research indicates that results based on such direct comparisons differ from results based on noncomparative studies, and may be better suited for evaluating comparative diagnostic test performance.[36]

We did not perform meta-analysis on staging accuracy and intermediate or clinical outcomes due to the small number of studies. Rather, we synthesized these studies qualitatively, using the methods described below for assessing the strength of evidence.

Approaches to Data Analysis

We conducted meta-analysis to quantitatively synthesize data and obtain summary estimates of test performance. We used a bivariate logistic mixed effects model[37] to analyze sensitivity and specificity, incorporating the correlation between sensitivity and specificity. We assumed random effects across studies with a bivariate normal distribution for sensitivity and specificity, and heterogeneity among the studies was measured based on the random effect variance (τ^2). The advantage of using a logistic mixed effects model is that it handles sparse data better and does not need to assume an ad hoc continuity correction when a study has zero events.[37] When few studies were available for an analysis, we used the moment estimates of correlation between sensitivity and specificity in the bivariate model. We calculated positive likelihood ratio (LR+) and negative likelihood ratio (LR-) using the summarized sensitivity and specificity.[38,39] We did not attempt to plot summary receiver operating characteristic (ROC) because many studies were missing data necessary to estimate ROC curves (due to failure to report specificity or number of true-negatives).[40] In addition, the "threshold effect" assumption required for valid summary ROC curves did not appear to be met, as the estimated correlation between sensitivity and specificity was often positive. Finally, when a confidence rating scale was used to diagnose HCC, the cutoffs used in the included studies did not vary enough to demonstrate a potential threshold effect.

The data were synthesized by each imaging modality. To address possible source of heterogeneity among studies and produce meaningful summary estimates, we stratified analyses by Key Questions and the unit of analysis. We also conducted extensive subgroup and sensitivity analyses based on study-level, patient, tumor, technical, and other factors. When data were available, we performed separate meta-analyses for within-study comparisons based on technical factors, lesion size, and degree of tumor differentiation.

To assess the comparative effectiveness of alternative imaging modalities, we also conducted head-to-head comparisons between imaging modalities when data were available, using the same bivariate logistic mixed effects model as described above, but adding an indicator variable for imaging modalities (equivalent to a meta-regression approach). These analyses only included studies that directly compared two imaging modalities, in order to restrict the comparison to direct evidence. Again we stratified the comparisons by Key Questions and unit of analysis, and we conducted subgroup analyses by methodological and lesion characteristics when the data allowed. All analyses were conducted using SAS 9.3 (SAS institute Inc., Cary, NC).

Grading the Strength of Evidence for Individual Comparisons and Outcomes

The strength of evidence for each Key Question was assessed by one researcher for each outcome described in the PICOTS using the approach described in the AHRQ "Methods Guide for Effectiveness and Comparative Effectiveness Reviews."[24] The strength of evidence pertains to the overall quality of each body of evidence, and is based on the risk of bias (graded low, moderate, or high); the consistency of results between studies (graded consistent, inconsistent, or unknown/not applicable when only one study was available); the directness of the evidence linking the intervention and health outcomes (graded direct or indirect); and the precision of the estimate of effect, based on the number and size of studies and confidence intervals for the estimates (graded precise or imprecise). We did not downgrade a body of evidence for directness that evaluated an intermediate outcome, if the intermediate outcome (such as diagnostic accuracy or effects on clinical decisionmaking) was the specific focus of the Key Question. We did not grade supplemental domains for cohort studies evaluating intermediate and clinical outcomes because too few studies were available for these factors to impact the strength of evidence grades. We did not assess studies of diagnostic test performance for publication bias using graphical or statistical methods because research indicates that such methods can be misleading. Rather, we searched for unpublished studies through searches of clinical trials registries and regulatory documents and by soliciting SIPs.

We graded the strength of evidence for each Key Question using the four key categories recommended in the AHRQ Methods Guide.[24] A "high" grade indicates high confidence that the evidence reflects the true effect and that further research is very unlikely to change our confidence in the estimate of effect. A "moderate" grade indicates moderate confidence that the evidence reflects the true effect and further research may change our confidence in the estimate of effect and may change the estimate. A "low" grade indicates low confidence that the evidence reflects the true effect and further research is likely to change the confidence in the estimate of effect and is likely to change the estimate. An "insufficient" grade indicates evidence either is unavailable or is too limited to permit any conclusion.

Assessing Applicability

We recorded factors important for understanding the applicability of studies, such as whether the publication adequately described the study population, the country in which the study was conducted, the prevalence of HCC in the patients who underwent imaging, the magnitude of differences in measures of diagnostic accuracy and clinical outcomes, and whether the imaging techniques were reasonably representative of standard practice.[41] We also recorded the funding source and role of the sponsor. We did not assign a rating of applicability (such as high or low) because applicability may differ based on the user of the report.

Peer Review and Public Commentary

Experts in gastroenterology, hepatology, and radiology, along with individuals representing stakeholder and user communities, were invited to provide external peer review of the draft report; AHRQ and an EPC associate editor also provided comments. The draft report was posted on the AHRQ Web site for 4 weeks to elicit public comment. All comments were reviewed and addressed in a disposition of comments report that will be made available 3 months after the Agency posts the final report of the systematic review on the AHRQ Web site.

Table 4. Search strategy—Ovid MEDLINE® (1998–2013)

1	Carcinoma, Hepatocellular/
2	Liver Neoplasms/
3	("hepatocellular cancer" or "hepatocellular carcinoma" or "HCC").ti,ab.
4	Diagnostic Imaging/
5	Ultrasonography/
6	Magnetic Resonance Imaging/
7	exp Tomography, Emission-Computed/ or exp Positron-Emission Tomography/ or exp Tomography, Spiral Computed/
8	("CT" or "dynamic multidetector computed tomography" or "MDCT" or "spiral CT" or "dual source CT" or "contrast CT" or "MRI" or "FDG-PET").ti,ab.
9	or/1-3
10	or/4-8
11	9 and 10
12	"Sensitivity and Specificity"/
13	"Predictive Value of Tests"/
14	ROC Curve/
15	"Reproducibility of Results"/
16	(sensitiv$ or "predictive value" or accurac$).ti,ab.
17	or/12-16
18	11 and 17
19	limit 18 to yr="1998 - 2013"

Table 5. Inclusion and exclusion criteria by Key Question

All Key Questions	Inclusion Criteria	Exclusion Criteria
Interventions	<ul><li>Ultrasound (with or without contrast)</li><li>Contrast-enhanced spiral CT (including nonmultidetector or multidetector CT, and CT using dual energy and spectral methods)</li><li>Contrast-enhanced MRI using a 1.5 or 3.0 T scanner</li><li>Diffusion-weighted MRI</li><li>PET or PET/CT (including use of ^{18}F-fluorodeoxyglucose, ^{18}F-fluorothymidine, ^{11}C-acetate, and ^{11}C-choline tracers)</li></ul>	<ul><li>Outdated imaging techniques (e.g., conventional, nonspiral/nonmultidetector CT, MRI using a ≤1.0 T scanner)</li><li>CT and MRI without contrast, with the exception of studies of diffusion-weighted MRI without contrast</li><li>CT arterial portography and CT hepatic arteriography</li><li>C-arm CT</li><li>Intraoperative ultrasound</li><li>MRI with ferucarbotran, ferumoxides, or mangafodipir contrast</li></ul>
Comparisons	For studies of diagnostic accuracy (comparative test performance):<ul><li>Reference standard comparators: Histopathology (based on explanted liver specimens or biopsy), clinical followup, and imaging followup</li><li>Imaging comparators: Alternative imaging tests or strategies.</li></ul>For studies of comparative effectiveness:<ul><li>No imaging or an alternative imaging strategy</li></ul>	Does not meet inclusion criteria
Timing	No restrictions	None
Setting	All care settings (e.g., primary and secondary care)	None
Study Designs	<ul><li>Controlled randomized and nonrandomized trials</li><li>Cohort studies on effects of imaging on diagnostic thinking or clinical decisionmaking</li><li>Studies of diagnostic accuracy</li></ul>	<ul><li>Studies of diagnostic accuracy that did not report the reference standard used, or in which the reference standard included the results of the test being investigated</li><li>Case reports, case series, letters to the editor, and nonsystematic reviews</li><li>Studies published prior to 1998 or in which imaging was performed prior to 1995, unless technical details were reported and studies met minimum technical criteria as described in the Interventions section above</li></ul>

Table 5. Inclusion and exclusion criteria by Key Question (continued)

Key Questions 1 and 2	Inclusion Criteria	Exclusion Criteria
Populations	Key Question 1 • Patients at high risk for HCC undergoing surveillance, including: Asian male HBV carriers over age 40, Asian female HBV carriers over age 50, HBV carriers with a family history of HCC, African/North American black HBV carriers, all individuals with cirrhosis (including alcoholic cirrhosis), HBV or HCV carriers with cirrhosis, and patients with stage 4 primary biliary cirrhosis • Other high-risk patients undergoing surveillance as defined by the primary studies • Patients enrolled in studies designed to determine detection rates of imaging for HCC, including patients who underwent liver transplantation or surgery for HCC or other reasons. Key Question 2 • Patients in whom a suspicious lesion(s) for HCC has been detected by surveillance or by other means, including patients who underwent liver transplantation for HCC or other reasons • Patients enrolled in studies designed to distinguish HCC from another type of liver lesion (benign or malignant)	• Patients with cholangiocarcinoma, unless they comprised <10% of the study population • Patients with nonprimary (metastatic) lesions to the liver • Patients undergoing imaging to evaluate response to ablative or other treatments • Children.
Outcomes	• Diagnostic outcomes: test performance, types of HCC lesions detected • Intermediate outcomes: effects on diagnostic thinking, effects on clinical decisionmaking. • Clinical and patient-centered outcomes: overall mortality or survival, recurrence of HCC, including rates of seeding by fine-needle aspiration; quality of life as measured with scales such as the Short-Form Health Survey or EuroQol 5D; and psychosocial effects of diagnostic testing on patients, patients' caregivers, and other family members • Resource utilization and patient burden (e.g., costs associated with the imaging procedure, the number of imaging procedures, and other procedures conducted) • Harms: adverse effects or harms associated with the imaging techniques (e.g., test-related anxiety, adverse events secondary to venipuncture, contrast allergy, exposure to radiation) and adverse effects or harms associated with test-associated diagnostic workup (e.g., harms of biopsy or harms associated with workup of other incidental tumors discovered on imaging).	• Nonclinical and nondiagnostic outcomes.

Table 5. Inclusion and exclusion criteria by Key Question (continued)

	Inclusion Criteria	Exclusion Criteria
Key Question 3		
Populations	• Patients diagnosed with HCC undergoing staging before initial treatment.	• Patients with cholangiocarcinoma, unless they comprised <10% of the study population • Patients with nonprimary (metastatic) lesions to the liver • Patients undergoing imaging to evaluate response to ablative or other treatments • Children.
Outcomes	• Measures of stage-specific accuracy of imaging (e.g., proportion correctly staged, understaged, and overstaged) • Intermediate and clinical outcomes as described for Key Questions 1 and 2.	• Nonclinical and nondiagnostic outcomes.

CT = computed tomography; HBV = hepatitis B virus; HCC = hepatocellular carcinoma; HCV = hepatitis C virus; MRI = magnetic resonance imaging; PET = positron emission tomography

Results

Introduction

The bulk of the available evidence addresses diagnostic accuracy of imaging techniques for hepatocellular carcinoma (HCC)—ultrasound (US), computed tomography (CT), magnetic resonance imaging (MRI), and positron emission tomography (PET). Few studies compared effects of different imaging modalities or strategies on clinical decisionmaking, clinical outcomes, and almost no studies reported harms.

Results of Literature Searches

The search and selection of articles are summarized in the study flow diagram (Figure 4). Of the 4846 citations identified at the title and abstract level, 851 articles appeared to meet inclusion criteria and were selected for further full-text review. Following review at the full-text level, a total of 281studies met inclusion criteria (Appendix A); primary reasons for exclusion of the articles reviewed at the full-text level were (Appendix B). We rated three studies low risk of bias,[42-44] 189 moderate risk of bias, and 89 high risk of bias (Appendix C).

Three cohort studies[45-47] and three randomized trials reported patient outcomes of imaging for staging.[48-50] We identified 274 studies that evaluated diagnostic accuracy of imaging tests.

Of the diagnostic accuracy studies, 70 evaluated US (Appendix D),[43,51-119] 134 evaluated CT (Appendix E),[42-44,51,53-56,58,60-62,66,69,74,75,81,82,87,89,91,92,96,99,101-103,110-112,117-220] 129 evaluated MRI (Appendix F),[43,44,51,56,59,61,65,69,74,75,82,99,100,103,105,106,108,110,118,121,123,126,129,131,134-136,138,140,141,144,145,150,158,163,164,166,168,176,179,184,190,191,193,195,198,200,203,206,207,209,211,212,218,221-295] and 32 evaluated PET (Appendix G).[110,111,127,152,154,171,189,296-320] Twenty-eight studies evaluated use of more than one imaging technique in combination or sequentially.[43,44,51,55,59,61,69,75,79,96,127,134,152,171,189,296,297,300,302,305,309,310,312-314,317,320,321] Almost all studies reported sensitivity, but only 130 reported specificity or provided data to calculate specificity. We found 119 studies avoided use of a case-control design, 151 used blinded ascertainment, and 75 used a prospective design. More studies were conducted in Asia (182 studies) than in Australia, Canada, the United States or Europe combined (92 studies). In 155 studies, imaging was conducted starting in or after 2003.

Twenty-seven studies evaluated CT using methods that met minimum technical specifications (≥8-row multidetector CT; contrast rate ≥3 ml/s; at least arterial, portal venous, and delayed phase imaging; delayed phase imaging performed >120 s following administration of contrast; and enhanced imaging section thickness ≤5 mm)[42,43,56,69,75,87,92,96,131,135,141,147,158,162-164,168,177,178,183,184,195,200,206,210,212,215] and 59 studies evaluated MRI using methods that met minimum technical specifications (1.5 or 3.0 T MRI; at least arterial, portal venous, and delayed phase imaging; delayed phase imaging performed >120 s following administration of contrast; and enhanced imaging section thickness ≤5 mm).[43,56,59,69,74,105,106,121,123,131,134,135,141,145,150,158,162,163,168,184,191,195,198,203,206,207,212,221,223-225,227,231,232,238,241,243-256,262-265,271,272,274,278,282] Sixty-three MRI studies evaluated use of hepatic-specific contrast (e.g., gadoxetic acid or gadobenate).[43,51,56,65,69,74,75,79,105,106,108,121,123,131,135,136,141,144,145,150,158,163,168,184,191,195,203,206,207,212,221-225,227,230-232,241,242,244,246-251,253-255,264,265,269-272,274,278,282,287,295,321] Forty-six US studies evaluated use of microbubble contrast agents.[43,51,53,55,57-60,63,65-69,71,73-75,78,79,81,85-89,91-93,95-98,100,101,104-109,113-117] 30 studies evaluated PET using FDG,[110,111,127,152,154,171,189,296-298,300-305,307-320] eight studies using ^{11}C-

21

acetate,[127,297,300-302,306,309,319] and three studies evaluated use of other tracers (^{18}F-fluorothymidine or ^{18}F-fluorocholine).[299,313,314]

Data for outcomes other than measures of test performance were sparse. Eight studies reported comparative effects on clinical decisionmaking,[82,102,122,127,179,202,208,322] four studies reported comparative clinical and patient-centered outcomes,[48-50,322] and three studies reported harms associated with imaging for HCC.[91,144,204]

Figure 4. Study flow diagram

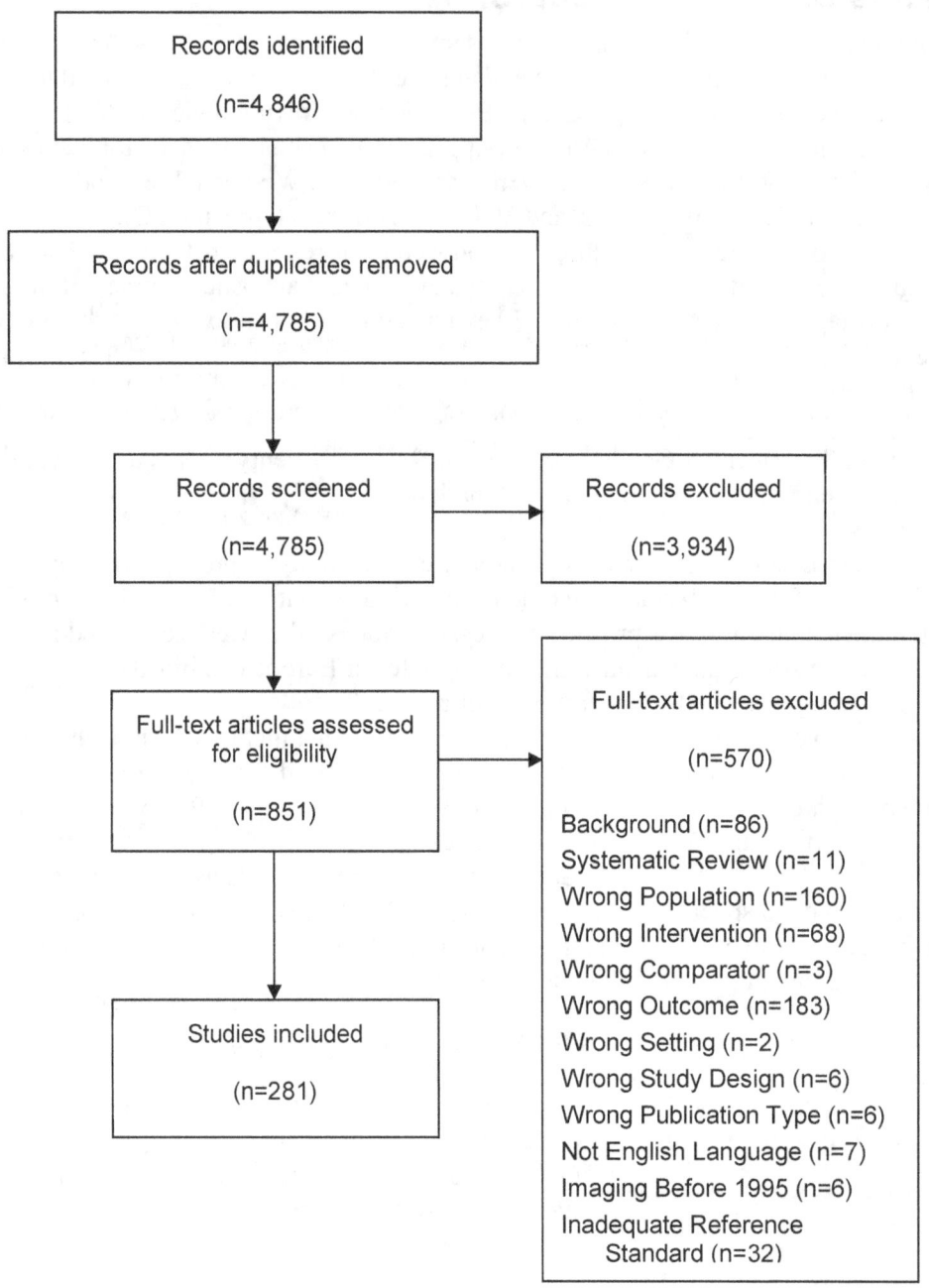

Key Question 1. What is the comparative effectiveness of available imaging-based strategies, used singly or in sequence, for detection of HCC among individuals in surveillance and nonsurveillance settings?

Description of Included Studies

Six studies[54,62,90,94,103,112] evaluated diagnostic accuracy of imaging techniques for surveillance and 182 studies[42,51,52,56,61,64,67,69-71,74,76-79,82-84,92,99,106,110,111,118-121,123-127,129-133,135-141,143-146,148-151,153-155,157-170,172-180,182-188,190-205,207-212,215-227,234-238,241,244,246,248-252,254-264,267,268,270,271,273-277,280,281,283-286,288,290,292,294,295,297,299,301-303,306-310,313-319,321] reported diagnostic accuracy in nonsurveillance settings (e.g., imaging performed to assess detection rates in a series of patients undergoing treatment for HCC or patients with otherwise known prevalence of HCC prior to imaging). Four studies of PET evaluated accuracy specifically for identification of recurrent HCC.[296,305,312,318]

One randomized trial (rated high risk of bias)[50] evaluated clinical outcomes associated with imaging-based surveillance versus no screening, and two trials[48,49] evaluated clinical outcomes associated with different US surveillance intervals. One study compared effects of different imaging surveillance strategies on diagnostic thinking or clinical decisionmaking.[322] Two studies reported harms associated with imaging for HCC.[144,204]

Key Points

Test Performance

- In surveillance settings, using patients with HCC as the unit of analysis:
  - US without contrast: Sensitivity was 0.78 (95% CI 0.60 to 0.89, 4 studies) and specificity was 0.89 (95% CI 0.80 to 0.94, 3 studies), for a LR+ of 6.8 (95% CI 4.2 to 11) and LR- of 0.25 (0.13 to 0.46). (Strength of Evidence: low for sensitivity and specificity)
  - CT: Sensitivity was 0.84 (95% CI 0.59 to 0.95, 2 studies) and specificity 0.99 (95% CI 0.86 to 0.999, 2 studies), for a LR+ of 60 (95% CI 5.9 to 622) and LR- of 0.16 (0.06 to 0.47). (Strength of Evidence: low for sensitivity and specificity).
  - MRI and PET were not evaluated in surveillance settings. (Strength of Evidence: insufficient)

- In surveillance settings, using HCC lesions as the unit of analysis:
  - US without contrast: Sensitivity was 0.60 (95% CI 0.24 to 0.87, 1 study); specificity was not reported. (Strength of Evidence: low for sensitivity, insufficient for specificity)
  - CT: Sensitivity was 0.62 (95% CI 0.46 to 0.76, 1 study). (Strength of Evidence: low for sensitivity, insufficient for specificity).

- In nonsurveillance settings (e.g., imaging performed in patients who underwent liver transplantation or resection, or in patients in whom the prevalence of HCC is already known), using patients with HCC as the unit of analysis:
  - US without contrast: Sensitivity was 0.73 (95% CI 0.46 to 0.90, 8 studies) and specificity was 0.93 (95% CI 0.85 to 0.97, 6 studies), for a LR+ of 11 (95% CI 5.4 to

21) and LR- of 0.29 (95% CI 0.13 to 0.65). (Strength of Evidence: low for sensitivity and specificity)
- CT: Sensitivity was 0.83 (95% CI 0.75 to 0.89, 16 studies) and specificity was 0.92 (95% CI 0.86 to 0.96, 11 studies), for a LR+ of 11 (95% CI 5.6 to 20) and LR- of 0.19 (95% CI 0.12 to 0.28). (Strength of Evidence: moderate for sensitivity and specificity)
- MRI: Sensitivity was 0.85 (95% CI 0.76 to 0.91, 10 studies) and specificity was 0.90 (95% CI 0.81 to 0.94, 8 studies), for a LR+ of 8.1 (95% CI 4.3 to 15) and LR- of 0.17 (95% CI 0.10 to 0.28). (Strength of Evidence: moderate for sensitivity and specificity)
- PET: For FDG PET, sensitivity was 0.52 (95% CI 0.39 to 0.66, 15 studies) and specificity was 0.95 (95% CI 0.82 to 0.99, 5 studies), for a LR+ of 11 (95% CI 2.6 to 49) and LR- of 0.50 (95% CI 0.37 to 0.68). For ^{11}C-acetate PET or PET/CT, sensitivity was 0.85 (95% CI 0.67 to 0.94, 4 studies); specificity was not reported. (Strength of Evidence: moderate for sensitivity, low for specificity)

- In nonsurveillance settings, using HCC lesions as the unit of analysis:
  - US without contrast: Sensitivity was 0.59 (95% CI 0.42 to 0.74, 11 studies). Only two studies reported specificity, with inconsistent results (0.63, 95% CI 0.53 to 0.73, and 0.95, 95% CI 0.85 to 0.99). (Strength of Evidence: moderate for sensitivity and low for specificity)
  - US with contrast: Sensitivity was 0.73 (95% CI 0.52 to 0.87, 8 studies). No study evaluated specificity. (Strength of Evidence: low for sensitivity, insufficient for specificity)
  - CT: Sensitivity was 0.77 (95% CI 0.72 to 0.80, 79 studies) and specificity was 0.89 (95% CI 0.84 to 0.93, 21 studies), for a LR+ of 7.1 (95% CI 4.7 to 11) and LR- of 0.26 (95% CI 0.22 to 0.31). (Strength of Evidence: moderate for sensitivity and specificity)
  - MRI: Sensitivity was 0.82 (95% CI 0.79 to 0.85, 75 studies) and specificity was 0.87 (95% CI 0.77 to -0.93, 16 studies), for a LR+ of 6.4 (95% CI 3.5 to 12) and LR- of 0.20 (95% CI 0.16 to 0.25). (Strength of Evidence: moderate for sensitivity and specificity)
  - PET: For FDG PET, sensitivity was 0.53 (95% CI 0.41 to 0.65, 5 studies) and specificity was 0.91 (95% CI 0.76 to 0.98, 1 study). For ^{11}C-acetate PET, sensitivity was 0.78 (95% CI 0.61 to 0.89, 4 studies); specificity was not reported. (Strength of Evidence: moderate for sensitivity, low for specificity)

- Direct (within-study) comparisons of imaging modalities, using patients with HCC as the unit of analysis:
  - US without contrast versus CT: Sensitivity was 0.68 (95% CI 0.54 to 0.80) versus 0.80 (95% CI 0.68 to 0.88), for a difference of -0.12 (95% CI -0.20 to -0.03), based on six studies. Two studies were performed in surveillance settings and rated as low strength of evidence for sensitivity and specificity. (Strength of Evidence: moderate for sensitivity and specificity for the 6 studies)
  - US without contrast versus MRI: Sensitivity was 0.61 (95% CI 0.48 to 0.74) versus 0.81 (95% CI 0.69 to 0.89), for a difference of -0.19 (95% CI -0.30 to -0.08), based

on three studies, none of which were performed in surveillance settings. (Strength of Evidence: moderate for sensitivity and specificity)
- MRI versus CT: Sensitivity was 0.88 (95% CI 0.53 to 0.98) versus 0.82 (95% CI 0.41 to 0.97), for a difference of 0.06 (95% CI -0.05 to 0.17), based on four studies, none of which were performed in surveillance settings. (Strength of Evidence: moderate for sensitivity and specificity)

- Direct (within-study) comparisons of imaging modalities, using HCC lesions as the unit of analysis (no study performed in a surveillance setting):
  - US without contrast versus CT: Sensitivity was 0.55 (95% CI 0.43 to 0.66) versus 0.66 (95% CI 0.54 to 0.76) for a difference of -0.11 (95% CI -0.18 to -0.04), based on three studies. (Strength of Evidence: moderate for sensitivity and specificity)
  - US without contrast versus MRI: Sensitivity was 0.57 (95% CI 0.42 to 0.71) versus 0.79 (95% CI 0.67 to 0.88), for a difference of -0.22 (95% -0.31 to -0.14), based on three studies. (Strength of Evidence: moderate for sensitivity and specificity)
  - US with contrast versus CT: Sensitivity was 0.51 (95% CI 0.29 to 0.74) versus 0.61 (95% CI 0.38 to 0.81), for a difference of -0.10 (95% CI -0.20 to 0.00), based on four studies. (Strength of Evidence: moderate for sensitivity, insufficient for specificity)
  - US with contrast versus MRI: Sensitivity was 0.65 (95% CI 0.41 to 0.84) versus 0.73 (95% CI 0.50 to 0.88), for a difference of -0.08 (95% CI -0.19 to 0.02), based on 3 studies. (Strength of Evidence: moderate for sensitivity, insufficient for specificity)
  - MRI versus CT: Sensitivity was 0.81 (95% CI 0.76 to 0.84) versus 0.71 (95% CI 0.66 to 0.76), for a difference of 0.09 (95% CI 0.07 to 0.12), based on 31 studies. Findings were similar when studies were stratified according to use of nonhepatic-specific or hepatic-specific contrast, and when the analysis was restricted to HCC lesions <2-3 cm. For HCC lesions <2-3 cm, the difference in sensitivity was greater for studies of hepatic-specific MRI contrast (0.23, 95% CI 0.17 to 0.29, 12 studies) than for studies of non-hepatic specific MRI contrast (0.06, 95% CI -0.01 to 0.13, 6 studies). (Strength of Evidence: moderate for sensitivity and specificity)

- Multiple imaging modalities
  - One study found sensitivity of imaging with various combinations of two imaging modalities was similar or lower than single modality imaging, based on concordant positive findings on two imaging modalities. The other study reported higher sensitivity with multiple imaging modalities than with single modality imaging, but criteria for positive results based on multiple imaging modalities were unclear. (Strength of Evidence: low for sensitivity and insufficient for specificity)

- Sensitivity of US, CT, and MRI was lower in studies that used explanted liver as the reference standard than in studies that used other histopathological reference standards, clinical or imaging criteria, or a mixed reference standard.
  - US without contrast: Using HCC lesions as the unit of analysis, sensitivity was 0.34 (95% CI 0.22 to 0.47) in 5 studies that used explanted liver as the reference standard and ranged from 0.72 to 0.75 in studies that used other reference standards. (Strength of Evidence: moderate for sensitivity, insufficient for specificity)
  - US with contrast: No study using HCC lesions as the unit of analysis used an explanted liver reference standard. Sensitivity was 0.58 (95% CI 0.39 to 0.75) using a nonexplant histopathological reference standard and 0.98 (95% CI 0.88 to 0.997)

using a mixed reference standard. (Strength of Evidence: low for sensitivity, insufficient for specificity)
- o CT: Using HCC lesions as the unit of analysis, sensitivity was 0.67 (95% CI 0.59 to 0.75) in 23 studies that used explanted liver as the reference standard and ranged 0.65 to 0.86 in studies that used other reference standards. (Strength of Evidence: moderate for sensitivity and specificity).
- o MRI: Using HCC lesions as the unit of analysis, sensitivity was 0.69 (95% CI 0.60 to 0.76) in 18 studies that used explanted liver as the reference standard and ranged from 0.86 to 0.88 in studies that used a nonexplant histopathological reference standard or mixed reference standard; only three studies evaluated an imaging/clinical reference standard (sensitivity 0.65, 95% CI 0.43 to 0.83). (Strength of Evidence: moderate for sensitivity and specificity)
- o PET: No study of FDG PET used an explanted liver reference standard. Four of the five studies that used HCC lesions as the unit of analysis used a nonexplant histological reference standard (sensitivity 0.49, 95% CI 0.37 to 0.61). Specificity was reported in too few studies to draw strong conclusions. (Strength of Evidence: low for sensitivity, insufficient for specificity)

- Across imaging modalities, based on within-study comparisons, sensitivity increased as HCC lesion size increased.
  - o US without contrast: Sensitivity was 0.82 (95% CI 0.68 to 0.91) for lesions ≥2 cm and 0.34 (95% CI 0.19 to 0.53) for lesions <2 cm, for a difference o 0.48 (95% CI 0.39 to 0.57). Sensitivity was 0.09 (95% CI 0.02 to 0.29, 4 studies) for lesions <10 mm, 0.50 (95% CI 0.23 to 0.78, 4 studies) for lesions 10-20 mm and 0.88 (95% CI 0.66 to 0.96, 4 studies) for lesions >20 mm , for a difference of 0.37 (95% CI 0.18 to 0.57) for lesions >20 mm versus 10-20 mm, and 0.41 (95% CI 0.19 to 0.63) for lesions 10-20 mm versus <10 mm. (Strength of Evidence: moderate for sensitivity, low for specificity)
  - o US with contrast: Sensitivity was 0.94 (95% CI 0.83 to 0.98) for lesions ≥2 cm and 0.77 (95% CI 0.53 to 0.91) for lesions <2 cm for a difference of 0.17 (95% CI 0.03 to 0.32), based on 5 studies. Three studies found sensitivity of 0.64 (95% CI 0.33 to 0.87) for lesions 10-20 mm and 0.91 (95% CI 0.71 to 0.98) for lesions >20 mm, for a difference of 0.26 (95% CI 0.04 to 0.48). (Strength of Evidence: low for sensitivity and specificity)
  - o CT: Sensitivity was 0.94 (95% CI 0.92 to 0.95) for lesions ≥2 cm and 0.63 (95% CI 0.57 to 0.69) for lesions <2 cm, for an absolute difference in sensitivity of 0.31 (95% CI 0.26 to 0.36), based on 34 studies. Sensitivity was 0.32 (95% CI 0.25 to 0.41, 21 studies) for lesions <10 mm, 0.74 (95% CI 0.67 to 0.80, 23 studies) for lesions 10-20 mm, and 0.95 (95% CI 0.92 to 0.97, 20 studies), for a difference of 0.21 (95% CI 0.15 to 0.26) for lesions >20 versus 10-20 mm and 0.42 (95% CI 0.36 to 0.48) for lesions 10-20 versus <10 mm. (Strength of Evidence: moderate for sensitivity, low for specificity)
  - o MRI: Sensitivity was 0.96 (95% CI 0.93 to 0.97) for lesions ≥2 cm and 0.66 (95% CI 0.58 to 0.74) for lesions <2 cm, for an absolute difference in sensitivity of 0.29 (95% CI 0.23 to 0.36), based on 29 studies. Sensitivity was 0.45 (95% CI 0.34 to 0.56, 20 studies) for lesions <10 mm, 0.78 (95% CI 0.69 to 0.85, 21 studies) for lesions 10-20 mm, and 0.97 (95% CI 0.94 to 0.98, 14 studies) for lesions >20 mm (0.97, 95% CI

0.94 to 0.98, 18 studies), for a difference of 0.19 (95% CI 0.12 to 0.26) for >20 versus 10-20 mm and 0.33 (95% CI 0.26 to 0.40) for 10-20 versus <10 mm. (Strength of Evidence: moderate for sensitivity and specificity)
- PET: For FDG PET, sensitivity was consistently higher for larger lesions, based on five studies. Data were not pooled due to differences in the tumor size categories evaluated. Two studies of ^{11}C-acetatate PET found inconsistent effects of lesion size on sensitivity. (Strength of Evidence: low for sensitivity, insufficient for specificity)

- Across imaging modalities, based on within-study comparisons, sensitivity was higher for moderately or poorly differentiated HCC lesions than for well-differentiated HCC lesions.
  - US with contrast: Sensitivity was 0.83 (95% CI 0.55 to 0.95) for moderately- or poorly-differentiated HCC lesions and 0.43 (95% CI 0.15 to 0.76) for well-differentiated lesions, for an absolute difference in sensitivity of 0.40 (95% CI 0.17 to 0.64), based on three studies. (Strength of Evidence: low for sensitivity, insufficient for specificity)
  - CT: Sensitivity was 0.82 (95% CI 0.66 to 0.91) for moderately- or poorly-differentiated HCC lesions and 0.50 (95% CI 0.29 to 0.70) for well-differentiated lesions, for an absolute difference in sensitivity of 0.32 (95% CI 0.19 to 0.45), based on five studies. (Strength of Evidence: low for sensitivity, insufficient for specificity).
  - MRI: Sensitivity was 0.68 (95% CI 0.44 to 0.86) for moderately- or poorly-differentiated HCC lesions and 0.37 (95% CI 0.17 to 0.62) for well-differentiated lesions, for an absolute difference in sensitivity of 0.31 (95% CI 0.13 to 0.49), based on three studies. (Strength of Evidence: low for sensitivity, insufficient for specificity)
  - PET: For FDG PET, sensitivity was 0.72 (95% CI 0.59 to 0.83) for moderately- or poorly-differentiated HCC lesions and 0.39 (95% CI 0.26 to 0.55) for well differentiated lesions, for an absolute difference in sensitivity of 0.33 (95% CI 0.20 to 0.46), based on six studies. In three studies of ^{11}C-acetate PET and one study of ^{18}F-fluorochlorine, sensitivity for more well-differentiated lesions was not lower than for more poorly-differentiated lesions. (Strength of Evidence: low for sensitivity, insufficient for specificity)

- Effects of other factors on estimates of test performance
  - US: In two studies that directly compared US with contrast versus without contrast, there was no clear difference in sensitivity (-0.04, 95% CI -0.11 to 0.04). One study that directly compared use of Doppler versus no Doppler showed no clear effect on estimates of sensitivity. Lesion depth and body mass index had no effect on estimates of sensitivity. (Strength of Evidence: low)
  - CT: Using patients with HCC as the unit of analysis, studies with a contrast rate ≥3 ml/s reported a higher sensitivity (0.87, 95% CI 0.77 to 0.93, 8 studies) than studies with a contrast rate <3 ml/s (0.71, 95% CI 0.50 to 0.85, 4 studies). Studies with delayed phase imaging reported somewhat higher sensitivity (0.89, 95% CI 0.81 to 0.94, 7 studies) than studies without delayed phase imaging (0.74, 95% CI 0.66 to 0.87, 7 studies). However, both of these technical parameters had no clear effects in studies that used HCC lesions as the unit of analysis. (Strength of Evidence: low)

- MRI: There were no clear differences in estimates of diagnostic accuracy when studies were stratified according to MRI scanner type (1.5 vs. 3.0 T), imaging phases evaluated (with or without delayed phase imaging), timing of delayed phase imaging (>120 seconds vs. <120 seconds), section thickness (≤5 mm for enhanced images vs. >5 mm), or use of diffusion-weighted imaging. In studies that directly compared diagnostic accuracy with different types of contrast, hepatic-specific contrast agents (gadoxetic acid or gadobenate) were associated with slightly higher sensitivity than nonhepatic-specific contrast agents (gadopentetate or gadodiamide) (0.83, 95% CI 0.75 to 0.90 vs. 0.74, 95% CI 0.62 to 0.83, difference 0.10, 95% CI 0.04 to 0.15, 6 studies). (Strength of Evidence: low)
- PET: FDG PET was associated with lower sensitivity that ^{11}C-acetate PET when either patients (0.58 vs. 0.81, for a difference of -0.23, 95% CI -0.34 to -0.13, 3 studies) or HCC lesions (0.52 vs. 0.79, for a difference of -0.27, 95% CI -0.36 to -0.17, 3 studies) were the unit of analysis. FDG PET was also associated with lower sensitivity than dual tracer PET with FDG and ^{11}C-acetate or ^{18}F-choline PET, but evidence was limited to 1 or 2 studies for each of these comparisons. Using patients as the unit of analysis, sensitivity of FDG PET (0.39, 95% CI 0.24 to 0.56, 8 studies) was lower than sensitivity of FDG PET/CT (0.65, 95% CI 0.50 to 0.78, 7 studies). (Strength of Evidence: low)

Clinical Decisionmaking

- One randomized controlled trial (n=163) found no clear differences between surveillance with US without contrast versus CT in HCC detection rates, subsequent imaging, or cost per HCC detected. (Strength of Evidence: low)

Clinical and Patient-Centered Outcomes

- One cluster randomized controlled trial (n=18,816) conducted in China found screening every 6 months with noncontrast US plus serum AFP versus no screening in persons 35 to 79 years of age (mean 42 years) with HBV infection or chronic hepatitis without HBV infection associated with lower risk of HCC-related mortality (32 vs. 54 deaths, rate ratio 0.63, 95% CI 0.41 to 0.98) at 5-year followup, but was rated high risk of bias due to multiple methodological shortcomings. (Strength of Evidence: low)

- Two trials found no clear differences in mortality with US screening at 4-month versus 12-month intervals, or at 3-month versus 6-month intervals. One trial found no difference in HCC mortality between surveillance with US without contrast versus CT, but was underpowered to detect differences. (Strength of Evidence: moderate)

Harms

- One study reported no serious adverse events associated with administration of gadoxetic acid for MRI and one study reported no clear differences in adverse events between CT with contrast at 3 ml/s versus 5 ml/s. No study reported rates of adverse events associated with use of microbubble contrast agents in US, and harms were not reported in randomized trials of screening with imaging. (Strength of Evidence: insufficient)

Detailed Synthesis

KQ1.a. What is the comparative test performance of imaging-based strategies for detecting HCC?

Ultrasound

In surveillance settings, using patients with HCC as the unit of analysis, sensitivity of US without contrast was 0.78 (95% CI 0.60 to 0.89, 4 studies) and specificity was 0.89 (95% CI 0.80 to 0.94, 3 studies), for a LR+ of 6.8 (95% CI 4.2 to 11) and LR- of 0.25 (0.13 to 0.46) (Figure 5; Appendix D).[54,90,94,112] Using HCC lesions as the unit of analysis, sensitivity was 0.60 (95% CI 0.24 to 0.87) in one study; specificity was not reported.[62]

In nonsurveillance settings, using patients with HCC as the unit of analysis, the sensitivity of US without contrast was 0.73 (95% CI 0.46 to 0.90, 8 studies) and specificity was 0.93 (95% CI 0.85 to 0.97, 6 studies), for a LR+ of 11 (95% CI 5.4 to 21) and LR- of 0.29 (95% CI 0.13 to 0.65) (Figure 6).[52,64,76,82,83,110,111,118] Restricting the analysis to studies that avoided a case-control design resulted in lower sensitivity (0.54, 95% CI 0.38 to 0.70, 6 studies). Other sensitivity analyses had little effect on estimates (e.g., restricted to studies conducted in United States and Europe, excluded high risk of bias studies, or restricted to studies with blinded interpretation of imaging) or resulted in imprecise estimates due to small numbers of studies (analysis restricted to prospective studies).

Using HCC lesions as the unit of analysis, the sensitivity of US without contrast was 0.59 (95% CI 0.42 to 0.74, 11 studies) and specificity 0.83 (95% CI 0.53 to 0.95, 2 studies), for a LR+ of 3.4 (95% CI 1.2 to 9.4) and LR- of 0.50 (95% CI 0.37 to 0.66) (Figure 7).[52,56,70,76,77,79,83,84,99,111,118] Only two studies reported specificity, with inconsistent results (0.63, 95% CI 0.52 to 0.73[56] and 0.95, 95% CI 0.85 to 0.99[99]). Excluding two studies[77,79] restricted to HCC lesions <2-3 cm resulted in similar estimates (Table 6). Sensitivity was higher in studies that used a prospective design (0.78, 95% CI 0.55 to 0.91, 3 studies), but confidence intervals were wide. Other sensitivity analyses had little effect on estimates (Table 6).

Using HCC lesions as the unit of analysis, the sensitivity of US with contrast was 0.73 (95% CI 0.52 to 0.87, 8 studies); no study reported specificity (Figure 8).[51,69,71,74,79,92,106,119] Excluing three studies restricted to HCC lesions 2-3 cm[74,79,92] resulted in slightly higher sensitivity (0.78, 95% CI 0.5 to 0.92, 5 studies). Seven of the eight contrast-enhanced studies used perflubutane.[51,71,74,79,92,106,119] The usefulness of sensitivity analyses was limited by the small number of studies (Table 6).

Figure 5. Test performance of ultrasound without contrast for detection of patients with hepatocellular carcinoma in surveillance settings

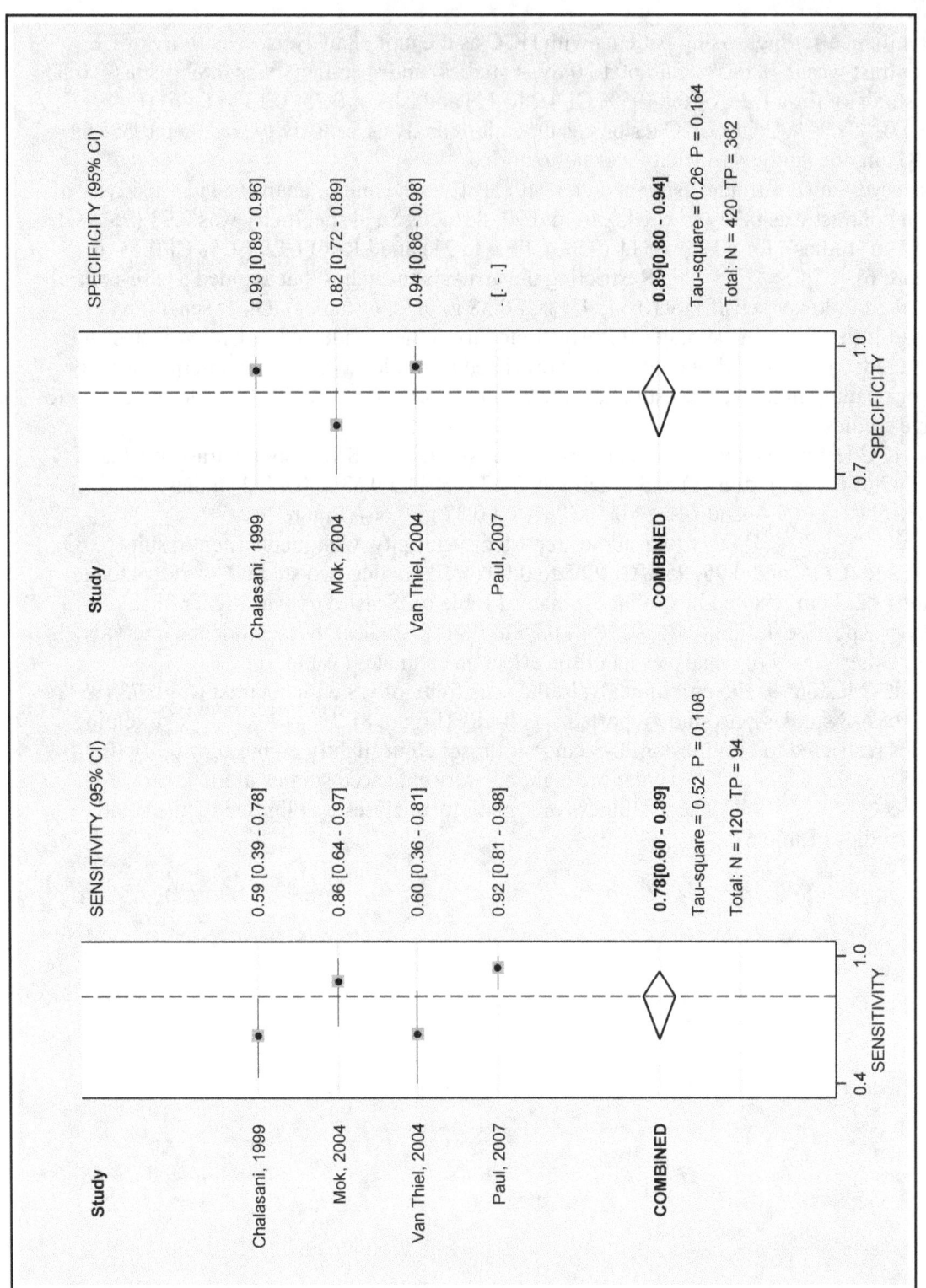

Figure 6. Test performance of ultrasound without contrast for detection of patients with hepatocellular carcinoma in nonsurveillance settings

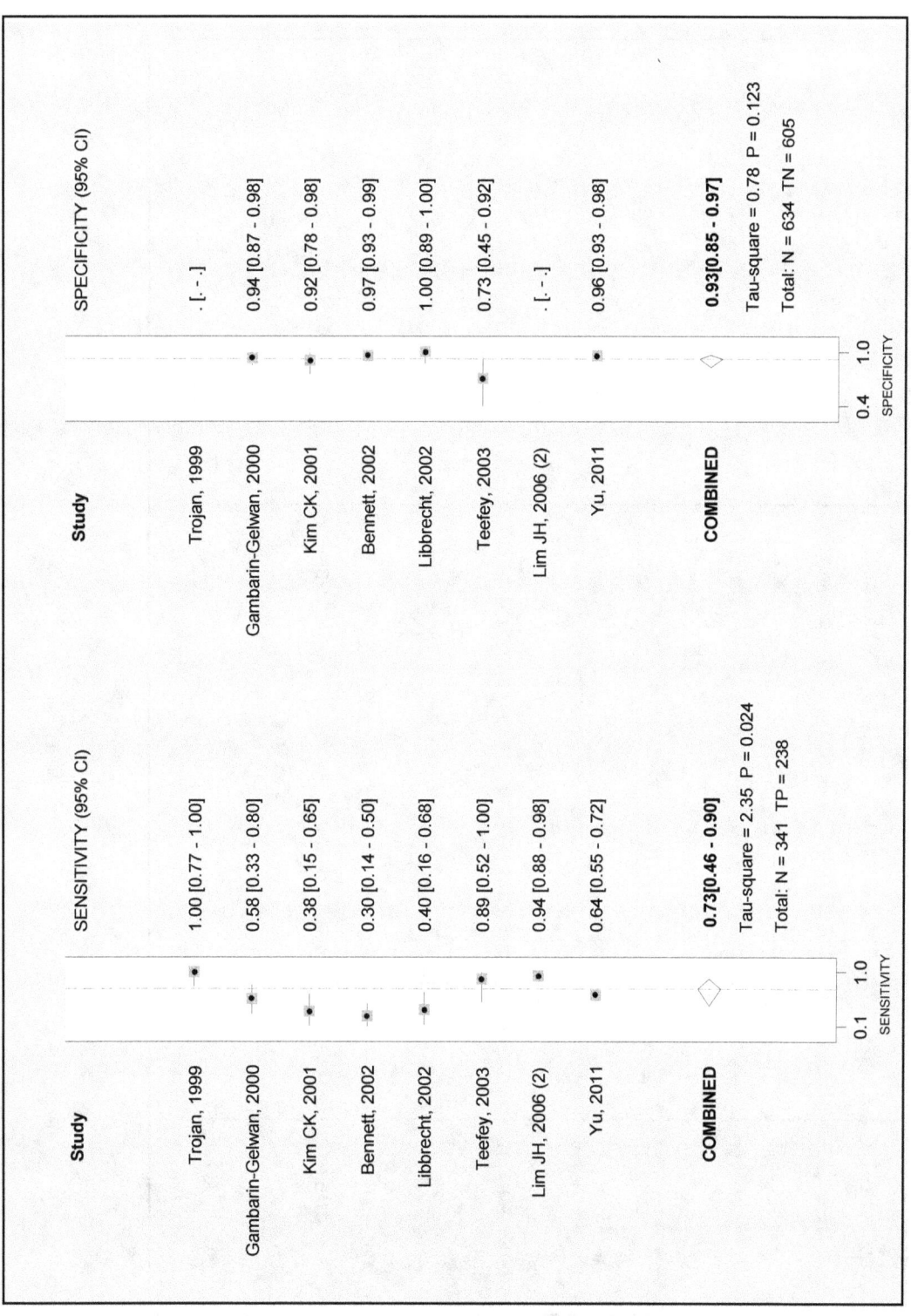

Figure 7. Sensitivity of ultrasound without contrast for detection of hepatocellular carcinoma lesions in nonsurveillance settings

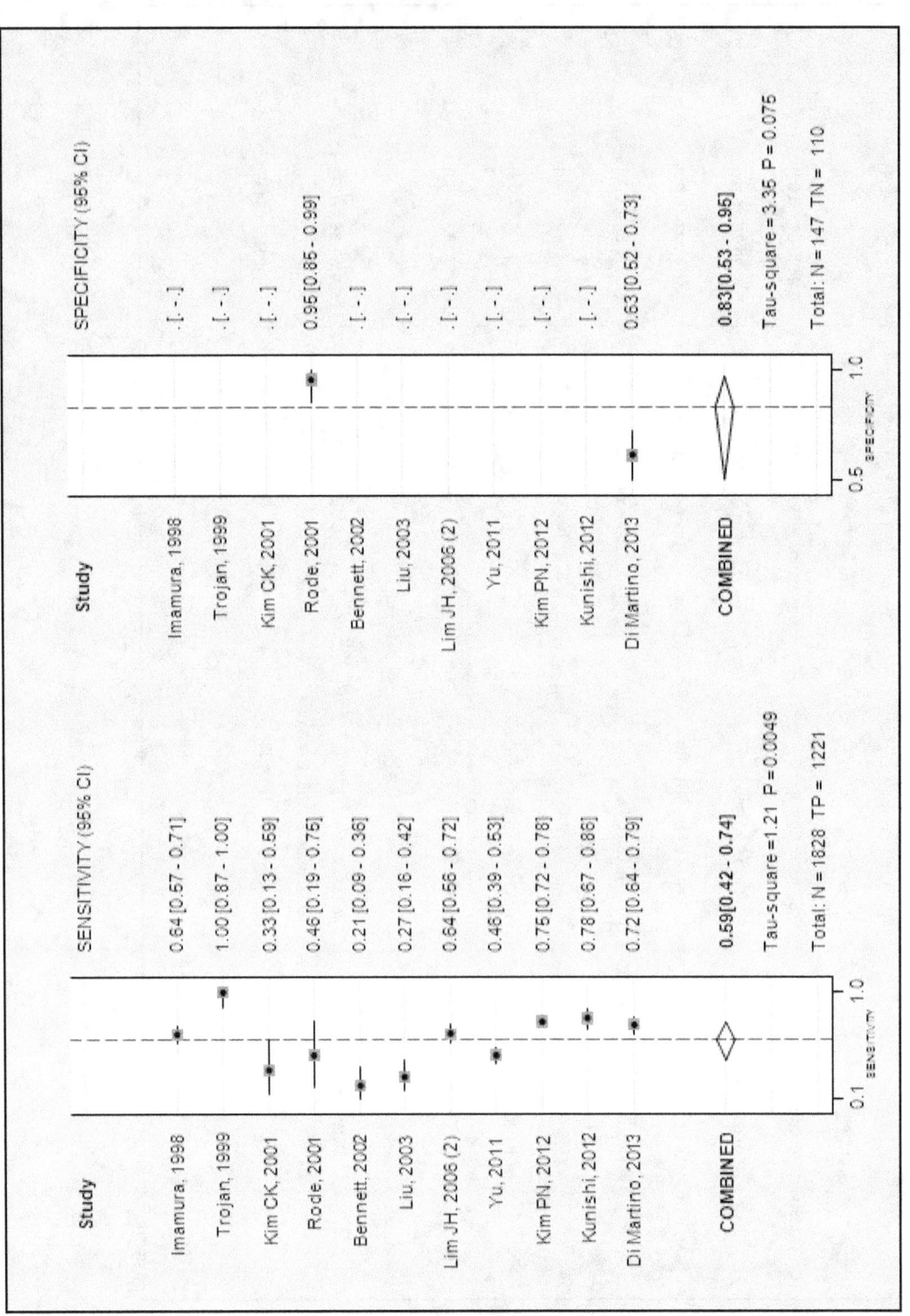

Figure 8. Sensitivity of ultrasound with contrast for detection of hepatocellular carcinoma lesions in nonsurveillance settings

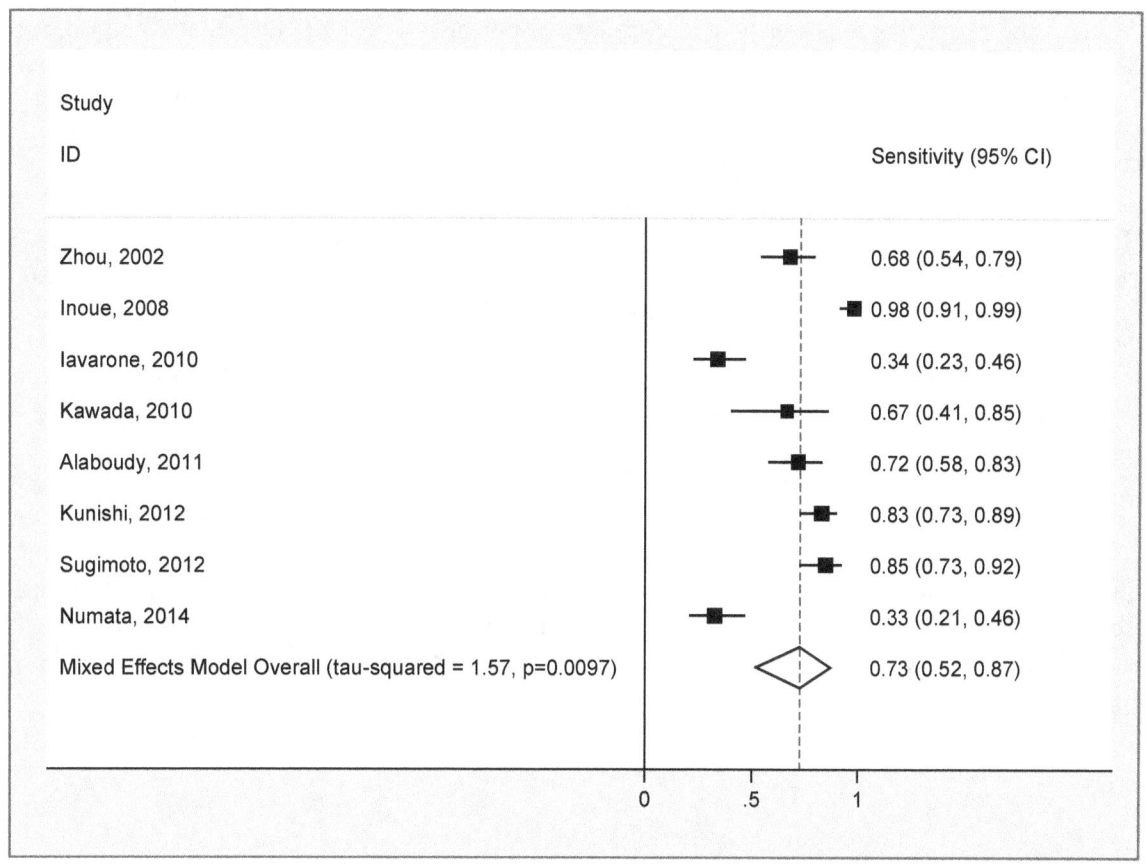

Computed Tomography

Few studies evaluated CT in surveillance settings. Using patients with HCC as the unit of analysis, sensitivity was 0.84 (95% CI 0.59 to 0.95) and specificity 0.99 (95% CI 0.86 to 0.999), based on two studies (Table 7.).[54,112] In one study that used HCC lesions as the unit of analysis, sensitivity was 0.62 (95% CI 0.46 to 0.76).[62]

In nonsurveillance settings, using patients with HCC as the unit of analysis, sensitivity of CT was 0.83 (95% CI 0.75 to 0.89, 16 studies) and specificity 0.92 (95% CI 0.86 to 0.96, 11 studies), for a LR+ of 11 (95% CI 5.6 to 20) and LR- of 0.19 (95% CI 0.12 to 0.28) (Figure 9).[82,110,111,118,126,129,130,133,154,155,164,175,186,197,201,202] Using HCC lesions as the unit of analysis, sensitivity was 0.77 (95% CI 0.72 to 0.80, 79 studies) and specificity 0.89 (95% CI 0.84 to 0.93, 21 studies), for a LR+ of 7.1 (95% CI 4.7 to 11) and LR- of 0.26 (95% CI 0.22 to 0.31) (Figure 10).[42,56,69,92,99,118-121,123-127,129-131,133,135-141,143-146,148,149,153,155,157,158,161-169,172,175-180,182-185,188,190-195,198,200,202-204,207-212,215-220] Using liver segments with HCC as the unit of analysis, sensitivity was 0.88 (95% CI 0.78 to 0.94, 8 studies) and specificity was 0.97 (95% CI 0.94 to 0.98, 8 studies), for a LR+ of 26 (95% CI 15 to 42) and LR- of 0.13 (95% CI 0.07 to 0.23).[132,150,151,159,160,174,205,216]

Excluding high risk of bias studies, studies limited to hypervascular HCC, or HCC lesions <2-3 cm, and restricting analyses to studies that were performed in the United States and Europe, used a prospective design, avoided a case-control design, or used blinded imaging interpretation had little impact on estimates of sensitivity and specificity or measures of heterogeneity.

Magnetic Resonance Imaging

No study evaluated MRI in surveillance settings.

In nonsurveillance settings, using patients with HCC as the unit of analysis, sensitivity was 0.85 (95% CI 0.76 to 0.91, 10 studies) and specificity was 0.90 (95% CI 0.81 to 0.94, 8 studies), for a LR+ of 8.1 (95% CI 4.3 to 15) and LR- of 0.17 (95% CI 0.10 to 0.28) (Table 8; Figure 11).[82,110,118,126,129,259,260,263,273,280]

Using HCC lesions as the unit of analysis, sensitivity was 0.82 (95% CI 0.79 to 0.85, 75 studies) and specificity was 0.87 (95% CI 0.77 to 0.93, 16 studies), for a LR+ of 6.4 (95% CI 3.5 to 12) and LR- of 0.20 (95% CI 0.16 to 0.25) (Figure 12).[56,69,99,106,118,121,123,126,129,131,135,136,138,140,141,144,145,158,163,164,166,168,179,184,190,191,193,195,198,200,203,207,209,211,212,218,221,224,227,234,236,238,244,246,248-252,254-257,259,260,262-264,267,268,270,271,274-277,281,283-286,288,290,292,295]

Excluding high risk of bias studies, studies limited to hypervascular HCC, or HCC lesions <2-3 cm, and restricting analyses to studies that were performed in the United States and Europe, used a prospective design, avoided a case-control design, or used blinded imaging interpretation had little impact on estimates of sensitivity and specificity or measures of heterogeneity.

Figure 9. Test performance of CT for detection of patients with hepatocellular carcinoma in nonsurveillance settings

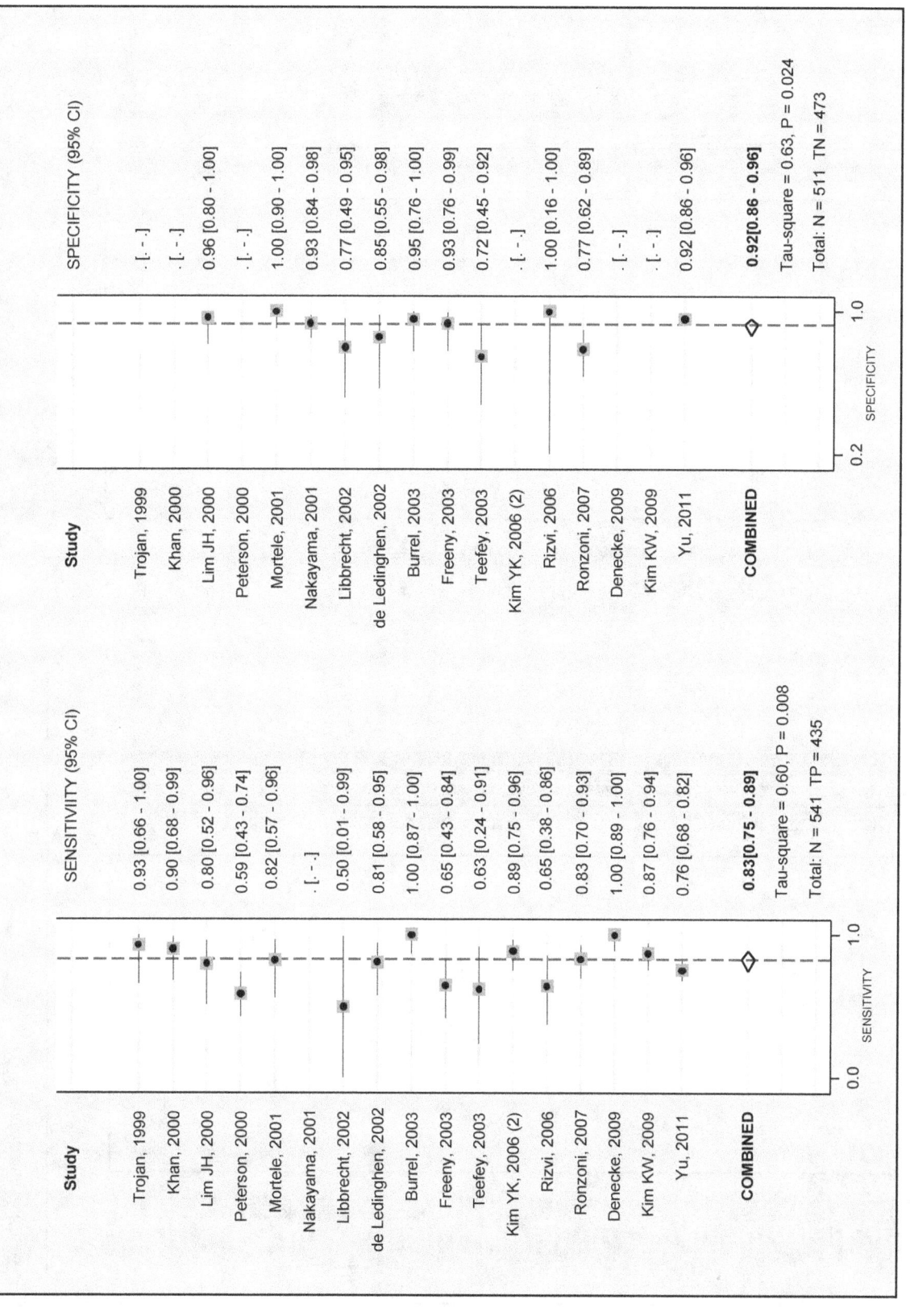

CT = computed tomography

Figure 10. Test performance of CT for detection of hepatocellular carcinoma lesions in nonsurveillance settings

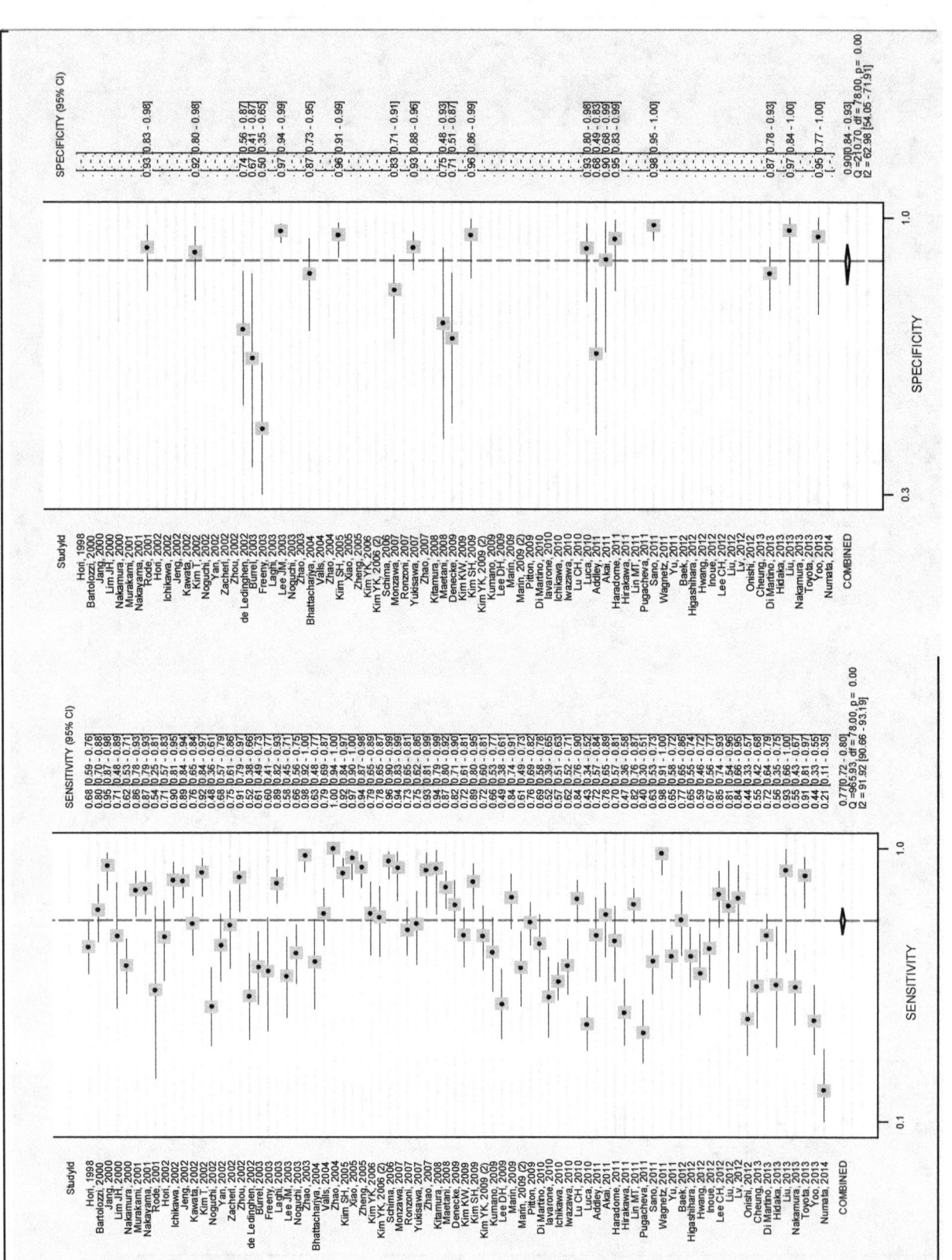

CT = computed tomography

Figure 11. Test performance of MRI for detection of patients with hepatocellular carcinoma in nonsurveillance settings

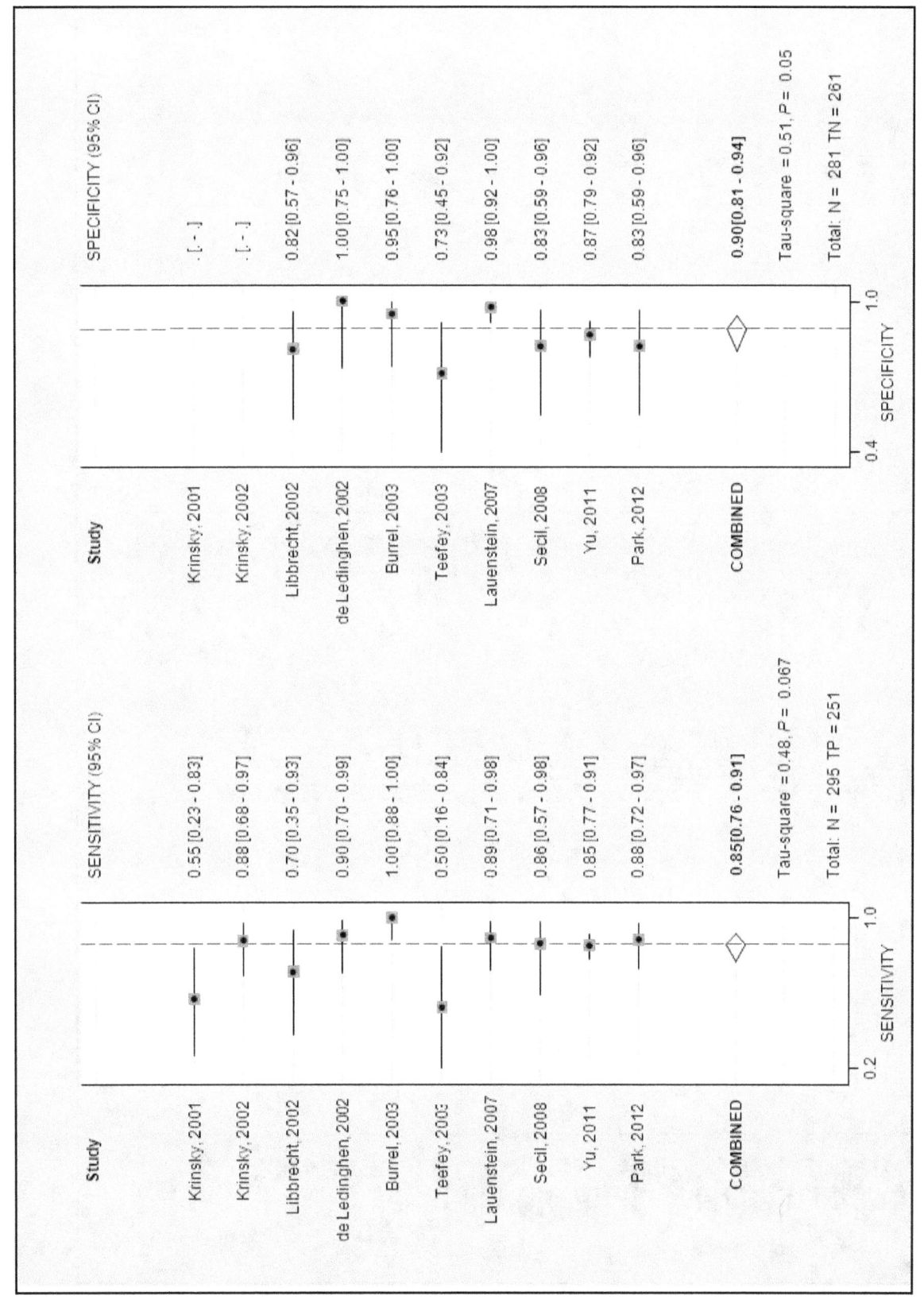

MRI = magnetic resonance imaging

Figure 12. Test performance of MRI for detection of hepatocellular carcinoma lesions in nonsurveillance settings

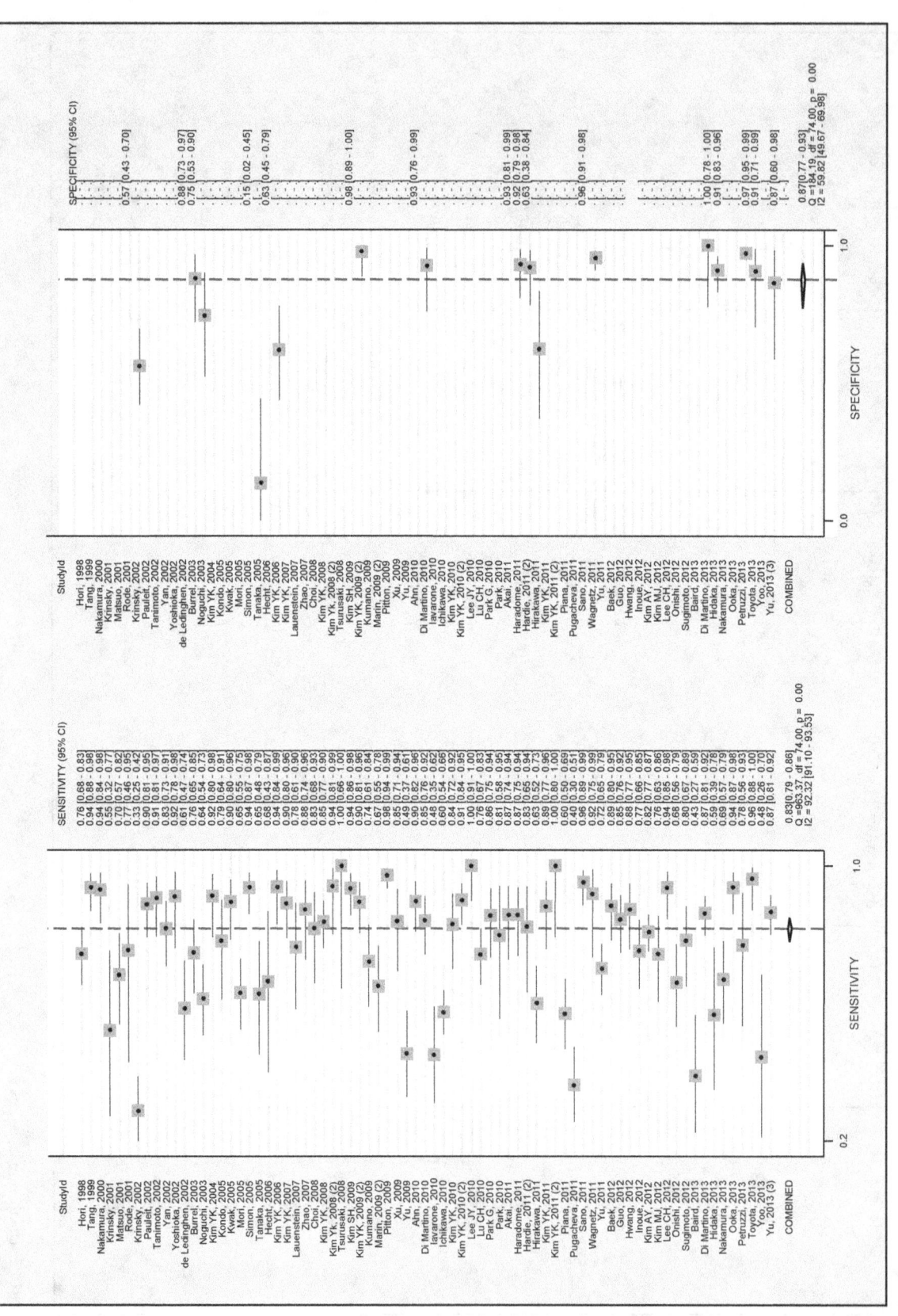

MRI = magnetic resonance imaging

Positron Emission Tomography

No study evaluated PET in surveillance settings.

In nonsurveillance settings, using patients with HCC as the unit of analysis, sensitivity of FDG PET was 0.52 (95% CI 0.39 to 0.66, 15 studies) and specificity was 0.95 (95% CI 0.82 to 0.99, 5 studies) (Table 9; Figure 13; Appendix G).[110,111,154,297,302,307-310,313-318] Using HCC lesions as the unit of analysis, sensitivity was 0.53 (95% CI 0.41 to 0.65, 5 studies) and specificity 0.91 (95% CI 0.76 to 0.98, 1 study) (Figure 14).[297,303,309,313,319] Results were similar when analyses excluded high risk of bias studies, or when analyses were restricted to studies that used a prospective design or were conducted in the United States or Europe.

Using patients with HCC as the unit of analysis, sensitivity of ^{11}C-acetate PET was 0.85 (95% CI 0.67 to 0.94, 4 studies) (Figure 15).[297,302,306,309] Using HCC lesions as the unit of analysis, sensitivity was 0.78 (95% CI 0.61 to 0.89, 4 studies) (Figure 16).[127,306,309,319] Sensitivities of around 0.90 were reported for PET with dual tracers (FDG plus ^{11}C-acetate)[127,317] and alternative tracers such as ^{18}F-fluorothymidine[299] or ^{18}F-fluorochlorine,[313,314] but evidence was limited to one or two studies each.

Three studies found FDG PET associated with sensitivity of 0.70 (95% CI 0.32 to 0.92, 3 studies) for detection of recurrent intrahepatic HCC, with a specificity of 0.71 (95% CI 0.29 to 0.96).[305,312,318]

Figure 13. Test performance of FDG PET for detection of patients with hepatocellular carcinoma in nonsurveillance settings

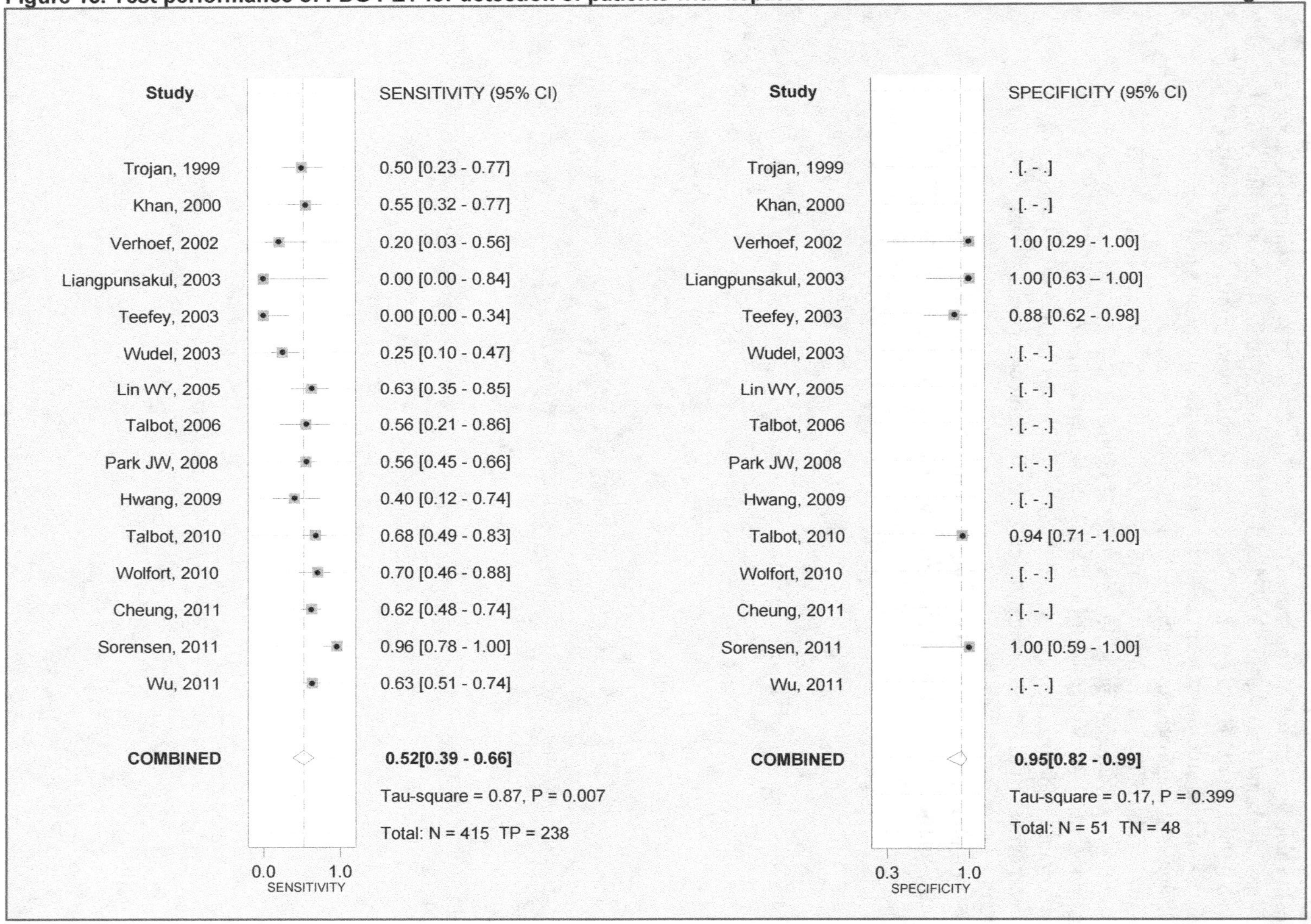
Study
SENSITIVITY (95% CI)
Trojan, 1999
0.50 [0.23 - 0.77]
Khan, 2000
0.55 [0.32 - 0.77]
Verhoef, 2002
0.20 [0.03 - 0.56]
Liangpunsakul, 2003
0.00 [0.00 - 0.84]
Teefey, 2003
0.00 [0.00 - 0.34]
Wudel, 2003
0.25 [0.10 - 0.47]
Lin WY, 2005
0.63 [0.35 - 0.85]
Talbot, 2006
0.56 [0.21 - 0.86]
Park JW, 2008
0.56 [0.45 - 0.66]
Hwang, 2009
0.40 [0.12 - 0.74]
Talbot, 2010
0.68 [0.49 - 0.83]
Wolfort, 2010
0.70 [0.46 - 0.88]
Cheung, 2011
0.62 [0.48 - 0.74]
Sorensen, 2011
0.96 [0.78 - 1.00]
Wu, 2011
0.63 [0.51 - 0.74]
COMBINED
0.52[0.39 - 0.66]
Tau-square = 0.87, P = 0.007
Total: N = 415 TP = 238
0.0
1.0
SENSITIVITY
Study
SPECIFICITY (95% CI)
Trojan, 1999
. [. - .]
Khan, 2000
. [. - .]
Verhoef, 2002
1.00 [0.29 - 1.00]
Liangpunsakul, 2003
1.00 [0.63 – 1.00]
Teefey, 2003
0.88 [0.62 - 0.98]
Wudel, 2003
. [. - .]
Lin WY, 2005
. [. - .]
Talbot, 2006
. [. - .]
Park JW, 2008
. [. - .]
Hwang, 2009
. [. - .]
Talbot, 2010
0.94 [0.71 - 1.00]
Wolfort, 2010
. [. - .]
Cheung, 2011
. [. - .]
Sorensen, 2011
1.00 [0.59 - 1.00]
Wu, 2011
. [. - .]
COMBINED
0.95[0.82 - 0.99]
Tau-square = 0.17, P = 0.399
Total: N = 51 TN = 48
0.3
1.0
SPECIFICITY

FDG = ^{18}F-fluorodeoxyglucose; PET = positron emission tomography

Figure 14. Test performance of FDG PET for detection of hepatocellular carcinoma lesions in nonsurveillance settings

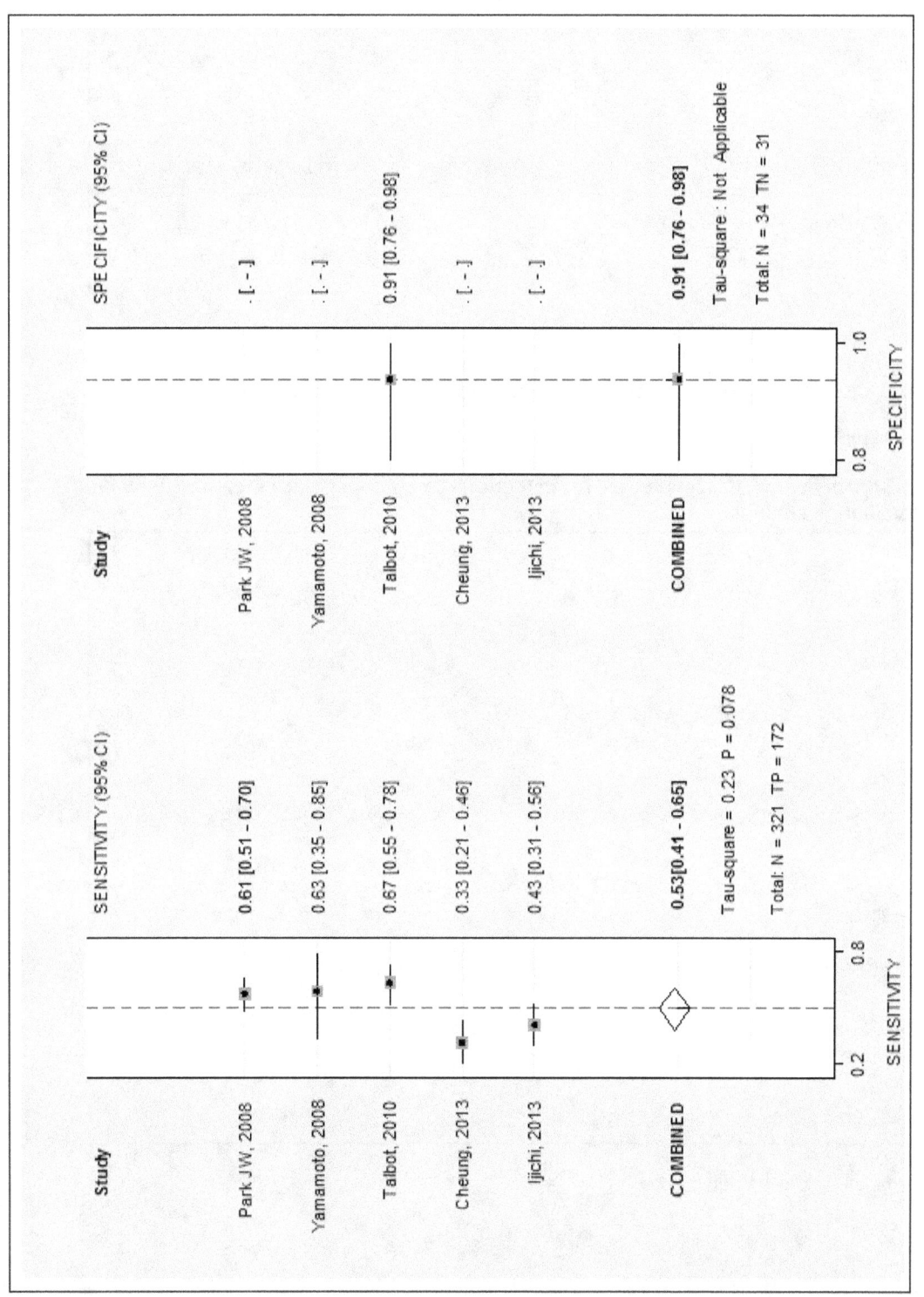

Figure 15. Sensitivity of ^{11}C-acetate PET for detection of patients with hepatocellular carcinoma in nonsurveillance settings*

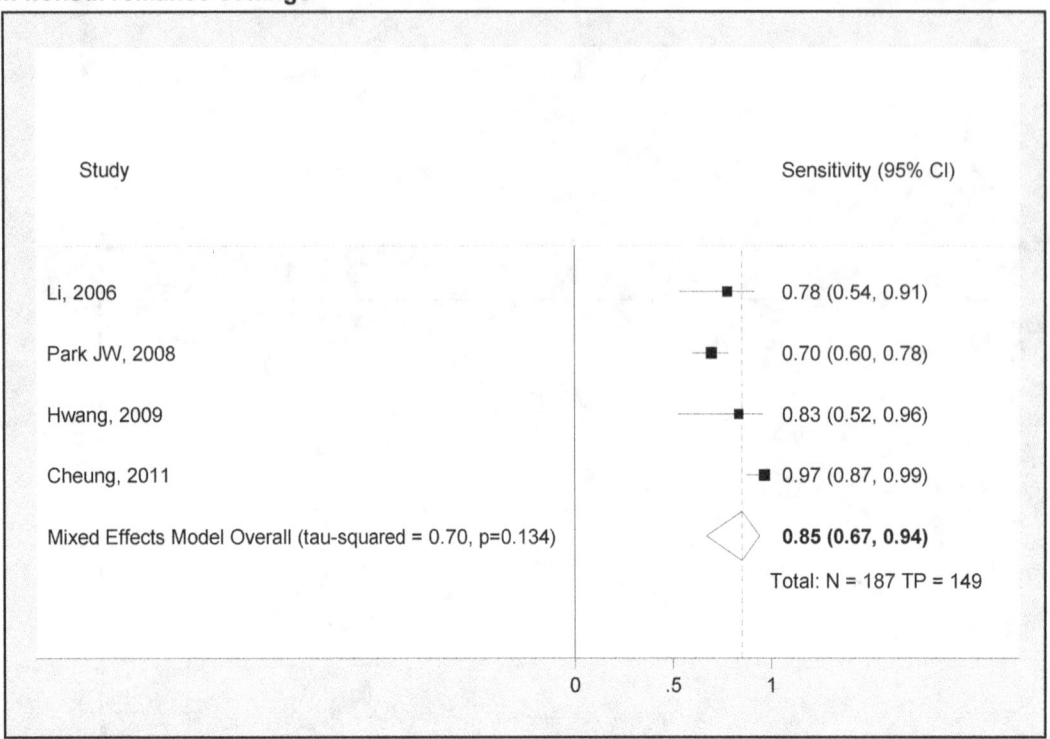

*Specificity not available
PET = positron emission tomography

Figure 16. Sensitivity of ^{11}C-acetate PET for detection of hepatocellular carcinoma lesions in nonsurveillance settings*

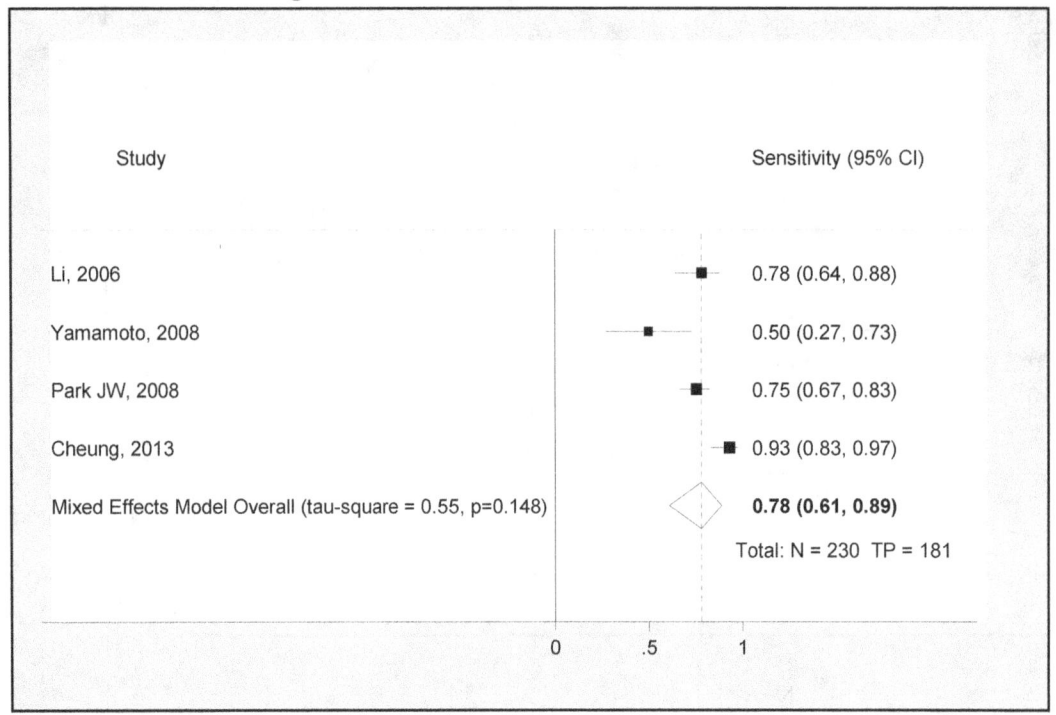

*Specificity not available
PET = positron emission tomography

Ultrasound Versus Computed Tomography

Using patients with HCC as the unit of analysis, sensitivity was lower for US without contrast (0.68, 95% CI 0.54 to 0.80) than for CT (0.80, 95% CI 0.68 to 0.88), for a difference of -0.12 (95% CI -0.20 to -0.03), based on six studies conducted in surveillance or nonsurveillance settings (Table 10.).[54,82,110-112,118] Findings were similar when one high risk of bias study [82] was excluded. Two of the studies were conducted in surveillance settings; both found US associated with lower sensitivity than CT (0.59 vs. 0.91[54] and 0.60 vs. 0.70[112]), with similar specificity.

Using HCC lesions as the unit of analysis, US without contrast was associated with lower sensitivity than CT (0.55, 95% CI 0.43 to 0.66 versus 0.66, 95% CI 0.54 to 0.76, for a difference of -0.11 95% CI -0.18 to -0.04), based on three studies.[56,99,118] Four studies reported similar findings for US with contrast versus CT (sensitivity 0.51, 95% CI 0.29 to 0.74 vs. 0.61, 95% CI 0.38 to 0.81, for a difference of -0.10, 95% CI -0.20 to 0.00).[51,69,92,119] There were no clear differences in sensitivity of US with or without contrast versus CT when analyses were restricted to HCC lesions <2 cm, but analyses were imprecise and based on small numbers of studies (Table 10).[56,62,69,92,118] None of the studies were performed in surveillance settings.

Ultrasound Versus Magnetic Resonance Imaging

No study evaluated MRI versus CT in surveillance settings.

In nonsurveillance settings, using patients with HCC as the unit of analysis, three studies found US without contrast associated with lower sensitivity than MRI (0.61, 95% CI 0.48 to 0.74 vs. 0.81, 95% CI 0.69 to 0.89, for a difference of -0.19, 95% CI -0.30 to -0.08), but higher specificity (0.94, 95% CI 0.87 to 0.97 vs. 0.82, 95% CI 0.66 to 0.91, for a difference of 0.13, 95% CI 0.03 to 0.22) (Table 10).[82,110,118] Using HCC lesions as the unit of analysis, three studies found US without contrast associated with lower sensitivity than MRI (0.57, 95% CI 0.42 to 0.71 versus 0.79, 95% CI 0.67 to 0.88, for a difference of -0.22, 95% CI -0.31 to -0.14).[56,99,118]

Three studies found US with contrast associated with lower sensitivity than MRI (0.65, 95% CI 0.41 to 0.84 vs. 0.73, 95% CI 0.50 to 0.88, for a difference of -0.08, 95% CI -0.19 to 0.02).[51,69,106] There were no clear differences between US with contrast versus MRI for HCC lesions <2 cm or for well-differentiated HCC lesions, but estimates were imprecise and based on small numbers of studies.

Magnetic Resonance Imaging Versus Computed Tomography

No study evaluated MRI versus CT in surveillance settings. In nonsurveillance settings, using patients with HCC as the unit of analysis, four studies found no clear differences between MRI and CT in sensitivity or specificity (Table 10).[82,110,118,126] Results were similar when high risk of bias studies were excluded.

Using HCC lesions as the unit of analysis, 31 studies found MRI associated with higher sensitivity than CT (0.81, 95% CI 0.76 to 0.84 vs. 0.71, 95% CI 0.66 to 0.76, for a difference of 0.09 (95% CI 0.07 to 0.12), with no difference in specificity.[51,56,69,99,118,121,123,126,131,135,136,140,144,145,158,163,164,166,168,176,179,184,190,191,193,195,198,207,209,211,212] Results were similar when high risk of bias studies were excluded. Differences in sensitivity were also similar when studies were stratified according to use of nonhepatic-specific[99,118,126,140,164,166,179,193,198,209,211] or hepatic-specific contrast[51,56,69,121,123,131,135,136,144,145,158,163,168,184,191,195,207,212] with MRI. Specificity was lower with nonhepatic-specific MRI than CT (0.62, 95% CI 0.51 to 0.72 vs. 0.86, 95% CI 0.77 to 0.93, for a difference of -0.24, 95% CI -0.37 to -0.11), but only two studies of nonhepatic-specific contrast reported specificity.[99,126]

MRI was also associated with higher sensitivity than CT when the analysis was restricted to HCC lesions <2-3 cm (0.71, 95% CI 0.64 to 0.78 vs. 0.56, 95% CI 0.48 to 0.63, for an absolute difference of 0.16, 95% CI 0.11 to 0.20, based on 19 studies).[56,69,74,118,123,126,131,135,140,141,145,168,176,184,193,195,200,203,218] The difference in sensitivity was greater in studies that evaluated hepatic specific MRI contrast agents (0.23, 95% CI 0.17 to 0.29, 12 studies) than in studies that evaluated non-hepatic specific MRI contrast agents (0.06, 95% CI -0.01 to 0.13, 6 studies) (Table 10).

Multiple Imaging Modalities

One study found sensitivity of imaging with various combinations of two imaging modalities was similar or lower than single modality imaging, based on concordant positive findings on two imaging modalities (Table 11).[51] The other study reported higher sensitivity with multiple imaging modalities than with single modality imaging, but criteria for positive results based on multiple imaging modalities were not reported.[69] Specificity was not reported in either study.

KQ1.a.i. How is a particular technique's test performance modified by use of various reference standards?

Ultrasound

There were too few studies of US in surveillance settings to evaluate effects of using different reference standards on estimate of accuracy.

In nonsurveillance settings, using patients as the unit of analysis, the sensitivity of US without contrast was 0.48 (95% CI 0.35 to 0.61, 5 studies) with explanted liver as the reference standard[52,64,76,82,118] and 0.95 (0.87 to 0.98, 3 studies) using a nonexplant histopathological reference standard (Table 6).[83,110,111] Using HCC lesions as the unit of analysis, the sensitivity of US without contrast was 0.34 (95% CI 0.22 to 0.47, 5 studies) with explanted liver as the reference standard[52,76,84,99,118] and ranged from 0.72 to 0.75 with other reference standards (nonexplant histopathological, imaging or mixed histological and imaging or clinical criteria).[56,70,83,111] The sensitivity of US with contrast was 0.66 (95% CI 0.47 to 0.81, 4 studies) using a nonexplant histopathological reference standard;[51,69,106,119] one study evaluated a mixed reference standard (0.98, 95% CI 0.86 to 0.99).[71]

Computed Tomography

Using patients as the unit of analysis, there were no clear differences in diagnostic accuracy based on the use of different reference standards (explanted liver, other histopathological reference standard, or mixed histological and clinical/imaging), with sensitivity ranging from 0.81 to 0.88 (Table 7).[82,110,111,118,126,129,130,133,154,155,164,175,186,192,197,201,202] Using HCC lesions as the unit of analysis, studies using explanted livers as the reference standard reported a lower sensitivity (0.67, 95% CI 0.59 to -0.75, 23 studies)[42,99,118,120,121,125,126,129,130,133,136,138,169,175,177-179,182,191,202,208,212,216] than studies that used a nonexplant histopathological reference standard (0.86, 95% CI 0.78 to 0.91, 12 studies)[69,119,127,135,143,145,148,157,158,176,207,209] or studies that used a mixed histological and clinical/imaging reference standard (0.80, 95% CI 0.75 to 0.84, 34 studies).[56,123,124,131,139,144,146,149,153,155,161-168,172,183,184,188,192-195,198,204,210,211,215,217,219,220] Only three studies used a clinical/imaging reference standard (sensitivity 0.65, 95% CI 0.43 to

0.83).[137,140,190] Estimates of specificity stratified by the reference standard used were somewhat lower for studies that used an explanted liver reference standard (0.82, 95% CI 0.74 to 0.88) than a nonexplant histopathological reference standard (0.95, 95% CI 0.88 to 0.98) or mixed reference standard (0.92, 95% CI 0.83 to 0.96), but estimates for the nonexplant reference standards were imprecise due to small numbers of studies.

Magnetic Resonance Imaging

Too few studies with patients as the unit of analysis used a nonexplant reference standard to evaluate effects of different reference standards on estimates of diagnostic accuracy. Eight of 10 studies used an explanted liver reference standard, with a pooled sensitivity of 0.87 (95% CI 0.78 to 0.92).[82,118,126,129,259,260,263,273,276]

Using HCC lesions as the unit of analysis, studies using explanted livers as the reference standard reported a lower sensitivity (0.69, 95% CI 0.60 to 0.76, 18 studies)[99,118,121,126,129,136,138,179,191,212,224,227,236,238,259,260,263,276] than studies that used a nonexplant histopathological reference standard or mixed histological and imaging/clinical reference standard (sensitivity estimates ranged from 0.86 to 0.88) (Table 8). Estimates of specificity stratified by the reference standard were imprecise due to small numbers of studies.

Positron Emission Tomography

No study of FDG PET used explanted livers as the reference standard. Using patients as the unit of analysis, there were no clear differences in sensitivity between studies that used a nonexplant histological reference standard (0.46, 95% CI 0.28 to 0.65, 7 studies)[110,111,154,297,309,315,316] and studies that used a mixed histological and imaging/clinical criteria reference standard (0.58, 95% CI 0.40-0.75, 8 studies), based on relatively wide and overlapping confidence intervals (Table 9). Four of the five studies that used HCC lesions as the unit of analysis used a nonexplant histological reference standard; the pooled sensitivity from this subset of studies was similar to the overall pooled estimate.[297,303,309,319]

KQ1.a.ii. How is the comparative effectiveness modified by patient, tumor, technical, or other factors?

Ultrasound

In two studies that directly compared US with versus without contrast, there was no clear difference in sensitivity (-0.04, 95% CI -0.11 to 0.04) (Table 12).[67,79] Excluding studies that used Doppler had little effect on estimates of sensitivity and specificity, and one study[62] that directly compared use of Doppler versus no Doppler showed no clear effect on estimates of sensitivity.

In studies that reported accuracy stratified by HCC lesion size, sensitivity of US without contrast was greater for lesions ≥2 cm (0.82, 95% CI 0.68 to 0.91) than for lesions <2 cm (0.34, 95% CI 0.19 to 0.53), for an absolute difference in sensitivity of 0.48 (95% CI 0.39 to 0.51, 9 studies).[52,56,67,70,76,80,83,84,118] For US with contrast, sensitivity was 0.94 (95% CI 0.83 to 0.98) for lesions <2 cm and 0.77 (95% CI 0.53 to 0.91) for lesions <2 cm, for an absolute difference in sensitivity of 0.17 (95% CI 0.03 to 0.32, 5 studies)[63,66,69,115,117] For US without contrast, sensitivity progressively improved from 0.09 (95% CI 0.02 to 0.29, 4 studies) for lesions <10 mm to 0.50 (95% CI 0.23 to 0.78, 4 studies) for lesions 10-20 mm and 0.88 (95% CI 0.66 to 0.96, 4 studies) for lesions >20 mm, for a difference of 0.37 (95% CI 0.18 to 0.57) for lesions >20 mm vs. 10-20 mm, and 0.41 (95% CI 0.19 to 0.63) for lesions 10-20 mm vs. <10 mm

(Table 13).[52,56,80,83] For US with contrast, three studies found sensitivity lower for lesions 10-20 mm (0.64, 95% CI 0.33 to 0.87) than >20 mm (0.91, 95% CI 0.71 to 0.98), for a difference of 0.26 (95% CI 0.04 to 0.48).[63,69,115]

In three studies, sensitivity was 0.83 (95% CI 0.55 to 0.95) for moderately- or poorly-differentiated HCC lesions versus 0.43 (95% CI 0.15 to 0.76) for well-differentiated lesions, for an absolute difference in sensitivity of 0.40 (95% CI 0.17 to 0.64).[53,69,89] Lesion depth and body mass index had no effect on estimates of sensitivity (Table 6). Two studies reported conflicting results for effects of cirrhosis on estimates of sensitivity, with one study reporting presence of cirrhosis associated with lower sensitivity than in patients without cirrhosis[77] but the other with slightly higher sensitivity.[83] Evidence on effects of liver volume, subcapsular location, presence of ascites, and underlying condition on estimates of accuracy was very sparse and showed no clear differences.[77,84]

Computed Tomography

Using patients with HCC as the unit of analysis, studies with a contrast rate ≥3 ml/s reported a higher sensitivity (0.87, 95% CI 0.77 to 0.93, 8 studies)[110,126,129,130,133,164,175,192,202] than studies with a contrast rate <3 ml/s (0.71, 95% CI 0.50-0.85, 4 studies),[82,118,186,197] with similar specificity, but there was no clear difference in studies that used HCC lesions as the unit of analysis (0.78, 95% CI 0.74 to 0.82, 58 studies and 0.74, 95% CI 0.59 to 0.85, 7 studies, respectively) (Table 14).

Using patients with HCC as the unit of analysis, studies with delayed phase imaging reported somewhat higher sensitivity (0.89, 95% CI 0.81 to 0.94, 7 studies)[82,111,118,129,154,186,197] than studies without delayed phase imaging (0.78, 95% CI 0.66 to 0.87, 7 studies),[110,126,130,155,164,175,202] but there was no clear difference in studies that used HCC lesions as the unit of analysis (0.74, 95% CI 0.69 to 0.80, 42 studies and 0.81, 95% CI 0.75 to 0.86, 26 studies, respectively) (Table 7).

The type of CT scanner (≥8-row multidetector, <8-row multidetector, or nonmultidetector) had no clear effect on estimates of diagnostic accuracy. Based on two studies that directly compared spectral versus standard CT, there was no clear difference in estimates of diagnostic accuracy.[180,181] Three studies compared effects of quantitative versus qualitative methods for evaluation of CT imaging findings on estimates of diagnostic accuracy.[58,155,178] One study found use of quantitative arterial enhancement fraction mapping associated with higher sensitivity than qualitative assessment for all HCC lesions, as well as lesions ≤2 cm,[155] but another study found qualitative assessment and quantitative assessment based on the arterial enhancement fraction both associated with a sensitivity of 1.0.[58] In the other study, use of the percentage attention ratio threshold had no clear effect on sensitivity.[178]

In 34 studies that reported accuracy of CT stratified by HCC lesion size, sensitivity was greater for lesions ≥2 cm (0.94, 95% CI 0.92 to 0.95) than for lesions <2 cm (0.63, 95% CI 0.57 to 0.69), for an absolute difference in sensitivity of 0.31 (95% CI 0.26 to 0.36).[56,66,117,118,120,123,125,126,130,131,138,140,142,145,146,155,157-160,167,169,174,183,184,188,192-195,202,207,208,215] Estimates were similar when the analysis was restricted to seven studies that met minimum technical criteria.[56,131,158,183,184,195,215] Sensitivity progressively improved from 0.32 (95% CI 0.25 to 0.41, 21 studies) for lesions <10 mm, 0.74 (95% CI 0.67 to 0.80, 23 studies) for lesions 10-20 mm, and 0.95 (95% CI 0.92 to 0.97, 20 studies), for a difference of 0.21 (95% CI 0.15 to 0.26) for lesions >20 versus 10-20 mm and 0.42 (95% CI 0.36 to 0.48) for lesions 10-20 versus <10 mm (Table 13).[42,56,69,123,125,126,130,134,138,140,141,146,157-160,174,176,192,195,200,202,207,215]

In five studies that reported accuracy of CT stratified by degree of tumor differentiation, sensitivity was greater for moderately- or poorly-differentiated HCC lesions (0.82, 95% CI 0.66 to 0.91) than for well-differentiated lesions (0.50, 95% CI 0.29 to 0.70), for an absolute difference in sensitivity of 0.32 (95% CI 0.19 to 0.45).[53,62,69,169,192]

In two studies that directly compared sensitivity using a section thickness of 7.5 mm versus 5.0 mm, there was no clear difference (sensitivity 0.64, 95% CI 0.58 to 0.70 vs. 0.72, 95% CI 0.64 to 0.78, for a difference of -0.07, 95% CI -0.17 to 0.02) (Table 14).[118,153]

Magnetic Resonance Imaging

There were no clear differences in estimates of diagnostic accuracy when studies were stratified according to MRI scanner type (1.5 vs. 3.0 T), type of contrast (gadopentetate or gadodiamide vs. gadoxetic acid or gadobenate), imaging phases evaluated (with or without delayed phase imaging), timing of delayed phase imaging (>120 seconds vs. <120 seconds), or section thickness (≤5 mm vs. >5 mm) (Table 8). Relatively few studies evaluated 3.0 T MRI[123,141,145,158,168,195,212,221,234,244,246,264,271,276,295] or MRI without delayed phase imaging,[82,129,166,286] precluding strong conclusions regarding the effects of these technical factors on diagnostic accuracy.

In studies that directly compared diagnostic accuracy of MRI for HCC lesions using different types of contrast, hepatic specific contrast agents (gadoxetic acid or gadobenate) were associated with slightly higher sensitivity than nonhepatic-specific contrast agents (gadopentetate or gadodiamide) (0.83, 95% CI 0.75 to 0.90 vs. 0.74, 95% CI 0.62 to 0.83, difference 0.10, 95% CI 0.04 to 0.15, 6 studies), with no difference in specificity (Table 15).[123,131,135,184,195,221] In studies restricted to HCC lesions <2 cm in diameter, the difference was somewhat larger (sensitivity 0.77, 95% CI 0.68 to 0.84 vs. 0.62, 95% CI 0.52 to 0.71, difference 0.15, 95% CI 0.08 to 0.22, 7 studies).[56,123,135,184,195,221,241]

In eight studies that directly compared diagnostic accuracy of MRI with versus without diffusion-weighted imaging, there was no difference in sensitivity.[235,244,248,269,273,277,287,289] Restricted to HCC lesions <2 cm in diameter, diffusion-weighted imaging was associated with slightly higher sensitivity (0.78, 95% CI 0.62 to 0.88 vs. 0.67, 95% CI 0.50-0.81, difference 0.10, 95% CI 0.02 to 0.18, 5 studies).[245,246,273,277,287]

In 29 studies that reported accuracy of MRI stratified by HCC lesion size, sensitivity was greater for lesions 2 cm (0.96, 95% CI 0.93 to 0.97) than for lesions <2 cm (0.66, 95% CI 0.58 to 0.74), for an absolute difference in sensitivity of 0.29 (95% CI 0.23 to 0.36)[56,118,123,126,131,134,138,140,145,158,184,191,193,195,207,221,226,227,234,245,259,260,263,266,270,273,277,284,292]. The difference was greater in studies of nonhepatic-specific contrast (0.40, 95% CI 0.32-0.49, 16 studies)[118,126,138,140,193,226,234,245,259,260,263,266,273,277,284,292] than in studies of hepatic-specific contrast (0.19, 95% CI 0.13 to 0.25, 12 studies).[56,123,131,145,158,184,191,195,207,221,227,270] Sensitivity progressively improved from 0.45 (95% CI 0.34 to 0.56, 20 studies) for lesions <10 mm, 0.78 (95% CI 0.69 to 0.85, 21 studies) for lesions 10-20 mm, and 0.97 (95% CI 0.94 to 0.98, 18 studies) for lesions >20 mm, for a difference of 0.19 (95% CI 0.12 to 0.26) for >20 versus 10-20 mm and 0.33 (95% CI 0.26 to 0.40) for 10-20 versus <10 mm (Table 13).[69,123,126,131,134,138,140,141,158,191,195,200,207,221,226,227,246,259,260,273,292]

In three studies that reported accuracy of MRI stratified by degree of tumor differentiation, sensitivity was greater for moderately- or poorly-differentiated HCC lesions (0.68, 95% CI 0.44 to 0.86) than for well-differentiated lesions (0.37, 95% CI 0.17 to 0.62), for an absolute difference in sensitivity of 0.31 (95% CI 0.31 to 0.49).[69,136,191] In two studies, sensitivity decreased as Child-Pugh class increased (class A 0.97, 95% CI 0.90-0.99, class B 0.91, 95% CI 0.74 to 0.97, class C 0.79 (0.54 to 0.93).[244,284]

Positron Emission Tomography

In studies that directly compared accuracy of PET using different tracers, FDG PET was associated with lower sensitivity that ^{11}C-acetate PET when either patients (0.58 vs. 0.81, for a difference of -0.23, 95% CI -0.34 to -0.13, 3 studies[297,302,309]) or HCC lesions (0.52 vs. 0.79, for a difference of -0.27, 95 %CI -0.36 to -0.17, 3 studies[297,309,319]) were the unit of analysis. FDG PET was also associated with lower sensitivity than dual tracer PET with FDG and ^{11}C-acetate[127,317] or ^{18}F-choline PET,[313,314] but evidence was limited to 1 or 2 studies for each of these comparisons.

Using patients as the unit of analysis, sensitivity of FDG PET (0.39, 95% CI 0.24 to 0.56, 8 studies)[110,111,154,307,308,315,316,318] was lower than sensitivity of FDG PET/CT (0.65, 95% CI 0.50-0.78, 7 studies) (Table 16).[297,302,309,310,313,314,317]. Similar findings were seen in studies that used ^{11}C-acetate as the tracer and HCC lesions as the unit of analysis, but the number of studies was small (0.68, 95% CI 0.46 to 0.84, 2 studies[306,319] versus 0.85, 95% CI 0.67 to 0.94, 2 studies[127,309]).

In five studies that reported accuracy of FDG PET stratified by HCC lesion size, sensitivity was consistently higher for larger lesions (Table 17).[111,297,305,309,316] Data were not pooled due to differences in the tumor size categories evaluated, with small samples in some studies. One study reported a similar pattern for ^{11}C-acetate PET, although the difference was less pronounced, due to higher sensitivity for lesions 2 to 5 cm in diameter.[309] Another study reported high sensitivity of ^{11}C-acetate PET for lesions ≤5 cm or >5 cm.[297]

Six studies of FDG PET found lower sensitivity for more poorly-differentiated lesions than for more well-differentiated lesions (0.39, 95% CI 0.26 to 0.55 vs. 0.72, 95% CI 0.59 to 0.83, for a difference of -0.33, 95% CI -0.46 to -0.20) (Table 18).[111,309,313,316,317] In two studies of ^{11}C-acetate PET[306,309] and one study of ^{18}F-fluorochlorine,[313] this pattern was not observed, due in part to higher sensitivity for more well-differentiated lesions.

KQ1.b. What is the comparative effectiveness of imaging-based strategies on intermediate outcomes related to clinical decisionmaking?

One study (n=163) evaluated effects of US without contrast versus CT for HCC surveillance in veterans with cirrhosis.[322] It was rated moderate risk of bias due to unclear allocation concealment methods and open-label design. It found no clear difference between imaging strategies in rates of HCC detection. US without contrast was associated with more subsequent CT tests (17 vs. 8) but similar numbers of MRI (9 vs. 12); the total number of subsequent imaging tests was similar (28 vs. 25). The strategy of surveillance with US with contrast was associated with lower cost per HCC detected ($12,069 vs. $18,768).

KQ1.c. What is the comparative effectiveness of imaging-based strategies on clinical and patient-centered outcomes?

One cluster randomized controlled trial (n=18,816) conducted in China compared screening every 6 months with noncontrast US plus serum AFP versus no screening in persons 35 to 79 years of age (mean 42 years) with HBV infection (n=17,250) or chronic hepatitis without HBV infection (n=1566) (Appendix H).[50] Technical details regarding the US methods used were not reported. Patients with an AFP >20 g/l or solid liver lesion on US underwent repeat testing;

patients with repeatedly positive results underwent further diagnostic evaluation, including repeat US and CT or MRI "when necessary". Final diagnoses were based on liver biopsy or long-term followup. The trial was rated as high risk of bias; important methodological shortcomings included inadequate description of randomization or allocation concealment methods, unblended design, failure to report attrition, and failure to control for clustering affects (Appendix C). In addition, outcomes were based on physician reporting or data from the Shanghai Cancer Registry, but the completeness and accuracy of outcomes ascertainment could not be determined.

All screened patients underwent 5 to 10 cycles of screening; compliance with screening was 58 percent. The trial found screening associated with lower risk of HCC-related mortality (32 vs. 54 deaths, rate ratio 0.63, 95% CI 0.41 to 0.98) at 5-year followup. Screening was associated with a trend towards more HCC diagnoses (86 vs. 67, rate ratio 1.37, 95% CI 0.99 to 1.89), but also more Stage I (subclinical or early stage) cancers (52 vs. 0), with more patients undergoing surgical resection. All-cause mortality and harms were not reported.

One other randomized trial[323] compared screening versus no screening, but did not meet inclusion criteria because AFP testing was the primary mode of screening, with US only obtained to evaluate high AFP values. It found no difference between screening and no screening in risk of all-cause or HCC mortality.

Two trials compared different US screening intervals (Appendix H).[48,49] Technical details regarding the US methods used were not reported. One cluster randomized trial in Taiwan (n=744) found no difference between 4- versus 12-month intervals in risk of mortality after 4 years in patients with HBV or HCV infection (57% vs. 56%), even though more frequent screening was associated with higher likelihood of early stage disease (37.5 vs. 6.7%, p=0.017).[49] The second trial (n=1278) in France and Belgium found no difference between 3- versus 6-month intervals in all-cause mortality in patients with cirrhosis related to alcohol use or viral hepatitis.[48]

One randomized trial (n=163) of surveillance among veterans with cirrhosis found no difference between surveillance with US without contrast versus CT in risk of death due to HCC, but was underpowered to detect differences (6.0% or 5/83 vs. 8.8% or 7/80).[322]

KQ1.d. What are the adverse effects or harms associated with imaging-based surveillance strategies?

Two studies that met inclusion criteria reported harms associated with diagnostic imaging for HCC. One study reported 25 percent of patients (n=178) undergoing MRI experienced an adverse event following gadoxetic acid administration, with 56 events classified as mild and 6 as moderate.[144] There were two events classified as serious (anemia and hypotension); neither was considered related to the study drug. Twenty-one drug-related adverse events were reported in 10 percent of the patients, with nausea (1.7%) the most frequently reported event. One other study reported no clear differences between CT with contrast at 3 ml/s versus 5 ml/s in rate of overall adverse events (13% and 15%), discomfort (8% vs. 2%), or adverse events not related to contrast agents (5% vs. 3%).[204] No study reported rates of adverse events associated with use of microbubble contrast agents in US, and harms were not reported in randomized trials of screening with imaging.

Key Question 2. What is the comparative effectiveness of imaging techniques, used singly, in combination, or in sequence, in diagnosing hepatocellular carcinoma among individuals in whom a focal liver lesion has been detected?

Description of Included Studies

Fifty-four studies[43,44,53,55,57-60,63,65,66,68,72,73,75,80,81,85-89,91,93,96-98,100,101,104,107,109,113-117,128,134,142,147,228-230,232,233,245,247,266,279,282,291,298,304] evaluated diagnostic accuracy of imaging tests in diagnosing HCC among individuals in whom an abnormal lesion has been detected and 19 studies[95,105,108,156,181,206,213,214,231,239,240,243,265,269,272,278,287,289,293] evaluated the accuracy of imaging tests for distinguishing HCC from another specific type of liver lesion.

No study compared effects of different imaging modalities or strategies on clinical decisionmaking or on clinical or patient-centered outcomes. One study reported harms.[91]

Key Points

Test Performance

- For evaluation of focal liver lesions, using patients with HCC as the unit of analysis:
  o US with contrast: Sensitivity was 0.87 (95% CI 0.79 to 0.92, 12 studies) and specificity was 0.91 (95% CI 0.83 to 0.95, 8 studies), for a LR+ of 9.6 (95% CI 5.1 to 18) and LR- of 0.14 (95% CI 0.09 to 0.23). (Strength of Evidence: moderate for sensitivity and specificity)
  o US without contrast: Sensitivity was 0.78 (95% CI 0.69 to 0.86) in 1 study; specificity was not reported. (Strength of Evidence: low for sensitivity, insufficient for specificity)
  o CT: Sensitivity was 0.86 (95% CI 0.75 to 0.92, 8 studies) and specificity was 0.88 (95% CI 0.76 to 0.95, 5 studies), for a LR+ of 7.4 (95% CI 3.3 to 17) and LR- of 0.16 (95% CI 0.09 to 0.30). (Strength of Evidence: moderate for sensitivity, low for specificity)
  o MRI: Sensitivity was 0.77 (95% CI 0.66 to 0.84, 4 studies) and specificity was 0.81 (95% CI 0.52 to 0.94, 4 studies), for a LR+ of 4.0 (95% CI 1.4 to 12) and LR- of 0.29 (95% CI 0.21 to 0.39). (Strength of Evidence: low for sensitivity and specificity)

- For evaluation of focal liver lesions, using HCC lesions as the unit of analysis:
  o US with contrast: Sensitivity was 0.87 (95% CI 0.80 to 0.92, 21 studies) and specificity was 0.91 (95% CI 0.85 to 0.95, 10 studies) for a LR+ of 9.8 (95% CI 5.7 to 17) and LR- of 0.14 (95% CI 0.09 to 0.23). (Strength of Evidence: moderate for sensitivity and specificity)
  o CT: Sensitivity was 0.79 (95% CI 0.67 to 0.87, 13 studies) and specificity was 0.90 (95% CI 0.37 to 0.99, 6 studies), for a LR+ of 7.7 (95% CI 0.71 to 84) and LR- of 0.24 (95% CI 0.15 to 0.38). (Strength of Evidence: moderate for sensitivity and specificity)
  o MRI: Sensitivity was 0.81 (95% CI 0.72 to 0.87, 14 studies) and specificity was 0.93 (95% CI 0.80 to 0.98, 11 studies), for a LR+ of 12 (95% CI 3.8 to 39) and LR- of

0.21 (95% CI 0.15 to 0.30). (Strength of Evidence: moderate for sensitivity and specificity)
- o PET: Sensitivity was 0.56 to 0.57 and specificity was 1.0 in two studies of FDG PET. (Strength of Evidence: low for sensitivity and specificity)

- For distinguishing HCC lesions from non-HCC hepatic lesions:
  - o US with contrast: One study found US with sulfur hexafluoride contrast associated with a sensitivity of 0.94 (62/66) and a specificity of 0.68 (23/34) for distinguishing hypervascular HCC from focal nodular hyperplasia, using quantitative methods and one study found US with perflubutane contrast associated with a sensitivity of 0.59 (32/54) and specificity of 1.0 (13/13) for distinguishing small (<3 cm), well-differentiated HCC lesions from regenerative nodules. (Strength of Evidence: low for sensitivity and specificity)
  - o CT: Five studies evaluated accuracy of CT for distinguishing HCC from non-HCC lesions, but the non-HCC lesions varied in the studies, precluding strong conclusions. (Strength of Evidence: low for sensitivity and specificity)
  - o MRI: Four studies reported inconsistent results for distinguishing small (<2 to 3 cm) hypervascular HCC lesions from hypervascular pseudolesions, with sensitivity of 0.47 and 0.52 in two studies, and 0.91 and 0.92 in the other two. Specificity was 0.93 or higher in all four studies. Eight other studies evaluated accuracy of MRI for distinguishing HCC from other non-HCC lesions, but the non-HCC lesions varied in the studies, precluding strong conclusions. (Strength of Evidence: moderate for sensitivity and specificity)

- For direct (within-study) comparisons of imaging modalities, using patients with HCC as the unit of analysis:
  - o US without contrast versus CT: Sensitivity was 0.78 (95% CI 0.70 to 0.85) versus 0.89 (95% CI 0.84 to 0.95), for a difference of -0.12 (95% CI -0.21 to -0.02), based on one study. (Strength of Evidence: low for sensitivity, insufficient for specificity)
  - o US with contrast versus CT: Sensitivity was 0.91 (0.85 to 0.94) versus 0.88 (95% CI 0.81 to 0.92), for a difference of 0.03 (95% CI -0.02 to 0.08), based on five studies. (Strength of Evidence: moderate for sensitivity, low for specificity)
  - o MRI versus CT: Sensitivity was 0.81 (95% CI 0.70 to 0.92) versus 0.74 (95% CI 0.62 to 0.87), for a difference of 0.06 (-0.10 to 0.23), based on one study. (Strength of Evidence: low for sensitivity and specificity)

- Direct (within-study) comparisons of imaging modalities, using HCC lesions as the unit of analysis
  - o US with contrast versus CT: Sensitivity was 0.91 (95% CI 0.85 to 0.94) versus 0.88 (95% CI 0.81 to 0.92), for a difference of 0.03 (95% CI -0.02 to 0.08), based on five studies. (Strength of Evidence: moderate for sensitivity, insufficient for specificity)
  - o US with contrast versus MRI: Sensitivity was 0.79 (95% CI 0.65 to 0.94) versus 0.83 (95% CI 0.69 to 0.97), for a difference of -0.03 (95% CI -0.24 to 0.17), based on one study. (Strength of Evidence: low for sensitivity and specificity)
  - o MRI versus CT: One study found MRI associated with higher sensitivity (0.84, 95% CI 0.76 to 0.92 versus 0.62, 95% CI 0.52 to 0.72, for a difference of 0.22, 95% CI 0.09 to 0.35) but lower specificity (0.36, 95% CI 0.20 to 0.52 versus 0.72, 95% CI

0.58 to 0.87, for a difference of -0.36, 95% CI -0.58 to -0.15) than CT. (Strength of Evidence: low for sensitivity and specificity)
- Multiple imaging modalities
  - In four studies in which positive results with multiple modality imaging were defined as concordant typical findings for HCC on two imaging modalities, sensitivity was lower than with a single modality (difference in sensitivity ranged from 0.09 to 0.27), with no clear difference in specificity. In three studies in which positive results with multiple modality imaging were defined as typical findings for HCC on at least one of the imaging techniques, sensitivity was higher than with a single modality (increase in sensitivity ranged from 0.09 to 0.25), with no clear difference in specificity. One study found that a sequential imaging strategy, in which a second imaging test was only performed for indeterminant results on initial CT, increased sensitivity for HCC from 0.53 to 0.74 to 0.79. (Strength of Evidence: moderate)
- No study used explanted liver as the reference standard. There were no clear differences across imaging modalities in estimates of diagnostic accuracy in analyses stratified by use of different nonexplant reference standards. (Strength of Evidence: moderate for sensitivity and specificity)
- Effects of lesion size and degree of tumor differentiation: See Key Question 1
- Other factors
  - US: In two studies that directly compared US with versus without contrast, US with contrast was associated with sensitivity of 0.89 (95% CI 0.83 to 0.93) and US without contrast with a sensitivity of (0.39) 95% CI 0.32 to 0.47), for a difference in sensitivity of 0.50 (95% CI 0.41 to 0.58). Based on across-study comparisons, there were no clear differences in sensitivity between different US contrast agents; no study directly compared different contrast agents. There were no differences in sensitivity of US based on lesion depth (3 studies) or body mass index (2 studies). (Strength of Evidence: low)
  - CT: Evidence on effects of technical parameters (type of CT scanner, use of delayed phase imaging, section thickness) was limited by small numbers of studies, wide confidence intervals and methodological limitations, precluding reliable conclusions. Two studies found no clear difference in sensitivity of CT for HCC in patients with versus without cirrhosis. (Strength of Evidence: low)
  - MRI: There were no clear differences in estimates of sensitivity based on the type of MRI machine (3.0 T versus 1.5 T), type of contrast, use of delayed phase imaging, timing of delayed phase imaging, and section thickness. Estimates were similar when studies that used diffusion-weighted imaging were excluded. (Strength of Evidence: low)

Clinical Decisionmaking

- No study compared effects of different imaging modalities or strategies on clinical decisionmaking. (Strength of Evidence: insufficient)

Clinical and Patient-Centered Outcomes

- No study compared effects of different imaging modalities or strategies on clinical outcomes. (Strength of Evidence: insufficient)

Harms

- One study of US (with and without contrast) and CT reported harms, but did not stratify results by imaging technique. The overall rate of adverse drug-related events was 10 percent, with all events classified as mild. (Strength of Evidence: insufficient)

Detailed Synthesis

KQ2.a. What is the comparative test performance of imaging techniques for diagnosing HCC in patients with a focal liver lesion?

Ultrasound

For evaluation of focal liver lesions, using patients with HCC as the unit of analysis, sensitivity of US with contrast was 0.87 (95% CI 0.79 to 0.92, 12 studies) and specificity was 0.91 (95% CI 0.83 to 0.95, 8 studies), for a LR+ of 9.6 (95% CI 5.1 to 18) and LR- of 0.14 (95% CI 0.09 to 0.23) (Table 6; Figure 17).[53,58-60,63,73,87,88,97,100,101,113] Sensitivity was lower in studies restricted to HCC lesions <2-3 cm (0.79, 95% CI 0.56 to 0.92),[59,60,73,113] but excluding these studies had little effect on the pooled estimates (Table 6). Using HCC lesions as the unit of analysis, sensitivity of US with contrast was 0.87 (95% CI 0.80 to 0.92, 21 studies) and specificity was 0.91 (95% CI 0.85 to 0.95, 10 studies) for a LR+ of 9.8 (95% CI 5.7 to 17) and LR- of 0.14 (95% CI 0.09 to -0.23) (Figure 18).[43,53,55,57,63,65,66,68,75,81,85,86,89,93,96,104,107,109,114,116,117] Sensitivity was lower in studies restricted to HCC lesions <2- 3 cm (0.73, 95% CI 0.55 to 0.85, 7 studies),[43,55,65,75,89,96,116] but excluding these studies had little effect on the pooled estimates (Table 6). Sensitivity analyses based on study country, use of prospective design, use of Doppler, excluding high risk of bias studies, avoidance of case-control design, and interpretation of imaging blinded to the reference standard had little impact on estimates, and did not reduce heterogeneity.

One study found US with sulfur hexafluoride contrast associated with a sensitivity of 0.94 (62/66) and specificity of 0.68 (23/34) for distinguishing hypervascular HCC from focal nodular hyperplasia, based on quantitative analysis of US findings,[95] and one study found US with perflubutane contrast associated with a sensitivity of 0.59 (32/54) and specificity of 1.0 (13/13) for distinguishing small (<3 cm), well-differentiated HCC lesions from regenerative nodules.[108]

Figure 17. Test performance of ultrasound with contrast in evaluation of focal liver lesions for identification of patients with hepatocellular carcinoma

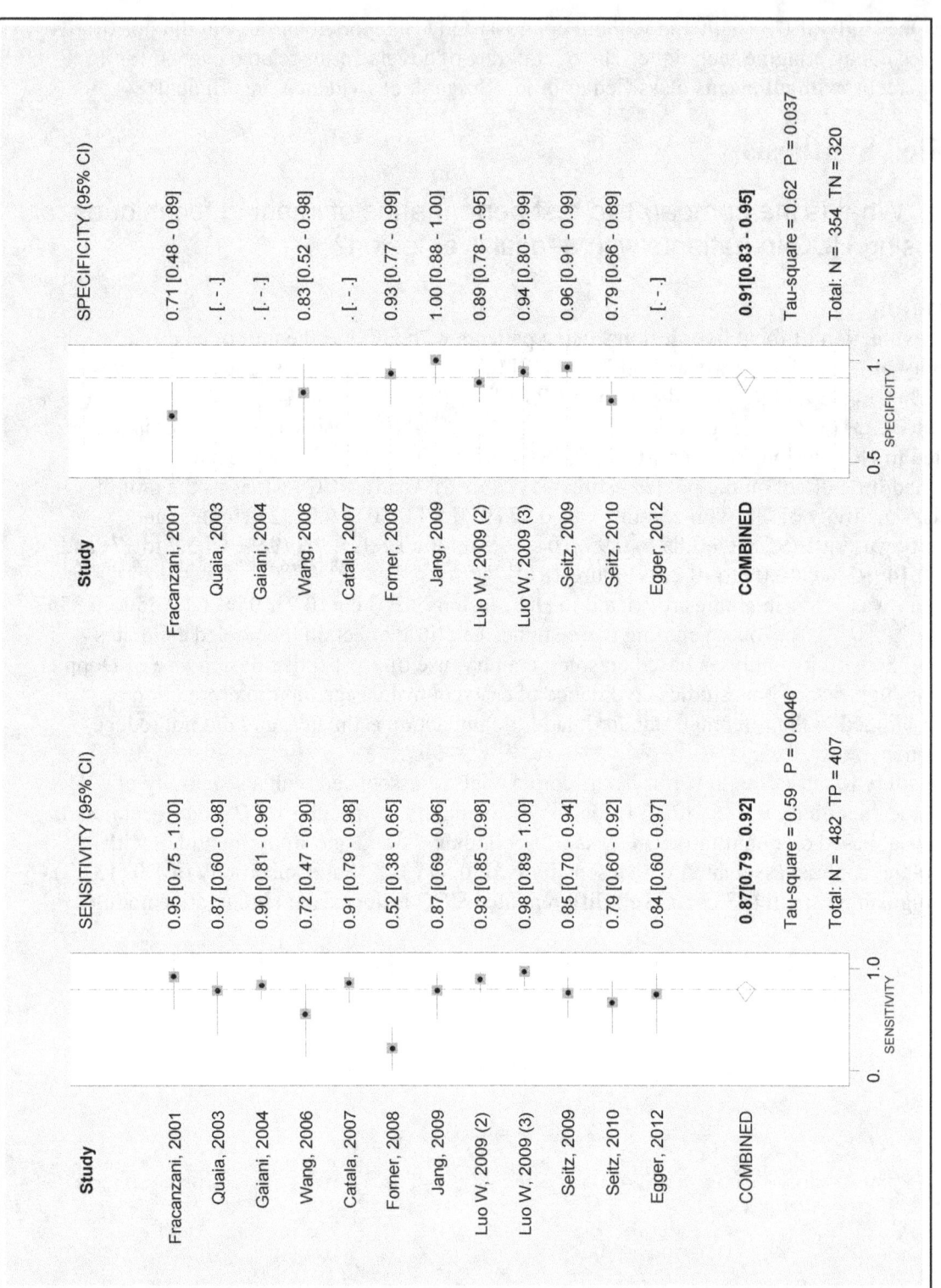

Figure 18. Test performance of ultrasound with contrast for evaluation of focal liver lesions for identification of hepatocellular carcinoma lesions

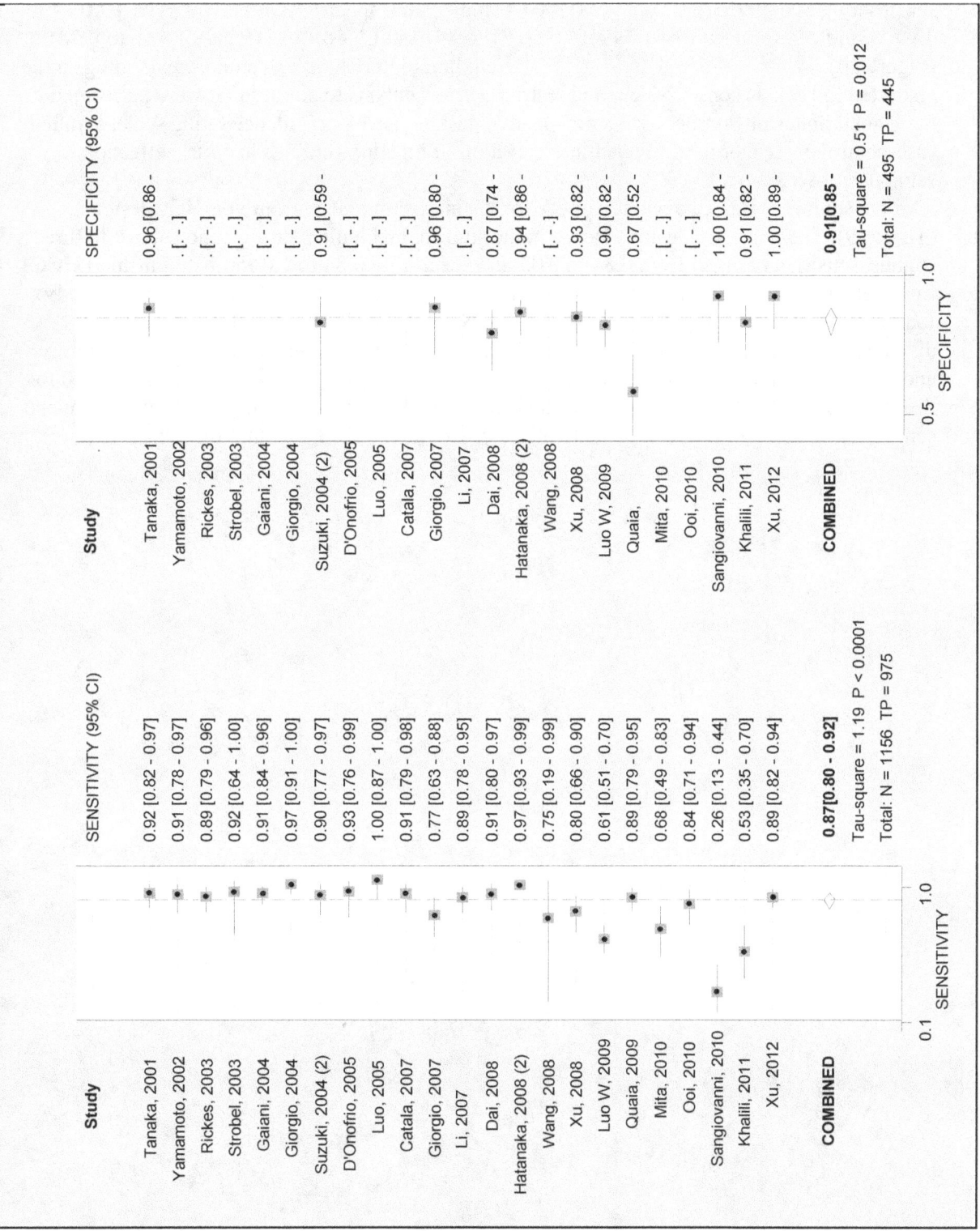

Computed Tomography

For evaluation of focal liver lesions, using patients with HCC as the unit of analysis, sensitivity of CT was 0.86 (95% CI 0.75 to 0.92, 8 studies) and specificity was 0.88 (95% CI 0.76 to 0.95, 5 studies), for a LR+ of 7.4 (95% CI 3.3 to 17) and LR- of 0.16 (95% CI 0.09 to 0.30) (Table 7; Figure 19).[44,53,58,60,87,91,101,134] Using HCC lesions as the unit of analysis, sensitivity was 0.79 (95% CI 0.67 to 0.87, 13 studies) and specificity was 0.90 (95% CI 0.37 to 0.99, 6 studies), for a LR+ of 7.7 (95% CI 0.71 to 84) and LR- of 0.24 (95% CI 0.15 to 0.38) (Figure 20).[43,53,55,66,75,81,89,96,117,128,134,142,147] Excluding high risk of bias studies, excluding studies restricted to HCC lesions <2-3 cm and restricting the analysis to studies that were performed in the United States or Europe, used a prospective design, used a confidence rating scale, avoided a case-control design, or used blinded interpretation of imaging findings had little effect on estimates of sensitivity.

Five studies evaluated accuracy of CT for distinguishing HCC from non-HCC lesions (Table 19). The non-HCC lesions varied in the studies, precluding strong conclusions. In three studies, sensitivity ranged from 0.84 to 0.95 and specificity 0.84 to 1.0 for distinguishing HCC from hemangioma,[181] focal nodular hyperplasia,[214] or various non-HCC lesions.[156] One study found CT associated with a sensitivity of 0.54 (18/33) and specificity of 0.96 (26/27) for distinguishing hypervascular HCC lesions <2 cm from hypervascular pseudolesions[206] and another study found spectral CT associated with a sensitivity of 0.84 and specificity of 0.50 for distinguishing HCC from angiomyolipma based on assessment of the enhancement pattern, and sensitivity of 0.91 to 1.0 and specificity of 1.0 based on various quantitative parameters.[213]

Figure 19. Test performance of CT in evaluation of focal liver lesions for identification of patients with hepatocellular carcinoma

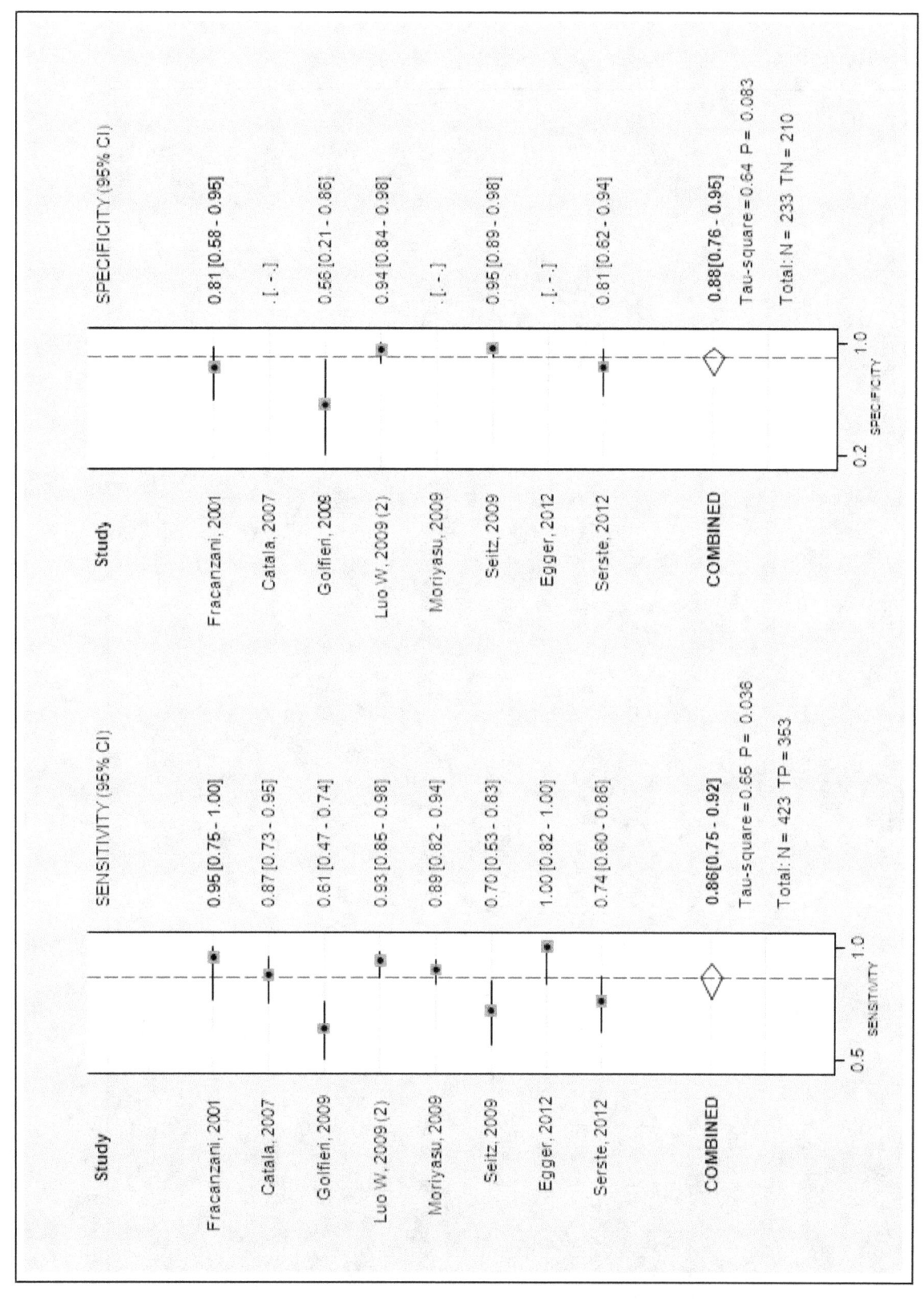

CT = computed tomography

Figure 20. Test performance of CT in evaluation of focal liver lesions for hepatocellular carcinoma lesions

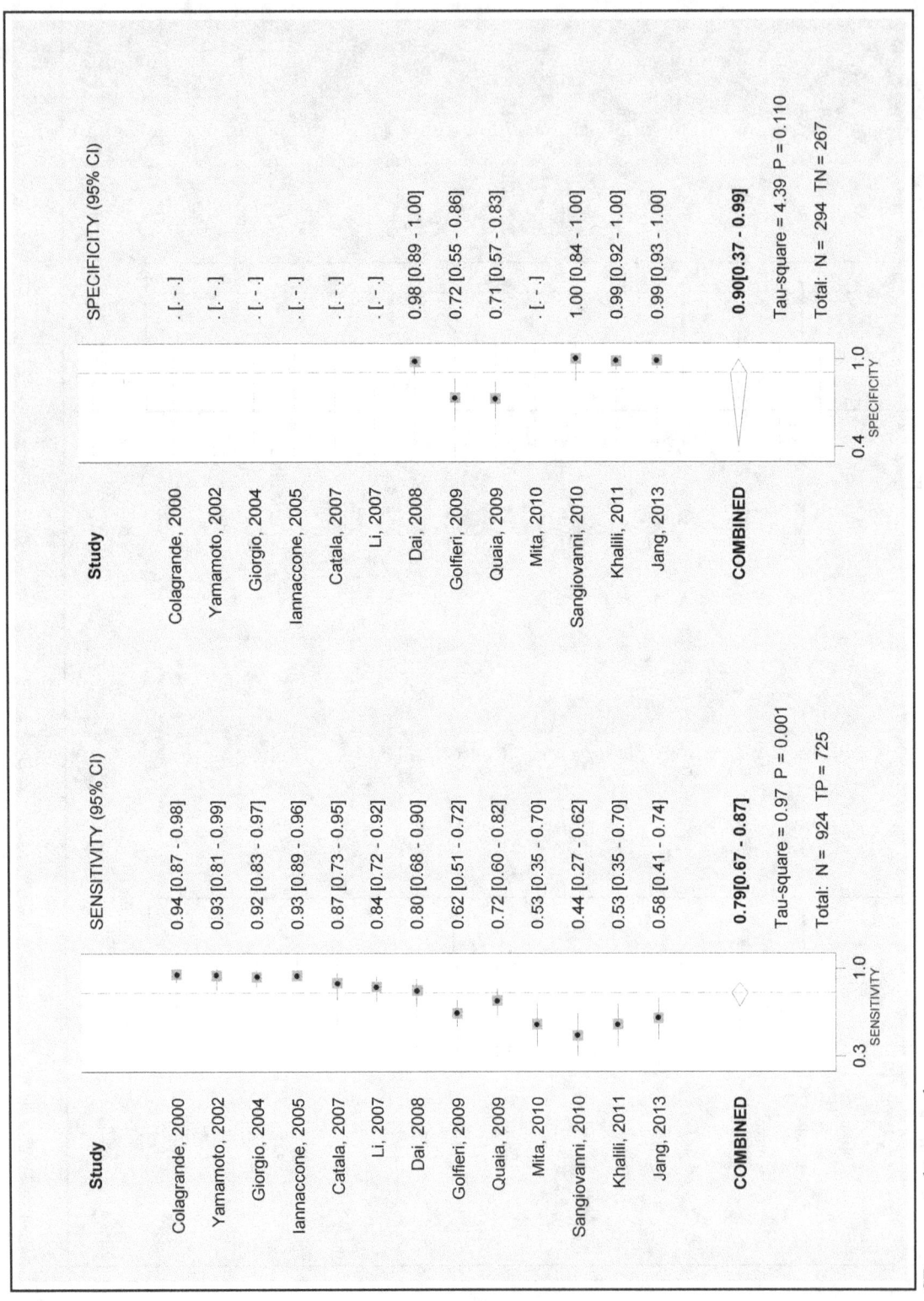

CT = computed tomography

Magnetic Resonance Imaging

For evaluation of focal liver lesions, using patients with HCC as the unit of analysis, sensitivity of MRI was 0.77 (95% CI 0.66 to 0.84, 4 studies) and specificity was 0.81 (95% CI 0.52 to -0.94, 4 studies), for a LR+ of 4.0 (95% CI 1.4 to 12) and LR- of 0.29 (95% CI 0.21 to 0.39) (Table 8; Figure 21).[44,59,100,134]

Using HCC lesions as the unit of analysis, sensitivity was 0.81 (95% CI 0.72 to 0.87, 14 studies and specificity was 0.93 (95% CI 0.80 to 0.98, 11 studies), for a LR+ of 12 (95% CI 3.8 to 39) and LR- of 0.21 (95% CI 0.15 to 0.30) (Figure 22).[43,65,75,134,229,230,232,245,247,253,266,279,282,291] Excluding studies that were restricted to HCC lesions <2 cm increased the sensitivity to 0.90 (95% C I 0.86 to 0.93, 5 studies)[229,230,266,282,291] and excluding studies that were restricted to hypervascular HCC lesions decreased the sensitivity (0.75, 95% CI 0.64 to 0.84, 9 studies).[43,65,75,134,232,247,253,279,291] No study was rated high risk of bias.

Twelve studies evaluated accuracy of MRI for distinguishing HCC from non-HCC lesions (Table 19).[108,206,231,239,240,243,265,269,272,287,289,293] Four studies reported inconsistent results for distinguishing small (<2 to 3 cm) hypervascular HCC lesions from hypervascular pseudolesions, with sensitivity 0.47 and 0.52 in two studies,[239,243] and 0.91 and 0.92 in the other two.[206,269] Specificity was 0.93 or higher in all four studies. There was no clear pattern based on factors such as risk of bias, the diagnostic criteria applied, the reference standard, or the unit of analysis to account for the observed heterogeneity.

One study found MRI associated with poor specificity (0.15, 31/207) for distinguishing HCC lesions from cavernous hemangioma, with sensitivity of 0.88 (137/155), based on the absence of transient peritumoral enhancement.[293] Another study reported a sensitivity of 0.94 (31/33) and specificity of 0.82 (15/18) for distinguishing hypervascular HCC from hemangioma, based on quantitative evaluation of contrast-to-noise ratio.[240] One study reported high (>0.90) sensitivity and specificity of MRI with hepatobiliary phase imaging for distinguishing HCC from dysplastic nodules[231] and one study reported high sensitivity and specificity of MRI with diffusion-weighted imaging for distinguishing small HCC from various benign lesions.[272] Four other studies reported high sensitivity (0.81 to 0.87) but low specificity (0.42 to 0.65) for distinguishing HCC from dysplastic nodules,[289] regenerative nodules,[108] or various benign lesions.[265,287]

Positron Emission Tomography

For evaluation of focal liver lesions, using patients with HCC as the unit of analysis, two studies reported similar sensitivity of FDG PET (0.56 to 0.57) and specificity of 1.0.[298,304]

Ultrasound Versus Computed Tomography

Using patients with HCC as the unit of analysis, based on five studies that directly compared diagnostic accuracy of imaging modalities, sensitivity was similar for US with contrast and CT (0.91, 95% CI 0.85 to 0.94 versus 0.88, 95% CI 0.81 to 0.92) (Table 20).[53,58,87,91,101] Using HCC lesions as the unit of analysis, US with contrast and CT were also associated with similar sensitivity (0.92, 95% CI 0.88 to 0.96 versus 0.89, 95% CI 0.83 to 0.93, for a difference of 0.04, 95% CI -0.02 to 0.09), based on four studies.[53,66,81,117] There were also no differences between US with contrast and CT for HCC lesions <2 cm (0.78, 95% CI 0.61 to 0.89 versus 0.71, 95% CI 0.52 to 0.85, for a difference of 0.07, 95% CI -0.01 to 0.15), based on seven studies,[43,55,66,75,89,96,117] or for well-differentiated HCC lesions, based on two studies.[53,89]

Figure 21. Test performance of MRI in evaluation of focal liver lesions for patients with hepatocellular carcinoma

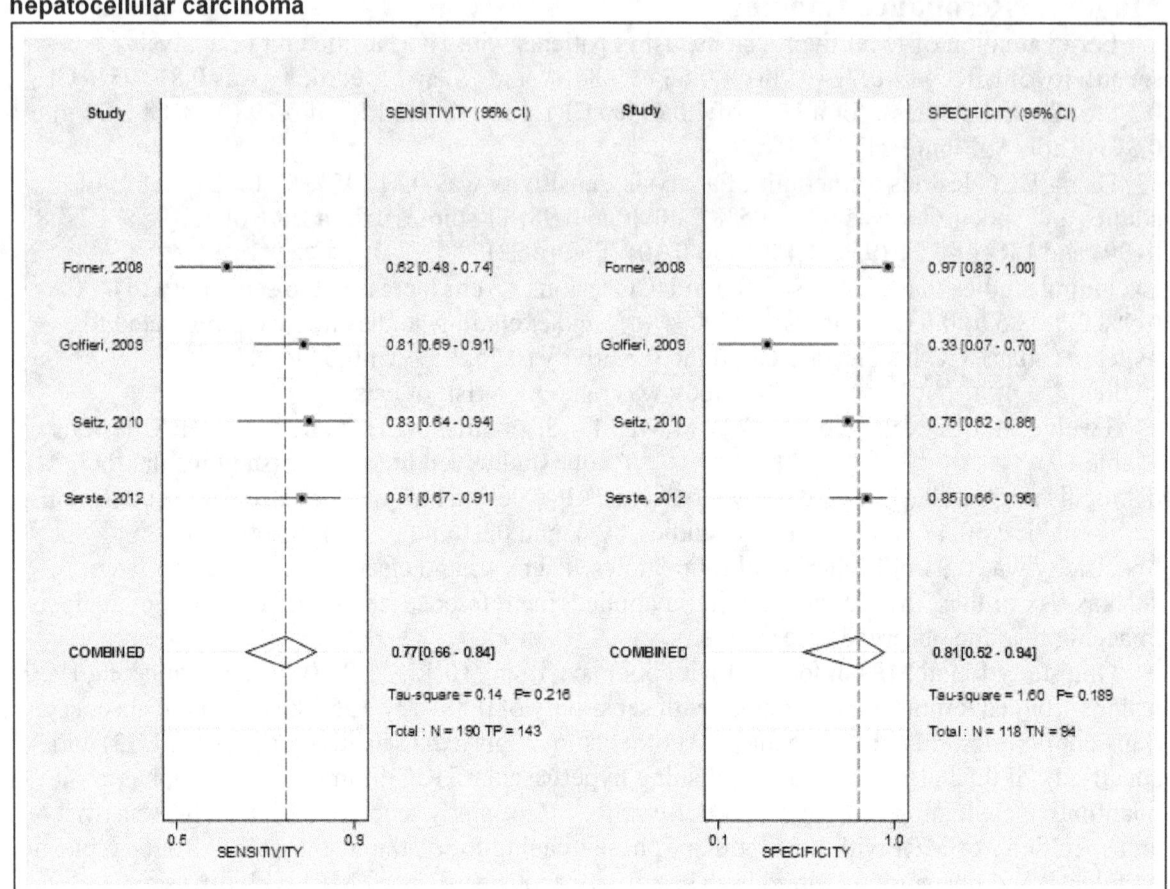

MRI = magnetic resonance imaging

Figure 22. Test performance of MRI in evaluation of focal liver lesions for hepatocellular carcinoma lesions

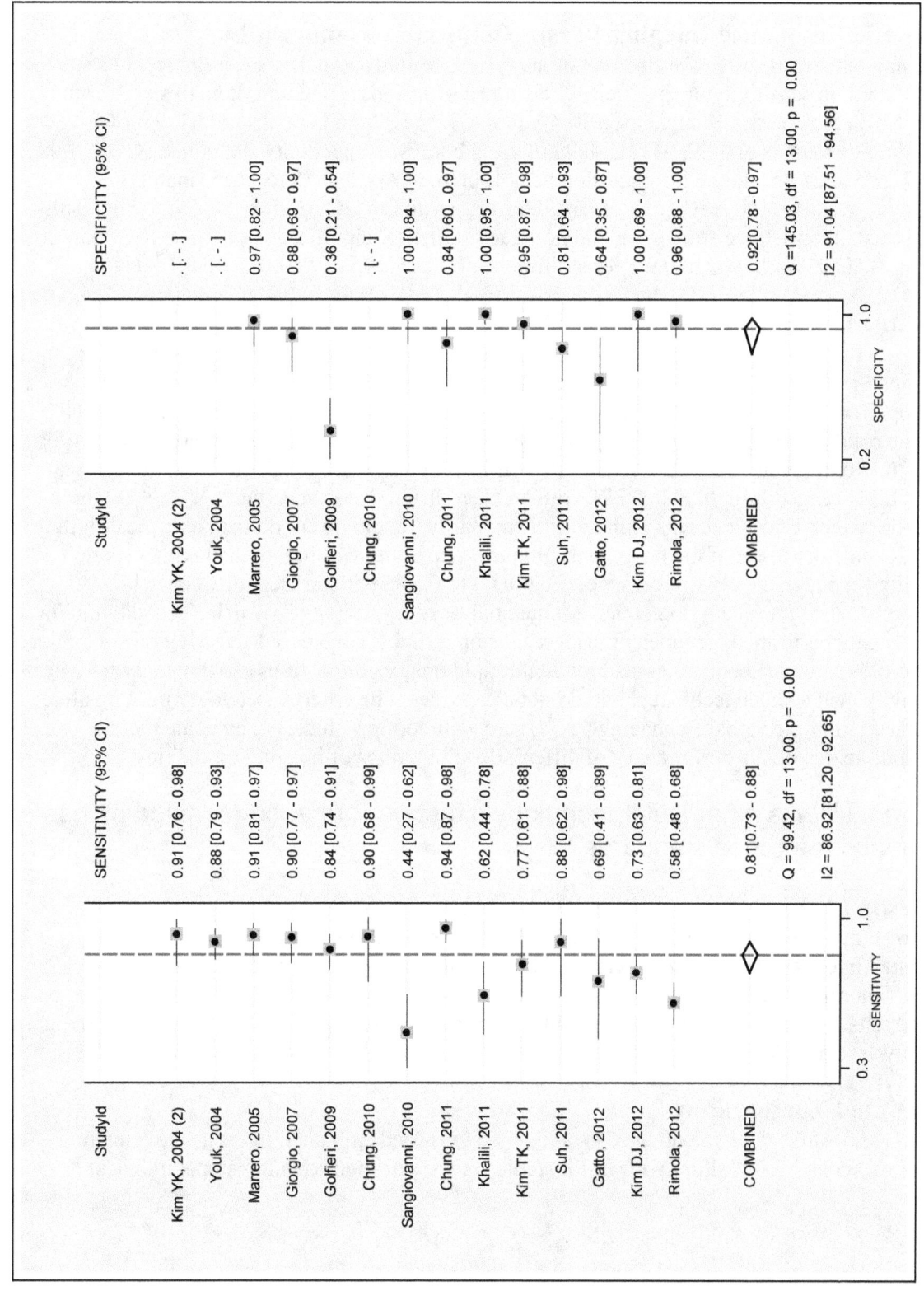

MRI = magnetic resonance imaging

Ultrasound Versus Magnetic Resonance Imaging

Using patients with HCC as the unit of analysis, one study found no difference in sensitivity between US with contrast and MRI (0.79, 95% CI 0.65 to 0.94 versus 0.83, 95% CI 0.69 to 0.97).[100]

Magnetic Resonance Imaging Versus Computed Tomography

Using patients with HCC as the unit of analysis, one study found no clear difference between MRI and CT in sensitivity or specificity.[44] Using HCC lesions as the unit of analysis, one study found MRI associated with higher sensitivity (0.84, 95% CI 0.76 to 0.92 vs. 0.62, 95% CI 0.52 to 0.72, for a difference of 0.22, 95% CI 0.09 to 0.35) but lower specificity (0.36, 95% CI 0.20-0.52 vs. 0.72, 95% CI 0.58 to 0.87, for a difference of -0.36, 95% CI -0.58 to -0.15) than CT.[134] Sensitivity was also lower when the analysis was restricted to HCC lesions <2-3 cm, but results were based on only three studies and did not reach statistical significance (0.65, 95% CI 0.04 to 0.99 vs. 0.50, 95% CI 0.02 to 0.98, for a difference of 0.15, 95% CI 0.00 to 0.30).[43,75,134]

Multiple Imaging Modalities

Seven studies compared diagnostic performance of single versus multiple modality imaging for diagnosis of HCC in patients with focal liver lesions (Table 11).[43,44,55,59,75,96,134] Five reported diagnostic accuracy for small (<2 or <3 cm) HCC lesions.[43,59,75,96,134] In four studies in which positive results with multiple modality imaging were defined as concordant typical findings for HCC on two imaging modalities, sensitivity was lower than with a single modality (decrease insensitivity ranged from 0.09 to 0.27), with no clear difference in specificity.[43,44,59,75] In three studies in which positive results with multiple modality imaging were defined as typical findings for HCC on at least one of the imaging techniques, sensitivity was higher than with a single modality (increases in sensitivity ranged from 0.09 to 0.25), with no clear difference in specificity.[43,44,96] One study found that a sequential imaging strategy in which a second imaging test was only performed for indeterminant results on initial CT increased sensitivity from 0.53 to 0.74 to 0.79.[75] Two other studies also found multiple imaging modalities associated with higher sensitivity than a single technique, but did not clearly describe criteria used to define a positive result with multiple modality imaging.[55,134] There were too few studies to evaluate the comparative diagnostic performance of different combinations of imaging modalities.

KQ2.a.i. How is a particular technique's test performance modified by use of various reference standards?

Ultrasound

No study evaluated diagnostic accuracy of US for evaluation of focal liver lesions using explanted livers as the reference standard. There were no clear differences in sensitivity for nonexplant reference standards (histopathological, imaging/clinical criteria, or mixed) based on pooled sensitivity (range 0.89 to 0.94), using either patients with HCC or HCC lesions as the unit of analysis (Table 6).

Computed Tomography

No study of CT for evaluation of focal liver lesions used explanted livers as the reference standard. Accuracy was slightly lower for studies that used a nonexplant histopathological reference standard (0.83, 95% CI 0.73 to 0.90, 6 studies)[53,66,81,89,96,128] than a mixed (histological with clinical/imaging criteria) reference standard (0.93, 95% CI 0.82 to 0.98),[117,142] but only two studies used a mixed reference standard (Table 7).

Magnetic Resonance Imaging

No study of MRI for evaluation of focal liver lesions used explanted livers as the reference standard. Using HCC lesions as the unit of analysis, sensitivity was the same for one study that used a nonexplant histopathological reference standard (0.91, 95% CI 0.81 to 0.96), 95% CI 0.53 to 0.85)[266] and four studies that used a mixed (histological with clinical/imaging criteria) reference standard (0.90, 95% CI 0.86 to 0.94),[229,230,282,291] (Table 8).

KQ2.a.ii. How is the comparative effectiveness modified by patient, tumor, technical, or other factors?

Ultrasound

Using HCC lesions as the unit of analysis, studies of US with contrast reported higher sensitivity (0.87, 95% CI 0.80 to 0.92, 21 studies)[43,53,55,57,63,65,66,68,75,81,85,86,89,93,96,104,107,109,114,116,117] than studies of US without contrast (0.62, 95% CI 0.18 to 0.93, 4 studies)[72,98,115,116] (Table 6). Using patients with HCC as the unit of analysis, all studies except for one[80] evaluated US with contrast. Two studies that directly compared US with versus without contrast using HCC lesions as the unit of analysis found US with contrast associated with higher sensitivity (0.89, 95% CI 0.83 to 0.93) than US without contrast (0.39, 95% CI 0.32 to 0.47), for a difference in sensitivity of 0.50 (95% CI 0.41 to 0.58) (Table 12).[115,116] Based on patients as the unit of analysis, sensitivity was similar in studies that used perflubutane (0.95, 95% CI 0.89 to 0.97, 2 studies)[86,87] or sulfur hexafluoride contrast (0.87, 95% CI 0.82 to 0.91, 6 studies).[53,58,63,97,100,101] Using HCC lesions as the unit of analysis, sensitivity was similar for sulfur hexafluoride (0.91, 95% CI 0.84 to 0.96, 7 studies),[53,57,63,66,81,93,114] perflubutane (0.86, 95% CI 0.67 to 0.95, 2 studies),[68,86] and galactose (0.94, 95% CI 0.85 to 0.97, 4 studies).[85Suzuki, 2004 #4467,109,117] No study directly compared different types of contrast agents.

One study using patients with HCC as the unit of analysis compared US with contrast versus without contrast (sensitivity 0.93, 95% CI 0.88 to 0.97 vs. 0.78, 95% CI 0.70-0.85, for a difference of 0.15, 95% CI 0.06 to 0.23), but results were potentially confounded by use of Doppler in the contrast group.[91] One study that used HCC lesions as the unit of analysis that directly compared US with versus without Doppler found no clear difference in sensitivity.[104] Effects of lesion size, tumor differentiation, lesion depth, and body mass index are presented in the results for Key Question 1.

Computed Tomography

Using HCC lesions as the unit of analysis, there were no clear differences in sensitivity between studies of multidetector CT with ≥8 or <8 rows, studies with versus without delayed phase imaging, or studies with section thickness ≤5 vs. >5 mm (Table 7). However, several estimates based on these technical parameters were imprecise.

Two studies found no clear difference in sensitivity of CT for HCC in patients with versus without cirrhosis.[156,181] Effects of lesion size and tumor differentiation on accuracy are presented in the results for Key Question 1.

Magnetic Resonance Imaging

Using HCC lesions as the unit of analysis, sensitivity was the same for studies that used non-hepatobiliary[229,266,291] or hepatobiliary[230,282] contrast (Table 8). Effects of lesion size and tumor differentiation on accuracy are presented in the results for Key Question 1. Among five studies that were not restricted to HCC lesions <2-3 cm, all used 1.5 T MRI, included delayed or hepatobiliary phase imaging, and had section thickness of ≤5 mm.

KQ2.b. What is the comparative effectiveness of the various imaging techniques on intermediate outcomes related to clinical decisionmaking?

No study evaluated the comparative effectiveness of different imaging techniques on clinical decisionmaking.

KQ2.c. What is the comparative effectiveness of the various imaging techniques on clinical and patient-centered outcomes?

No study evaluated the comparative effectiveness of different imaging techniques on clinical and patient-centered outcomes.

KQ2.d. What are the adverse effects or harms associated with imaging-based diagnostic strategies?

One study of US (with and without contrast) and CT reported harms, but did not stratify results by imaging technique. The overall rate of adverse drug-related events was 10 percent, with all events classified as mild.[91]

Key Question 3. What is the comparative effectiveness of imaging techniques used singly, in combination, or in sequence, in staging HCC among patients diagnosed with HCC?

Description of Included Studies

Six studies reported test performance of various imaging techniques for staging of patients with HCC based on TNM criteria.[42,61,122,126,127,216] Ten studies reported test performance of PET for detection of metastatic disease.[152,171,189,300,309-311,316,317,320]

Seven studies reported effects of imaging on transplant decisions[82,102,122,127,179,202,208] and one study reported comparative effects of imaging on clinical and patient-centered outcomes.[152,171,189,300,309-311,316,317,320] No study reported harms associated with imaging for HCC staging.

Key Points

Test Performance

- For staging, using TNM criteria, using explanted liver or surgical resection reference standard:
    - CT: The proportion correctly staged ranged from 28 to 58 percent, the proportion overstaged from 2 to 27 percent, and the proportion understaged from 25 to 52 percent, based on six studies. (Strength of Evidence: moderate)

- o MRI: The proportion correctly staged was 40 to 75 percent, the proportion overstaged 3.1 to 31 percent, and the proportion understaged 19 to 31 percent, based on three studies. (Strength of Evidence: low)
- o PET: One study found 26 percent of patients were correctly staged with FDG PET and 91 percent with ^{11}C-choline PET. (Strength of Evidence: low)
- o MRI versus CT: Two studies reported similar staging accuracy. (Strength of Evidence: low)

- For identification of metastatic disease, using patients with metastatic HCC as the unit of analysis:
  - o PET: Sensitivity of FDG PET was 0.85 (95% CI 0.71 to 0.93, 6 studies) and specificity was 0.93 (95% CI 0.89 to 0.95, 5 studies), for a LR+ of 11 (95% CI 7.8 to 17) and LR- of 0.16 (95% CI 0.08 to 0.33). One study that directly compared sensitivity of FDG PET to ^{11}C-acetate PET reported comparable sensitivity (0.79 vs. 0.71), although sensitivity was higher when both tracers were used (0.98). (Strength of Evidence: low for sensitivity and specificity)
  - o PET/CT versus CT: Three studies found no difference in sensitivity (0.82, 95% CI 0.61 to 0.93 vs. 0.85, 95% CI 0.66 to 0.95). (Strength of Evidence: low)

- For identification of metastatic disease, using metastatic HCC lesions as the unit of analysis:
  - o PET: Sensitivity of FDG PET was 0.82 (95% CI 0.72 to 0.90, 5 studies). One study that directly compared sensitivity of FDG to ^{11}C-acetate PET reported comparable sensitivity (0.86 vs. 0.77, respectively). (Strength of Evidence: low for sensitivity, insufficient for specificity)

- Evidence was insufficient to determine effects of different reference standards on test performance:
  - o For accuracy of staging using TNM criteria, all but one study used explanted livers as the reference standard. (Strength of Evidence: insufficient for sensitivity and specificity)
  - o For accuracy of PET for identifying metastatic HCC, five of the six studies that used patients with metastatic HCC as the reference standard used mixed histological and imaging/clinical criteria as the reference standard. For studies that used metastatic HCC lesions as the unit of analysis, different reference standards were each evaluated in only one or two studies. (Strength of Evidence: insufficient for sensitivity and specificity)

- Effects of patients, tumor, or technical factors on test performance:
  - o For accuracy of staging using TNM criteria, no study evaluated effects of patient-level characteristics or other factors on accuracy of imaging techniques for staging. (Strength of Evidence: insufficient)
  - o For identifying metastatic HCC, estimates for sensitivity were too imprecise to determine how use of PET versus PET/CT affected test performance. In one study that directly compared sensitivity of PET versus PET/CT for identifying metastatic HCC lesions, there was no clear difference in sensitivity. (Strength of Evidence: low)
  - o Four studies of PET with FDG found sensitivity increased as lesion size increased, but the number of lesions <1 cm was small (total of 20). (Strength of Evidence: low)

- o Eight studies reported test performance of FDG PET stratified by location of metastasis. In most studies, sensitivity was higher for lymph and bone metastasis than for lung metastasis, but samples were small, precluding strong conclusions. (Strength of Evidence: low)

Clinical Decisionmaking

- Transplant eligibility, using Milan criteria
  - o CT: The proportion correctly assessed for transplant eligibility ranged from 40 to 96 percent. Three studies reported that the proportion of patients who met transplant criteria based on CT but exceeded criteria based on the reference standard was 3.5 to 7.8 percent. Two studies found that 2.3 and 16 percent of patients who underwent transplantation based on Milan criteria had no HCC lesions on examination of explanted livers. (Strength of Evidence: moderate)
  - o CT versus MRI: One study reported similar accuracy. (Strength of Evidence: low)
  - o PET versus CT: One study found ^{11}C-choline PET more accurate than CT (95% vs. 40%). (Strength of Evidence: low)
  - o MRI versus CT: One study reported that the proportion of decisions to perform resection or ablative therapies that were classified as correct were similar for MRI (90% and 90%, respectively) and CT (80% and 77%, respectively). (Strength of Evidence: low)

Clinical and Patient-Centered Outcomes

- US with contrast versus US without contrast plus CT: One cohort study found that contrast enhanced US identified more small (≤2 cm) HCC lesions than noncontrast US plus CT (36 vs. 31), and was associated with a higher complete necrosis rate following ablation (92% or 106/115 vs. 83% or 93/112 lesions, p=0.036), but was rated high risk of bias. Another study that appeared to be performed in the same series of patients found US with contrast prior to radiofrequency ablation associated with lower local tumor progression rate (7.2% vs. 18%, RR 0.40, 95% CI 0.16 to 0.87) and longer tumor-free survival (38 vs. 26 months), but was also rated high risk of bias. (Strength of Evidence: low)

Harms

- No evidence. (Strength of Evidence: insufficient)

Detailed Synthesis

KQ3.a. What is the comparative test performance of imaging techniques to predict HCC tumor stage?

Accuracy of Imaging for Staging

Seven studies evaluated accuracy of imaging techniques for staging using TNM criteria (six studies), BCLC criteria (one study), or UNOS criteria (one study) (Table 21).[42,47,61,122,126,127,216] Six studies used an explanted liver reference standard and the other[127] used an explanted liver or surgical resection reference standard. CT was evaluated in six studies, MRI in three studies, and PET in one study. For CT, the proportion correctly staged ranged from 28 to 58 percent, the proportion overstaged from 2 to 27 percent, and the proportion understaged from 25 to 52 percent.[42,61,122,126,127,216] For MRI, the TNM, BCLC, and UNOS criteria were used in one study each, with estimates of the proportion correctly staged ranging from 40 to 75 percent, the proportion overstaged from 3.1 to 31 percent, and the proportion understaged from 19 to 31 percent.[47,61,126] One study found 26 percent of patients correctly staged with FDG PET and 91 percent with ^{11}C-choline PET.[127]

Two studies that directly compared staging accuracy of imaging modalities found similar staging accuracy for MRI versus CT.[61,126]

PET for Detection of Metastatic Hepatocellular Carcinoma Disease

Using patients with metastatic HCC as the unit of analysis, sensitivity of FDG PET was 0.85 (95% CI 0.71 to 0.93, 6 studies) and specificity was 0.93 (95% CI 0.89 to 0.95, 5 studies), for a LR+ of 11 (95% CI 7.8 to 17) and LR- of 0.16 (95% CI 0.08 to 0.33) (Table 9; Figure 23).[152,171,300,311,317,320] Estimates were similar when high risk of bias studies were excluded and when the analysis was restricted to studies that used a prospective design. All studies were conducted in Asia. One study that directly compared sensitivity of FDG PET to ^{11}C-acetate PET reported comparable sensitivity (0.79 vs. 0.71), although sensitivity was higher when both tracers were used (0.98).[300]

Using metastatic HCC lesions as the unit of analysis, sensitivity of FDG PET was 0.82 (95% CI 0.72 to 0.90, 5 studies) (Figure 24).[189,305,309,311,316] No study reported specificity. All studies except one were rated high risk of bias. In the one moderate risk of bias study, sensitivity was 0.86 (95% CI 0.70-0.95).[309] All studies were conducted in Asia except for one small study (n=5) conducted in the United States.[316] One study that directly compared sensitivity of FDG to ^{11}C-acetate PET reported comparable sensitivity (0.86 vs. 0.77, respectively) (Table 16. PET direct comparisons).[309]

Figure 23. Test performance of FDG PET for detection of patients with metastatic hepatocellular carcinoma

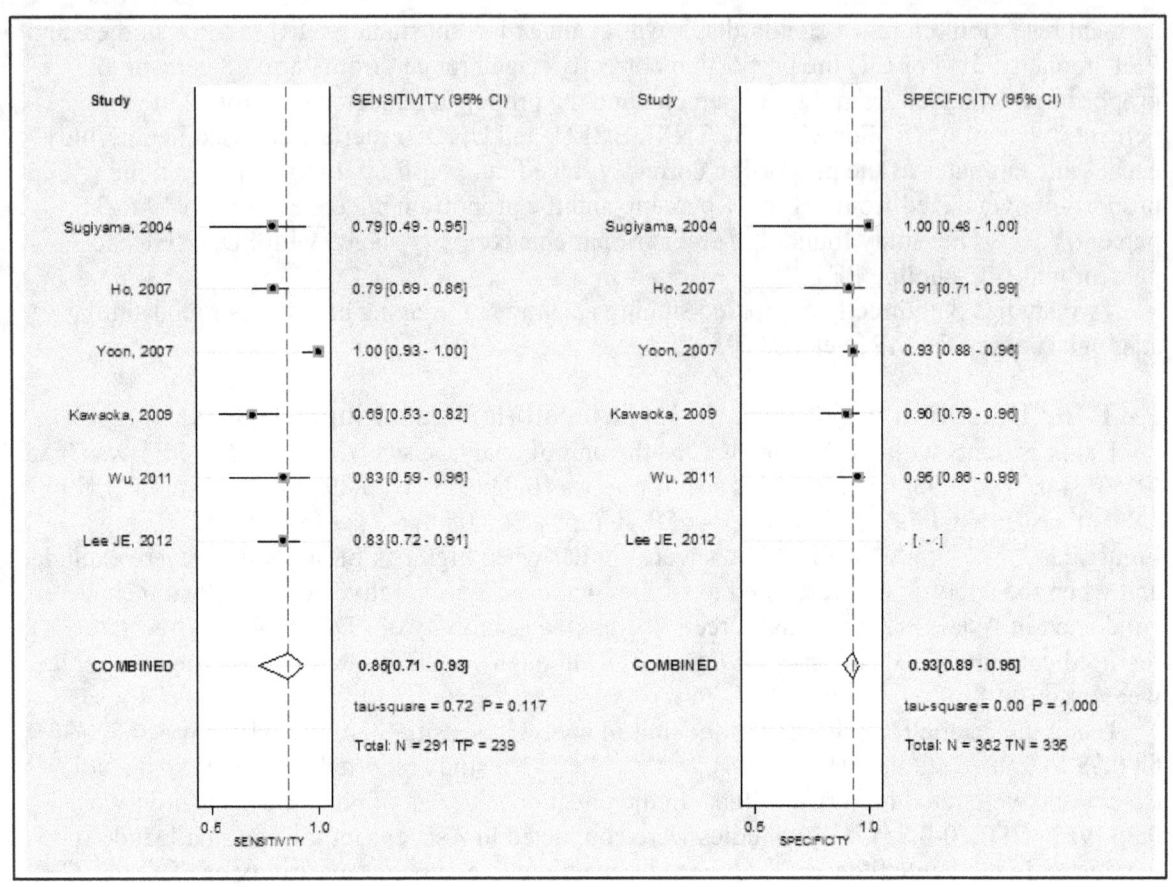

FDG = ^{18}F-fluorodeoxyglucose; PET = positron emission tomography

Figure 24. Test performance of FDG PET for detection of metastatic hepatocellular carcinoma lesions

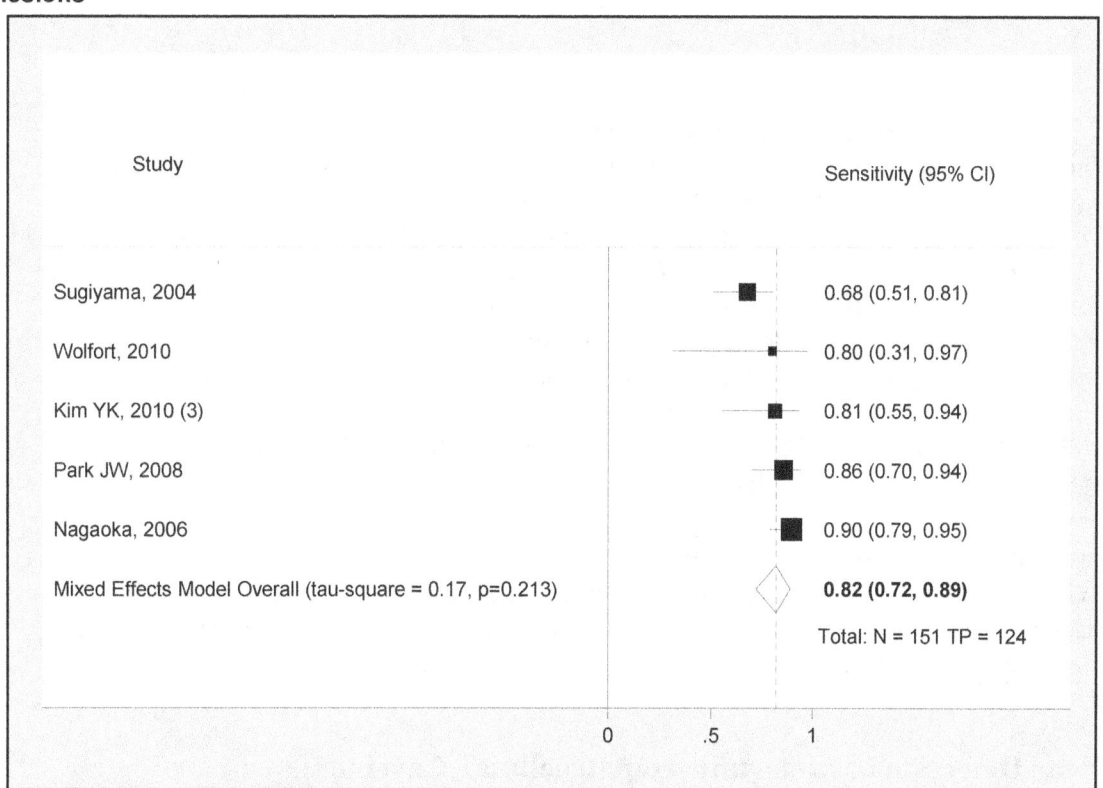

*Only sensitivity available

PET Versus Other Imaging Modalities

Three studies found no difference in sensitivity between PET/CT versus CT for metastatic HCC (0.82, 95% CI 0.61 to 0.93 vs. 0.85, 95% CI 0.66 to 0.95).[152,171,189]

One study found FDG PET associated with higher sensitivity than conventional imaging with CT, MRI, and chest x-ray for identifying HCC metastatic to lymph node (1.0 vs. 0.79) or bone (1.0 vs. 0.46), with no difference in specificity.[320] Both imaging methods identified all 12 patients with lung metastases. However, one other study found FDG PET associated with lower sensitivity than imaging with chest x-ray and CT for identifying lung metastases (1.0 vs. 0.61).[171]

KQ3.a.i. How is a particular technique's test performance modified by use of various reference standards?

Accuracy of Imaging for Staging

Evidence was insufficient to determine effects of the use of different reference standards on accuracy of imaging techniques for staging. All studies used explanted livers as the reference standard except for one, which used explanted livers or surgical resection as the reference standard.[42,47,61,122,126,127,216]

PET for Detection of Metastatic Hepatocellular Carcinoma Disease

Evidence was too limited to determine effects of the use of different reference standards on accuracy of FDG PET for detection of metastatic HCC. Five of the six studies that used patients with metastatic HCC as the unit of analysis used mixed histological and imaging/clinical criteria as the reference standard.[152,171,300,311,317,320] For studies that used metastatic HCC lesions as the reference standard, different reference standards (nonexplant histological reference standard, imaging and clinical criteria, or mixed) were each evaluated in only one or two studies.[189,305,309,311,316]

KQ3.a.ii. How is the comparative effectiveness modified by patient, tumor, technical, or other factors?

Accuracy of Imaging for Staging

No study evaluated effects of patient-level characteristics or other factors on accuracy of imaging techniques for staging.

PET for Detection of Metastatic Hepatocellular Disease

Estimates of sensitivity stratified by use of PET or PET/CT showed no clear differences, with overlapping confidence intervals (Table 9). In one study that directly compared sensitivity of PET versus PET/CT for identifying metastatic HCC lesions, there was no clear difference in sensitivity (0.90 vs. 0.98, respectively, difference of -0.09, 95% CI -0.17 to 0.0) (Table 16).[189]

One study found PET with FDG associated with higher sensitivity than ^{11}C-acetate (0.79 vs. 0.64, for a difference of 0.15, 95% CI 0.03 to 0.28), but lower sensitivity than the combination of FDG and ^{11}C-acetate (0.98, difference -0.19, 95% CI -0.28 to -0.11).

Four studies of FDG PET that stratified analyses by metastatic lesion size found higher sensitivity as lesion size increased, but the number of lesions <1 cm was small (total of 20), precluding strong conclusions (Table 17).[171,305,309,311]

Eight studies reported test performance of FDG PET stratified by location of metastasis (Table 22).[152,171,189,305,309,311,317,320] In most studies, sensitivity was higher for lymph and bone metastasis than for lung metastasis, but samples were small, precluding strong conclusions.

KQ3.b. What is the comparative test performance of imaging techniques on intermediate outcomes related to clinical decisionmaking?

Seven studies evaluated accuracy of imaging techniques for assessing transplant eligibility based on Milan criteria (Table 21).[82,102,122,127,179,202,208] Two studies also evaluated University of California, San Francisco (UCSF) liver transplantation criteria.[122,179] Six studies used explanted liver as the reference standard and the seventh[127] used an explanted liver or surgical resection. Five studies evaluated CT, one study evaluated MRI, one study evaluated PET, and two studies evaluated use of more than one imaging modality (US or CT and US, CT, or MRI). For CT, the proportion correctly assessed for transplant eligibility ranged from 40 to 96 percent using Milan criteria;[122,127,179,202,208] estimates from two studies that used UCSF criteria were similar to estimates based on Milan criteria. The proportion that met transplant criteria based on CT but exceeded criteria based on the reference standard was 3.5 to 7.8 percent in three studies[179,202,208] and 26 percent in the fourth.[122] In two studies, the proportion of patients who underwent transplantation based on CT but had no HCC lesion on examination of explanted livers was 2.3 percent and 16 percent.[122,202] In two studies not restricted to a single imaging modality (e.g., CT or MRI, or CT, MRI, or US), the proportion correctly assessed were 38 percent and 57 percent.[82,102]

Two studies directly compared accuracy of two or more imaging modalities for assessing transplant eligibility. One study reported similar accuracy for CT and MRI.[179] The other study found ^{11}C-choline PET more accurate than CT (95% vs. 40%).[127]

One study reported that the proportion of decisions to perform resection or ablative therapies that were classified as correct were similar for MRI (90% and 90%, respectively) and CT (80% and 77%, respectively).[126]

KQ3.c. What is the comparative effectiveness of imaging techniques on clinical and patient-centered outcomes?

One high risk of bias cohort study (n=167) of patients with HCC who underwent radiofrequency ablation compared effects of preprocedure US with contrast versus US without contrast plus CT on clinical outcomes (Appendix I).[46] US with contrast was performed within 10 minutes prior to the ablation procedure by two experienced radiologists using sulfur hexafluoride microbubble contrast; technical information for US without contrast was not reported. Contrast-enhanced CT with arterial and portal venous phase imaging was performed within one month prior to ablation, with followup one month after ablation. The study found that contrast enhanced US identified more small (≤2 cm) HCC lesions than US without contrast plus CT (36 vs. 31), and was associated with a higher complete necrosis rate following ablation (92% or 106/115 vs. 83% or 93/112 lesions, p=0.036). An important methodological shortcoming of this study was failure to adjust for potential confounders (Appendix C). Furthermore, additional lesions identified on US with contrast and cases classified as complete necrosis (treatment response) did not undergo histopathological or other confirmation prior to ablation. Another cohort study that appeared to be performed in the same patient population found US with contrast prior to radiofrequency ablation associated with a lower likelihood of local tumor progression (7.2% vs. 18.3%, RR 0.40, 95% CI 0.16 to 0.87), and longer progression-free (40 vs. 33 months, p=0.015) and tumor-free survival (38 vs. 26 months, p<0.001) than US without contrast, but also failed to adjust for confounders.[45]

KQ3.d. What are the adverse effects or harms associated with imaging-based staging strategies?

No study evaluated harms associated with use of imaging techniques for staging in patients diagnosed with HCC.

Table 6. Test performance of ultrasound imaging for identification and diagnosis of hepatocellular carcinoma

Detection of HCC (KQ 1)	Unit of Analysis	Sensitivity (95% CI); τ^2 (p value)	Number of Studies	Specificity (95% CI); τ^2 (p value)	Number of Studies	LR+	LR-
Surveillance settings							
Ultrasound without contrast	Patient	0.78 (0.60 to 0.89); 0.52 (p=0.11)	4	0.89 (0.80 to 0.94); 0.26 (p=0.16)	3	6.8 (4.2 to 11)	0.25 (0.13 to 0.46)
	Lesion	0.60 (0.24 to 0.87)	1	No data	--	--	--
Nonsurveillance settings							
Ultrasound without contrast	Patient	0.73 (0.46 to 0.90); 2.3 (p=0.02)	8	0.93 (0.85 to 0.97); 0.78 (p=0.12)	6	11 (5.4 to 21)	0.29 (0.13 to 0.65)
• Excluding Doppler		0.77 (0.48 to 0.93); 2.5 (p=0.04)	7	0.92 (0.82 to 0.97); 0.70 (p=0.14)	5	9.8 (4.7 to 21)	0.25 (0.09 to 0.64)
• Prospective design		0.97 (0.68 to 0.998); 1.3 (p=0.02)	2	0.73 (0.45 to 0.90)	1	3.6 (1.5 to 8.5)	0.04 (0.003 to 0.59)
• Reference standard: Explanted liver		0.48 (0.35 to 0.61); 0.17 (p=0.08)	5	0.96 (0.94 to 0.97); <0.0001 (p=0.97)	5	12 (7.4 to 19)	0.54 (0.42 to 0.70)
• Reference standard: Histopathological, non-explant		0.95 (0.87 to 0.98)	3	0.73 (0.47 to 0.90)	1	3.6 (1.5 to 8.2)	0.07 (0.03 to 0.19)
• United States or Europe		0.70 (0.37 to 0.91); 1.9 (p=0.02)	5	0.93 (0.84 to 0.97); 0.51 (p=0.13)	4	10 (4.9 to 21)	0.32 (0.12 to 0.83)
• Excluding poor quality studies		0.77 (0.48 to 0.93); 2.5 (p=0.04)	7	0.92 (0.82 to 0.97); 0.70 (p=0.14)	5	9.8 (4.7 to 21)	0.25 (0.09 to 0.64)
• Avoided case-control design		0.54 (0.38 to 0.70); 0.44 (p=0.09)	6	0.95 (0.91 to 0.97); 0.41 (p=0.16)	6	11 (6.1 to 19)	0.48 (0.34 to 0.68)
• Blinded interpretation of imaging		0.75 (0.33 to 0.95); 2.0 (p=0.02)	3	0.94 (0.81 to 0.98); 0.51 (p=0.13)	2	12 (4.4 to 33)	0.27 (0.07 to 0.97)
	Lesion	0.59 (0.42 to 0.74); 1.2 (p=0.005)	11	0.83 (0.53 to 0.95); 3.4 (p=0.07)	2	3.4 (1.2 to 9.4)	0.50 (0.37 to 0.66)
• HCC lesions <2-3 cm		0.75 (0.72 to 0.78); <0.0001 (p=1.0)	2	No data	--	--	--
• Excluding studies restricted to HCC lesions <2-3 cm		0.54 (0.35 to 0.73); 1.3 (p=0.01)	9	0.86 (0.55 to 0.97); 3.5 (p=0.09)	2	4.0 (1.2 to 13)	0.53 (0.38 to 0.73)
• Excluding Doppler		0.50 (0.30 to 0.71); 1.2 (p=0.02)	7	0.95 (95% CI 0.85 to 0.99)	1	Not calculated	Not calculated
• Reference standard: Explanted liver		0.34 (0.22 to 0.47); 0.28 (p=0.06)	5	Insufficient data	--	--	--

73

Table 6. Test performance of ultrasound imaging for identification and diagnosis of hepatocellular carcinoma (continued)

	Unit of Analysis	Sensitivity (95% CI); τ^2 (p value)	Number of Studies	Specificity (95% CI); τ^2 (p value)	Number of Studies	LR+	LR-
• Reference standard: Histopathological, non-explant		0.75 (0.58 to 0.86)	3	Insufficient data	--	--	--
• Reference standard: Mixed histological and imaging/clinical criteria		0.72 (0.46 to 0.88)	1	Insufficient data	--	--	--
• Prospective		0.78 (0.55 to 0.91); 0.61 (p=0.02)	3	Insufficient data	--	--	--
• U.S. or Europe		0.66 (0.35 to 0.87); 1.3 (p=0.01)	4	Insufficient data	--	--	--
• Avoided case-control design		0.43 (0.22 to 0.68); 1.2 (p=0.01)	5	Insufficient data	--	--	--
• Blinded interpretation of imaging		0.67 (0.44 to 0.84); 1.0 (p=0.02)	5	Insufficient data	--	--	--
Ultrasound with contrast	Lesion	0.73 (0.52 to 0.87); 1.6 (p=0.01)	8	No data	--	--	--
• All HCC lesions <2-3 cm		0.63 (0.35 to 0.84); 0.89 (p=0.16)	3	No data	--	--	--
• No Doppler		0.78 (0.50 to 0.92); 1.9 (p=0.05)	5	No data	--	--	--
• Excluding studies restricted to HCC lesions <2-3 cm		0.78 (0.50 to 0.92); 1.9 (p=0.05)	5	No data	--	--	--
• Contrast: Perflubutane		0.85 (0.65 to 0.94); 1.1 (p=0.11)	4	No data	--	--	--
• Reference standard: Histopathological, non-explant		066 (0.47 to 0.81); 0.58 (p=0.06)	4	No data	--	--	--
• Reference standard: Mixed histological and imaging/clinical		0.98 (0.86 to 0.998)	1	No data	--	--	--
• Prospective		0.34 (95% CI 0.11 to 0.68); 0.48 (p=0.10)	1	No data	--	--	--
• United States or Europe		0.34 (95% CI 0.08 to 0.75); 0.76 (p=0.08)	1	No data	--	--	--
• Excluding high risk of bias studies		0.66 (0.33 to 0.88); 1.4 (p=0.05)	3	No data	--	--	--
• Avoided case-control design		No data	0	No data	--	--	--
• Blinded interpretation of imaging		0.80 (0.50 to 0.94); 1.8 (p=0.05)	4	No data	--	--	--

Table 6. Test performance of ultrasound imaging for identification and diagnosis of hepatocellular carcinoma (continued)

	Unit of Analysis	Sensitivity (95% CI); τ^2 (p value)	Number of Studies	Specificity (95% CI); τ^2 (p value)	Number of Studies	LR+	LR-
	Liver segment	0.79 (0.62 to 0.89); 1.6 (p=0.0006)	2	0.95 (0.84 to 0.99); 0.74 (p=0.04)	2	17 (4.7 to 60)	0.22 (0.12 to 0.42)
Evaluation of focal liver lesions (KQ 2)							
Ultrasound without contrast	Patient	0.78 (0.69 to 0.86)	1	No data	--	--	--
Ultrasound with contrast	Patient	0.87 (0.79 to 0.92); 0.59 (p=0.005)	12	0.91 (0.83 to 0.95); 0.62 (p=0.04)	8	9.6 (5.1 to 18)	0.14 (0.09 to 0.23)
• HCC lesions <2-3 cm		0.79 (0.56 to 0.92); 0.90 (p=0.18)	4	0.91 (0.74 to 0.97); 0.88 (p=0.26)	4	8.6 (2.9 to 26)	0.23 (0.10 to 0.53)
• Excluding Doppler		0.90 (0.85 to 0.93); 0.02 (p=0.60)	6	0.91 (0.83 to 0.96); 0.41 (p=0.10)	4	10 (5.0 to 21)	0.11 (0.07 to 0.16)
• Excluding studies restricted to hypervascular HCC		0.87 (0.78 to 0.92); 0.65 (p=0.007)	11	0.91 (0.83 to 0.95); 0.62 (p=0.04)	8	9.6 (5.1 to 18)	0.15 (0.09 to 0.25)
• Excluding studies restricted to HCC lesions <2-3 cm		0.90 (0.86 to 0.93); 0.02 (p=0.76)	8	0.91 (0.83 to 0.96); 0.41 (p=0.10)	4	10 (5.0 to 21)	0.11 (0.08 to 0.16)
• Contrast: sulfur hexafluoride		0.87 (0.82 to 0.91); 0.02 (p=0.59)	6	0.92 (0.78 to 0.97); 0.42 (p=0.10)	2	11 (3.7 to 31)	0.14 (0.10 to 0.20)
• Contrast: perflubutane		0.95 (0.89 to 0.97)	2	0.92 (0.78 to 0.97)	2	12 (3.9 to 35)	0.06 (0.03 to 0.13)
• Reference standard: Histopathological, non-explant		0.91 (0.84 to 0.95); 0.06 (p=0.39)	4	0.87 (0.61 to 0.97); 0.41 (p=0.09)	1	7.0 (1.9 to 25)	0.11 (0.06 to 0.20)
• Reference standard: Mixed histological and imaging/clinical criteria		0.89 (0.83 to 0.93)	4	0.93 (0.83 to 0.97)	3	12 (5.0 to 29)	0.12 (0.07 to 0.19)
• Prospective Design		0.87 (0.82 to 0.91); 0.02 (p=0.59)	6	0.92 (0.78 to 0.97); 0.42 (p=0.10)	2	11 (3.7 to 31)	0.14 (0.10 to 0.20)
• United States or Europe		0.87 (0.82 to 0.91); 0.02 (p=0.59)	6	0.92 (0.78 to 0.97); 0.42 (p=0.10)	2	11 (3.7 to 31)	0.14 (0.10 to 0.20)
• Excluding high risk of bias studies		0.89 (0.84 to 0.93); 0.03 (p=0.73)	6	0.91 (0.83 to 0.96); 0.41 (p=0.10)	4	10 (4.9 to 21)	0.12 (0.07 to 0.18)
• Avoided case-control design		0.90 (0.86 to 0.93); 0.02 (p=0.61)	6	0.91 (0.83 to 0.96); 0.41 (p=0.10)	4	11 (5.1 to 22)	0.11 (0.07 to 0.16)
• Blinded interpretation of imaging		0.92 (0.87 to 0.95); 0.03 (p=0.54)	5	0.94 (0.89 to 0.96); 0.05 (p=0.51)	3	14 (8.1 to 26)	0.09 (0.06 to 0.14)
• Used confidence rating scale		0.93 (0.83 to 0.97)	1	0.89 (0.65 to 0.97)	1	8.5 (2.2 to 33)	0.08 (0.03 to 0.21)
Ultrasound without contrast	Lesion	0.62 (0.18 to 0.93); 3.7 (p=0.19)	4	0.92 (0.84 to 0.96); 0.16 (p=0.34)	3	8.1 (3.6 to 18)	0.41 (0.12 to 1.4)
• Excluding studies restricted to HCC lesions <2-3 cm		0.76 (0.14 to 0.98); 5.4 (p=0.36)	3	0.91 (0.78 to 0.97); 0.14 (p=0.54)	2	8.5 (3.2 to 22)	0.26 (0.03 to 2.4)

Table 6. Test performance of ultrasound imaging for identification and diagnosis of hepatocellular carcinoma (continued)

	Unit of Analysis	Sensitivity (95% CI); τ^2 (p value)	Number of Studies	Specificity (95% CI); τ^2 (p value)	Number of Studies	LR+	LR-
Ultrasound with contrast		0.87 (0.80 to 0.92); 1.2 (p<0.0001)	21	0.91 (0.85 to 0.95); 0.51 (p=0.01)	10	9.8 (5.7 to 17)	0.14 (0.09 to 0.23)
• HCC lesions <2-3 cm		0.73 (0.55 to 0.85); 0.997 (p=0.02)	7	0.92 (0.81-0.97); 0.95 (p=0.07)	6	8.7 (4.1 to 18)	0.30 (0.18 to 0.51)
• Excluding studies restricted to hypervascular HCC		0.87 (0.79 to 0.92); 1.3 (p<0.0001)	20	0.91 (0.85 to 0.95); 0.52 (p=0.01)	10	9.8 (5.7 to 17)	0.15 (0.09 to 0.24)
• Excluding studies restricted to HCC lesions <2-3 cm		0.91 (0.86 to 0.95); 0.59 (p=0.002)	14	0.93 (0.88 to 0.96); 0.05 (p=0.38)	4	14 (7.7 to 24)	0.09 (0.06 to 0.15)
• Contrast: sulfur hexafluoride		0.91 (0.84 to 0.96); 0.53 (p=0.003)	7	No data; 0.03 (p=0.34)	--	--	--
• Contrast: perflubutane		0.86 (0.67 to 0.95)	2	0.92 (0.87 to 0.96)	2	11 (5.8 to 22)	0.15 (0.06 to 0.40)
• Contrast: galactose		0.94 (0.85 to 0.97)	4	0.95 (0.86 to 0.98)	2	19 (6.2 to 61)	0.07 (0.03 to 0.17)
• Reference standard: Histological specimen		0.94 (0.88 to 0.97); 0.54 (p=0.002)	6	0.95 (0.86 to 0.98); 0.03 (p=0.34)	2	20 (6.3 to 61)	0.06 (0.03 to 0.13)
• Reference standard: Mixed histological and imaging/clinical criteria		0.89 (0.81 to 0.94)	8	0.93 (0.87 to 0.96)	2	12 (6.5 to 23)	0.12 (0.07 to 0.22)
• Prospective design		0.91 (0.85 to 0.95); 0.58 (p=0.002)	8	0.93 (0.88 to 0.96); 0.05 (p=0.36)	2	14 (7.7 to 24)	0.09 (0.05 to 0.17)
• United States or Europe		0.94 (0.87 to 0.97); 0.53 (p=0.002)	5	No data	--	--	--
• Excluding Doppler		0.90 (0.85 to 0.94); 0.57 (p=0.002)	12	0.93 (0.88 to 0.96); 0.05 (p=0.38)	4	13 (7.6 to 24)	0.10 (0.06 to 0.17)
• Excluding high risk of bias studies		0.91 (0.85 to 0.95); 0.59 (p=0.002)	10	0.93 (0.88 to 0.96); 0.05 (p=0.38)	4	14 (7.7 to 24)	0.09 (0.05 to 0.17)
• Avoided case-control design		0.90 (0.83 to 0.94); 0.55 (p=0.002)	10	0.92 (0.87 to 0.96); 0.03 (p=0.49)	3	12 (6.6 to 21)	0.11 (0.06 to 0.19)
• Blinded interpretation of imaging		0.92 (0.84 to 0.96); 0.60 (p=0.002)	7	0.93 (0.86 to 0.96); 0.03 (p=0.48)	2	12 (6.5 to 23)	0.09 (0.05 to 0.18)
• Used confidence rating scale		No studies	0	No studies	0	--	--
Lesion depth <53, <60, or <85 mm		0.87 (0.80-0.92); <0.0001 (p=1.0)	3	Insufficient data	--	--	--
• >53, >60, or >85 mm		0.83 (0.74 to 0.90)	3	Insufficient data	--	--	--
Body mass index <23 or <25		0.80 (0.70-0.88); 0.11 (p=0.37)	2	Insufficient data	--	--	--
• >23 or >25		0.80 (0.70-0.87)	2	Insufficient data	--	--	--

HCC = hepatocellular carcinoma; KQ = Key Question

Table 7. Test performance of computed tomography imaging for identification of intrahepatic and extrahepatic hepatocellular carcinoma

	Unit of Analysis	Sensitivity (95% CI); τ^2 (p value)	Number of Studies	Specificity (95% CI); τ^2 (p value)	Number of Studies	LR+	LR-
Detection of HCC (KQ 1)							
Surveillance settings	Patient	0.84 (0.59 to 0.95); 0.50 (p=0.74)	2	0.99 (0.86 to 0.999); 1.1 (p=0.97)	2	60 (5.9 to 622)	0.16 (0.06 to 0.47)
	Lesion	0.62 (0.46 to 0.76)	1	Insufficient data	--	--	--
Nonsurveillance settings	Patient	0.83 (0.75 to 0.89); 0.60 (p=0.008)	16	0.92 (0.86 to 0.96); 0.63 (p=0.02)	11	11 (5.6 to 20)	0.19 (0.12 to 0.28)
• Excluding studies restricted to hypervascular HCC		0.84 (0.77 to 0.90); 0.46 (p=0.03)	15	0.92 (0.85 to 0.96); 0.62 (p=0.02)	11	11 (5.6 to 21)	0.17 (0.11 to 0.26)
• Excluding studies restricted to HCC lesions <2-3 cm		0.83 (0.75 to 0.89); 0.60 (p=0.008)	16	0.92 (0.86 to 0.96); 0.63 (p=0.02)	11	11 (5.6 to 20)	0.19 (0.12 to 0.28)
• CT type: Multidetector, ≥8 rows		0.88 (0.69 to 0.96); 0.55 (p=0.01)	2	Insufficient data; 0.48 (p=0.07)	--	--	--
• CT type: Multidetector, <8 rows		0.89 (0.69 to 0.97)	2	0.98 (0.87 to 0.996)	1	37 (6.1 to 222)	0.11 (0.03 to 0.37)
• CT type: Non-multidetector		0.82 (0.71 to 0.89)	11	0.90 (0.83 to 0.95)	9	8.3 (4.5 to 15)	0.20 (0.12 to 0.34)
• Contrast rate: ≥3 ml/s		0.87 (0.77 to 0.93); 0.48 (p=0.04)	8	0.90 (0.81 to 0.94); 0.38 (p=0.08)	7	8.4 (4.5 to 16)	0.15 (0.08 to 0.27)
• Contrast rate: <3 ml/s		0.71 (0.50-0.85)	4	0.95 (0.87 to 0.98)	3	13 (4.8 to 37)	0.31 (0.17 to 0.58)
• Imaging phases: Arterial, portal venous, and delayed		0.89 (0.81 to 0.94); 0.33 (p=0.06)	7	0.88 (0.74 to 0.95); 0.41 (p=0.09)	4	7.3 (3.2 to 17)	0.13 (0.07 to 0.22)
• Imaging phases: Missing delayed phase imaging		0.78 (0.66 to 0.87)	7	0.94 (0.87 to 0.97)	5	13 (5.8 to 27)	0.23 (0.14 to 0.38)
• Delayed phase ≥120 s		0.87 (0.79 to 0.92); 0.17 (p=0.12)	6	0.87 (0.74 to 0.94); 0.40 (p=0.10)	4	6.8 (3.1 to 15)	0.15 (0.09 to 0.25)
• Section thickness: ≤5 mm		0.84 (0.73 to 0.91); 0.57 (p=0.02)	9	0.87 (0.76 to 0.93); 0.19 (p=0.19)	6	6.3 (3.4 to 12)	0.19 (0.11 to 0.33)
• Section thickness: >5 mm		0.83 (0.67 to 0.92)	5	0.95 (0.90-0.98)	4	17 (8.3 to 34)	0.18 (0.09 to 0.37)
• Reference standard: Explanted liver		0.81 (0.71 to 0.88); 0.47 (p=0.02)	11	0.93 (0.87 to 0.96); 0.36 (p=0.05)	9	11 (6.0-20)	0.21 (0.13 to 0.32)
• Reference standard: Histopathological, non-explant		0.85 (0.64 to 0.95)	3	0.73 (0.31 to 0.94)	1	3.1 (0.83 to 12)	0.20 (0.07 to 0.62)
• Reference standard: Histological and clinical/imaging reference standard		0.88 (0.70-0.96)	2	0.93 (0.75 to 0.98)	1	13 (3.2 to 52)	0.13 (0.05 to 0.35)
• Prospective		0.72 (0.57 to 0.84); 0.30 (p=0.03)	5	0.85 (0.67 to 0.94); 0.43 (p=0.03)	3	4.9 (2.0-12)	0.33 (0.20-0.54)
• United States or Europe		0.83 (0.73 to 0.90); 0.60 (p=0.008)	12	0.89 (0.80-0.94); 0.32 (p=0.11)	8	7.3 (3.9 to 14)	0.19 (0.12 to 0.32)
• Used confidence rating scale		0.85 (0.70-0.93); 0.53 (p=0.01)	4	0.73 (0.31 to 0.94); 0.36 (p=0.05)	1	3.1 (0.84 to 12)	0.20 (0.08 to 0.51)
• Excluding high risk of bias studies		0.85 (0.75 to 0.91); 0.55 (p=0.01)	9	0.92 (0.83 to 0.97); 0.63 (p=0.02)	6	11 (4.6 to 26)	0.16 (0.10-0.28)

Table 7. Test performance of computed tomography imaging for identification of intrahepatic and extrahepatic hepatocellular carcinoma (continued)

	Unit of Analysis	Sensitivity (95% CI); τ² (p value)	Number of Studies	Specificity (95% CI); τ² (p value)	Number of Studies	LR+	LR−
• Avoided case-control design		0.75 (0.63 to 0.84); 0.44 (p=0.007)	9	0.91 (0.83 to 0.95); 0.59 (p=0.03)	9	8.1 (4.1 to 16)	0.28 (0.18 to 0.43)
• Blinded interpretation of imaging		0.83 (0.74 to 0.89); 0.55 (p=0.01)	13	0.94 (0.88 to 0.97); 0.49 (p=0.02)	8	13 (6.5 to 27)	0.19 (0.12 to 0.29)
	Lesion	0.77 (0.72 to 0.80); 0.92 (p<0.0001)	79	0.89 (0.84 to 0.93); 0.92 (p<0.0001)	21	7.1 (4.7 to 11)	0.26 (0.22 to 0.31)
• HCC lesions <2-3 cm		0.70 (0.45 to 0.87); 1.8 (p=0.02)	7	0.97 (0.88 to 0.99); 2.2 (p=0.08)	2	24 (6.6 to 85)	0.31 (0.15 to 0.62)
• Excluding studies restricted to hypervascular HCC		0.75 (0.71 to 0.80); 0.79 (p<0.0001)	55	0.87 (0.80 to 0.91); 0.64 (p<0.0001)	16	5.6 (4.0 to 8.5)	0.28 (0.23 to 0.35)
• Excluding studies restricted to HCC lesions <2-3 cm		0.77 (0.73 to 0.81); 0.81 (p<0.0001)	72	0.89 (0.83 to 0.93); 0.83 (p<0.0001)	19	7.0 (4.5 to 11)	0.26 (0.21 to 0.31)
• CT type: Multidetector, ≥8 rows		0.77 (0.71 to 0.82); 0.81 (p<0.0001)	36	0.91 (0.84 to 0.95); 0.79 (p<0.0001)	10	8.5 (4.6 to 16)	0.26 (0.20 to 0.33)
• CT type: Multidetector, <8 rows		0.79 (0.59 to 0.91)	4	Insufficient data	—	—	—
• CT type: Non-multidetector		0.75 (0.67 to 0.82)	22	0.86 (0.73 to 0.93)	7	5.3 (2.7 to 10)	0.29 (0.21 to 0.40)
• Contrast rate: ≥3 ml/s		0.78 (0.74 to 0.82); 0.79 (p<0.0001)	58	0.90 (0.84 to 0.94); 0.82 (p<0.0001)	18	7.7 (4.8 to 12)	0.24 (0.20 to 0.30)
• Contrast rate: <3 ml/s		0.74 (0.59 to 0.85)	7	0.71 (0.22 to 0.95)	1	2.5 (0.54 to 12)	0.37 (0.16 to 0.85)
• Imaging phases: Arterial, portal venous, and delayed		0.74 (0.69 to 0.80); 0.78 (p<0.0001)	42	0.90 (0.85 to 0.94); 0.51 (p<0.0001)	13	7.8 (4.9 to 12)	0.28 (0.23 to 0.35)
• Imaging phases: Missing delayed phase imaging		0.81 (0.75 to 0.86)	26	0.88 (0.75 to 0.95)	5	6.7 (3.0 to 15)	0.22 (0.16 to 0.30)
• Delayed phase ≥120 s		0.75 (0.69 to 0.80); 0.78 (p<0.0001)	38	0.92 (0.88 to 0.95); 0.39 (p=0.002)	10	9.6 (5.9 to 16)	0.27 (0.22 to 0.35)
• Section thickness: ≤5 mm		0.75 (0.70 to 0.79); 0.78 (p<0.0001)	53	0.90 (0.85 to 0.94); 0.76 (p<0.0001)	16	7.5 (4.7 to 12)	0.28 (0.23 to 0.34)
• Section thickness: >5 mm		0.83 (0.75 to 0.89)	14	0.83 (0.53 to 0.96)	2	4.9 (1.4 to 17)	0.21 (0.13 to 0.34)
• Reference standard: Explanted liver		0.67 (0.59 to 0.75); 0.63 (p<0.0001)	23	0.82 (0.74 to 0.88); 0.46 (p=0.0001)	12	3.8 (2.6 to 5.6)	0.40 (0.31 to 0.50)
• Reference standard: Histopathological, non-explant		0.86 (0.78 to 0.91)	12	0.95 (0.88 to 0.98)	3	19 (7.1 to 49)	0.15 (0.10 to 0.23)
• Reference standard: Imaging/clinical		0.65 (0.43 to 0.83)	3	Insufficient data	—	—	—
• Reference standard: Mixed histological and imaging/clinical		0.80 (0.75 to 0.84)	34	0.84 (0.74 to 0.91); 0.58 (p<0.0001)	4	11 (5.3 to 21)	0.22 (0.17 to 0.27)
• Prospective		0.73 (0.63 to 0.81); 0.71 (p<0.0001)	16	0.81 (0.70 to 0.88); 0.46 (p=0.0002)	8	4.5 (2.6 to 7.8)	0.32 (0.23 to 0.46)
• United States or Europe		0.76 (0.69 to 0.83); 0.81 (p<0.0001)	23	0.81 (0.70 to 0.88); 0.46 (p=0.0002)	10	3.9 (2.5 to 6.3)	0.29 (0.21 to 0.40)
• Used confidence rating scale		0.74 (0.67 to 0.80); 0.80 (p<0.0001)	31	0.92 (0.86 to 0.96); 0.63 (p<0.0001)	9	9.3 (5.2 to 17)	0.28 (0.22 to 0.36)
• Excluding high risk of bias		0.75 (0.70 to 0.80);	47	0.91 (0.87 to 0.94); 0.51	15	8.5 (5.6 to 13)	0.27 (0.22 to 0.34)

Table 7. Test performance of computed tomography imaging for identification of intrahepatic and extrahepatic hepatocellular carcinoma (continued)

studies	Unit of Analysis	Sensitivity (95% CI); τ^2 (p value)	Number of Studies	Specificity (95% CI); τ^2 (p value)	Number of Studies	LR+	LR-
		0.79 (p<0.0001)		(p<0.0001)			
• Avoided case-control design		0.74 (0.66 to 0.81); 0.80 (p<0.0001)	21	0.87 (0.78 to 0.93); 0.78 (p<0.0001)	10	5.7 (3.2 to 10)	0.30 (0.21 to 0.41)
• Blinded interpretation of imaging		0.78 (0.72 to 0.82); 0.81 (p<0.0001)	42	0.86 (0.77 to 0.92); 0.79 (p<0.0001)	10	5.7 (3.3 to 9.7)	0.26 (0.20 to 0.33)
	Liver segment	0.88 (0.78 to 0.94); 0.81 (p=0.02)	8	0.97 (0.94 to 0.98); 0.29 (p=0.06)	8	26 (15 to 42)	0.10 (0.94 to 0.98)
• Excluding studies restricted to hypervascular HCC		0.87 (0.75 to 0.93); 0.86 (p=0.03)	7	0.97 (0.95 to 0.98); 0.31 (p=0.08)	7	29 (16 to 51)	0.14 (0.07 to 0.27)
• Excluding studies restricted to HCC lesions <2 cm		0.87 (0.76 to 0.94); 0.87 (p=0.02)	7	0.97 (0.94 to 0.98); 0.39 (p=0.06)	7	28 (15 to 51)	0.13 (0.07 to 0.25)
Evaluation of focal liver lesions (KQ 2)							
	Patient	0.86 (0.75 to 0.92); 0.65 (p=0.04)	8	0.88 (0.76 to 0.95); 0.64 (p=0.08)	5	7.4 (3.3 to 17)	0.16 (0.09 to 0.30)
• Excluding studies restricted to HCC lesions <2-3 cm		0.87 (0.78 to 0.93); 0.42 (p=0.11)	6	0.93 (0.85 to 0.96); 0.11 (p=0.57)	3	12 (5.7 to 24)	0.14 (0.08 to 0.25)
	HCC lesion	0.79 (0.67 to 0.87); 0.97 (p=0.001)	13	0.90 (0.37 to 0.99); 4.4 (p=0.11)	6	7.7 (0.71 to 84)	0.24 (0.15 to 0.38)
• HCC lesions <2-3 cm		0.61 (0.49 to 0.71); 0.19 (p=0.14)	5	0.98 (0.87 to 0.996); 2.5 (p=0.11)	5	25 (4.5 to 138)	0.40 (0.30 to 0.53)
• Excluding studies restricted to HCC lesions <2-3 cm		0.87 (0.78 to 0.92); 0.67 (p=0.01)	8	0.71 (0.57 to 0.83)	1	Not calculated	Note calculated
• CT type: Multidetector, ≥8 rows		0.79 (0.56 to 0.91); 0.49 (p=0.02)	2	Insufficient data		--	--
• CT type: Non-multidetector		0.87 (0.77 to 0.93)	5	Insufficient data		--	--
• Contrast rate: ≥3 ml/s		0.87 (0.78 to 0.92); 0.67 (p=0.01)	8	Insufficient data		--	--
• Imaging phases: Arterial, portal venous, and delayed		0.83 (0.73 to 0.90); 0.48 (p=0.15)	6	Insufficient data		--	--
• Imaging phases: Missing delayed phase imaging		0.94 (0.82 to 0.98)	2	Insufficient data		--	--
• Delayed phase imaging >120 s		0.88 (0.81 to 0.92); 0.17 (p=0.03)	4	Insufficient data		--	--
• Section thickness: ≤5 mm		0.78 (0.61 to 0.89); 0.45 (p=0.01)	3	Insufficient data		--	--
• Section thickness: >5 mm		0.91 (0.78 to 0.97); 0.45	2	Insufficient data		--	--
• Reference standard: Histopathological, non-explant		0.83 (0.73 to 0.90); 0.48 (p=0.02)	6	Insufficient data		--	--
• Reference standard: Histological and clinical/imaging		0.93 (0.82 to 0.98)	2	Insufficient data		--	--
• Prospective		0.90 (0.80 to 0.95);	4	Insufficient data		--	--

Table 7. Test performance of computed tomography imaging for identification of intrahepatic and extrahepatic hepatocellular carcinoma (continued)

Unit of Analysis	Sensitivity (95% CI); τ^2 (p value)	Number of Studies	Specificity (95% CI); τ^2 (p value)	Number of Studies	LR+	LR-
	0.48 (p=0.02)					
• United States or Europe	0.89 (0.80 to 0.94); 0.53 (p=0.02)	5	Insufficient data	--	--	--
• Used confidence rating scale	0.86 (0.64 to 0.95); 0.66 (p=0.01)	2	Insufficient data	--	--	--
• Excluding high risk of bias studies	00.83 (0.71 to 0.90); 0.51 (p=0.01)	5	Insufficient data	--	--	--
• Avoided case-control design	0.88 (0.74 to 0.95); 0.66 (p=0.01)	4	Insufficient data	--	--	--
• Blinded interpretation of imaging	0.86 (0.75 to 0.93); 0.65 (p=0.01)	6	Insufficient data	--	--	--

CT = computed tomography; HCC = hepatocellular carcinoma

Table 8. Test performance of magnetic resonance imaging for identification of intrahepatic and extrahepatic hepatocellular carcinoma

	Unit of Analysis	Sensitivity (95% CI); τ^2 (p value)	Number of Studies	Specificity (95% CI); τ^2 (p value)	Number of Studies	LR+	LR-
Detection of HCC (KQ 1)							
Nonsurveillance settings							
	Patient	0.85 (0.76 to 0.91); 0.47 (p=0.07)	10	0.90 (0.81 to 0.94); 0.51 (p=0.05)	8	8.1 (4.3 to 15)	0.17 (0.10 to 0.28)
• Excluding studies restricted to hypervascular HCC		0.85 (0.75 to 0.91); 0.58 (p=0.06)	9	0.90 (0.81 to 0.95); 0.62 (p=0.06)	7	8.7 (4.2 to 18)	0.17 (0.10 to 0.30)
• Excluding studies restricted to HCC lesions <2-3 cm		0.85 (0.76 to 0.91); 0.47 (p=0.07)	10	0.90 (0.81 to 0.94); 0.51 (p=0.05)	8	8.1 (4.3 to 15)	0.17 (0.10 to 0.28)
• MRI type: 1.5 T		0.85 (0.76 to 0.91); 0.45 (p=0.10)	10	0.90 (0.82 to 0.95); 0.48 (p=0.08)	8	8.3 (4.5 to 15)	0.17 (0.10 to 0.27)
• Contrast: Gadopentetate or gadodiamide		0.85 (0.76 to 0.91); 0.45 (p=0.10)	10	0.90 (0.82 to 0.95); 0.48 (p=0.08)	8	8.3 (4.5 to 15)	0.17 (0.10 to 0.27)
• Imaging phases: Arterial, portal venous, and delayed		0.85 (0.75 to 0.91); 0.45 (p=0.10)	8	0.89 (0.80 to 0.95); 0.49 (p=0.08)	6	8.0 (4.1 to 15)	0.17 (0.10 to 0.29)
• Imaging phases: Missing delayed phase imaging		0.84 (0.57 to 0.95)	2	0.92 (0.69 to 0.98)	2	10 (2.2 to 47)	0.18 (0.06 to 0.56)
• Delayed phase ≥120 s		0.79 (0.58 to 0.91); 0.11 (p=0.45)	2	0.92 (0.77 to 0.97); 0.41 (p=0.13)	2	9.7 (3.1 to 30)	0.23 (0.10 to 0.51)
• Section thickness: ≤5 mm		0.88 (0.76 to 0.94); 0.31 (p=0.18)	4	0.95 (0.89 to 0.98); <0.0001 (p=1.0)	3	17 (8.1 to 37)	0.13 (0.06 to 0.27)
• Section thickness: >5 mm		0.76 (0.54 to 0.90)	3	0.84 (0.70 to 0.92)	3	4.7 (2.3 to 9.4)	029 (0.13 to 0.62)
• Reference standard: Explanted liver		0.87 (0.78 to 0.92); 0.32 (p=0.24)	8	0.92 (0.84 to 0.96); 0.46 (p=0.14)	6	11 (5.3 to 23)	0.15 (0.09 to 0.24)
• Prospective		0.78 (0.59 to 0.89); 0.42 (p=0.12)	4	0.94 (0.84 to 0.98); 0.29 (p=0.23)	3	12 (4.5 to 34)	0.24 (0.12 to 0.48)
• United States or Europe		0.87 (0.77 to 0.93); 0.70 (p=0.05)	11	0.88 (0.79 to 0.93); 0.58 (p=0.04)	9	7.2 (3.9 to 13)	0.15 (0.08 to 0.27)
• Used confidence rating scale		0.53 (0.23 to 0.81); <0.0001 (p=1.0)	1	0.72 (0.37 to 0.92); 0.27 (p=0.14)	1	1.9 (0.55 to 6.8)	0.72 (0.37 to 0.92)
• Excluding high risk of bias studies		0.83 (0.74 to 0.90); 0.35 (p=0.18)	8	0.90 (0.80 to 0.95); 0.48 (p=0.08)	6	8.0 (4.1 to 16)	0.19 (0.12 to 0.30)
• Avoided case-control design		0.82 (0.73 to 0.88); 0.19 (p=0.34)	8	0.89 (0.80 to 0.94); 0.43 (p=0.08)	7	7.4 (4.0 to 13)	0.20 (0.13 to 0.32)
• Blinded interpretation of imaging		0.90 (0.82 to 0.95); 0.18 (p=0.19)	5	0.94 (0.87 to 0.97); 0.18 (p=0.15)	4	15 (6.9 to 32)	0.11 (0.06 to 0.20)
	Lesion	0.82 (0.79 to 0.85); 0.80 (p<0.0001)	75	0.87 (0.77 to 0.93); 1.6 (p<0.0001)	16	6.4 (3.5 to 12)	0.20 (0.16 to 0.25)
• HCC lesions <2-3 cm		0.82 (0.78 to 0.85); 0.85 (p=0.001)	12	Insufficient data	--	--	--
• Excluding studies that used diffusion-weighted imaging		0.82 (0.78 to 0.85); 0.81 (p<0.0001)	69	0.86 (0.75 to 0.92); 1.6 (p<0.0001)	15	5.8 (3.2 to 11)	0.21 (0.17 to 0.26)

Table 8. Test performance of magnetic resonance imaging for identification of intrahepatic and extrahepatic hepatocellular carcinoma (continued)

Unit of Analysis	Sensitivity (95% CI); τ^2 (p value)	Number of Studies	Specificity (95% CI); τ^2 (p value)	Number of Studies	LR+	LR-
• Excluding studies restricted to hypervascular HCC	0.84 (0.80 to 0.87); 0.72 (p<0.0001)	64	0.87 (0.77 to 0.93); 1.6 (p<0.0001)	16	6.6 (3.6 to 12)	0.18 (0.15 to 0.23)
• Excluding studies restricted to HCC lesions <2-3 cm	0.82 (0.79 to 0.86); 0.78 (p<0.0001)	63	0.86 (0.75 to 0.93); 1.7 (p<0.0001)	15	6.0 (3.2 to 11)	0.20 (0.16 to 0.25)
• MRI type: 3.0 T	0.87 (0.78 to 0.93); 0.76 (p<0.0001)	8	0.94 (0.66 to 0.99); 1.5 (p<0.0001)	2	14 (2.1 to 100)	0.14 (0.07 to 0.25)
• MRI type: 1.5 T	0.82 (0.77 to 0.85) (p<0.0001)	50	0.83 (0.69 to 0.91) (p<0.0001)	11	4.8 (2.5 to 9.1)	0.22 (0.17 to 0.28)
• Contrast: Gadopentetate or gadodiamide	0.81 (0.75 to 0.85); 0.75 (p<0.0001)	32	0.62 (0.48 to 0.74); 0.44 (p=0.005)	6	2.1 (1.5 to 3.0)	0.31 (0.23 to 0.42)
• Contrast: Gadobenate disodium or gadobenate	0.84 (0.78 to 0.88)	29	0.95 (0.91 to 0.97)	8	18 (9.5 to 32)	0.17 (0.13 to 0.23)
• Imaging phases: Arterial, portal venous, and delayed	0.82 (0.78 to 0.86); 0.76 (p<0.0001)	59	0.86 (0.74 to 0.93); 1.7 (p<0.0001)	14	6.0 (3.1 to 12)	0.20 (0.16 to 0.26)
• Imaging phases: Missing delayed phase imaging	0.77 (0.52 to 0.91)	3	0.88 (0.30 to 0.99)	1	6.6 (0.52 to 83)	0.26 (0.10 to 0.66)
• Delayed phase ≥120 s	0.83 (0.79 to 0.87); 0.74 (p<0.0001)	49	0.90 (0.84 to 0.94); 0.66 (p=0.0002)	10	8.6 (5.1 to 14)	0.19 (0.15 to 0.24)
• Section thickness: ≤5 mm	0.85 (0.81 to 0.88); 0.68 (p<0.0001)	39	0.87 (0.72 to 0.94); 1.7 (p<0.0001)	10	6.3 (2.9 to 14)	0.17 (0.13 to 0.23)
• Section thickness: >5 mm	0.81 (0.73 to 0.87)	15	0.88 (0.61 to 0.97)	3	6.6 (1.7 to 25)	0.21 (0.14 to 0.32)
• Reference standard: Explanted liver	0.69 (0.60 to 0.76); 0.54 (p<0.0001)	18	0.85 (0.70 to 0.93); 1.5 (p=0.002)	9	4.6 (2.3 to 9.3)	0.37 (0.29 to 0.47)
• Reference standard: Histopathological, non-explant	0.88 (0.82 to 0.93)	11	0.97 (0.89 to 0.99)	3	31 (7.7 to 123)	0.12 (0.08 to 0.19)
• Reference standard: Imaging/clinical reference standard	0.86 (0.67 to 0.95)	2	Insufficient data	--	--	--
• Reference standard: Mixed histological and imaging/clinical	0.86 (0.82 to 0.89)	32	0.84 (0.56 to 0.96)	3	5.4 (1.6 to 18)	0.17 (0.13 to 0.23)
• Prospective	0.82 (0.74 to 0.89); 0.78 (p<0.0001)	15	0.89 (0.71 to 0.97); 1.7 (p<0.0001)	5	7.6 (2.6 to 23)	0.20 (0.13 to 0.31)
• United States or Europe	0.78 (0.70 to 0.85); 0.71 (p<0.0001)	19	0.73 (0.58 to 0.84); 0.73 (p=0.0004)	8	2.9 (1.8 to 4.8)	0.30 (0.21 to 0.43)
• Used confidence rating scale	0.86 (0.82 to 0.89)); 0.68 (p<0.0001)	36	0.90 (0.78 to 0.96); 1.8 (p=0.0005)	9	8.6 (3.7 to 20)	0.16 (0.12 to 0.20)
• Excluding high risk of bias studies	0.81 (0.76 to 0.85); 0.74 (p<0.0001)	47	0.88 (0.76 to 0.94); 1.7 (p<0.0001)	12	6.6 (3.2 to 13)	0.22 (0.17 to 0.28)
• Avoided case-control design	0.80 (0.73 to 0.86); 0.77 (p<0.0001)	22	0.83 (0.69 to 0.92); 1.4 (p<0.0001)	11	4.7 (2.4 to 9.1)	0.24 (0.17 to 0.34)
• Blinded interpretation of imaging	0.84 (0.79 to 0.87); 0.77 (p<0.0001)	38	0.88 (0.73 to 0.95); 1.7 (p<0.0001)	8	7.1 (2.9 to 17)	0.19 (0.14 to 0.25)

Table 8. Test performance of magnetic resonance imaging for identification of intrahepatic and extrahepatic hepatocellular carcinoma (continued)

	Unit of Analysis	Sensitivity (95% CI); τ^2 (p value)	Number of Studies	Specificity (95% CI); τ^2 (p value)	Number of Studies	LR+	LR-
	Liver segment	0.77 (0.56 to 0.90); 0.56 (p=0.31)	3	0.97 (0.87 to 0.99); 1.6 (p=0.29)	3	28 (5.6 to 0.90)	0.97 (0.87 to 0.99)
Evaluation of focal liver lesions (KQ 2)							
	Patient	0.77 (0.66 to 0.84); 0.14 (p=0.22)	4	0.81 (0.52 to 0.94); 1.6 (p=0.19)	4	4.0 (1.4 to 12)	0.29 (0.21 to 0.39)
• HCC lesions <2-3 cm		0.82 (0.71 to 0.89); <0.0001 (p=1.0)	2	0.79 (0.68 to 0.86); <0.0001 (p=1.0)	2	3.8 (2.5 to 5.9)	0.23 (0.14 to 0.38)
• Excluding studies restricted to HCC lesions <2-3 cm		0.72 (0.55 to 0.85); 0.22 (p=0.14)	2	0.79 (0.16 to 0.99); 3.9 (p=0.09)	2	3.5 (0.38 to 31)	0.35 (0.23 to 0.53)
	HCC lesion	0.81 (0.72 to 0.87); 0.64 (p=0.001)	14	0.93 (0.80 to 0.98); 3.7 (p=0.006)	11	12 (3.8 to 39)	0.21 (0.15 to 0.30)
• HCC lesions <2-3 cm		0.73 (0.62 to 0.82); 0.44 (p=0.01)	9	0.95 (0.73 to 0.99); 5.8 (p=0.03)	8	14 (2.5 to 76)	0.29 (0.21 to 0.39)
• Excluding studies that used diffusion-weighted imaging		0.79 (0.70 to 0.85); 0.53 (p=0.002)	13	0.94 (0.78 to 0.98); 4.3 (p=0.01)	10	13 (3.3 to 47)	0.23 (0.16 to 0.32)
• Excluding studies restricted to hypervascular HCC lesions		0.75 (0.64 to 0.84); 0.56 (p=0.01)	9	0.92 (0.62 to 0.99); 6.3 (p=0.03)	7	9.2 (1.7 to 49)	0.27 (0.20 to 0.37)
• Excluding studies restricted to HCC lesions <2-3 cm		0.90 (0.86 to 0.93); 0.0006 (p=0.95)	5	0.88 (0.76 to 0.94); 0.10 (p=0.64)	3	7.5 (3.6 to 16)	0.11 (0.08 to 0.16)
• MRI type: 1.5 T		0.90 (0.86 to 0.93); 0.0006 (p=0.95)	5	0.88 (0.76 to 0.94); 0.10 (p=0.64)	3	7.5 (3.6 to 16)	0.11 (0.08 to 0.16)
• Contrast: Gadopentetate or gadodiamide		0.91 (0.86 to 0.94); <0.0001 (p=1.0)	3	0.92 (0.80 to 0.97); <0.0001 (p=1.0)	2	11 (4.3 to 28)	0.10 (0.07 to 0.15)
• Contrast: Gadoxetic acid or gadobenate		0.88 (0.73 to 0.95)	2	0.81 (0.64 to 0.91)	1	4.7 (2.3 to 9.7)	0.15 (0.06 to 0.36)
• Imaging phases: Arterial, portal venous, and delayed		0.90 (0.86 to 0.93); 0.0006 (p=0.95)	5	0.88 (0.77 to 0.94); 0.10 (p=0.64)	3	7.5 (3.6 to 16)	0.11 (0.08 to 0.16)
• Delayed phase imaging >120 s		0.91 (0.86 to 0.94); <0.0001 (p=0.99)	4	0.88 (0.77 to 0.94); 0.10 (p=0.64)	3	7.5 (3.7 to 15)	0.11 (0.07 to 0.16)
• Section thickness: ≤5 mm		0.90 (0.86 to 0.93); 0.0006 (p=0.95)	5	0.88 (0.76 to 0.94); 0.10 (p=0.64)	3	7.5 (3.6 to 16)	0.11 (0.08 to 0.16)
• Reference standard: Histopathological, non-explant		0.91 (0.81 to 0.96); <0.0001 (p=1.0)	1	0.97 (0.79 to 0.995); <0.0001 (p=1.0)	1	26 (3.8 to 181)	0.10 (0.04 to 0.21)
• Reference standard: Histological and clinical/imaging		0.90 (0.86 to 0.94)	4	0.82 (0.69 to 0.91)	2	5.1 (2.8 to 9.3)	0.12 (0.08 to 0.18)
• Excluding high risk of bias studies		0.90 (0.86 to 0.93); 0.0006 (p=0.95)	5	0.88 (0.76 to 0.94); 0.10 (p=0.64)	3	7.5 (3.6 to 16)	0.11 (0.08 to 0.16)

HCC = hepatocellular carcinoma; MRI = magnetic resonance imaging

Table 9. Test performance of positron emission tomography for identification of intrahepatic and extrahepatic hepatocellular carcinoma

	Unit of Analysis	Sensitivity (95% CI); τ^2 (p value)	Number of Studies	Specificity (95% CI); τ^2 (p value)	Number of Studies	LR+	LR-
Detection of intrahepatic HCC (KQ 1)							
FDG PET for intrahepatic HCC	Patient	0.52 (0.39 to 0.66); 0.87 (p=0.01)	15	0.95 (0.82 to 0.99); 0.17 (p=0.40)	5	11 (2.6 to 49)	0.50 (0.37 to 0.68)
• Excluding high risk of bias studies		0.42 (0.26 to 0.60); 0.65 (p=0.01)	7	0.92 (0.76 to 0.98); 0.04 (p=0.73)	3	5.3 (1.5 to 18)	0.63 (0.45 to 0.87)
• PET type: PET		0.39 (0.24 to 0.56); 0.54 (p=0.01)	8	0.94 (0.68 to 0.99); 0.11 (p=0.68)	3	6.6 (0.92 to 47)	0.65 (0.48 to 0.88)
• PET type: PET/CT		0.65 (0.50–0.78)	7	0.96 (0.74 to 0.99)	2	15 (2.0-111)	0.36 (0.24 to 0.56)
• Prospective		0.46 (0.31 to 0.62); 0.46 (p=0.02)	8	0.94 (0.80–0.98); 0.06 (p=0.62)	4	7.6 (2.0-30)	0.6 (0.41 to 0.79)
• United States or Europe		0.49 (0.32 to 0.66); 0.84 (p=0.01)	10	0.95 (0.82 to 0.99); 0.16 (p=0.41)	5	10 (2.3 to 43)	0.54 (0.37 to 0.77)
• Reference standard: Histopathological, non-explant		0.46 (0.28 to 0.65); 0.81 (p=0.01)	7	0.91 (0.42 to 0.99); 0.02 (p=0.86)	2	5.2 (0.45 to 60)	0.59 (0.38 to 0.91)
• Reference standard: Mixed histological and imaging/clinical		0.58 (0.40–0.75)	8	0.97 (0.79 to 0.996)	3	18 (2.4 to 132)	0.43 (0.28 to 0.67)
	HCC lesion	0.53 (0.41 to 0.65); 0.23 (p=0.08)	5	0.91 (0.76 to 0.98)	1	Not calculated	Not calculated
• Excluding high risk of bias studies		0.58 (0.46 to 0.68); 0.11 (p=0.26)	3	0.91 (0.76 to 0.98)	1	Not calculated	Not calculated
• PET type: PET/CT		0.51 (0.38 to 0.65); 0.26 (p=0.11)	4	0.91 (0.76 to 0.98)	1	Not calculated	Not calculated
• Reference standard: Histopathological, non-explant		0.49 (0.37 to 0.61); 0.25 (p=0.15)	4	No data	No data	--	--
• United States or Europe		0.67 (0.55 to 0.78)	1	0.91 (0.76 to 0.98)	1	Not calculated	Not calculated
¹¹C-acetate PET for intrahepatic HCC	Patient	0.85 (0.67 to 0.94); 0.70 (p=0.13)	4	No data	No data	--	--
	HCC lesion	0.78 (0.61 to 0.89); 0.55 (p=0.15)	4	No data	No data	--	--
• Excluding high risk of bias studies		0.76 (0.69 to 0.82); <0.0001 (p=1.0)	2	No data	No data	--	--

84

Table 9. Test performance of positron emission tomography for identification of intrahepatic and extrahepatic hepatocellular carcinoma (continued)

	Unit of Analysis	Sensitivity (95% CI); τ^2 (p value)	Number of Studies	Specificity (95% CI); τ^2 (p value)	Number of Studies	LR+	LR-
• PET type: PET		0.68 (0.46 to 0.84); 0.22 (p=0.49)	2	No data	No data	--	--
• PET type: PET/CT		0.85 (0.67 to 0.94); 0.42 (p=0.39)	2	No data	No data	--	--
• Reference standard: Histopathological, non-explant		0.78 (0.61 to 0.89); 0.55 (p=0.15)	4	No data	No data	--	--
• United States or Europe	Patient	0.78 (0.64 to 0.89)	1	No data	No data	--	--
FDG + ^{11}C-acetate PET for intrahepatic HCC	HCC lesion	0.89 (0.80 to 0.95)	1	No data	No data	--	--
^{18}F-fluorothymidine PET for intrahepatic HCC	Patient	0.95 (0.86 to 0.99)	1	No data	No data	--	--
		0.69 (0.41 to 0.89)	1	No data	No data	--	--
^{18}F-fluorochlorine PET for intrahepatic HCC	Patient	0.91 (0.78 to 0.96); <0.0001 (p=1.0)	2	0.47 (0.23 to 0.72)	1	Not calculated	Not calculated
	HCC lesion	0.84 (0.74 to 0.92)	1	0.62 (0.44 to 0.78)	1	Not calculated	Not calculated
FDG PET for recurrent intrahepatic HCC	Patient	0.70 (0.32 to 0.92); 1.5 (p=0.29)	3	0.71 (0.29 to 0.96)	1	Not calculated	Not calculated
	HCC lesion	0.07 (2/27) and 0.73 (22/30)	2	1.0 (1/0)	1	Not calculated	Not calculated
Staging of HCC (KQ 3)							
FDG PET for metastatic HCC	Patient with metastatic HCC	0.85 (0.71 to 0.93); 0.12 (p=0.13)	6	0.93 (0.89 to 0.95); 1.0 (p=0.17)	5	11 (7.8 to 17)	0.16 (0.08 to 0.33)
• PET type: PET		0.98 (0.29 to 0.9998); 6.1 (p=0.30)	2	0.93 (0.86 to 0.97); 0.005 (p=0.85)	2	14 (7.1 to 29)	0.02 (0.0003 to 2.2)
• PET type: PET/CT		0.78 (0.72 to 0.83); <0.0001 (p=1.0)	4	0.92 (0.86 to 0.96); <0.0001 (p=1.0)	4	9.8 (5.5 to 17)	0.24 (0.18 to 0.30)
• Excluding high risk of bias studies		0.90 (0.71 to 0.97); 1.1 (p=0.26)	4	0.93 (0.89 to 0.95); <0.0001 (p=1.0)	3	13 (8.3 to 20)	0.11 (0.04 to 0.34)
• Reference standard: Mixed histological and imaging/clinical		0.78 (0.73 to 0.83); <0.0001 (p=1.0)	5	0.92 (0.87 to 0.96); <0.0001(p=1.0)	4	10 (5.7 to 18)	0.24 (0.18 to 0.30)

Table 9. Test performance of positron emission tomography for identification of intrahepatic and extrahepatic hepatocellular carcinoma (continued)

	Unit of Analysis	Sensitivity (95% CI); τ^2 (p value)	Number of Studies	Specificity (95% CI); τ^2 (p value)	Number of Studies	LR+	LR-
• Prospective		0.96 (0.87 to 0.99); <0.0001 (p=1.0)	2	0.93 (0.90-0.96); <0.0001 (p=1.0)	2	14 (9.0-22)	0.05 (0.02 to 0.14)
• United States or Europe		No data	--	No data	--	--	--
• Avoided case-control design		0.88 (0.63 to 0.97); 1.6 (p=0.23)	4	0.92 (0.88 to 0.95); <0.0001 (p=1.0)	3	11 (7.1 to 17)	0.14 (0.04 to 0.47)
• Blinded interpretation of imaging		0.92 (0.80-0.97); 0.26 (p=0.23)	2	0.93 (0.88 to 0.95)	1	13 (7.8 to 20)	0.08 (0.03 to 0.23)
	Metastatic HCC lesion	0.82 (0.72 to 0.90); 0.17 (p=0.21)	5	No data	--	--	--
• PET type: PET		0.81 (0.64 to 0.91); 0.31 (p=0.28)	3	No data	--	--	--
• PET type: PET/CT		0.92 (0.77 to 0.97); 0.63 (p=0.31)	3	No data	--	--	--
• Reference standard: Histopathological, non-explant		0.85 (0.70-0.93); <0.0001 (p=1.0)	2	No data	--	--	--
• Reference standard: Imaging and clinical criteria		0.90 (0.79 to 0.95)	1	No data	--	--	--
• Reference standard: Mixed histological and imaging/clinical		0.72 (0.58 to 0.82)	2	No data	--	--	--
• Excluding high risk of bias studies		0.86 (0.70-0.95)	1	No data	--	--	--
• Blinded interpretation of imaging		0.87 (0.78 to 0.93); <0.0001 (p=1.0)	3	No data	--	--	--
• United States or Europe		No data[a]	--	No data	--	--	--

CT = computed tomography; FDG = fluorodeoxyglucose; HCC = hepatocellular carcinoma; KQ = Key Question; PET = positron emission tomography

[a] 1 study with 5 patients

Table 10. Pooled direct (within-study) comparisons of test performance of imaging modalities for identification and diagnosis of hepatocellular carcinoma

	Unit of Analysis	Sensitivity A (95% CI)	Sensitivity B (95% CI)	Difference (95% CI); τ^2 (p value)	Number of Studies	Specificity A (95% CI)	Specificity B (95% CI)	Difference (95% CI); τ^2 (p value)	Number of Studies
Detection of HCC (KQ 1)									
US without contrast (A) vs. CT (B)	Patient	0.68 (0.54 to 0.80)	0.80 (0.68 to 0.88)	-0.12 (-0.20 to -0.03); 0.36 (p=0.15)	6	0.92 (0.84 to 0.96)	0.94 (0.87 to 0.97)	-0.01 (-0.05 to 0.02); 0.62 (p=0.07)	5
• Excluding high risk of bias studies	Patient	0.71 (0.58 to 0.82)	0.82 (0.71 to 0.89)	-0.10 (-0.18 to -0.02); 0.19 (p=0.25)	5	0.91 (0.81 to 0.96)	0.94 (0.86 to 0.98)	-0.03 (-0.07 to 0.01); 0.73 (p=0.11)	4
US without contrast (A) vs. CT (B)	Lesion	0.55 (0.43 to 0.66)	0.66 (0.54 to 0.76)	-0.11 (-0.18 to -0.04); 0.11 (p=0.28)	3	0.83 (0.65 to 0.93)	0.93 (0.83 to 0.98)	-0.10 (-0.20 to -0.008); 0.44 (p=0.29)	2
• HCC lesions <2 cm	Lesion	0.46 (0.30-0.63)	0.54 (0.37 to 0.70)	-0.07 (-0.17 to 0.02); 0.31 (p=0.27)	3	0.72 (0.61 to 0.80)	0.80 (0.71 to 0.86)	-0.08 (-0.20 to 0.04); 0.002 (p=0.85)	2
US with contrast (A) vs. CT (B)	Lesion	0.58 (0.37 to 0.77)	0.74 (0.54 to 0.87)	-0.16 (-0.32 to -0.01); 0.50 (p=0.15)	3	No data	No data	--	--
• HCC lesions <2 cm	Lesion	0.30 (0.17 to 0.43)	0.44 (0.30-0.58)	-0.14 (-0.32 to 0.05)	1	No data	No data	--	--
US without contrast (A) vs. MRI (B)	Patient	0.61 (0.48 to 0.74)	0.81 (0.69 to 0.89)	-0.19 (-0.30 to -0.08); 0.01 (p=0.79)	3	0.94 (0.87 to 0.97)	0.82 (0.66 to 0.91)	0.13 (0.03 to 0.22); 0.01 (p=0.40)	3
US without contrast (A) vs. MRI (B)	Lesion	0.57 (0.42 to 0.71)	0.79 (0.67 to 0.88)	-0.22 (-0.31 to -0.14); 0.22 (p=0.28)	3	0.75 (0.66 to 0.82)	0.78 (0.70-0.85)	-0.03 (-0.13 to 0.06); 0.001 (p=0.89)	2
• HCC lesions <2 cm	Lesion	0.40 (0.18 to 0.67)	0.65 (0.38 to 0.85)	-0.26 (-0.36 to -0.15); 0.60	2	0.71 (0.60-0.80)	0.84 (0.76 to 0.89)	-0.13 (-0.25 to -0.01); 0.006	2
US with contrast (A) vs. MRI (B)	Lesion	0.65 (0.41 to 0.84)	0.73 (0.50 to 0.88)	-0.08 (-0.19 to 0.02); 0.69 (p=0.15)	3	No data	No data	--	--

Table 10. Pooled direct (within-study) comparisons of test performance of imaging modalities for identification and diagnosis of hepatocellular carcinoma (continued)

	Unit of Analysis	Sensitivity A (95% CI)	Sensitivity B (95% CI)	Difference (95% CI); τ^2 (p value)	Number of Studies	Specificity A (95% CI)	Specificity B (95% CI)	Difference (95% CI); τ^2 (p value)	Number of Studies
• HCC lesions <2 cm	Lesion	0.30 (0.17 to 0.43)	0.42 (0.28 to 0.56)	-0.12 (-0.31 to 0.07)	1	No data	No data	--	--
• Well-differentiated HCC lesions	Lesion	0.43 (0.14 to 0.77)	0.36 (0.11 to 0.72)	0.07 (-0.19 to 0.33); 0.87 (p=0.34)	2	No data	No data	--	--
MRI (A) vs. CT (B)	Patient	0.88 (0.53 to 0.98)	0.82 (0.41 to 0.97)	0.06 (-0.05 to 0.17); 3.0 (p=0.21)	4	0.84 (0.70 to 0.92)	0.91 (0.82 to 0.96)	-0.08 (-0.16 to 0.00); 0.40 (p=0.21)	4
• Excluding high risk of bias studies	Patient	0.82 (0.75 to 0.88)	0.75 (0.68 to 0.81)	0.07 (-0.02 to 0.17); <0.0001 (p=0.10)	2	0.80 (0.57 to 0.92)	0.91 (0.77 to 0.97)	-0.11 (-0.23 to 0.01); 0.44 (p=0.11)	2
MRI (A) vs. CT (B)	Lesion	0.81 (0.76 to 0.84)	0.71 (0.66 to 0.76)	0.09 (0.07 to 0.12); 0.48 (p<0.0001)	31	0.86 (0.78 to 0.91)	0.91 (0.85 to 0.95)	-0.05 (-0.10 to 0.002); 0.42 (p=0.006)	7
• Excluding high risk of bias studies	Lesion	0.79 (0.73 to 0.85)	0.72 (0.65 to 0.79)	0.07 (0.04 to 0.10); 0.64 (p<0.0001)	22	0.87 (0.79 to 0.92)	0.92 (0.87 to 0.96)	-0.06 (-0.11 to -0.01)	6
• MRI contrast type: Non-hepatic specific	Lesion	0.81 (0.74 to 0.87)	0.74 (0.65 to 0.81)	0.08 (0.04 to 0.11); 0.39 (p=0.006)	11	0.62 (0.51 to 0.72)	0.86 (0.77 to 0.93)	-0.24 (-0.37 to -0.11)	2
• MRI contrast type: Hepatic specific	Lesion	0.80 (0.73 to 0.85)	0.70 (0.62 to 0.77)	0.10 (0.06 to 0.14); 0.56 (p<0.0001)	11	0.92 (0.87 to 0.95)	0.90 (0.85 to 0.94)	0.01 (-0.04 to 0.07); 0.03 (p=0.40)	2
• HCC lesions <2 cm	Lesion	0.71 (0.64 to 0.78)	0.56 (0.48 to 0.63)	0.16 (0.11 to 0.20); 0.42 (p<0.0001)	19	0.91 (0.80 to 0.96)	0.91 (0.80 to 0.96)	0.001 (-0.04 to 0.05); 0.74 (p=0.02)	4
• Excluding high risk of bias studies	Lesion	0.71 (0.62 to 0.78)	0.54 (0.45 to 0.63)	0.17 (0.12 to 0.22); 0.38 (p=0.0008)	13	0.91 (0.80 to 0.96)	0.91 (0.80 to 0.96)	0.00 (-0.05 to 0.05); 0.74 (p=0.03)	4
• MRI contrast: Non-hepatic contrast	Lesion	0.61 (0.44 to 0.75)	0.55 (0.38 to 0.70)	0.06 (0.00 to 0.13); 0.65 (p=0.04)	6	0.77 (0.64 to 0.86)	0.74 (0.61 to 0.84)	0.03 (-0.13 to 0.19); <0.0001 (p=1.0)	1

88

Table 10. Pooled direct (within-study) comparisons of test performance of imaging modalities for identification and diagnosis of hepatocellular carcinoma (continued)

	Unit of Analysis	Sensitivity A (95% CI)	Sensitivity B (95% CI)	Difference (95% CI); τ^2 (p value)	Number of Studies	Specificity A (95% CI)	Specificity B (95% CI)	Difference (95% CI); τ^2 (p value)	Number of Studies
• MRI contrast: Hepatic specific contrast	Lesion	0.77 (0.70 to 0.83)	0.54 (0.45 to 0.62)	0.23 (0.17 to 0.29); 0.29 (p=0.002)	12	0.94 (0.86 to 0.979)	0.94 (0.87 to 0.98)	-0.01 (-0.05 to 0.04); 0.37 (p=0.10)	3
• Restricted to studies meeting all CT and MRI technical criteria*	Lesion	0.75 (0.66 to 0.82)	0.55 (0.44 to 0.65)	0.29 (0.13 to 0.27); 0.30 (p=0.02)	8	0.93 (0.82 to 0.98)	0.90 (0.77 to 0.96)	0.03 (-0.05 to 0.11); 0.21 (p=0.40)	2
Evaluation of focal liver lesion (KQ 2)									
US without contrast (A) vs. CT (B)	Patient	0.78 (0.70 to 0.85)	0.89 (0.84 to 0.95)	-0.12 (-0.21 to -0.02)	1	No data	No data	--	--
• US with contrast (A) vs. CT (B)	Patient	0.91 (0.85 to 0.94)	0.88 (0.81 to 0.92)	0.03 (-0.02 to 0.08); 0.15 (p=0.13)	5	0.93 (0.87 to 0.96)	0.94 (0.88 to 0.97)	-0.01 (-0.06 to 0.05); 0.07 (p=0.32)	2
• Excluding high risk of bias studies	Patient	0.90 (0.79 to 0.95)	0.87 (0.76 to 0.94)	0.02 (-0.05 to 0.10); 0.28 (p=0.31)	3	0.93 (0.87 to 0.97)	0.94 (0.88 to 0.97)	-0.01 (-0.06 to 0.05); 0.08 (p=0.45)	2
US with contrast (A) vs. CT (B)	Lesion	0.92 (0.88 to 0.96)	0.89 (0.83 to 0.93)	0.04 (-0.02 to 0.09); 0.07 (p=0.33)	4	No data	No data	--	--
• HCC lesions <2 cm	Lesion	0.78 (0.61 to 0.89)	0.71 (0.52 to 0.85)	0.07 (-0.01 to 0.15); 1.1 (p-0.02)	7	0.87 (0.62 to 0.97)	0.94 (0.77 to 0.98)	-0.06 (-0.15 to 0.03); 2.4 (p=0.09)	4
• HCC lesions <2 cm	Patient	0.95 (0.85 to 1.0)	0.95 (0.85 to 1.0)	0.0 (-0.14 to 0.14)	1	0.71 (0.52 to 0.91)	0.81 (0.64 to 0.98)	0.10 (-0.35 to 0.16)	1
• Well-differentiated HCC lesions	Lesion	0.55 (0.25 to 0.82)	0.55 (0.25 to 0.82)	0.00 (-0.30 to 0.30); 0.48 (p=0.40)	2	No data	No data	--	--
US with contrast (A) vs. MRI (B)	Patient	0.79 (0.65 to 0.94)	0.83 (0.69 to 0.97)	-0.03 (-0.24 to 0.17)	1	0.79 (0.68 to 0.90)	0.75 (0.64 to 0.87)	0.04 (-0.12 to 0.20)	1
• HCC lesions <2 cm	Patient	0.52 (0.39 to 0.64)	0.62 (0.49 to 0.74)	-0.10 (-0.27 to 0.08)	1	0.93 (0.84 to 1.0)	0.97 (0.90-1.0)	-0.03 (-0.15 to 0.08)	1
US with contrast (A) vs. MRI (B)	Lesion	0.79 (0.65 to 0.94)	0.83 (0.69 to 0.97)	-0.03 (-0.24 to 0.17)	1	0.79 (0.68 to 0.90)	0.75 (0.64 to 0.87)	0.04 (-0.12 to 0.20)	1
• HCC lesions <2 cm	Lesion	0.53 (0.28 to 0.76)	0.68 (0.43 to 0.86)	-0.16 (-0.30 to -0.02); 0.72 (p=0.25)	3	0.95 (0.85 to 0.98)	0.98 (0.91 to 0.99)	-0.03 (-0.08 to 0.02); 0.38 (p=0.43)	3

89

Table 10. Pooled direct (within-study) comparisons of test performance of imaging modalities for identification and diagnosis of hepatocellular carcinoma (continued)

	Unit of Analysis	Sensitivity A (95% CI)	Sensitivity B (95% CI)	Difference (95% CI); τ^2 (p value)	Number of Studies	Specificity A (95% CI)	Specificity B (95% CI)	Difference (95% CI); τ^2 (p value)	Number of Studies
MRI (A) vs. CT (B)	Patient	0.81 (0.70 to 0.92)	0.74 (0.62 to 0.87)	0.06 (-0.10 to 0.23)	1	0.85 (0.72 to 0.99)	0.81 (0.66 to 0.96)	0.04 (-0.16 to 0.24)	1
MRI (A) vs. CT (B)	Lesion	0.84 (0.76 to 0.92)	0.62 (0.52 to 0.72)	0.22 (0.09 to 0.35)	1	0.36 (0.20-0.52)	0.72 (0.58 to 0.87)	-0.36 (-0.58 to -0.15)	1
• HCC lesion <2 cm	Lesion	0.65 (0.04 to 0.99)	0.50 (0.02 to 0.98)	0.15 (-0.002 to 0.30); 11 (p=0.26)	3	0.93 (0.21 to 0.998)	0.98 (0.48 to 0.9996)	-0.05 (-0.23 to 0.13); 11 (p=0.24)	3
Detection of metastatic HCC (KQ 4)									
PET/CT (A) vs. CT (B)	Patient (2), lesion (1)	0.82 (0.61 to 0.93)	0.85 (0.66 to 0.95)	-0.03 (-0.12 to 0.060); 0.75 (p=0.17)	3	Insufficient data	Insufficient data	--	--

*Defined for CT as multidetector CT≥8 rows, contrast rate ≥3 ml/s, includes arterial, portal venous and delayed phase imaging, delayed phase imaging >120 s after administration of contrast, and section thickness ≤5 mm; for MRI includes arterial, portal venous and delayed phase imaging, delayed phase imaging >120 s after administration of contrast, and section thickness ≤5 mm

CT = computed tomography; HCC = hepatocellular carcinoma; MRI = magnetic resonance imaging; PET = positron emission tomography; US = ultrasound

Table 11. Comparisons of test performance for hepatocellular carcinoma of single compared with multiple modality imaging[a]

Study, Year	Unit of Analysis	Single Imaging Modalities	Sensitivity	Specificity	Multiple Imaging Modalities	Criteria for Positive Results with Multiple Imaging Modalities	Sensitivity	Specificity
Detection of HCC (KQ 1)								
Alaboudy, 2011[51]	Lesion	A: US B: CT C: MRI	A: 0.72 B: 0.74 C: 0.86	Not reported	A: US + MRI B: US + CT C: CT + MRI	Unclear	A: 0.90 B: 0.82 C: 0.88	Not reported
Iavarone, 2010[69]	Lesion (1 to 2 cm)	A: MRI B: CT C: US	A: 0.42 B: 0.45 C: 0.32	Not reported	A: US + MR B: US + CT C: MRI + CT D: Any dual combination of MRI, CT, and US	Concordant positive findings on 2 imaging modalities	A: 0.16 B: 0.19 C: 0.29 D: 0.40	
Evaluation of focal liver lesions (KQ 2)								
Dai, 2008[55]	Lesion	A: US B: CT	A: 0.91 B: 0.80	A: 0.87 B: 0.98	CT + US	Unclear	0.80	0.87
Forner, 2008[59]	Lesion (<2 cm)	MRI	0.62	0.97	MRI + US	1: Definite positive findings on 2 imaging modalities 2: "At least suspicious" on 2 imaging modalities	1: 0.33 2: 0.67	1: 1.0 2: 1.0
Golfieri, 2009[134]	Lesion (<3 cm)	CT	0.62	0.72	MRI + CT	Unclear	0.89	0.22
Khalili, 2011[75]	Lesion (1 to 2 cm)	CT	0.53	0.99	A: US + MRI B: CT + MRI C: CT + US D: MRI then US E: MRI then CT F: CT then US	A-C: Concordant positive results on 2 imaging modalities D-F: Positive findings on initial imaging modality or positive findings on second imaging modality for indeterminate findings on first scan	A: 0.35 B: 0.41 C: 0.29 D: 0.79 E: 0.74 F: 0.76	A: 1.0 B: 1.0 C: 0.99 D: 0.91 E: 0.99 F: 0.91

Table 11. Comparisons of test performance for hepatocellular carcinoma of single compared with multiple modality imaging[a] (continued)

Study, Year	Unit of Analysis	Single Imaging Modalities	Sensitivity	Specificity	Multiple Imaging Modalities	Sensitivity	Specificity	Criteria for Positive Results with Multiple Imaging Modalities
Quaia, 2009[96]	Lesion (<3 cm)	A: CT B: US	A: 0.72 B: 0.88	A: 0.71 B: 0.66	CT + US	0.97	0.70	Positive findings from at least one imaging technique
Sangiovanni, 2010[43]	Lesion (1 to 2 cm)	A: US B: CT C: MRI	A: 0.26 B: 0.44 C: 0.44	A: 1.0 B: 1.0 C: 1.0	US, CT, and MRI	1: 0.35 2: 0.65	Not reported	1: Concordant positive findings on two imaging techniques 2: Positive findings from at least one imaging technique
Serste, 2012[44]	Patient	CT	0.74	0.81	CT + MRI	1: 0.57 2: 0.98	1: 0.85 2: 0.81	1: Concordant positive findings on two imaging techniques 2: Positive findings from at least one imaging technique

CT = computed tomography; HCC = hepatocellular carcinoma; MRI = magnetic resonance imaging; US = ultrasound
[a] Ultrasound contrast-enhanced in all studies except Forner 2008 and Iavarone 2010

Table 12. Pooled direct (within-study) comparisons of ultrasound for identification and diagnosis of hepatocellular carcinoma

	Unit of Analysis	Sensitivity A (95% CI)	Sensitivity B (95% CI)	Difference (95% CI); τ^2 (p value)	Number of Studies	Specificity A (95% CI)	Specificity B (95% CI)	Difference (95% CI); τ^2 (p value)	Number of Studies
Detection of HCC (KQ 1)									
Contrast (A) vs. no contrast (B)	Lesion (1), liver segment (1)	0.79 (0.72 to 0.76))	0.81 (0.76 to 0.86)	-0.04 (-0.11 to 0.04); -0.04 (p=1.0)	2	0.98 (0.96 to 0.997)	0.92 (0.89 to 0.95)	0.06 (0.02 to 0.10)	1
Doppler (A) vs. no Doppler (B)	Lesion	0.67 (0.52 to 0.81)	0.60 (0.45 to 0.74)	0.07 (-0.13 to 0.28)	1	No data	No data	--	--
Evaluation of focal liver lesions (KQ 2)									
Contrast (A) vs. no contrast (B)	Lesion	0.89 (0.83 to 0.93)	0.39 (0.32 to 0.47)	0.50 (0.41 to 0.58); <0.0001 (p=1.0)	2	1.0 (1.0-1.0)	0.94 (0.85 to 1.0)	0.06 (-0.02 to 0.15)	1
Doppler (A) vs. no Doppler (B)	Lesion	0.69 (0.29 to 0.93)	0.68 (0.28 to 0.92)	-0.01 (-0.15 to 0.13); 1.2 (p=0.34)	2	No data	No data	--	--
Doppler (A) vs. no Doppler (B) (also contrast vs. no contrast)	Patient	0.93 (0.88 to 0.97)	0.78 (0.70-0.85)	0.15 (0.06 to 0.23)	1	No data	No data	--	--
Moderately or poorly-differentiated (A) vs. well-differentiated HCC lesion (B), with contrast	Lesion	0.83 (0.55 to 0.95)	0.43 (0.15 to 0.76)	0.40 (0.17 to 0.64); 1.2 (p=0.17)	3	No data	No data	--	--
HCC lesion ≥20 mm (A) vs. <20 mm (B)									
• No contrast	Patient (1), lesion (7), liver segment (1)	0.82 (0.68 to 0.91)	0.34 (0.19 to 0.53)	0.48 (0.39 to 0.57); 1.3 (p=0.005)	9	0.80 (0.61 to 0.91)	0.81 (0.62 to 0.92)	-0.01 (-0.13 to 0.11); 0.51 (p=0.08)	2
• With contrast	Lesion	0.94 (0.83 to 0.98)	0.77 (0.53 to 0.91)	0.17 (0.03 to 0.32); 1.3 (p=0.05)	5	1.0 (26/26)	1.0 (2/2)	Not calculated	1

HCC = hepatocellular carcinoma

Table 13. Direct comparisons of diagnostic accuracy according to lesion size <10, 10-20, and >20 mm

	Sensitivity (95% CI); τ^2 (p value)	Number of Studies	Specificity (95% CI); τ^2 (p value)	Number of Studies	LR+	LR-
Ultrasound without contrast						
• <10 mm	0.09 (0.02 to 0.29); 1.5 (p=0.08)	4	0.93 (0.79 to 1.0)	1	1.3	0.98
• 10-20 mm	0.50 (0.23 to 0.78)	4	0.60 (0.46 to 0.74)	1	1.2	0.83
• >20 mm	0.88 (0.66 to 0.96)	4	0.53 (0.35 to 0.71)	1	1.9	0.23
• Difference >20 mm vs. 10-20 mm	0.37 (0.18 to 0.57)	4	-0.33 (-0.53 to -0.14)	1	--	--
• Difference 10-20 mm vs. <10 mm	0.41 (0.19 to 0.63)	4	-0.06 (-0.29 to 0.16)	1	--	--
Ultrasound with contrast						
• 10-20	0.64 (0.33 to 0.87); 1.2 (p=0.15)	3	1.0 (26/26)	1	--	--
• >20 mm	0.91 (0.71 to 0.98)	3	1.0 (2/2)	1	--	--
• Difference >20 mm vs. 10-20 mm	0.26 (0.04 to 0.48)	3	0.0	0	--	--
Computed Tomography (CT)						
• <10 mm	0.32 (0.25 to 0.41); 0.51 (p<0.0001)	21	0.69 (0.52 to 0.82); <0.0001 (p=0.9993)	2	1.0 (0.59 to 1.8)	0.99 (0.77 to 1.3)
• 10-20 mm	0.74 (0.67 to 0.80)	23	0.86 (0.74 to 0.93)	2	5.3 (2.8 to 10)	0.30 (0.23 to 0.40)
• >20 mm	0.95 (0.92 to 0.97)	20	0.90 (0.73 to 0.97)	1	9.5 (3.2 to 28)	0.06 (0.04 to 0.09)
• Difference >20 mm vs. 10-20 mm	0.21 (0.15 to 0.26)	20	0.04 (-0.10 to 0.18)	2	--	--
• Difference 10-20 mm vs. <10 mm	0.42 (0.36 to 0.48)	21	0.17 (-0.004 to 0.35)	1	--	--
Magnetic Resonance Imaging (MRI)						
• <10 mm	0.45 (0.34 to 0.56); 0.86 (p<0.0001)	20	0.68 (0.23 to 0.94); 1.9 (p=0.08)	2	1.4 (0.37 to 5.3)	0.81 (0.43 to 1.5)
• 10-20 mm	0.78 (0.69 to 0.85)	21	0.83 (0.41 to 0.97)	2	4.6 (0.93 to 23)	0.26 (0.17 to 0.41)
• >20 mm	0.97 (0.94 to 0.98)	18	0.92 (0.56 to 0.99)	2	12 (1.6 to 93)	0.03 (0.02 to 0.06)
• Difference >20 mm vs. 10-20 mm	0.19 (0.12 to 0.26)	18	0.09 (-0.10 to 0.28)	2	--	--
• Difference 10-20 mm vs. <10 mm	0.33 (0.26 to 0.40)	20	0.15 (-0.10 to 0.41)	2	--	--

Table 14. Pooled direct (within-study) comparisons of computed tomography for identification and diagnosis of hepatocellular carcinoma

	Unit of Analysis	Sensitivity A (95% CI)	Sensitivity B (95% CI)	Difference (95% CI); τ^2 (p value)	Number of Studies	Specificity A (95% CI)	Specificity B (95% CI)	Difference (95% CI); τ^2 (p value)	Number of Studies
Section thickness 7.5 mm (A) vs. 5 mm (B)	Lesion	0.64 (0.58 to 0.70)	0.72 (0.64 to 0.78)	-0.07 (-0.17 to 0.02); <0.0001 (p=1.0)	2	No data	No data	--	--
Section thickness 7.5 mm (A) vs. 5 mm (B), restricted to lesions <2 cm	Lesion	0.39 (0.27 to 0.52)	0.41 (0.22 to 0.59)	-0.01 (-0.24 to 0.21)	1	No data	No data	--	--
Spectral CT (A) vs. standard CT (B)	Lesion	0.97 (0.89 to 0.99)	0.91 (0.80-0.97)	0.05 (-0.02 to 0.12); 0.33 (p=0.39)	3	0.98 (0.80-0.998)	0.92 (0.64 to 0.99)	0.06 (-0.06 to 0.18); 0.99 (p=0.59)	2
Moderately or poorly (A) vs. well differentiated (B) HCC lesion	Lesion	0.82 (0.66 to 0.91)	0.50 (0.29 to 0.70)	0.32 (0.19 to 0.45); 0.77 (p=0.05)	5	No data	No data	--	--
HCC lesion ≥20 mm (A) vs. <20 mm (B)	Lesion (32); liver segment (3)	0.94 (0.92 to 0.95)	0.63 (0.57 to 0.69)	0.31 (0.26 to 0.36); 0.50 (p<0.0001)	34	0.92 (0.85 to 0.96)	0.80 (0.71 to 0.86)	0.12 (0.03 to 0.21); <0.0001 (p=1.0)	2
HCC lesion ≥20 mm (A) vs. <20 mm (B), restricted to studies meeting minimum technical criteria*	Lesion	0.94 (0.89 to 0.97)	0.60 (0.49 to 0.70)	0.35 (0.25 to 0.44); 0.26 (p=0.04)	7	0.90 (0.73 to 0.97)	0.85 (0.74 to 0.92)	0.05 (-0.09 to 0.19); <0.0001 (p=0.999)	1
Cirrhosis (A) vs. no cirrhosis (B)	Lesion	0.85 (0.77 to 0.91)	0.81 (0.74 to 0.87)	0.04 (-0.05 to 0.14); <0.0001 (p=1.0)	2	No data	No data	--	--

*Defined as multidetector CT with ≥8 rows, contrast rate ≥3 ml/s, imaging phases include arterial, portal venous and delayed phase imaging >120 s after administration of contrast, and section thickness for enhanced images ≤5 mm; HCC = hepatocellular carcinoma

Table 15. Pooled direct (within-study) comparisons of magnetic resonance imaging for identification and diagnosis of hepatocellular carcinoma

	Unit of Analysis	Sensitivity A (95% CI)	Sensitivity B (95% CI)	Difference (95% CI); τ^2 (p value)	Number of Studies	Specificity A (95% CI)	Specificity B (95% CI)	Difference (95% CI); τ^2 (p value)	Number of Studies
Gadoxetic acid or gadobenate (A) vs. gadopentetate or gadodiadmide (B)	Lesion	0.83 (0.75 to 0.90)	0.74 (0.62 to 0.83)	0.10 (0.04 to 0.15); 0.36 (p=0.04)	6	0.91 (0.86 to 0.95)	0.89 (0.83 to 0.93)	0.02 (-0.04 to 0.09); 0.002 (p=0.88)	3
Gadoxetic acid or gadobenate (A) vs. gadopentetate or gadodiadmide (B), for HCC lesions <2 cm	Lesion	0.77 (0.68 to 0.84)	0.62 (0.52 to 0.71)	0.15 (0.08 to 0.22); 0.20 (p=0.05)	7	0.93 (0.82 to 0.98)	0.91 (0.79 to 0.97)	0.02 (-0.05 to 0.09); 0.14 (p=0.51)	2
Diffusion-weighted imaging (A) vs. no diffusion-weighted imaging (B)	Lesion (7), patient (1)	0.81 (0.74 to 0.86)	0.81 (0.75 to 0.86)	-0.01 (-0.05 to 0.03); 0.14 (p=0.05)	8	0.92 (0.83 to 0.97)	0.81 (0.65 to 0.91)	0.11 (0.02 to 0.20); 0.73 (p=0.13)	5
Diffusion-weighted imaging (A) vs. no diffusion-weighted imaging (B) for HCC lesion <2 cm	Lesion	0.78 (0.62 to 0.88)	0.67 (0.50-0.81)	0.10 (0.02 to 0.18); 0.75 (p=0.03)	5	0.97 (0.31 to 0.9995)	0.91 (0.15 to 0.999)	0.06 (-0.16 to 0.28); 4.4 (p=0.37)	2
Moderately or poorly (A) vs. well differentiated (B) HCC lesion	Lesion	0.68 (0.44 to 0.86)	0.37 (0.17 to 0.62)	0.31 (0.13 to 0.49)	3	No data	No data	–	–

Table 15. Pooled direct (within-study) comparisons of magnetic resonance imaging for identification and diagnosis of hepatocellular carcinoma (continued)

Unit of Analysis	Sensitivity A (95% CI)	Sensitivity B (95% CI)	Difference (95% CI); τ^2 (p value)	Number of Studies	Specificity A (95% CI)	Specificity B (95% CI)	Difference (95% CI); τ^2 (p value)	Number of Studies
HCC lesion ≥20 mm (A) vs. <20 mm (B)	Lesion (28); liver segment (1)	0.96 (0.93 to 0.97)	0.66 (0.58 to 0.74)	0.29 (0.23 to 0.36); 0.74 (p<0.0001)	29	0.94 (0.77 to 0.99)	0.80 (0.50 to 0.94)	0.14 (-0.01 to 0.30); 1.9 (p=0.03)	4
HCC lesion ≥20 mm (A) vs. <20 mm (B), gadopentetate or gadodiamide contrast	Lesion (15); liver segment (1)	0.94 (0.90 to 0.96)	0.54 (0.43 to 0.63)	0.40 (0.32 to 0.49); 0.58 (p=0.0003)	16	0.96 (0.82 to 0.99)	0.85 (0.61 to 0.95)	0.11 (-0.01 to 0.23); 0.46 (p=0.45)	2
HCC lesion ≥20 mm (A) vs. <20 mm (B), gadoxetic acid or gadobenate contrast	Lesion	0.97 (0.95 to 0.99)	0.78 (0.71 to 0.84)	0.19 (0.13 to 0.25); 0.29 (p=0.01)	12	0.93 (0.77 to 0.98)	0.90 (0.80 to 0.96)	0.03 (-0.08 to 0.15); <0.0001 (p=1.0)	1
HCC lesion ≥20 mm (A) vs. <20 mm (B), restricted to studies meeting minimum technical criteria*	Lesion	0.97 (0.95 to 0.99)	0.73 (0.65 to 0.79)	0.25 (0.18 to 0.31); 0.30 (p=0.004)	13	0.93 (0.76 to 0.98)	0.90 (0.79 to 0.96)	0.03 (-0.09 to 0.15); <0.0001 (p=1.0)	1

*Defined as 1.5 or 3.0 T MRI with contrast, imaging phases included arterial, portal venous, and delayed or hepatobiliary phases; delayed phase imaging >~120 s following contrast administration, and section thickness for enhanced images ≤5 mm

HCC = hepatocellular carcinoma

Table 16. Pooled direct (within-study) comparisons of positron emission tomography for identification and diagnosis of hepatocellular carcinoma

Detection of intrahepatic HCC (KQ 1)	Unit of Analysis	Sensitivity A (95% CI)	Sensitivity B (95% CI)	Difference (95% CI); τ^2 (p value)	Number of Studies	Specificity A (95% CI)	Specificity B (95% CI)	Difference (95% CI); τ^2 (p value)	Number of Studies
FDG (A) vs. ^{11}C-acetate (B) PET	Patient	0.58 (0.44 to 0.70)	0.81 (0.70-0.89)	-0.23 (-0.34 to -0.13) ; 0.13 (p=0.23)	3	No data	No data	--	--
	Lesion	0.52 (0.45 to 0.59)	0.79 (0.72 to 0.84)	-0.27 (-0.36 to -0.17)	3	No data	No data	--	--
FDG (A) vs. FDG + ^{11}C-acetate (B) PET	Patient	0.63 (0.52 to 0.74)	0.89 (-0.83 to 0.96)	-0.26 (-0.39 to -0.13)	1	No data	No data	--	--
	Lesion	0.33 (0.21 to 0.45)	0.95 (0.89 to 1.0)	-0.62 (-0.75 to -0.49)	1	No data	No data	--	--
FDG (A) vs. ^{18}F-fluorocholine (B)	Patient	0.65 (0.50-0.78)	0.91 (0.78 to 0.96)	-0.26 (-0.42 to -0.09)	2	0.94 (0.83 to 1.0)	0.47 (0.23 to 0.71)	0.47 (0.23 to 0.71)	1
	Lesion	0.67 (0.56 to 0.78)	0.84 (0.76 to 0.93)	-0.17 (-0.31 to -0.03)	1	0.91 (0.82 to 1.0)	0.62 (0.45 to 0.78)	0.29 (0.10-0.48)	1
Moderately- or poorly-differentiated (A) vs. well-differentiated (B) HCC lesion, FDG PET	Patient (2), lesion (4)	0.72 (0.59 to 0.83)	0.39 (0.26 to 0.55)	0.33 (0.20 to 0.46); 0.32 (p=0.05)	6	No data	No data	--	--
Moderately- or poorly-differentiated (A) vs. well-differentiated (B) HCC lesion, ^{11}C-acetate PET	Lesion (2)	0.80 (0.65 to 0.89)	0.76 (0.67 to 0.83)	0.04 (-0.11 to 0.18); <0.0001 (p=1.0)	2	No data	No data	--	--

Table 16. Pooled direct (within-study) comparisons of positron emission tomography for identification and diagnosis of hepatocellular carcinoma (continued)

	Unit of Analysis	Sensitivity A (95% CI)	Sensitivity B (95% CI)	Difference (95% CI); τ^2 (p value)	Number of Studies	Specificity A (95% CI)	Specificity B (95% CI)	Difference (95% CI); τ^2 (p value)	Number of Studies
Detection of metastatic HCC (KQ 3)									
FDG (A) vs. ^{11}C-acetate (B) PET	Patient	0.79 (0.71 to 0.87)	0.64 (0.54 to 0.73)	0.15 (0.03 to 0.28)	1	0.91 (0.79 to 1.0)	0.95 (0.87 to 1.0)	-0.05 (-0.19 to 0.10)	1
FDG (A) vs. FDG + ^{11}C-acetate (B) PET	Patient	0.79 (0.71 to 0.87)	0.98 (0.95 to 1.0)	-0.19 (-0.28 to -0.11)	1	0.91 (0.79 to 1.0)	0.86 (0.72 to 1.0)	0.05 (-0.14 to 0.23)	1
PET vs. PET/CT	Metastatic HCC lesion	0.90 (0.82 to 0.97)	0.98 (0.95 to 1.0)	-0.09 (-0.17 to 0.0)	1	No data	No data	--	--

CT = computed tomography; FDG = 18F-fluorodeoxyglucose; HCC = hepatocellular carcinoma; PET = positron emission tomography

Table 17. Test performance of ^{18}F-fluorodeoxyglucose positron emission tomography for hepatocellular carcinoma, stratified by lesion size

Study, Year	HCC Location	Unit of Analysis	Sensitivity: FDG	Sensitivity: ^{11}C-acetate
Cheung, 2011[297]	Intrahepatic	Patient	≤5 cm: 0.24 (7/29) >5 cm: 0.62 (18/29)	≤5 cm: 0.97 (28/29) >5 cm: 0.97 (28/29)
Kim YK, 2010 (3)[305]	Intrahepatic	Lesion	<1 cm: 0.0 (0/21) ≥1 cm: 0.33 (2/6)	--
Park JW, 2008[309]	Intrahepatic	Lesion	≥1 to 2 cm: 0.27 (6/22) ≥2 to 5 cm: 0.48 (22/46) ≥5 cm: 0.93 (39/42)	≥1 to 2 cm: 0.32 (7/22) ≥2 to 5 cm: 0.78 (36/46) ≥5 cm: 0.95 (40/42)
Trojan, 1999[111]	Intrahepatic	Patient	<5 cm: 0.12 (1/8) ≥5 cm: 1.0 (6/6)	--
Wolfort, 2010[316]	Intrahepatic	Lesion	≤5 cm: 0.25 (2/8) >5 cm: 1.0 (5/5)	--
Kim YK, 2010 (3)[305]	Extrahepatic	Lesion	<1 cm: 0.0 (0/2) ≤1 cm: 0.93 (13/14)	--
Lee JE, 2012[171]	Lung	Patient	<1 cm: 0.20 (2/10) ≥1 cm: 0.92 (12/13)	--
Park JW, 2008[309]	Extrahepatic	Lesion	≤1 to 2 cm: 0.80 (16/20) ≥2 cm: 0.93 (14/15)	≤1 to 2 cm: 0.65 (13/20) ≥2 cm: 0.93 (14/15)
Sugiyama, 2004[311]	Extrahepatic	Lesion	<1 cm: 0.12 (1/8) ≥1 cm: 0.83 (24/29)	--

FDG = ^{18}F-fluorodeoxyglucose; HCC = hepatocellular carcinoma

Table 18. Test performance of ^{18}F-fluorodeoxyglucose positron emission tomography for hepatocellular carcinoma, stratified by degree of tumor differentiation

Study, Year	Unit of Analysis	Sensitivity: FDG	Sensitivity: 11C-Acetate
Li, 2006	Lesion	--	Well- or moderately differentiated: 0.67 (8/12) Poorly differentiated: 0.62 (8/13)
Park JW, 2008	Lesion	Grade I or II: 0.50 (35/70) Grade III or IV: 0.87 (27/31)	Grade I or II: 0.71 (50/70) Grade III or IV: 0.87 (27/31)
Talbot, 2010	Lesion	Well-differentiated: 0.59 (19/32) Poorly-differentiated: 0.74 (28/38)	--
Trojan, 1999	Patient	Well-differentiated: 0.0 (0/6) Moderately or poorly differentiated: 0.88 (7/8)	--
Wolfort, 2010	Lesion	Well-differentiated: 0.67 (4/6) Moderately or poorly differentiated: 0.75 (6/8)	--
Wu, 2011	Patient	Well differentiated: 0.36 (5/14) Moderately or poorly differentiated: 0.74 (23/31)	--
Yamamoto, 2008	Lesion	Moderately differentiated: 0.42 (5/12) Poorly differentiated: 0.75 (3/4)	Moderately differentiated: 0.75 (9/12) Poorly differentiated: 0.25 (1/4)

FDG = ^{18}F-fluorodeoxyglucose

Table 19. Studies on accuracy of imaging for differentiating hepatocellular carcinoma from other hepatic lesions

Study, Year	Imaging Modality	HCC Lesion	Lesion for Differentiation	Unit of Analysis	Reference Standard	Sensitivity	Specificity	Diagnostic Criteria
Pei, 2012[95]	US with contrast	Hypervascular HCC	Focal nodular hyperplasia	Patient	Histological	0.94 (62/66)	0.68 (23/34)	Based on quantitative analysis of contrast-enhanced US findings
Kim SE, 2011[156]	CT	HCC	Non-HCC lesion (including cholangiocarcinoma, metastasis, and FNH)	Lesion	Histological	0.85 (140/164)	0.90 (38/42)	Based on arterial enhancement and venous washout
Lv, 2011[181]	CT	Hypervascular HCC lesion <3 cm	Hemangioma	Lesion	Mixed histological and clinical/imaging	0.91 (32/35)	0.87 (26/30)	Based on enhancement pattern on standard CT images
Sun, 2010[206]	CT	Hypervascular HCC lesion <2 cm	Hypervascular pseudolesion	Patient	Mixed histological and clinical/imaging	0.54 (18/33)	0.96 (26/27)	Confidence level score of 4-5 on 1 to 5 scale, based on enhancement pattern
Yu, 2013[214]	CT	HCC	Focal nodular hyperplasia	Lesion	Histological	0.95 (40/42)	1.0 (16/16)	Criteria for diagnosis not defined
Yu, 2013[213]	CT (spectral)	HCC	Angiomyolipoma	Lesion	Histological	0.84-1.0 (n=45)	0.50-1.0 (n=8)	Specificity 0.50 based on enhancement pattern, 0.91 to 1.0 based on various quantitative parameters
Filippone, 2010[231]	MRI	HCC	Dysplastic nodule	Lesion	Mixed histological and clinical/imaging	0.92 (36/39)	0.93 (14/15)	Confidence level score 3-4 on 1 to 4 scale, based on enhancement pattern including hepatobiliary phase imaging
Ito, 2004[239]	MRI	Hypervascular HCC lesion <3 cm	Hypervascular pseudolesion	Lesion	Mixed histological and clinical/imaging	0.52 (21/40)	1.0 (30/30)	Based on rapid central washout after early enhancement and peritumoral coronal enhancement
Jeong, 1999[240]	MRI	Hypervascular HCC lesion	Hemangioma	Lesion	Mixed histological and clinical/imaging	0.94 (31/33)	0.82 (15/18)	Based on contrast to noise ratio of 7.00 on imaging 60 s after administration of contrast

Table 19. Studies on accuracy of imaging for differentiating hepatocellular carcinoma from other hepatic lesions (continued)

Study, Year	Imaging Modality	HCC Lesion	Lesion for Differentiation	Unit of Analysis	Reference Standard	Sensitivity	Specificity	Diagnostic Criteria
Kamura, 2002[243]	MRI	Hypervascular HCC lesion <2 cm	Hypervascular pseudolesion	Lesion	Mixed histological and clinical/imaging	0.47 (9/19)	0.93 (13/14)	Based on hyperintensity on T2 to weighted images
Lee MH, 2011[265]	MRI	Well-differentiated HCC lesion	Benign nodule (regenerative nodule or dysplastic nodule)	Lesion	Histological	0.85 (39/46)	0.42 (10/24)	Based on hypointensity on hepatobiliary phase imaging
Motosugi, 2010[269]	MRI	Hypervascular HCC lesion (mean 16 mm)	Hypervascular pseudolesion (mean 11 mm)	Lesion	Mixed histological and clinical/imaging	0.91 (112/123)	0.91 (29/32)	Based on hepatocyte-phase signal intensity ratio of 0.84 on gadoxetic-enhanced images
Park, 2013[272]	MRI	HCC lesion <2 cm	Benign lesions (dysplastic nodules, regenerative nodules, hemangiomas, arterioportal shunts)	Lesion	Histological	0.97-0.98 (100-101/103)	0.97 (30/33)	Based on meeting one or more of 5 categories based on enhanced and diffusion-weighted imaging
Sun, 2010[206]	MRI	Hypervascular HCC lesion <2 cm	Hypervascular pseudolesion	Patient	Mixed histological and clinical/imaging	0.92 (30.5/33)	0.94 (25/27)	Confidence level score 4-5 on 1 to 5 scale, based on enhancement pattern
Takahashi, 2013[108]	MRI	Well-differentiated HCC lesion <3 cm	Regenerative nodules	Lesion	Histological	0.87 (47/54)	0.46 (6/13)	Based on enhancement pattern with hepatobiliary phase imaging
Vandecaveye, 2009[287]	MRI	HCC lesion[a]	Benign lesions (regenerative nodules, low-grade dysplastic nodules, stable lesions, or other benign lesions)	Lesion	Mixed histological and clinical/imaging	0.81 (50/62)	0.65 (34/52)	Based on T2- and T1-signal intensity ratio and enhancement pattern
Xu, 2010[289]	MRI	HCC lesion	Dysplastic nodule	Lesion	Histological	0.82 (33/40)	0.58 (11/18)	Confidence level score 4-5 on 1 to 5 scale, based on enhancement pattern
Yu, 2002[293]	MRI	HCC lesion <4 cm	Cavernous hemangioma	Lesion	Mixed histological and clinical/imaging	0.88 (137/155)	0.15 (31/207)	Based on absence of transient peritumoral enhancement

Table 19. Studies on accuracy of imaging for differentiating hepatocellular carcinoma from other hepatic lesions (continued)

Study, Year	Imaging Modality	HCC Lesion	Lesion for Differentiation	Unit of Analysis	Reference Standard	Sensitivity	Specificity	Diagnostic Criteria
Takahashi, 2013[108]	US	Well-differentiated HCC lesion <3 cm	Regenerative nodules	Lesion	Histological	0.44 (24/54)	1.0 (13/13)	Based on enhancement pattern with hepatobiliary phase imaging

CT = computed tomography; HCC = hepatocellular carcinoma; MRI = magnetic resonance imaging; US = ultrasound
[a] Including two cholangiocarcinomas and two high-grade dysplastic nodules

Table 20. Pooled direct (within-study) comparisons of test performance of one imaging modality versus another imaging modality for identification and diagnosis of hepatocellular carcinoma

	Unit of Analysis	Sensitivity A (95% CI)	Sensitivity B (95% CI)	Difference (95% CI); τ^2 (p value)	Number of Studies	Specificity A (95% CI)	Specificity B (95% CI)	Difference (95% CI); τ^2 (p value)	Number of Studies
Identification of lesions (KQ 1)									
US without contrast (A) vs. CT (B)	Patient	0.68 (0.54 to 0.80)	0.80 (0.68 to 0.88)	-0.12 (-0.20 to -0.03); 0.36 (p=0.15)	6	0.92 (0.84 to 0.96)	0.94 (0.87 to 0.97)	-0.01 (-0.05 to 0.02); 0.62 (p=0.07)	5
• Excluding high risk of bias studies	Patient	0.71 (0.58 to 0.82)	0.82 (0.71 to 0.89)	-0.10 (-0.18 to -0.02); 0.19 (p=0.25)	5	0.91 (0.81 to 0.96)	0.94 (0.86 to 0.98)	-0.03 (-0.07 to 0.01); 0.73 (p=0.11)	4
US without contrast (A) vs. CT (B)	Lesion	0.55 (0.43 to 0.66)	0.66 (0.54 to 0.76)	-0.11 (-0.18 to -0.04); 0.11 (p=0.28)	3	0.83 (0.65 to 0.93)	0.93 (0.83 to 0.98)	-0.10 (-0.20 to -0.008); 0.44 (p=0.29)	2
• HCC lesions <2 cm	Lesion	0.46 (0.30-0.63)	0.54 (0.37 to 0.70)	-0.07 (-0.17 to 0.02); 0.31 (p=0.27)	3	0.72 (0.61 to 0.80)	0.80 (0.71 to 0.86)	-0.08 (-0.20 to 0.04); 0.002 (p=0.85)	2
US with contrast (A) vs. CT (B)	Lesion	0.58 (0.37 to 0.77)	0.74 (0.54 to 0.87)	-0.16 (-0.32 to -0.01); 0.50 (p=0.15)	3	No data	No data	--	--
• HCC lesions <2 cm	Lesion	0.30 (0.17 to 0.43)	0.44 (0.30-0.58)	-0.14 (-0.32 to 0.05)	1	No data	No data	--	--
US without contrast (A) vs. MRI (B)	Patient	0.61 (0.48 to 0.74)	0.81 (0.69 to 0.89)	-0.19 (-0.30 to -0.08); 0.01 (p=0.79)	3	0.94 (0.87 to 0.97)	0.82 (0.66 to 0.91)	0.13 (0.03 to 0.22); 0.01 (p=0.40)	3
US without contrast (A) vs. MRI (B)	Lesion	0.57 (0.42 to 0.71)	0.79 (0.67 to 0.88)	-0.22 (-0.31 to -0.14); 0.22 (p=0.28)	3	0.75 (0.66 to 0.82)	0.78 (0.70-0.85)	-0.03 (-0.13 to 0.06); 0.001 (p=0.89)	2
• HCC lesion <2 cm	Lesion	0.40 (0.18 to 0.67)	0.65 (0.38 to 0.85)	-0.26 (-0.36 to -0.15); 0.60	2	0.71 (0.60-0.80)	0.84 (0.76 to 0.89)	-0.13 (-0.25 to -0.01); 0.006	2
US with contrast (A) vs. MRI (B)	Lesion	0.54 (0.25 to 0.80)	0.70 (0.40-0.89)	-0.16 (-0.30 to -0.02); 0.71 (p=0.31)	2	No data	No data	--	--
• HCC lesions <2 cm	Lesion	0.30 (0.17 to 0.43)	0.42 (0.28 to 0.56)	-0.12 (-0.31 to 0.07)	1	No data	No data	--	--

Table 20. Pooled direct (within-study) comparisons of test performance of one imaging modality versus another imaging modality for identification and diagnosis of hepatocellular carcinoma (continued)

	Unit of Analysis	Sensitivity A (95% CI)	Sensitivity B (95% CI)	Difference (95% CI); τ²□ (p value)	Number of Studies	Specificity A (95% CI)	Specificity B (95% CI)	Difference (95% CI); τ²□ (p value)	Number of Studies
• Well-differentiated HCC Lesion	Lesion	0.43 (0.14 to 0.77)	0.36 (0.11 to 0.72)	0.07 (-0.19 to 0.33); 0.87 (p=0.34)	2	No data	No data	--	1
MRI (A) vs. CT (B)	Patient	0.88 (0.53 to 0.98)	0.82 (0.41 to 0.97)	0.06 (-0.05 to 0.17); 3.0 (p=0.21)	4	0.84 (0.70-0.92)	0.91 (0.82 to 0.96)	-0.08 (-0.16 to 0.00); 0.40 (p=0.21)	4
• Excluding high risk of bias studies	Patient	0.82 (0.75 to 0.88)	0.75 (0.68 to 0.81)	0.07 (-0.02 to 0.17); <0.0001	2	0.80 (0.57 to 0.92)	0.91 (0.77 to 0.97)	-0.11 (-0.23 to 0.01); 0.44 (p=0.44)	2
MRI (A) vs. CT (B)	Lesion	0.81 (0.77 to 0.84)	0.72 (0.67 to 0.77)	0.09 (0.06 to 0.12); 0.37 (p<0.0001)	28	0.85 (0.76 to 0.92)	0.90 (0.82 to 0.95)	-0.05 (-0.10 to 0.01); 0.43 (p=0.01)	6
• Excluding high risk of bias studies	Lesion	0.80 (0.73 to 0.85)	0.73 (0.66 to 0.79)	0.07 (0.04 to 0.10); 0.50 (p<0.0001)	19	0.87 (0.78 to 0.93)	0.93 (0.86 to 0.96)	-0.05 (-0.10 to 0.00); 0.37 (p=0.03)	5
• Non-hepatic specific contrast	Lesion	0.81 (0.74 to 0.87)	0.74 (0.65 to 0.81)	0.08 (0.04 to 0.11); 0.39 (p=0.01)	11	0.62 (0.51 to 0.72)	0.86 (0.77 to 0.93)	-0.24 (-0.37 to -0.11); <0.0001 (p=1.0)	2
• Hepatic specific contrast	Lesion	0.80 (0.74 to 0.85)	0.70 (0.62 to 0.77)	0.10 (0.06 to 0.14); 0.41 (p=0.0003)	15	0.93 (0.88 to 0.96)	0.91 (0.85 to 0.94)	0.02 (-0.03 to 0.07); 0.01 (p=0.78)	4
• HCC lesions <2 cm	Lesion	0.59 (0.43 to 0.73)	0.46 (0.32 to 0.62)	0.12 (0.03 to 0.22); 0.25 (p=0.27)	3	0.84 (0.73 to 0.91)	0.80 (0.67 to 0.89)	0.04 (-0.06 to 0.14); 0.12 (p=0.41)	2
Evaluation of previously identified lesion (KQ 2)									
US without contrast (A) vs. CT (B)	Patient	0.78 (0.70-0.85)	0.89 (0.84 to 0.95)	-0.12 (-0.21 to -0.02)	1	No data	No data	--	1
US with contrast (A) vs. CT (B)	Patient	0.91 (0.85 to 0.94)	0.88 (0.81 to 0.92)	0.03 (-0.02 to 0.08); 0.15 (p=0.13)	5	0.93 (0.87 to 0.96)	0.94 (0.88 to 0.97)	-0.01 (-0.06 to 0.05); 0.07 (p=0.32)	2
• Excluding high risk of bias studies	Patient	0.90 (0.79 to 0.95)	0.87 (0.76 to 0.94)	0.02 (-0.05 to 0.10); 0.28 (p=0.31)	3	0.93 (0.87 to 0.97)	0.94 (0.88 to 0.97)	-0.01 (-0.06 to 0.05); 0.08 (p=0.45)	2

Table 20. Pooled direct (within-study) comparisons of test performance of one imaging modality versus another imaging modality for identification and diagnosis of hepatocellular carcinoma (continued)

	Unit of Analysis	Sensitivity A (95% CI)	Sensitivity B (95% CI)	Difference (95% CI); τ^2 (p value)	Number of Studies	Specificity A (95% CI)	Specificity B (95% CI)	Difference (95% CI); τ^2 (p value)	Number of Studies
US with contrast (A) vs. CT (B)	Lesion	0.94 (0.89 to 0.97)	0.91 (0.85 to 0.94)	0.03 (-0.03 to 0.09); <0.0001 (p=1.0)	3	No data	No data	--	--
• HCC lesion <2 cm	Lesion	0.78 (0.61 to 0.89)	0.71 (0.52 to 0.85)	0.07 (-0.01 to 0.15); 1.1 (p-0.02)	7	0.87 (0.62 to 0.97)	0.94 (0.77 to 0.98)	-0.06 (-0.15 to 0.03); 2.4 (p=0.09)	4
• Well-differentiated HCC Lesion	Lesion	0.55 (0.25 to 0.82)	0.55 (0.25 to 0.82)	0.00 (-0.30 to 0.30); 0.48 (p=0.40)	2	No data	No data	--	--
US with contrast (A) vs. MRI (B)	Patient	0.79 (0.65 to 0.94)	0.83 (0.69 to 0.97)	-0.03 (-0.24 to 0.17)	1	0.79 (0.68 to 0.90)	0.75 (0.64 to 0.87)	0.04 (-0.12 to 0.20)	1
• HCC lesion <2 cm	Patient	0.52 (0.39 to 0.64)	0.62 (0.49 to 0.74)	-0.10 (-0.27 to 0.08)	1	0.93 (0.84 to 1.0)	0.97 (0.90-1.0)	-0.03 (-0.15 to 0.08)	1
US with contrast (A) vs. MRI (B)	Lesion	0.79 (0.65 to 0.94)	0.83 (0.69 to 0.97)	-0.03 (-0.24 to 0.17)	1	0.79 (0.68 to 0.90)	0.75 (0.64 to 0.87)	0.04 (-0.12 to 0.20)	1
• HCC lesion <2 cm	Lesion	0.53 (0.28 to 0.76)	0.68 (0.43 to 0.86)	-0.16 (-0.30 to -0.02); 0.72 (p=0.25)	3	0.95 (0.85 to 0.98)	0.98 (0.91 to 0.99)	-0.03 (-0.08 to 0.02); 0.38 (p=0.43)	3
MRI (A) vs. CT (B)	Patient	0.81 (0.70-0.92)	0.74 (0.62 to 0.87)	0.06 (-0.10 to 0.23)	1	0.85 (0.72 to 0.99)	0.81 (0.66 to 0.96)	0.04 (-0.16 to 0.24)	1
MRI (A) vs. CT (B)	Lesion	0.84 (0.76 to 0.92)	0.62 (0.52 to 0.72)	0.22 (0.09 to 0.35)	1	0.36 (0.20-0.52)	0.72 (0.58 to 0.87)	-0.36 (-0.58 to -0.15)	1
Identification of metastatic HCC (KQ 4)									
PET/CT (A) vs. CT (B)	Patient (2), lesion (1)	0.82 (0.61 to 0.93)	0.85 (0.66 to 0.95)	-0.03 (-0.12 to 0.060); 0.75 (p=0.17)	3	Insufficient data	Insufficient data	--	--

CT = computed tomography; HCC = hepatocellular carcinoma; MRI = magnetic resonance imaging; PET = positron emission tomography; US = ultrasound

Table 21. Accuracy of imaging for staging of hepatocellular carcinoma

Author, Year	Diagnostic Test	Dates of Imaging	Reference Standard	Country	Sample Size	Patient Population	Staging System	Stage Analysis	Correctly Staged	Over-staged	Under-staged
Baccarini, 2006[122]	CT	1996-2005	Explant	Italy	50	Liver transplant	TNM	0, 1, 2, 3, 4a	28%	20%	52%
Burrel, 2003[126]	MRI	2000-2001	Explant	Spain	50	Liver transplant	BCLC	A, B, C	59%	10%	31%
Cheung, 2013[127]	CT	2004-2010	Explant or surgical resection	China	43	Liver transplant or surgical resection	TNM	1, 2, 3	58%	4%	38%
	FDG PET								26%	NR	NR
	^{11}C-choline PET								91%	NR	NR
	Dual tracer PET								91%	NR	NR
	CT								42%	NR	NR
Freeman, 2006[61]	MRI	2003-2005	Explant	United States	285	Liver transplant	TNM	0, 1, 2, 3, 4a, 4b	40%	31%	29%
	CT				357				47%	27%	25%
	US				10				30%	30%	40%
	Two or more imaging methods				117				49%	29%	22%
Libbrecht, 2002[82]	US, CT, or MRI	2000-2001	Explant	Belgium	13	Liver transplant	NR	NR	NR	NR	NR
Lu CH, 2010[179]	CT	2006-2008	Explant	Taiwan	57	Liver transplant	NR	NR	NR	NR	NR
	MRI										
Luca, 2010[42]	CT	2004-2006	Explant	Italy	57	Liver transplant	TNM	1, 2, 3	46%	2%	52%
Ronzoni, 2007[202]	CT	2003-2006	Explant	Italy	88	Liver transplant	NR	NR	NR	NR	NR
Shah, 2006[102]	US or CT	1991-2004	Explant	Canada	118	Liver transplant	TNM	NR	NR	NR	NR
Valls, 2004[208]	CT	1995-2002	Explant	Spain	85	Liver transplant	NR	NR	NR	NR	NR
Zacherl, 2002[216]	CT	1998-2000	Explant	Austria	23	Liver transplant	TNM	1, 2, 3, 4	39%	NR	NR

BCLC = Barcelona Clinic Liver Cancer; NR = not reported; TNM = tumor nodule metastasis

Table 22. Test performance of ^{18}F-fluorodeoxyglucose positron emission tomography for metastatic hepatocellular carcinoma, stratified by location of metastasis

Study, Year	Unit of Analysis	Sensitivity: Lung Metastasis	Sensitivity: Lymph Node Metastasis	Sensitivity: Bone Metastasis	Specificity: Lung Metastasis	Specificity: Lymph Node Metastasis	Specificity: Bone Metastasis
Kawaoka, 2009[a,152]	Patient	0.59 (10.7/18)	0.67 (10.7/16)	0.83 (10/12)	0.92 (14.7/16)	0.92 (16.7/18)	0.86 (20.7/24)
Kim YK, 2010 (3)[305]	Lesion	0.60 (3/5)	1.0 (3/3)	1.0 (5/5)	Not reported	Not reported	Not reported
Lee JE, 2012[171]	Patient	0.61 (14/23)	0.91 (20/22)	1.0 (11/11)	0.99[b]	0.96[b]	1.0[b]
Nagaoka, 2006[189]	Lesion	0.70 (7/10)	0.95 (21/22)	1.0 (16/16)	Not reported	Not reported	Not reported
Park JW, 2008[309]	Lesion	0.80 (16/20)	Not reported	1.0 (6/6)	Not reported	Not reported	Not reported
Sugiyama, 2004[311]	Lesion	0.42 (5/12)	1.0 (9/9)	0.80 (8/10)	Not reported	Not reported	Not reported
Wu, 2011[317]	Patient	0.80 (8/10)	Not reported	0.75 (3/4)	Not reported	Not reported	Not reported
Yoon, 2007[320]	Patient	1.0 (12/12)	1.0 (19/19)	1.0 (11/11)	0.84 (63/75)	0.94 (64/68)	1.0 (76/76)

[a] Based on average from three readers
[b] Unable to determine number of true-negatives from information provided in study

Discussion

Key Findings and Strength of Evidence

The key findings of this review, including strength of evidence grades, are summarized in Tables 23–40. Details about factors assessed to determine the overall strength of evidence grades are shown in Appendix J. No body of evidence was rated high strength of evidence, due to methodological shortcomings, imprecision, and/or inconsistency. Moderate strength of evidence ratings were primarily limited to estimates of diagnostic accuracy for CT and MRI, and some direct comparisons involving US versus CT or MRI.

The great preponderance of evidence on imaging for HCC addressed diagnostic test performance. However, few studies evaluated test performance of imaging for HCC in true surveillance settings (i.e., in patients at high risk for but without a prior diagnosis of HCC), resulting in low strength of evidence ratings. Among the limited evidence available in this setting, two studies that directly compared sensitivity of US without contrast and CT did report lower sensitivity with US for detection of patients with HCC (low strength of evidence). [54,112]

Many more studies evaluated test performance of imaging for detection of HCC in nonsurveillance settings, such as populations of patients undergoing treatment such as liver transplantation, hepatic resection, or ablation therapy, or in series of patients previously diagnosed with HCC who underwent additional imaging. Although these patients were known to have HCC lesions, the purpose of these studies was not to further characterize previously identified HCC lesions. Rather, their purpose was to evaluate test performance for detection of HCC lesions. We analyzed these studies separately from studies conducted in true surveillance settings, given the differences in the reason for imaging and the populations evaluated (including a generally much higher prevalence of HCC—some studies were restricted to only patients with HCC). In these studies, sensitivity was lower for US without contrast than for CT or MRI, with a difference in sensitivity based on within-study (direct) comparisons of 0.11 to 0.22, using HCC lesions as unit of analysis (moderate strength of evidence). MRI and CT performed similarly when patients with HCC were the unit of analysis, but sensitivity of MRI was higher than CT when HCC lesions were the unit of analysis (pooled difference 0.09. 95% CI 0.07 to 12) (moderate strength of evidence).

Ultrasound with contrast did not perform better than ultrasound without contrast for detection of HCC (low strength of evidence).[67,79] This is probably related to the short duration in which microbubble contrast is present within the liver, such that it is not possible to perform a comprehensive contrast-enhanced examination of the liver.[20] Rather, the main use of ultrasound with contrast appears to be for evaluation of previously identified focal liver lesions.

For characterization of previously identified lesions, we found no clear differences in sensitivity between US with contrast, CT, and MRI (moderate strength of evidence). Although some evidence was available on the accuracy of imaging modalities for distinguishing between HCC and other (non-HCC) liver lesions, it was not possible to draw strong conclusions due to variability in the types of non-HCC lesions evaluated (regenerative nodules, dysplastic nodules, hypervascular pseudolesions, hemangiomas, etc.), small numbers of studies, and some inconsistency in findings.

Several factors appeared to affect estimates of test performance across different imaging modalities. Studies of patients with HCC were generally associated with somewhat higher sensitivity than studies that used HCC lesions as the unit of analysis. In addition, use of multiple reference standards poses a challenge to assessment of diagnostic accuracy.[324] Studies that used explanted livers as the reference standard reported lower sensitivity than studies that used a nonexplant reference standard (moderate strength of evidence). The explanted liver reference standard is probably associated with lower sensitivity because additional lesions not detectable on imaging—and therefore not targets for percutaneous or surgical biopsy—are identified on examination of the entire liver. However, explanted livers are also an imperfect reference standard, as lesions may still be missed. In addition, the clinical significance of small lesions seen on explant but not by other methods is unclear. Across imaging modalities, sensitivity was markedly lower for HCC lesions <2 cm versus those ≥2 cm (differences in sensitivity ranged from 0.30 to 0.39), and further declined for lesions <10 mm in diameter (moderate strength of evidence). Evidence also consistently indicated substantially lower sensitivity for well-differentiated lesions than moderately- or poorly-differentiated lesions (low strength of evidence).

Evidence on the effects of other patient, tumor, and technical factors on test performance was more limited (low strength of evidence). For US, there was no clear effect of use of Doppler, lesion depth, or body mass index on test performance. For CT, limited evidence indicated higher sensitivity for studies that used a contrast rate of ≥3 ml/s than those with a contrast rate <3 ml/s, and for studies that used delayed phase imaging. For MRI, there were no clear effects of magnetic field strength (3.0 vs. 1.5 T), use of delayed phase imaging, type of contrast (hepatic specific vs. non-hepatic specific), timing of delayed phase imaging (≥120 seconds after administration of contrast of <120 s), section thickness (≤5 mm vs. >5 mm), or use of diffusion-weighted imaging. For identification of intrahepatic HCC lesions, limited evidence found PET with ^{11}C-acetate and other alternative tracers such as ^{18}F-fluorocholine and ^{18}F-fluorothymidine associated with substantially higher sensitivity than FDG PET. Sensitivity of FDG PET was lower than sensitivity of FDG PET/CT.

Few studies evaluated the comparative test performance of multiple imaging modalities, either in combination or sequentially as part of a diagnostic algorithm. The available evidence suggests that using multiple imaging tests and defining a positive test as typical imaging findings on at least one imaging modality increases sensitivity without substantively reducing specificity (moderate strength of evidence).

Conclusions were generally robust on sensitivity and stratified analyses based on study factors such as setting (Asia vs. United States or Europe), prospective collection of data, interpretation of imaging findings blinded to results of the reference standard, avoidance of case-control design, and overall risk of bias.

Across analyses, specificity was generally high, with most pooled estimates around 0.85 or higher, and few clear differences between imaging modalities. However, many studies did not report specificity and pooled estimates were frequently imprecise, precluding strong conclusions regarding comparative test performance. Since likelihood ratios are sensitive to small changes in estimates when the specificity is high, it was also difficult to draw strong conclusions regarding comparative diagnostic test performance based on differences in positive or negative likelihood ratios. Most likelihood ratio estimates fell into or near the "moderately useful" range (positive likelihood ratio of 5 to 10 and negative likelihood ratio of 0.1 to 0.2), with the exception of FDG PET for identification of intrahepatic HCC lesions, which was associated with a negative likelihood ratio of 0.50.

Evidence regarding the accuracy of imaging modalities for staging was primarily limited to CT, with 28 to 58 percent of patients correctly staged based on TNM criteria and somewhat more understaging (25% to 52%) than overstaging (2% to 27%) (moderate strength of evidence).

Studies on the accuracy of imaging for identifying metastatic HCC disease were primarily limited to FDG PET or PET/CT, with a pooled sensitivity of 0.82 to 0.85 (low strength of evidence).

Evidence on the comparative effectiveness of imaging for HCC on clinical decisionmaking (including use of subsequent tests, procedures, or interventions) was extremely limited. In studies that compared the accuracy of transplant decisions based on CT against primarily explanted livers as the reference standard, the proportion correctly assessed for transplant eligibility based on Milan criteria ranged from 40 to 96 percent (moderate strength of evidence). Evidence on the effects of surveillance with imaging versus no surveillance on clinical outcomes was limited to a single randomized trial[50] (low strength of evidence). Although it found an association between surveillance with US and AFP and decreased liver-specific mortality, it had important methodological shortcomings, and the trial was conducted in China, potentially limiting applicability to screening to the United States. The trial primarily enrolled patients with HBV infection, who are more likely to develop HCC in the absence of cirrhosis and therefore more likely to be candidates for surgical resection, potentially overestimating survival benefits compared to a United States population.

Evidence on comparative harms associated with imaging was also extremely limited, with no study measuring downstream harms related to false-positive tests or subsequent workup, or potential harms related to labeling or psychological effects. A handful of studies reported low rates of serious direct harms (e.g., allergic reactions) associated with imaging. However, evidence on administration of contrast for radiological procedures in general also suggests a low rate of serious adverse events. For example, a retrospective analysis of over 450,000 doses of low-osmolar iodinated or gadolinium contrast administered at a single center identified a total of 522 adverse events (0.11% of total), with the most frequent adverse events being urticaria (52%) and nausea (18%).[325] Fewer than 100 of the events required further treatment, with use of epinephrine in nine instances. The rate of adverse events was 0.15 percent for iodinated contrast and 0.04 percent for gadolinium, consistent with estimates from other studies.[326-328]

No study of US with contrast reported harms. Potential harms associated with use of microbubble contrast agents were highlighted when the FDA issued a black box warning in 2007 regarding use of perflutren microbubble contrast for cardiac imaging, due to reports of four fatalities due to cardiopulmonary events within 30 minutes of perflutren administration and 11 fatalities within 12 hours.[329] Other studies have attempted to quantify rates of harms associated with microbubble contrast. One study of sulfur hexafluoride contrast for various abdominal applications (23,188 imaging studies) reported 29 adverse events, with two rated serious (0.01%); there were no deaths.[330] A study of 16,025 patients who received perflutren contrast in cardiac imaging reported an overall adverse event rate of 0.12 percent, with a rate of serious adverse events of 0.04 percent and no deaths.[331]

Although PET and CT are associated with risk of radiation exposure, no study of imaging for HCC was designed to evaluate potential long-term clinical outcomes associated with radiation exposure. According to the Radiological Society of North American and the American College of Radiology, abdominal CT with and without contrast is associated with an approximate effective radiation dose of 20 mSv and PET/CT with 25 mSV.[332]

Table 23. Summary of evidence for Key Question 1.a (detection): Test performance

Subquestion	Imaging Modality or Comparison	Strength of Evidence	Summary
Surveillance settings *Unit of analysis: patients with HCC*	US without contrast	Sensitivity: Low Specificity: Low	Sensitivity was 0.78 (95% CI, 0.60 to 0.89; 4 studies) and specificity 0.89 (95% CI, 0.80 to 0.94; 3 studies), for an LR+ of 6.8 (95% CI, 4.2 to 11) and LR- of 0.25 (95% CI, 0.13 to -0.46).
Surveillance settings *Unit of analysis: patients with HCC*	CT	Sensitivity: Low Specificity: Low	Sensitivity was 0.84 (95% CI, 0.59 to 0.95; 2 studies) and specificity 0.999 (95% CI, 0.86 to 0.99; 2 studies), for an LR+ of 60 (95% CI, 5.9 to 622) and LR- of 0.16 (95% CI, 0.06 to 0.47).
Surveillance settings *Unit of analysis: patients with HCC*	MRI or PET	Insufficient	No evidence
Surveillance settings *Unit of analysis: HCC lesions*	US without contrast	Sensitivity: Low Specificity: Insufficient	Sensitivity was 0.60 (95% CI, 0.24 to 0.87; 1 study); specificity was not reported.
Surveillance settings *Unit of analysis: HCC lesions*	CT	Sensitivity: Low Specificity: Insufficient	Sensitivity was 0.62 (95% CI, 0.46 to 0.76; 1 study).
Surveillance settings *Unit of analysis: HCC lesions*	MRI or PET	Insufficient	No evidence
Nonsurveillance settings *Unit of analysis: patients with HCC*	US without contrast	Sensitivity: Low Specificity: Low	Sensitivity was 0.73 (95% CI, 0.46 to 0.90; 8 studies) and specificity 0.93 (95% CI, 0.85 to 0.97; 6 studies), for an LR+ of 11 (95% CI, 5.4 to 21) and LR- of 0.29 (95% CI, 0.13 to 0.65).
Nonsurveillance settings *Unit of analysis: patients with HCC*	CT	Sensitivity: Moderate Specificity: Moderate	Sensitivity was 0.83 (95% CI, 0.75 to 0.89; 16 studies) and specificity 0.92 (95% CI, 0.86 to 0.96; 11 studies), for an LR+ of 11 (95% CI, 5.6 to 20) and LR- of 0.19 (95% CI, 0.12 to 0.28).
Nonsurveillance settings *Unit of analysis: patients with HCC*	MRI	Sensitivity: Moderate Specificity: Moderate	Sensitivity was 0.85 (95% CI, 0.76 to 0.91; 10 studies) and specificity 0.90 (95% CI, 0.81 to 0.94; 8 studies), for an LR+ of 8.1 (95% CI, 4.3 to 15) and LR- of 0.17 (95% CI, 0.10 to 0.28).
Nonsurveillance settings *Unit of analysis: patients with HCC*	PET	Sensitivity: Moderate Specificity: Low	For FDG PET, sensitivity was 0.52 (95% CI, 0.39 to 0.66; 15 studies) and specificity was 0.95 (95% CI, 0.82 to 0.99; 5 studies), for an LR+ of 11 (95% CI, 2.6 to 49) and LR- of 0.50 (95% CI, 0.37 to 0.68). For ^{11}C-acetate PET or PET/CT, sensitivity was 0.85 (95% CI, 0.67 to 0.94; 4 studies); specificity was not reported.
Nonsurveillance settings *Unit of analysis: HCC lesions*	US without contrast	Sensitivity: Moderate Specificity: Low	Sensitivity was 0.59 (95% CI, 0.42 to 0.74; 11 studies). Only 2 studies reported specificity, with inconsistent results (0.63; 95% CI, 0.53 to 0.73, and 0.95; 95% CI, 0.85 to 0.99).

Table 23. Summary of evidence for Key Question 1.a (detection): Test performance (continued)

Subquestion	Imaging Modality or Comparison	Strength of Evidence	Summary
Nonsurveillance settings *Unit of analysis: HCC lesions*	US with contrast	Sensitivity: Low Specificity: Insufficient	Sensitivity was 0.73 (95% CI, 0.52 to 0.87; 8 studies). No study evaluated specificity.
Nonsurveillance settings *Unit of analysis: HCC lesions*	CT	Sensitivity: Moderate Specificity: Moderate	Sensitivity was 0.77 (95% CI, 0.72 to 0.80; 79 studies) and specificity 0.89 (95% CI, 0.84 to 0.93; 21 studies), for an LR+ of 7.1 (95% CI, 4.7 to 11) and LR- of 0.26 (95% CI, 0.22 to 0.31).
Nonsurveillance settings *Unit of analysis: HCC lesions*	MRI	Sensitivity: Moderate Specificity: Moderate	Sensitivity was 0.82 (95% CI, 0.79 to 0.85; 75 studies) and specificity 0.87 (95% CI, 0.77 to -0.93; 16 studies), for an LR+ of 6.4 (95% CI, 3.5 to 12) and LR- of 0.20 (95% CI, 0.16 to 0.25).
Nonsurveillance settings *Unit of analysis: HCC lesions*	PET	Sensitivity: Moderate Specificity: Low	For FDG PET, sensitivity was 0.53 (95% CI, 0.41 to 0.65; 5 studies) and specificity 0.91 (95% CI, 0.76 to 0.98; 1 study). For ^{11}C-acetate PET, sensitivity was 0.78 (95% CI, 0.61 to 0.89; 4 studies); specificity was not reported.
Direct (within-study) comparisons of imaging modalities *Unit of analysis: patients with HCC*	US without contrast vs. CT	Sensitivity: Moderate Specificity: Moderate	Sensitivity was 0.68 (95% CI, 0.54 to 0.80) vs. 0.80 (95% CI, 0.68 to 0.88), for a difference of -0.12 (95% CI, -0.20 to -0.03), based on 6 studies. Two studies were performed in surveillance settings. (Low strength of evidence for sensitivity and specificity.)
Direct (within-study) comparisons of imaging modalities *Unit of analysis: patients with HCC*	US without contrast vs. MRI	Sensitivity: Moderate Specificity: Moderate	Sensitivity was 0.61 (95% CI, 0.48 to 0.74) vs. 0.81 (95% CI, 0.69 to 0.89), for a difference of -0.19 (95% CI, -0.30 to -0.08), based on 3 studies, none of which were performed in surveillance settings.
Direct (within-study) comparisons of imaging modalities *Unit of analysis: patients with HCC*	MRI vs. CT	Sensitivity: Moderate Specificity: Moderate	Sensitivity was 0.88 (95% CI, 0.53 to 0.98) vs. 0.82 (95% CI, 0.41 to 0.97), for a difference of 0.06 (95% CI, -0.05 to 0.17), based on 4 studies, none of which were performed in surveillance settings.
Direct (within-study) comparisons of imaging modalities *Unit of analysis: HCC lesions*	US without contrast vs. CT	Sensitivity: Moderate Specificity: Moderate	Sensitivity was 0.55 (95% CI, 0.43 to 0.66) vs. 0.66 (95% CI, 0.54 to 0.76), for a difference of -0.11 (95% CI, -0.18 to -0.04), based on 3 studies, none of which were performed in surveillance settings.
Direct (within-study) comparisons of imaging modalities *Unit of analysis: HCC lesions*	US without contrast vs. MRI	Sensitivity: Moderate Specificity: Moderate	Sensitivity was 0.57 (95% CI, 0.42 to 0.71) vs. 0.79 (95% CI, 0.67 to 0.88), for a difference of -0.22 (95% CI, -0.31 to 0.14), based on 3 studies, none of which were performed in surveillance settings.

Table 23. Summary of evidence for Key Question 1.a (detection): Test performance (continued)

Subquestion	Imaging Modality or Comparison	Strength of Evidence	Summary
Direct (within-study) comparisons of imaging modalities *Unit of analysis: HCC lesions*	US with contrast vs. CT	Sensitivity: Moderate Specificity: Insufficient	Sensitivity was 0.51 (95% CI, 0.29 to 0.74) vs. 0.61 (95% CI, 0.38 to 0.81), for a difference of -0.10 (95% CI, -0.20 to -0.00), based on 4 studies, none of which were performed in surveillance settings.
Direct (within-study) comparisons of imaging modalities *Unit of analysis: HCC lesions*	US with contrast vs. MRI	Sensitivity: Moderate Specificity: Insufficient	Sensitivity was 0.65 (95% CI, 0.41 to 0.84) vs. 0.73 (95% CI, 0.50 to 0.88), for a difference of -0.08 (95% CI, -0.19 to 0.02), based on 3 studies, none of which were performed in surveillance settings.
Direct (within-study) comparisons of imaging modalities *Unit of analysis: HCC lesions*	MRI vs. CT	Sensitivity: Moderate Specificity: Moderate	Sensitivity was 0.81 (95% CI, 0.76 to 0.84) vs. 0.71 (95% CI, 0.66 to 0.76), for a difference of 0.09 (95% CI, 0.07 to 0.12), based on 31 studies, none of which were performed in surveillance settings. Findings were similar when studies were stratified according to use of nonhepatic-specific or hepatic-specific contrast and when the analysis was restricted to HCC lesions <2–3 cm. For HCC lesions <2–3 cm, the difference in sensitivity was greater for studies of hepatic-specific MRI contrast (0.23; 95% CI, 0.17 to 0.29; 12 studies) than for studies of nonhepatic-specific MRI contrast (0.06; 95% CI, -0.01 to 0.13; 6 studies).
Multiple imaging modalities	Various combinations	Sensitivity: Insufficient Specificity: Insufficient	One study found sensitivity of imaging with various combinations of 2 imaging modalities was similar or lower than with single-modality imaging, based on concordant positive findings on 2 imaging modalities. The other study reported higher sensitivity with multiple imaging modalities than with single-modality imaging, but criteria for positive results based on multiple imaging modalities were unclear.

CI = confidence interval; CT = computed tomography; FDG = ^{18}F-fluorodeoxyglucose; HCC = hepatocellular carcinoma; LR+ = positive likelihood ratio; LR- = negative likelihood ratio; MRI = magnetic resonance imaging; PET = positron emission tomography; US = ultrasound.

Table 24. Summary of evidence for Key Question 1.a.i (detection): Effects of reference standard on test performance (based on HCC lesions as the unit of analysis)

Imaging Modality or Comparison	Strength of Evidence	Summary
US without contrast	Sensitivity: Moderate Specificity: Insufficient	Using HCC lesions as the unit of analysis, sensitivity was 0.34 (95% CI, 0.22 to 0.47) in 5 studies that used explanted liver as the reference standard and ranged from 0.72 to 0.75 in studies that used other reference standards.
US with contrast	Sensitivity: Low Specificity: Insufficient	No study using HCC lesions as the unit of analysis used an explanted liver reference standard. Sensitivity was 0.58 (95% CI, 0.39 to 0.75) using a nonexplant histopathological reference standard and 0.98 (95% CI, 0.88 to 0.997) using a mixed reference standard.
CT	Sensitivity: Moderate Specificity: Moderate	Using HCC lesions as the unit of analysis, sensitivity was 0.67 (95% CI, 0.59 to 0.75) in 23 studies that used explanted liver as the reference standard and ranged from 0.65 to 0.86 in studies that used other reference standards.
MRI	Sensitivity: Moderate Specificity: Moderate	Using HCC lesions as the unit of analysis, sensitivity was 0.69 (95% CI, 0.59 to 0.77) in 15 studies that used explanted liver as the reference standard and ranged from 0.85 to 0.88 in studies that used a nonexplant histopathological reference standard or mixed reference standard; only 3 studies evaluated an imaging/clinical reference standard (sensitivity, 0.65; 95% CI, 0.43 to 0.83).
PET	Sensitivity: Low Specificity: Insufficient	No study of FDG PET used an explanted liver reference standard. Four of the 5 studies that used HCC lesions as the unit of analysis used a nonexplant histological reference standard (sensitivity, 0.49; 95% CI, 0.37 to 0.61).

CI = confidence interval; CT = computed tomography; FDG = ^{18}F-fluorodeoxyglucose; HCC = hepatocellular carcinoma; MRI = magnetic resonance imaging; PET = positron emission tomography; US = ultrasound.

Table 25. Summary of evidence for Key Question 1.a.ii (detection): Effects of patient, tumor, technical, and other factors on test performance

Subquestion	Imaging Modality or Comparison	Strength of Evidence	Summary
Lesion size	US without contrast	Sensitivity: Moderate Specificity: Low	Sensitivity was 0.82 (95% CI, 0.68 to 0.91) for lesions ≥2 cm and 0.34 (95% CI, 0.19 to 0.53) for lesions <2 cm, for a difference of 0.48 (95% CI, 0.39 to 0.57). Sensitivity was 0.09 (95% CI, 0.02 to 0.29; 4 studies) for lesions <10 mm, to 0.50 (95% CI, 0.23 to 0.78; 4 studies) for lesions 10–20 mm and 0.88 (95% CI, 0.66 to 0.96; 4 studies) for lesions >20 mm, for a difference of 0.37 (95% CI, 0.18 to 0.57) for lesions >20 mm vs. 10–20 mm and 0.41 (95% CI, 0.19 to 0.63) for lesions 10–20 mm vs. <10 mm.
Lesion size	US with contrast	Sensitivity: Low Specificity: Low	Sensitivity was 0.94 (95% CI, 0.83 to 0.98) for lesions ≥2 cm and 0.77 (95% CI, 0.53 to 0.91) for lesions <2 cm, for a difference of 0.17 (95% CI, 0.03 to 0.32), based on 5 studies. Three studies found sensitivity of 0.64 (95% CI, 0.33 to 0.87) for lesions 10–20 mm and 0.91 (95% CI, 0.71 to 0.98) for lesions >20 mm, for a difference of 0.26 (95% CI, 0.04 to 0.48).
Lesion size	CT	Sensitivity: Moderate Specificity: Low	Sensitivity was 0.94 (95% CI, 0.92 to 0.95) for lesions ≥2 cm and 0.63 (95% CI, 0.57 to 0.69) for lesions <2 cm, for an absolute difference in sensitivity of 0.31 (95% CI, 0.26 to 0.36), based on 34 studies. Sensitivity was 0.32 (95% CI, 0.25 to 0.41; 21 studies) for lesions <10 mm, 0.74 (95% CI, 0.67 to 0.80; 23 studies) for lesions 10–20 mm, and 0.95 (95% CI, 0.92 to 0.97; 20 studies), for a difference of 0.21 (95% CI, 0.15 to 0.26) for lesions >20 vs. 10–20 mm and 0.42 (95% CI, 0.36 to 0.48) for lesions 10–20 vs. <10 mm.

Table 25. Summary of evidence for Key Question 1.a.ii (detection): Effects of patient, tumor, technical, and other factors on test performance (continued)

Subquestion	Imaging Modality or Comparison	Strength of Evidence	Summary
Lesion size	MRI	Sensitivity: Moderate Specificity: Moderate	Sensitivity was 0.96 (95% CI, 0.93 to 0.97) for lesions ≥2 cm and 0.66 (95% CI, 0.58 to 0.74) for lesions <2 cm, for an absolute difference in sensitivity of 0.29 (95% CI, 0.23 to 0.36), based on 29 studies. Sensitivity was 0.45 (95% CI, 0.34 to 0.56; 20 studies) for lesions <10 mm, 0.78 (95% CI, 0.69 to 0.85; 21 studies) for lesions 10–20 mm, and 0.97 (95% CI, 0.94 to 0.98, 14 studies) for lesions >20 mm (95% CI, 0.94 to 0.98; 18 studies), for a difference of 0.19 (95% CI, 0.12 to 0.26) for >20 vs. 10–20 mm and 0.33 (95% CI, 0.26 to 0.40) for 10–20 vs. <10 mm.
Lesion size	PET	Sensitivity: Low Specificity: Insufficient	For FDG PET, sensitivity was consistently higher for larger lesions, based on 5 studies. Data were not pooled due to differences in the tumor size categories evaluated. Two studies of ^{11}C-acetate PET found inconsistent effects of lesion size on sensitivity.
Degree of tumor differentiation	US with contrast	Sensitivity: Low Specificity: Insufficient	Sensitivity was 0.83 (95% CI, 0.55 to 0.95) for moderately or poorly differentiated HCC lesions and 0.43 (95% CI, 0.15 to 0.76) for well differentiated lesions, for an absolute difference in sensitivity of 0.40 (95% CI, 0.17 to 0.64), based on 3 studies.
Degree of tumor differentiation	CT	Sensitivity: Low Specificity: Insufficient	Sensitivity was 0.82 (95% CI, 0.66 to 0.91) for moderately or poorly differentiated HCC lesions and 0.50 (95% CI, 0.29 to 0.70) for well differentiated lesions, for an absolute difference in sensitivity of 0.32 (95% CI, 0.19 to 0.45), based on 5 studies.
Degree of tumor differentiation	MRI	Sensitivity: Low Specificity: Insufficient	Sensitivity was 0.68 (95% CI, 0.44 to 0.86) for moderately or poorly differentiated HCC lesions and 0.37 (95% CI, 0.17 to 0.62) for well differentiated lesions, for an absolute difference in sensitivity of 0.31 (95% CI, 0.13 to 0.49), based on 3 studies.
Degree of tumor differentiation	PET	Sensitivity: Low Specificity: Insufficient	For FDG PET, sensitivity was 0.72 (95% CI, 0.59 to 0.83) for moderately or poorly differentiated HCC lesions and 0.39 (95% CI, 0.26 to 0.55) for well differentiated lesions, for an absolute difference in sensitivity of 0.33 (95% CI, 0.20 to 0.46), based on 6 studies. In 3 studies of ^{11}C-acetate PET and 1 study of ^{18}F-fluorochorine PET, sensitivity for more well differentiated lesions was not lower than for more poorly differentiated lesions.
Other factors	US	Low	In 2 studies that directly compared US with vs. without contrast, there was no clear difference in sensitivity (-0.04; 95% CI, -0.11 to 0.04). One study that directly compared use of Doppler vs. no Doppler showed no clear effect on estimates of sensitivity. Lesion depth and body mass index had no effect on estimates of sensitivity.
Other factors	CT	Low	Using patients with HCC as the unit of analysis, studies with a contrast rate ≥3 ml/s reported a higher sensitivity (0.87; 95% CI, 0.77 to 0.93; 8 studies) than studies with a contrast rate <3 ml/s (0.71; 95% CI, 0.50 to -0.85; 4 studies). Studies with delayed phase imaging reported somewhat higher sensitivity (0.89; 95% CI, 0.81 to 0.94; 7 studies) than studies without delayed phase imaging (0.74; 95% CI, 0.66 to 0.87; 7 studies). However, neither of these technical parameters had clear effects in studies that used HCC lesions as the unit of analysis.
Other factors	MRI	Low	There were no clear differences in estimates of diagnostic accuracy when studies were stratified according to MRI scanner type (1.5 vs. 3.0 T), imaging phases evaluated (with or without delayed phase imaging), timing of delayed phase imaging (≥120 seconds vs. <120 seconds), section thickness (≤5 mm for enhanced images vs. >5 mm), or use of diffusion-weighted imaging. In studies that directly compared diagnostic accuracy with different types of contrast, hepatic-specific contrast agents

Table 25. Summary of evidence for Key Question 1.a.ii (detection): Effects of patient, tumor, technical, and other factors on test performance (continued)

Subquestion	Imaging Modality or Comparison	Strength of Evidence	Summary
			were associated with slightly higher sensitivity than nonhepatic-specific contrast agents (0.83; 95% CI, 0.75 to 0.90, vs. 0.74; 95% CI, 0.62 to 0.83; difference 0.10; 95% CI, 0.04 to 0.15; 6 studies).
Other factors	PET	Low	FDG PET was associated with lower sensitivity that ^{11}C-acetate PET when either patients (0.58 vs. 0.81, for a difference of -0.23; 95% CI, -0.34 to -0.13; 3 studies) or HCC lesions (0.52 vs. 0.79, for a difference of -0.27; 95% CI, -0.36 to -0.17; 3 studies) were the unit of analysis. FDG PET was also associated with lower sensitivity that dual tracer PET with FDG and ^{11}C-acetate or ^{18}F-choline PET, but evidence was limited to 1 or 2 studies for each of these comparisons. Using patients as the unit of analysis, sensitivity of FDG PET (0.39; 95% CI, 0.24 to 0.56; 8 studies) was lower than sensitivity of FDG PET/CT (0.65; 95% CI, 0.50 to 0.78; 7 studies).

CI = confidence interval; CT = computed tomography; FDG = ^{18}F-fluorodeoxyglucose; HCC = hepatocellular carcinoma; MRI = magnetic resonance imaging; PET = positron emission tomography; US = ultrasound.

Table 26. Summary of evidence for Key Question 1.b (detection): Clinical decisionmaking

Imaging Modality or Comparison	Strength of Evidence	Summary
Effects of different imaging modalities or strategies on clinical decisionmaking	Low	One randomized controlled trial (n = 163) found no clear differences between surveillance with US without contrast vs. CT in HCC detection rates, subsequent imaging, or cost per HCC detected.

CT = computed tomography; HCC = hepatocellular carcinoma; US = ultrasound.

Table 27. Summary of evidence for Key Question 1.c (detection): Clinical and patient-centered outcomes

Imaging Modality or Comparison	Strength of Evidence	Summary
US plus serum AFP	Low	One cluster randomized controlled trial (n = 18,816) conducted in China found screening every 6 months with noncontrast US plus serum AFP vs. no screening in persons 35 to 79 years of age (mean, 42 years) with HBV infection or chronic hepatitis without HBV infection to be associated with lower risk of HCC-related mortality (32 vs. 54 deaths; rate ratio, 0.63; 95% CI, 0.41 to 0.98) at 5-year followup, but was rated high risk of bias due to multiple methodological shortcomings.
US screening at different intervals, mortality	Moderate	Two trials (n = 2,022) found no clear differences in mortality with US screening at 4- vs. 12-month intervals, or at 3- vs. 6-month intervals. One trial (n = 163) found no difference in HCC mortality between surveillance with US without contrast vs. CT, but was underpowered to detect differences.

AFP = alpha-fetoprotein; CI = confidence interval; CT = computed tomography; HBV = hepatitis B virus; HCC = hepatocellular carcinoma; US = ultrasound.

Table 28. Summary of evidence for Key Question 1.d (detection): Harms

Imaging Modality or Comparison	Strength of Evidence	Summary
MRI, CT, US	Insufficient	One study reported no serious adverse events associated with administration of gadoxetic acid for MRI, and 1 study reported no clear differences in adverse events between CT with contrast at 3 ml/s vs. 5 ml/s. No study reported rates of adverse events associated with use of microbubble contrast agents in US, and harms were not reported in randomized trials of screening with imaging.

CT = computed tomography; MRI = magnetic resonance imaging; US = ultrasound.

Table 29. Summary of evidence for Key Question 2.a (evaluation of focal liver lesions): Test performance

Subquestion	Imaging Modality or Comparison	Strength of Evidence	Summary
Evaluation of focal liver lesion *Unit of analysis: patients with HCC*	US with contrast	Sensitivity: Moderate Specificity: Moderate	Sensitivity was 0.87 (95% CI, 0.79 to 0.92; 12 studies) and specificity 0.91 (95% CI, 0.83 to 0.95; 8 studies), for an LR+ of 9.6 (95% CI, 5.1 to 18) and LR- of 0.14 (95% CI, 0.09 to 0.23).
Evaluation of focal liver lesion *Unit of analysis: patients with HCC*	US without contrast	Sensitivity: Low Specificity: Insufficient	Sensitivity was 0.78 (95% CI, 0.69 to 0.86) in 1 study; specificity was not reported.
Evaluation of focal liver lesion *Unit of analysis: patients with HCC*	CT	Sensitivity: Moderate Specificity: Low	Sensitivity was 0.86 (95% CI, 0.75 to 0.92; 8 studies) and specificity 0.88 (95% CI, 0.76 to 0.95; 5 studies), for an LR+ of 7.4 (95% CI, 3.3 to 17) and LR- of 0.16 (95% CI, 0.09 to 0.30).

Table 29. Summary of evidence for Key Question 2.a (evaluation of focal liver lesions): Test performance (continued)

Subquestion	Imaging Modality or Comparison	Strength of Evidence	Summary
Evaluation of focal liver lesion *Unit of analysis: patients with HCC*	MRI	Sensitivity: Low Specificity: Low	Sensitivity was 0.77 (95% CI, 0.66 to 0.84; 4 studies) and specificity was 0.81 (95% CI, 0.52 to 0.94; 4 studies), for an LR+ of 4.0 (95% CI, 1.4 to 12) and LR- of 0.29 (95% CI, 0.21 to 0.39).
Evaluation of focal liver lesion *Unit of analysis: HCC lesions*	US with contrast	Sensitivity: Moderate Specificity: Moderate	Sensitivity was 0.87 (95% CI, 0.80 to 0.92; 21 studies) and specificity 0.91 (95% CI, 0.85 to 0.95; 10 studies) for an LR+ of 9.8 (95% CI, 5.7 to 17) and LR- of 0.14 (95% CI, 0.09 to 0.23).
Evaluation of focal liver lesion *Unit of analysis: HCC lesions*	CT	Sensitivity: Moderate Specificity: Moderate	Sensitivity was 0.79 (95% CI, 0.67 to 0.87; 13 studies) and specificity 0.90 (95% CI, 0.37 to 0.99; 6 studies), for an LR+ of 7.7 (95% CI, 0.71 to 84) and LR- of 0.24 (95% CI, 0.15 to 0.38).
Evaluation of focal liver lesion *Unit of analysis: HCC lesions*	MRI	Sensitivity: Moderate Specificity: Moderate	Sensitivity was 0.81 (95% CI, 0.72 to 0.87; 14 studies) and specificity 0.93 (95% CI, 0.80 to 0.98; 11 studies), for an LR+ of 12 (95% CI, 3.8 to 39) and LR- of 0.21 (95% CI, 0.15 to 0.30).
Evaluation of focal liver lesion *Unit of analysis: HCC lesions*	PET	Sensitivity: Low Specificity: Low	Sensitivity was 0.56 to 0.57 and specificity 1.0 in 2 studies of FDG PET.
For distinguishing HCC lesions from non-HCC hepatic lesions	US with contrast	Sensitivity: Low Specificity: Low	One study found US with sulfur hexafluoride contrast associated with a sensitivity of 0.94 (62/66) and a specificity of 0.68 (23/34) for distinguishing hypervascular HCC from focal nodular hyperplasia using quantitative methods, and 1 study found US with perflubutane contrast associated with a sensitivity of 0.59 (32/54) and specificity of 1.0 (13/13) for distinguishing small (<3 cm) well differentiated HCC lesions from regenerative nodules.
For distinguishing HCC lesions from non-HCC hepatic lesions	CT	Sensitivity: Low Specificity: Low	Five studies evaluated accuracy of CT for distinguishing HCC from non-HCC lesions, but the non-HCC lesions varied in the studies, precluding strong conclusions.
For distinguishing HCC lesions from non-HCC hepatic lesions	MRI	Sensitivity: Moderate Specificity: Moderate	Four studies reported inconsistent results for distinguishing small (<2 to 3 cm) hypervascular HCC lesions from hypervascular pseudolesions, with sensitivity 0.47 and 0.52 in 2 studies, and 0.91 and 0.92 in the other 2. Specificity was 0.93 or higher in all 4 studies. Eight other studies evaluated accuracy of MRI for distinguishing HCC from non-HCC lesions, but the non-HCC hepatic lesions varied in the studies.

Table 29. Summary of evidence for Key Question 2.a (evaluation of focal liver lesions): Test performance (continued)

Subquestion	Imaging Modality or Comparison	Strength of Evidence	Summary
Direct (within-study) comparisons of imaging modalities *Unit of analysis: patients with HCC*	US without contrast vs. CT	Sensitivity: Low Specificity: Insufficient	Sensitivity was 0.78 (95% CI, 0.70 to 0.85) vs. 0.89 (95% CI, 0.84 to 0.95), for a difference of -0.12 (95% CI, -0.21 to -0.02), based on 1 study.
Direct (within-study) comparisons of imaging modalities *Unit of analysis: patients with HCC*	US with contrast vs. CT	Sensitivity: Moderate Specificity: Low	Sensitivity was 0.91 (95% CI, 0.85 to 0.94) vs. 0.88 (95% CI, 0.81 to 0.92), for a difference of 0.03 (95% CI, -0.02 to 0.08), based on 5 studies.
Direct (within-study) comparisons of imaging modalities *Unit of analysis: patients with HCC*	MRI vs. CT	Sensitivity: Low Specificity: Low	Sensitivity was 0.81 (95% CI, 0.70 to 0.92) vs. 0.74 (95% CI, 0.62 to 0.87), for a difference of 0.06 (-0.10 to 0.23), based on 1 study.
Direct (within-study) comparisons of imaging modalities *Unit of analysis: HCC lesions*	US with contrast vs. CT	Sensitivity: Moderate Specificity: Insufficient	Sensitivity was 0.92 (95% CI, 0.88 to 0.96) vs. 0.89 (95% CI, 0.83 to 0.93), for a difference of 0.04 (95% CI, -0.02 to 0.09), based on 4 studies.
Direct (within-study) comparisons of imaging modalities *Unit of analysis: HCC lesions*	US with contrast vs. MRI	Sensitivity: Low Specificity: Low	Sensitivity was 0.79 (95% CI, 0.65 to 0.94) vs. 0.83 (95% CI, 0.69 to 0.97), for a difference of -0.03 (95% CI, -0.24 to 0.17), based on 1 study.
Direct (within-study) comparisons of imaging modalities *Unit of analysis: HCC lesions*	MRI vs. CT	Sensitivity: Low Specificity: Low	One study found MRI associated with higher sensitivity (0.84; 95% CI, 0.76 to 0.92 vs. 0.62; 95% CI, 0.52 to 0.72, for a difference of 0.22; 95% CI, 0.09 to 0.35) but lower specificity (0.36; 95% CI, 0.20 to 0.52 vs. 0.72; 95% CI, 0.58 to 0.87, for a difference of -0.36; 95% CI, -0.58 to -0.15) than CT.
Multiple imaging modalities	Various combinations	Moderate	In 4 studies in which positive results with multiple modality imaging were defined as concordant typical findings for HCC on 2 imaging modalities, sensitivity was lower than with a single modality (difference in sensitivity ranged from 0.09 to 0.27), with no clear difference in specificity. In 3 studies in which positive

Table 29. Summary of evidence for Key Question 2.a (evaluation of focal liver lesions): Test performance (continued)

Subquestion	Imaging Modality or Comparison	Strength of Evidence	Summary
			results with multiple modality imaging were defined as typical findings for HCC on at least 1 of the imaging techniques, sensitivity was higher than with a single modality (increase in sensitivity ranged from 0.09 to 0.25), with no clear difference in specificity. One study found that a sequential imaging strategy in which a second imaging test was performed only for indeterminate results on initial CT increased sensitivity for HCC from 0.53 to 0.74 to 0.79.

CI = confidence interval; CT = computed tomography; FDG = ^{18}F-fluorodeoxyglucose;; LR+ = positive likelihood ratio; LR- = negative likelihood ratio; MRI = magnetic resonance imaging; PET = positron emission tomography; US = ultrasound.

Table 30. Summary of evidence for Key Question 2.a.i (evaluation of focal liver lesions): Effects of reference standard on test performance (based on HCC lesions as the unit of analysis)

Imaging Modality or Comparison	Strength of Evidence	Summary
All	Sensitivity: Moderate Specificity: Moderate	No study used explanted liver as the reference standard. There were no clear differences across imaging modalities in estimates of diagnostic accuracy in analyses stratified by use of different nonexplant reference standards.

HCC = hepatocellular carcinoma.

Table 31. Summary of evidence for Key Question 2.a.ii (evaluation of focal liver lesions): Effects of patient, tumor, technical, and other factors on test performance

Subquestion	Imaging Modality or Comparison	Strength of Evidence	Summary
Other factors	US	Low	In 2 studies that directly compared US with vs. without contrast, US with contrast was associated with sensitivity of 0.89 (95% CI, 0.83 to 0.93) and US without contrast with a sensitivity of 0.39 (95% CI, 0.32 to 0.47), for a difference in sensitivity of 0.50 (95% CI, 0.41 to 0.58). Based on across-study comparisons, there were no clear differences in sensitivity between different US contrast agents; no study directly compared different contrast agents. There were no differences in sensitivity of US based on lesion depth (3 studies) or body mass index (2 studies).
Other factors	CT	Low	Evidence on effects of technical parameters (type of CT scanner, use of delayed phase imaging, section thickness) was limited by small numbers of studies with wide CIs and methodological limitations, precluding reliable conclusions. Two studies found no clear difference in sensitivity of CT for HCC in patients with vs. without cirrhosis.
Other factors	MRI	Low	There were no clear differences in estimates of sensitivity based on the type of MRI machine (3.0 T vs. 1.5 T), type of contrast, use of delayed phase imaging, timing of delayed phase imaging, and section thickness. Estimates were similar when studies that used diffusion-weighted imaging were excluded.

CI = confidence interval; CT = computed tomography; HCC = hepatocellular carcinoma; MRI = magnetic resonance imaging; US = ultrasound.

Table 32. Summary of evidence for Key Question 2.b (evaluation of focal liver lesions): Clinical decisionmaking

Imaging Modality or Comparison	Strength of Evidence	Summary
All	Insufficient	No evidence

Table 33. Summary of evidence for Key Question 2.c (evaluation of focal liver lesions): Clinical and patient-centered outcomes

Imaging Modality or Comparison	Strength of Evidence	Summary
All	Insufficient	No evidence

Table 34. Summary of evidence for Key Question 2.d (evaluation of focal liver lesions): Harms

Imaging Modality or Comparison	Strength of Evidence	Summary
US and CT	Insufficient	One study of US (with and without contrast) and CT reported harms, but did not stratify results by imaging technique. The overall rate of adverse drug-related events was 10%, with all events classified as mild.

CT = computed tomography; US = ultrasound.

Table 35. Summary of evidence for Key Question 3.a (staging): Test performance

Subquestion	Imaging Modality or Comparison	Strength of Evidence	Summary
Staging accuracy, using TNM criteria	CT	Moderate	The proportion correctly staged using TNM or BCLC criteria ranged from 28% to 58%, the proportion overstaged from 2% to 27%, and the proportion understaged from 25% to 52%, based on 6 studies.
Staging accuracy, using TNM criteria	MRI	Low	The proportion correctly staged ranged from 40% to 75%, the proportion overstaged from 3.1% to 31%, and the proportion understaged from 19% to 31%, based on 3 studies.
Staging accuracy, using TNM criteria	PET	Low	One study found 26% of patients were correctly staged with FDG PET and 91% with ^{11}C-choline PET.
Staging accuracy, using TNM criteria	MRI vs. CT	Low	Two studies reported similar staging accuracy.
Identification of metastatic disease *Unit of analysis: patients with metastatic HCC*	PET	Sensitivity: Low Specificity: Low	Sensitivity of FDG PET was 0.85 (95% CI, 0.71 to 0.93; 6 studies) and specificity 0.93 (95% CI, 0.89 to 0.95; 5 studies), for an LR+ of 11 (95% CI, 7.8 to 17) and LR- of 0.16 (95% CI, 0.08 to 0.33). One study that directly compared sensitivity of FDG PET vs. ^{11}C-acetate PET reported comparable sensitivity (0.79 vs. 0.71), although sensitivity was higher when both tracers were used (0.98).
Identification of metastatic disease *Unit of analysis: patients with metastatic HCC*	PET/CT vs. CT	Low	Three studies found no difference in sensitivity (0.82; 95% CI, 0.61 to 0.93 vs. 0.85; 95% CI, 0.66 to 0.95).
Identification of metastatic disease *Unit of analysis: metastatic HCC lesions*	PET	Sensivity: Low Specificity: Insufficient	Sensitivity of FDG PET was 0.82 (95% CI, 0.72 to 0.90; 5 studies). One study that directly compared sensitivity of FDG vs. ^{11}C-acetate PET reported comparable sensitivity (0.86 vs. 0.77).

BCLC = Barcelona Clinic Liver Cancer; CI = confidence interval; CT = computed tomography; FDG = ^{18}F-fluorodeoxyglucose; HCC = hepatocellular carcinoma; LR+ = positive likelihood ratio; LR- = negative likelihood ratio; MRI = magnetic resonance imaging; PET = positron emission tomography; TNM = tumor, node, metastasis staging.

Table 36. Summary of evidence for Key Question 3.a.i (staging): Effects of reference standard on test performance

Imaging Modality or Comparison	Strength of Evidence	Summary
CT, MRI, PET	Sensitivity: Insufficient Specificity: Insufficient	Evidence was insufficient to determine effects of different reference standards on accuracy of staging using TNM criteria or accuracy of PET for identifying metastatic HCC because few studies evaluated alternative reference standards.

CT = computed tomography; HCC = hepatocellular carcinoma; MRI = magnetic resonance imaging; PET = positron emission tomography; TNM = tumor, node, metastasis staging.

Table 37. Summary of evidence for Key Question 3.a.ii (staging): Effects of patient, tumor, and technical factors on test performance

Imaging Modality or Comparison	Strength of Evidence	Summary
CT, MRI, PET	Insufficient	For accuracy of staging using TNM criteria, no study evaluated effects of patient-level characteristics or other factors on accuracy of imaging techniques for staging.
PET	Low	In 1 study that directly compared sensitivity of PET vs. PET/CT for identifying metastatic HCC lesions, there was no clear difference in sensitivity. Four studies of FDG PET found sensitivity increased as lesion size increased, but the number of lesions <1 cm was small (total of 20). Eight studies generally found sensitivity of FDG PET higher for lymph and bone metastasis than for lung metastasis, but samples were small, precluding strong conclusions.

CT = computed tomography; FDG = ^{18}F-fluorodeoxyglucose; HCC = hepatocellular carcinoma; MRI = magnetic resonance imaging; PET = positron emission tomography; TNM = tumor, node, metastasis staging.

Table 38. Summary of evidence for Key Question 3.b (staging): Clinical decisionmaking

Subquestion	Imaging Modality or Comparison	Strength of Evidence	Summary
Transplant eligibility, using Milan criteria	CT	Moderate	The proportion correctly assessed for transplant eligibility ranged from 40% to 96%. The proportion of patients who met transplant criteria based on CT but exceeded criteria based on the reference standard was 3.5% to 7.8%, based on 3 studies. Two studies found that 2.3% and 16% of patients who underwent transplantation based on Milan criteria had no HCC lesions on examination of explanted livers.
Transplant eligibility, using Milan criteria	CT vs. MRI	Low	One study reported similar accuracy.
Transplant eligibility, using Milan criteria	PET vs. CT	Low	One study found ^{11}C-choline PET more accurate than CT (95% vs. 40%).
Use of resection and ablative therapies	MRI vs. CT	Low	One study reported that the proportion of decisions to perform resection or ablative therapies that were classified as correct were similar for MRI (90% and 90%, respectively) and CT (80% and 77%, respectively).

CT = computed tomography; HCC = hepatocellular carcinoma; MRI = magnetic resonance imaging; PET = positron emission tomography.

Table 39. Summary of evidence for Key Question 3.c (staging): Clinical and patient-centered outcomes

Imaging Modality or Comparison	Strength of Evidence	Summary
US with contrast vs. US without contrast plus CT	Low	One cohort study found that contrast-enhanced US identified more small (≤2 cm) HCC lesions than noncontrast US plus CT (36 vs. 31) and was associated with a higher complete necrosis rate following ablation (92%, or 106/115, vs. 83%, or 93/112 lesions; p = 0.036) but was rated high risk of bias. Another study that appeared to be performed in the same series of patients found US with contrast prior to radiofrequency ablation associated with lower local tumor progression rate (7.2% vs. 18%; rate ratio, 0.40; 95% CI, 0.16 to 0.87) and longer tumor-free survival (38 vs. 26 months), but was also rated high risk of bias.

CI = confidence interval; CT = computed tomography; HCC = hepatocellular carcinoma; US = ultrasound.

Table 40. Summary of evidence for Key Question 3.d (staging): Harms

Imaging Modality or Comparison	Strength of Evidence	Summary
All	Insufficient	No evidence

Findings in Relationship to What Is Already Known

Unlike our review, several previously published reviews on detection of HCC and evaluation of focal liver lesions found no clear differences in test performance between US, CT, and MRI for HCC.[333-336] Factors that may explain these discrepancies are: we included more studies than any prior review, separately analyzed studies based on the reason for imaging, stratified studies according to the unit of analysis, and focused on within-study (direct) comparisons of two or more imaging modalities against a common reference standard instead of relying primarily or solely on across-study (indirect) estimates of test performance. Research on meta-analyses of diagnostic tests found that conclusions based on such direct comparisons are often different from conclusions based on indirect comparisons, and may therefore be more suitable for comparing diagnostic tests.[36] In fact, a recently published meta-analysis that focused on direct comparisons was consistent with our review in finding MRI with hepatic-specific contrast associated with higher sensitivity than CT.[337] Our review's findings are consistent with those of previous reviews regarding lower sensitivity of imaging for detection of small and well-differentiated HCC lesions.

Our findings regarding test performance of PET for detection of metastatic HCC are consistent with those from a recently published systematic review and meta-analysis that reported a pooled sensitivity of 0.77.[338] Like our review, a recent systematic review found insufficient evidence to determine effects of surveillance with imaging on clinical outcomes.[339] A systematic review on screening for HCC in chronic liver disease funded by the U.S. Department of Veterans Affairs was conducted at the same time as our review.[32]

Applicability

A number of potential issues could impact the applicability of our findings. Over half of the studies were conducted in Asia, where the prevalence, underlying causes, course, evaluation, and management of chronic liver disease may be different than in the United States. To mitigate potential effects of study country on applicability, we excluded invasive imaging techniques not typically used in the United States such as CT arterial portography and CT hepatic arteriography, as well as imaging techniques considered inadequate in the United States (such as C-arm CT). We also performed stratified analyses focusing on studies performed in the United States and Europe to evaluate effects on estimates of diagnostic accuracy and found no clear effects on estimates.

Imaging techniques are rapidly evolving, which is another factor that could affect applicability. To mitigate effects of outdated techniques on applicability, we excluded imaging technologies considered outdated, such as MRI with magnetic field strength <1.5 T and nonspiral CT, and included only studies published since 1998. We also performed additional analyses on technical factors such as contrast rate, imaging phases evaluated, timing of imaging phases, section thickness, use of hepatobiliary contrast (for MRI), use of diffusion-weighted imaging, and newer technologies such as dual-source or spectral CT. We included studies of US with microbubble contrast even though no agent is currently approved for abdominal imaging in the United States, because efforts to obtain U.S. Food and Drug Administration approval are ongoing and this technique is commonly used in other areas of the world, including Canada and Europe.

As noted above, few studies were performed in true surveillance settings, i.e., in patients at high risk for HCC but not previously diagnosed with this condition. Rather, most studies of test performance that were not performed specifically to evaluate or characterize previously identified lesions were conducted in patients undergoing imaging for other reasons, including series of patients undergoing liver transplantation, surgical resection, or other treatments for HCC. Although such studies are likely to provide some useful findings regarding diagnostic accuracy, results may not be directly applicable to patients undergoing surveillance. In particular, the high prevalence of HCC (many studies enrolled only patients with HCC) could overestimate test performance in true surveillance settings, in which the prevalence of HCC would be much lower.[340]

Implications for Clinical and Policy Decisionmaking

Our review has important potential implications for clinical and policy decisionmaking. Due to the lack of direct evidence regarding clinical benefits and downstream harms associated with different imaging tests for surveillance, diagnosis, and staging of HCC, most decisions regarding use of imaging tests must necessarily be made primarily on the basis of diagnostic test performance. Current guidelines from the AASLD recommend US without contrast for surveillance of HCC in at-risk individuals.[9] Evidence from true surveillance settings to evaluate the comparative test performance of different imaging modalities was very limited. Based primarily on studies conducted in nonsurveillance settings, our study suggests that US without contrast is less sensitive than MRI or CT for detecting HCC. However, findings may not be directly applicable to clinical and policy decisions related to surveillance, as the spectrum of patients evaluated in these studies could have affected estimates of sensitivity. In addition, decisions regarding choice of diagnostic tests to use in surveillance may depend on factors other than diagnostic testing accuracy (e.g., costs) and the weight placed on any gains in sensitivity.

In patients found to have a focal liver lesion on surveillance, our review found high sensitivity and specificity of CT and MRI to further characterize lesions >1 cm in size. The AASLD guideline recommends these modalities for evaluation of focal liver lesions. Evidence is very limited but appears consistent with the sequential diagnostic imaging algorithm as outlined in the AASLD guideline, in which typical findings for HCC on sequentially performed CT or MRI are considered sufficient to make a diagnosis.

Table 24 shows estimated probabilities for HCC following US, MRI, or CT in various scenarios, based on likelihood ratios calculated from pooled sensitivities and specificities. For detection of HCC, in populations with a pre-test probability of HCC of 1 percent, the post-test probability increased to 6 to 10 percent with a positive finding on US with contrast, CT, or MRI, and decreased to 0.17 to 0.29 percent with a negative test. In settings with a pre-test probability of 5 percent, post-test probabilities ranged from 25 to 37 percent following a positive imaging test, and decreased to about 1 percent following a negative imaging test. For evaluation of focal liver lesions, based on a pre-test probability of 10 percent, the post-test probability of HCC increased to 31 to 59 percent following a positive imaging test. Based on a pre-test probability of 25 percent, the post-test probability increased to 71 to 81 percent following a positive imaging test. The post-test probability following a negative test was <3 percent when the prevalence was 10 percent, and 5 to 10 percent when the pre-test probability was 25 percent.

Table 41. Post-test probability of HCC with different imaging modalities in detection of HCC or for evaluation of focal liver lesions for HCC

Imaging Modality	Unit of Analysis	Pretest Probability	Positive Likelihood Ratio	Post-Test Probability of HCC Following a Positive Test	Negative Likelihood Ratio	Post-Test Probability of HCC Following a Negative Test
Detection of HCC						
US without contrast*	Patient with HCC	1%	6.8 (4.2 to 11)	6.4%	0.25 (0.13 to 0.46)	0.25%
		5%		26%		1.3%
US without contrast^	Patient with HCC	1%	11 (5.4 to 21)	10%	0.29 (0.13 to 0.65)	0.29%
		5%		37%		1.5%
CT^	Patient with HCC	1%	11 (5.6 to 20)	10%	0.19 (0.12 to 0.28)	0.19%
		5%		37%		0.99%
CT^	HCC lesion	1%	7.1 (4.7 to 11)	6.7%	0.26 (0.22 to 0.31)	0.26%
		5%		27%		1.3%
MRI^	Patient with HCC	1%	8.1 (4.3 to 15)	7.6%	0.17 (0.10 to 0.28)	0.17%
		5%		30%		0.89%
MRI^	HCC lesions	1%	6.5 (3.5 to 12)	6.2%	0.20 (0.16 to 0.25)	0.20%
		5%		25%		1.0%
Evaluation of focal liver lesions						
US with contrast	Patient with HCC	10%	9.6 (5.1 to 18)	52%	0.14 (0.09 to 0.23)	1.5%
		25%		76%		4.5%
US with contrast	HCC lesion	10%	9.8 (5.7 to 17)	52%	0.14 (0.09 to 0.23)	1.5%
		25%		77%		4.5%
CT	Patient with HCC	10%	7.4 (3.3 to 17)	45%	0.16 (0.09 to 0.30)	1.7%
		25%		71%		5.1%

Table 41. Post-test probability of HCC with different imaging modalities in detection of HCC or for evaluation of focal liver lesions for HCC (continued)

Imaging Modality	Unit of Analysis	Pretest Probability	Positive Likelihood Ratio	Post-Test Probability of HCC Following a Positive Test	Negative Likelihood Ratio	Post-Test Probability of HCC Following a Negative Test
CT	HCC lesion	10%	7.7 (0.71 to 84)	46%	0.24 (0.15 to 0.38)	2.6%
		25%		72%		7.4%
MRI	Patient with HCC	10%	4.0 (1.4 to 12)	31%	0.29 (0.21 to 0.39)	3.1%
		25%		57%		8.8%
MRI	HCC lesion	10%	13 (3.9 to 42)	59%	0.22 (0.15 to 0.31)	2.4%
		25%		81%		6.8%

*Based on studies conducted in surveillance settings
^Based on studies conducted in nonsurveillance settings

Our findings also provide some support for minimal technical specifications for MRI and CT for HCC imaging as suggested in recent guidance, such as those regarding minimum contrast rates and use of delayed phase imaging.[15] Evidence on the potentially superior test performance of MRI with hepatic-specific versus nonhepatic-specific contrast appears promising, although differences were relatively small. Therefore, clinical and policy decisions around use of nonhepatic-specific contrast may be impacted by additional factors other than test performance, such as cost, harms, or convenience. For example, whereas delayed phase imaging with non-hepatic specific contrast should occur within several minutes of contrast administration, maximum increase in liver parenchyma signal intensity with hepatic-specific contrast agents is not achieved until 20 minutes to hours following contrast administration.[341]

Although US with contrast was associated with similar test performance as MRI and CT for evaluation of focal liver lesions, no microbubble contrast agents are currently approved for use in the United States. Although the role of PET is likely to remain focused on identification of metastatic HCC and staging, additional research could help clarify the role of PET with alternative tracers for identification and evaluation of intrahepatic HCC.

Clinicians and policymakers may consider modeling studies to help estimate potential benefits and harms of screening. For models to appropriately inform decisionmaking, however, requires reliable estimates of important input parameters such as subsequent testing, interventions, and associated benefits and harms that occur as a result of imaging. Such data are not currently available.

Limitations of the Review Process

Substantial statistical heterogeneity was present in most pooled analyses of diagnostic accuracy; this situation is common in meta-analyses of diagnostic accuracy.[342-344] As noted in the Cochrane Handbook for Systematic Reviews of Diagnostic Test Accuracy, "heterogeneity is to be expected in meta-analyses of diagnostic test accuracy."[344] To address the anticipated heterogeneity, we utilized random effects models to pool studies and stratified studies according to the reason that imaging was performed and the unit of analysis used. We also performed additional stratified and sensitivity analyses based on the reference standard used, study characteristics (such as country in which the study was conducted, factors related to risk of bias), patient characteristics, and technical factors related to the imaging tests under investigation. As noted previously, results were generally robust in sensitivity analyses, despite the heterogeneity. Due to the relatively small numbers of studies, we were unable to perform meaningful meta-regression. We also focused on evaluations of comparative test performance based on within-study comparisons of imaging modalities, which tended to be associated with less heterogeneity than pooled across-study estimates. A limitation of our analysis of within-group comparisons is that we had to treat the two compared groups as independent, because we had only aggregated data. Individual patient level data would be required to take into account the paired nature of the comparisons. However, such correlations are generally positive and would be expected to result in more narrow confidence intervals. Therefore, results are likely to be informative when differences are detected.

We did not construct summary receiver operating characteristic (ROC) curves. Many of the studies were missing data necessary to construct ROC curves, because they did not report specificity or numbers of true negatives. In addition, the "threshold effect" assumption necessary for valid ROC curves did not appear to be met, as the estimated correlation between sensitivity and specificity was often positive.[40] Also, most studies did not use a ratings scale to classify imaging tests as positive or negative, and the scales that were used differed across studies (e.g., 1-3, 0-4, 1-4, 1-5, and others). When a confidence rating scale was used, the cutoffs did not vary enough to demonstrate a potential threshold effect. We also did not attempt to pool summary measures of discrimination, for several reasons. Some studies reported the area under the receiver operating characteristic (AUROC) curve and others reported the alternate free response operating characteristic (AFROC) curve, and the suitability of pooling such measures is uncertain. In addition, a number of studies that reported the AUROC or AFROC did not report specificity, and it was unclear from the data provided in the studies how the measures were calculated. Finally, it was often unclear whether the AUROC or AFROC was constructed based on different cutoffs for sensitivity and specificity (representing a true area under a curve) or based on a single cutoff for sensitivity and specificity.

We excluded non-English-language articles and did not search for studies published only as abstracts. We did not formally assess for publication bias using statistical or graphical methods for assessing sample size effects, as research indicates that such methods can be seriously misleading.[345,346] Although we found no evidence of unpublished studies through searches on clinical trial registries and regulatory documents, the usefulness of such methods for identifying unpublished studies of test performance is likely to be limited.

Limitations of the Evidence Base

We identified a number of limitations of the evidence base on imaging for HCC. Only one clinical trial with important methodological shortcomings has evaluated clinical outcomes associated with surveillance for HCC in high-risk patients versus no screening,[50] and no trial has compared effects of different imaging modalities for screening. Evidence on effects of imaging on subsequent clinical decisionmaking is also extremely sparse. There is almost no evidence comparing harms associated with different imaging modalities or strategies.

Despite identifying over 200 studies on test performance, we also found important limitations related to these outcomes. Only three studies were rated low risk of bias and 89 studies were rated high risk of bias. Nearly half of the studies did not avoid use of a case-control design, which can result in spectrum bias and inflated estimates of diagnostic accuracy. In addition, nearly half of the studies did not clearly report interpretation of imaging findings blinded to the results of the reference standard test. Many studies did not report specificity, particularly for lesion-based analyses of diagnostic accuracy, perhaps due to the difficulty in defining a "true negative" lesion in such situations. Estimates for pooled specificity were therefore incomplete and typically imprecise, as were likelihood ratio estimates, which are calculated from pooled sensitivity and specificity. In addition, the estimated pooled specificity and likelihood ratios could be biased if studies that did not report specificity differed systematically from those that did.

Other limitations include relatively limited numbers of direct comparisons of diagnostic accuracy between different imaging modalities and techniques (i.e., studies that perform two or more imaging techniques in the same population and evaluate diagnostic accuracy of each technique against the same reference standard). Research has shown that results from such direct comparisons are often different from results based on indirect comparisons (i.e., comparisons of different tests in across studies performed in different populations). Therefore, we focused on results from direct comparisons when possible.

We were unable to evaluate a number of potentially important technical factors in the studies, such as the type of contrast injector and use of bolus-tracking methods for CT; type of contrast injector, use of bolus-tracking methods, spatial resolution, and length of breath hold for MRI; and effects of reader experience and training and transducer frequency for US. Evidence for newer techniques such as spectral or dual-source CT was also limited to only a few studies. For evaluation of the effects of patient and tumor characteristics on measures of diagnostic accuracy, most of the evidence focused on effects of tumor size and degree of differentiation, with very little evidence on patient characteristics such as age, race, sex, severity of liver disease, or underlying cause of liver disease.

Research Gaps

Significant research gaps limit the full understanding of the comparative effectiveness of imaging for surveillance, diagnosis, and staging of HCC. The only randomized trial of effects of surveillance for HCC with imaging on clinical outcomes had important methodological shortcomings and was performed in China, potentially limiting applicability to screening in the United States[50] Although conducting a randomized trial of surveillance versus no screening in the United States could be difficult because screening is recommended in clinical practice guidelines and routinely performed in high-risk patients, randomized trials that compare screening using different imaging modalities or combinations of modalities would be helpful for understanding optimal approaches. In particular, studies assessing clinical outcomes associated with application of the AASLD algorithm versus alternative strategies would be very informative. Potential challenges in conducting such studies include the need to enroll large samples with sufficient statistical power and with lengthy followup.

In lieu of such studies, evidence on effects of alternative imaging strategies on intermediate outcomes such as clinical decisionmaking, subsequent procedures, and resource utilization could also be informative. Such studies could potentially enroll smaller samples than randomized trials to compare screening using different imaging modalities and would probably not require the extended followup needed to assess clinical outcomes.

Although many studies are available on test performance of alternative imaging modalities and strategies, important research gaps remain. Notably, few studies evaluated imaging in true surveillance settings, and evidence on accuracy of imaging for identifying HCC lesions from nonsurveillance settings may not be directly applicable to surveillance due to spectrum effects.

More studies are also needed to clarify the role of promising alternative techniques, such as US with contrast, MRI with hepatic-specific contrast, and PET with alternative tracers, on estimates of accuracy. Research should focus on improving methods for identifying small or well-differentiated HCC lesions, for which imaging remains suboptimal. Two systems (the Liver Imaging Reporting and Data System and the Organ Procurement and Transplant Network/United Network for Organ Sharing Criteria) have been proposed to better standardize methods for scoring findings on CT and MRI to diagnose HCC; additional research is needed to determine how their use impacts estimates of accuracy and to identify potential opportunities for additional standardization.[47,347]

To be most informative it is important for studies to utilize methods for reducing bias in the conduct of studies of test performance, such as avoidance of case-control design and use of methods to insure interpretation of imaging tests blinded to results of the reference standard. Another important shortcoming of the available literature is the failure of many studies to report specificity, resulting in incomplete and less precise estimates. Given the difficulty in defining true negatives for studies that use HCC lesions as the unit of analysis, we suggest that investigators consider routinely reporting results using patients as the unit of analysis, although HCC lesion-based analyses may be reported in addition. Finally, additional studies that evaluate different imaging modalities, techniques, or strategies against a common reference standard in the same population would be more helpful for understanding comparative test performance than studies that evaluate a single imaging modality or technique.

Conclusions

Based on estimates of test performance, several imaging modalities appear to be reasonable options for detection of HCC, evaluation of focal liver lesions for HCC, or staging of HCC. Although there are some potential differences in test performance between different imaging modalities and techniques, more research is needed to understand the effects of such differences on clinical decisionmaking and clinical outcomes.

References

1. Parkin DM. Global cancer statistics in the year 2000. Lancet Oncol. 2001 Sep;2(9):533-43. PMID: 11905707.

2. National Cancer Institute. Liver Cancer. http://www.cancer.gov/cancertopics/types/liver. Accessed on September 21, 2011.

3. Howlader NN, A; Neyman, N; Altekruse, SF; Kosary, CL; Yu, M; Ruhl, J; Tatalovich, Z; Cho, H; Mariotto, A; Lewis, DR; Chen, HS; Feuer, EJ; Cronin, KA. SEER Cancer Statistics Review, 1975-2010. Bethesda, MD: National Cancer Institute; 2013. http://seer.cancer.gov/csr/1975_2010/.

4. Kohler BA, Ward E, McCarthy BJ, et al. Annual report to the nation on the status of cancer, 1975-2007, featuring tumors of the brain and other nervous system. J Natl Cancer Inst. 2011 May 4;103(9):714-36. PMID: 21454908.

5. McGlynn KA, London WT. Epidemiology and natural history of hepatocellular carcinoma. Best Pract Res Clin Gastroenterol. 2005 Feb;19(1):3-23. PMID: 15757802.

6. El-Serag HB. Epidemiology of hepatocellular carcinoma in USA. Hepatol Res. 2007 Sep;37 Suppl 2:S88-94. PMID: 17877502.

7. El-Serag HB. Hepatocellular carcinoma: an epidemiologic view. J Clin Gastroenterol. 2002 Nov-Dec;35(5 Suppl 2):S72-8. PMID: 12394209.

8. Zanetti AR, Van Damme P, Shouval D. The global impact of vaccination against hepatitis B: a historical overview. Vaccine. 2008 Nov 18;26(49):6266-73. PMID: 18848855.

9. Bruix J, Sherman M. Management of hepatocellular carcinoma: an update. Hepatology. 2011 Mar;53(3):1020-2. PMID: 21374666.

10. Cabibbo G, Enea M, Attanasio M, et al. A meta-analysis of survival rates of untreated patients in randomized clinical trials of hepatocellular carcinoma. Hepatology. 2010 Apr;51(4):1274-83. PMID: 20112254.

11. Pons F, Varela M, Llovet JM. Staging systems in hepatocellular carcinoma. HPB (Oxford). 2005;7(1):35-41. PMID: 18333159.

12. Forner A, Reig ME, de Lope CR, et al. Current strategy for staging and treatment: the BCLC update and future prospects. Semin Liver Dis. 2010 Feb;30(1):61-74. PMID: 20175034.

13. Mazzaferro V, Bhoori S, Sposito C, et al. Milan criteria in liver transplantation for hepatocellular carcinoma: An evidence-based analysis of 15 years of experience. Liver Transpl. 2011;17(S2):S44-S57. PMID:21695773.

14. Wilson SR, Greenbaum LD, Goldberg BB. Contrast-enhanced ultrasound: what is the evidence and what are the obstacles? AJR Am J Roentgenol. 2009 Jul;193(1):55-60. PMID: 19542395.

15. Wald C, Russo MW, Heimbach JK, et al. New OPTN/UNOS policy for liver transplant allocation: standardization of liver imaging, diagnosis, classification, and reporting of hepatocellular carcinoma. Radiology. 2013 Feb;266(2):376-82. PMID: 23362092.

16. Seale MK, Catalano OA, Saini S, et al. Hepatobiliary-specific MR contrast agents: role in imaging the liver and biliary tree. Radiographics. 2009 Oct 1;29(6):1725-48. PMID: 19959518.

17. Frydrychowicz A, Lubner MG, Brown JJ, et al. Hepatobiliary MR imaging with gadolinium-based contrast agents. J Magn Reson Imaging. 2012 Mar;35(3):492-511. PMID: 22334493.

18. Altenbernd J, Heusner TA, Ringelstein A, et al. Dual-energy-CT of hypervascular liver lesions in patients with HCC: investigation of image quality and sensitivity. Eur Radiol. 2011 Apr;21(4):738-43. PMID: 20936520.

19. Silva AC, Morse BG, Hara AK, et al. Dual-Energy (Spectral) CT: applications in abdominal imaging. Radiographics. 2011 July 1, 2011;31(4):1031-46. PMID: 21768237.

20. Lencioni R, Piscaglia F, Bolondi L. Contrast-enhanced ultrasound in the diagnosis of hepatocellular carcinoma. J Hepatol. 2008 May;48(5):848-57. PMID: 18328590.

21. Treglia G, Giovannini E, Di Franco D, et al. The role of positron emission tomography using carbon-11 and fluorine-18 choline in tumors other than prostate cancer: a systematic review. Ann Nucl Med. 2012 Jul;26(6):451-61. PMID: 22566040.

22. Li C, Zhang Z, Zhang P, et al. Diagnostic accuracy of des-gamma-carboxy prothrombin versus alpha-fetoprotein for hepatocellular carcinoma: A systematic review. Hepatol Res. 2013 Jul 9 [Epub ahead of print]. PMID: 23834468.

23. Di Tommaso L, Franchi G, Park YN, et al. Diagnostic value of HSP70, glypican 3, and glutamine synthetase in hepatocellular nodules in cirrhosis. Hepatology. 2007 Mar;45(3):725-34. PMID: 17326147.

24. Methods Guide for Effectiveness and Comparative Effectiveness Reviews. AHRQ Publication No. 10(14)-EHC063-EF. Rockville, MD: Agency for Healthcare Research and Quality; January 2014. Chapters available at www.effectivehealthcare.ahrq.gov.

25. Chang SM, Matchar DB, eds. Methods Guide for Medical Test Reviews. AHRQ Publication No. 12-EHC017-EF. Rockville, MD: Agency for Healthcare Research and Quality; June 2012. Available at http://effectivehealthcare.ahrq.gov/ehc/products/246/558/Methods-Guide-for-Medical-Test-Reviews_Full-Guide_20120530.pdf.

26. Imaging Techniques for the Surveillance, Diagnosis, and Staging of Hepatocellular Carcinoma. Research Protocol. Rockville, MD: Agency for Healthcare Research and Quality; 2013. http://effectivehealthcare.ahrq.gov/index.cfm/search-for-guides-reviews-and-reports/?productid=1600&pageaction=displayproduct. Accessed on November 11, 2013.

27. Imaging techniques for the surveillance, diagnosis, and staging of hepatocellular carcinoma. PROSPERO 2013: CRD42013005246 2013. Available from http://www.crd.york.ac.uk/PROSPERO/display_record.asp?ID=CRD42013005246. Accessed on November 11, 2013.

28. Submit Scientific Information Packets. Lencioni R, Piscaglia F, Bolondi L. Contrast-enhanced ultrasound http://effectivehealthcare.ahrq.gov/index.cfm/submit-scientific-information-packets/. Accessed on November 12, 2013.

29. Barr RG. Off-label use of ultrasound contrast agents for abdominal imaging in the United States. J Ultrasound Med. 2013 Jan;32(1):7-12. PMID: 23269705.

30. Greenbaum L, Burns P, Copel J, et al. American Institute of Ultrasound in Medicine recommendations for contrast-enhanced liver ultrasound imaging clinical trials. J Ultrasound Med. 2007 June 1, 2007;26(6):705-16. PMID: 17526602.

31. Nelson TR, Fowlkes JB. Contrast-enhanced ultrasound: an idea whose time has come. J Ultrasound Med. 2007 June 1, 2007;26(6):703-4. PMID: 17526601.

32. Kansagara D, Papak J, Pasha A, et al. Screening for Hepatocellular Cancer in Chronic Liver Disease: A Systematic Review. Washington: Department of Veterans Affairs; January 2014. www.ncbi.nlm.nih.gov/books/NBK222184.

33. Harris RP, Helfand M, Woolf SH, et al. Current methods of the U.S. Preventive Services Task Force: a review of the process. Am J Prev Med. 2001 Apr;20(3 Suppl):21-35. PMID: 11306229.

34. Whiting PF, Rutjes AW, Westwood ME, et al. QUADAS-2: a revised tool for the quality assessment of diagnostic accuracy studies. Ann Intern Med. 2011 Oct 18;155(8):529-36. PMID: 22007046.

35. Fu R, Gartlehner G, Grant M, et al. Conducting quantitative synthesis when comparing medical interventions. In: Methods Guide for Effectiveness and Comparative Effectiveness Reviews. AHRQ Publication No. 10(13)-EHC063-EF. Chapter 9 Agency for Healthcare Research and Quality. Rockville, MD: 2013. Chapter available at http://www.effectivehealthcare.ahrq.gov/.

36. Takwoingi Y, Leeflang MM, Deeks JJ. Empirical evidence of the importance of comparative studies of diagnostic test accuracy. Ann Intern Med. 2013 Apr 2;158(7):544-54. PMID: 23546566.

37. Chu H, Cole SR. Bivariate meta-analysis of sensitivity and specificity with sparse data: a generalized linear mixed model approach. J Clin Epidemiol. 2006 Dec;59(12):1331-2; author reply 2-3. PMID: 17098577.

38. Zwinderman AH, Bossuyt PM. We should not pool diagnostic likelihood ratios in systematic reviews. Stat Med. 2008 Feb 28;27(5):687-97. PMID: 17611957.

39. Trikalinos TA, Balion CM, Coleman CI, et al. Chapter 8: meta-analysis of test performance when there is a "gold standard". J Gen Intern Med. 2012 Jun;27 Suppl 1:S56-66. PMID: 22648676.

40. Chappell FM, Raab GM, Wardlaw JM. When are summary ROC curves appropriate for diagnostic meta-analyses? Stat Med. 2009 Sep 20;28(21):2653-68. PMID: 19591118.

41. Atkins D, Chang SM, Gartlehner G, et al. Assessing applicability when comparing medical interventions: AHRQ and the Effective Health Care Program. J Clin Epidemiol. 2011 Nov;64(11):1198-207. PMID: 21463926.

42. Luca A, Caruso S, Milazzo M, et al. Multidetector-row computed tomography (MDCT) for the diagnosis of hepatocellular carcinoma in cirrhotic candidates for liver transplantation: prevalence of radiological vascular patterns and histological correlation with liver explants.[Erratum appears in Eur Radiol. 2011 Jul;21(7):1574 Note: Grutttadauria, Salvatore [corrected to Gruttadauria, Salvatore]]. Eur Radiol. 2010 Apr;20(4):898-907. PMID: 19802612.

43. Sangiovanni A, Manini MA, Iavarone M, et al. The diagnostic and economic impact of contrast imaging techniques in the diagnosis of small hepatocellular carcinoma in cirrhosis. Gut. 2010 May;59(5):638-44. PMID: 19951909.

44. Serste T, Barrau V, Ozenne V, et al. Accuracy and disagreement of computed tomography and magnetic resonance imaging for the diagnosis of small hepatocellular carcinoma and dysplastic nodules: role of biopsy. Hepatology. 2012 Mar;55(3):800-6. PMID: 22006503

45. Chen MH, Wu W, Yang W, et al. The use of contrast-enhanced ultrasonography in the selection of patients with hepatocellular carcinoma for radio frequency ablation therapy. J Ultrasound Med. 2007;26(8):1055-63. PMID: 17646367.

46. Chen MH, Yang W, Yan K, et al. The role of contrast-enhanced ultrasound in planning treatment protocols for hepatocellular carcinoma before radiofrequency ablation. Clin Radiol. 2007 Aug;62(8):752-60. PMID: 17604763.

47. Fowler KJ, Karimova EJ, Arauz AR, et al. Validation of organ procurement and transplant network (OPTN)/united network for organ sharing (UNOS) criteria for imaging diagnosis of hepatocellular carcinoma. Transplantation. 2013;95(12):1506-11. PMID: 23778569.

48. Trinchet JC, Chaffaut C, Bourcier V, et al. Ultrasonographic surveillance of hepatocellular carcinoma in cirrhosis: a randomized trial comparing 3- and 6-month periodicities. Hepatology. 2011 Dec;54(6):1987-97. PMID: 22144108.

49. Wang JH, Chang KC, Kee KM, et al. Hepatocellular carcinoma surveillance at 4- vs. 12-month intervals for patients with chronic viral hepatitis: a randomized study in community. Am J Gastroenterol. 2013 Mar;108(3):416-24. PMID: 23318478.

50. Zhang BH, Yang BH, Tang ZY. Randomized controlled trial of screening for hepatocellular carcinoma. J Cancer Res Clin Oncol. 2004 Jul;130(7):417-22. PMID: 15042359.

51. Alaboudy A, Inoue T, Hatanaka K, et al. Usefulness of combination of imaging modalities in the diagnosis of hepatocellular carcinoma using Sonazoid(R)-enhanced ultrasound, gadolinium diethylene-triamine-pentaacetic acid-enhanced magnetic resonance imaging, and contrast-enhanced computed tomography. Oncology. 2011;81 Suppl 1:66-72. PMID: 22212939.

52. Bennett GL, Krinsky GA, Abitbol RJ, et al. Sonographic detection of hepatocellular carcinoma and dysplastic nodules in cirrhosis: correlation of pretransplantation sonography and liver explant pathology in 200 patients. AJR Am J Roentgenol. 2002 Jul;179(1):75-80. PMID: 12076908.

53. Catala V, Nicolau C, Vilana R, et al. Characterization of focal liver lesions: comparative study of contrast-enhanced ultrasound versus spiral computed tomography. Eur Radiol. 2007 Apr;17(4):1066-73. PMID: 17072617.

54. Chalasani N, Horlander JC, Sr., Said A, et al. Screening for hepatocellular carcinoma in patients with advanced cirrhosis. Am J Gastroenterol. 1999 Oct;94(10):2988-93. PMID: 10520857.

55. Dai Y, Chen MH, Fan ZH, et al. Diagnosis of small hepatic nodules detected by surveillance ultrasound in patients with cirrhosis: Comparison between contrast-enhanced ultrasound and contrast-enhanced helical computed tomography. Hepatol Res. 2008 Mar;38(3):281-90. PMID: 17908168.

56. Di Martino M, Marin D, Guerrisi A, et al. Intraindividual comparison of gadoxetate disodium-enhanced MR imaging and 64-section multidetector CT in the Detection of hepatocellular carcinoma in patients with cirrhosis. Radiology. 2010 Sep;256(3):806-16. PMID: 20720069.

57. D'Onofrio M, Rozzanigo U, Masinielli BM, et al. Hypoechoic focal liver lesions: characterization with contrast enhanced ultrasonography. J Clin Ultrasound. 2005 May;33(4):164-72. PMID: 15856516.

58. Egger C, Goertz RS, Strobel D, et al. Dynamic contrast-enhanced ultrasound (DCE-US) for easy and rapid evaluation of hepatocellular carcinoma compared to dynamic contrast-enhanced computed tomography (DCE-CT)--a pilot study. Ultraschall Med. 2012;33(6):587-92. PMID: 23154871.

59. Forner A, Vilana R, Ayuso C, et al. Diagnosis of hepatic nodules 20 mm or smaller in cirrhosis: Prospective validation of the noninvasive diagnostic criteria for hepatocellular carcinoma.[Erratum appears in Hepatology. 2008 Feb;47(2):769]. Hepatology. 2008 Jan;47(1):97-104. PMID: 18069697.

60. Fracanzani AL, Burdick L, Borzio M, et al. Contrast-enhanced Doppler ultrasonography in the diagnosis of hepatocellular carcinoma and premalignant lesions in patients with cirrhosis. Hepatology. 2001 Dec;34(6):1109-12. PMID: 11731999.

61. Freeman RB, Mithoefer A, Ruthazer R, et al. Optimizing staging for hepatocellular carcinoma before liver transplantation: A retrospective analysis of the UNOS/OPTN database. Liver Transpl. 2006 Oct;12(10):1504-11. PMID: 16952174.

62. Furuse J, Maru Y, Yoshino M, et al. Assessment of arterial tumor vascularity in small hepatocellular carcinoma. Comparison between color doppler ultrasonography and radiographic imagings with contrast medium: dynamic CT, angiography, and CT hepatic arteriography. Eur J Radiol. 2000 Oct;36(1):20-7. PMID: 10996754.

63. Gaiani S, Celli N, Piscaglia F, et al. Usefulness of contrast-enhanced perfusional sonography in the assessment of hepatocellular carcinoma hypervascular at spiral computed tomography. J Hepatol. 2004 Sep;41(3):421-6. PMID: 15336445.

64. Gambarin-Gelwan M, Wolf DC, Shapiro R, et al. Sensitivity of commonly available screening tests in detecting hepatocellular carcinoma in cirrhotic patients undergoing liver transplantation. Am J Gastroenterol. 2000 Jun;95(6):1535-8. PMID: 10894592.

65. Giorgio A, De Stefano G, Coppola C, et al. Contrast-enhanced sonography in the characterization of small hepatocellular carcinomas in cirrhotic patients: comparison with contrast-enhanced ultrafast magnetic resonance imaging. Anticancer Res. 2007 Nov-Dec;27(6C):4263-9. PMID: 18214030.

66. Giorgio A, Ferraioli G, Tarantino L, et al. Contrast-enhanced sonographic appearance of hepatocellular carcinoma in patients with cirrhosis: Comparison with contrast-enhanced helical CT appearance. AJR Am J Roentgenol. 2004;183(5):1319-26. PMID: 15505297.

67. Goto E, Masuzaki R, Tateishi R, et al. Value of post-vascular phase (Kupffer imaging) by contrast-enhanced ultrasonography using Sonazoid in the detection of hepatocellular carcinoma. J Gastroenterol. 2012;47(4):477-85. PMID: 22200940.

68. Hatanaka K, Kudo M, Minami Y, et al. Differential diagnosis of hepatic tumors: value of contrast-enhanced harmonic sonography using the newly developed contrast agent, Sonazoid. Intervirology. 2008;51 Suppl 1:61-9. PMID: 18544950.

69. Iavarone M, Sangiovanni A, Forzenigo LV, et al. Diagnosis of hepatocellular carcinoma in cirrhosis by dynamic contrast imaging: the importance of tumor cell differentiation. Hepatology. 2010 Nov;52(5):1723-30. PMID: 20842697.

70. Imamura M, Shiratori Y, Shiina S, et al. Power Doppler sonography for hepatocellular carcinoma: factors affecting the power Doppler signals of the tumors. Liver. 1998 Dec;18(6):427-33. PMID: 9869398.

71. Inoue T, Kudo M, Hatanaka K, et al. Imaging of hepatocellular carcinoma: Qualitative and quantitative analysis of postvascular phase contrast-enhanced ultrasonography with sonazoid. Oncology. 2008;75(SUPPL. 1):48-54. PMID: 19092272.

72. Inoue T, Kudo M, Maenishi O, et al. Value of liver parenchymal phase contrast-enhanced sonography to diagnose premalignant and borderline lesions and overt hepatocellular carcinoma. AJR Am J Roentgenol. 2009 Mar;192(3):698-705. PMID: 19234266.

73. Jang HJ, Kim TK, Wilson SR. Small nodules (1-2 cm) in liver cirrhosis: characterization with contrast-enhanced ultrasound. Eur J Radiol. 2009 Dec;72(3):418-24. PMID: 18834687.

74. Kawada N, Ohkawa K, Tanaka S, et al. Improved diagnosis of well-differentiated hepatocellular carcinoma with gadolinium ethoxybenzyl diethylene triamine pentaacetic acid-enhanced magnetic resonance imaging and Sonazoid contrast-enhanced ultrasonography. Hepatol Res. 2010;40(9):930-6. PMID: 20887598.

75. Khalili K, Kim TK, Jang H-J, et al. Optimization of imaging diagnosis of 1-2 cm hepatocellular carcinoma: an analysis of diagnostic performance and resource utilization. J Hepatol. 2011 Apr;54(4):723-8. PMID: 21156219.

76. Kim CK, Lim JH, Lee WJ. Detection of hepatocellular carcinomas and dysplastic nodules in cirrhotic liver: accuracy of ultrasonography in transplant patients. J Ultrasound Med. 2001 Feb;20(2):99-104. PMID: 11211142.

77. Kim PN, Choi D, Rhim H, et al. Planning ultrasound for percutaneous radiofrequency ablation to treat small (≤ 3 cm) hepatocellular carcinomas detected on computed tomography or magnetic resonance imaging: a multicenter prospective study to assess factors affecting ultrasound visibility. J Vasc Interv Radiol. 2012 May;23(5):627-34. PMID: 22387030.

78. Korenaga K, Korenaga M, Furukawa M, et al. Usefulness of Sonazoid contrast-enhanced ultrasonography for hepatocellular carcinoma: Comparison with pathological diagnosis and superparamagnetic iron oxide magnetic resonance images. J Gastroenterol. 2009;44(7):733-41. PMID: 19387532.

79. Kunishi Y, Numata K, Morimoto M, et al. Efficacy of fusion imaging combining sonography and hepatobiliary phase MRI with Gd-EOB-DTPA to detect small hepatocellular carcinoma. AJR Am J Roentgenol. 2012 Jan;198(1):106-14. PMID: 22194485.

80. Lee MW, Kim YJ, Park HS, et al. Targeted sonography for small hepatocellular carcinoma discovered by CT or MRI: factors affecting sonographic detection. AJR Am J Roentgenol. 2010 May;194(5):W396-400. PMID: 20410384.

81. Li R, Guo Y, Hua X, et al. Characterization of focal liver lesions: comparison of pulse-inversion harmonic contrast-enhanced sonography with contrast-enhanced CT. J Clin Ultrasound. 2007 Mar-Apr;35(3):109-17. PMID: 17295272.

82. Libbrecht L, Bielen D, Verslype C, et al. Focal lesions in cirrhotic explant livers: pathological evaluation and accuracy of pretransplantation imaging examinations. Liver Transpl. 2002 Sep;8(9):749-61. PMID: 12200773.

83. Lim JH, Kim SH, Lee WJ, et al. Ultrasonographic detection of hepatocellular carcinoma: Correlation of preoperative ultrasonography and resected liver pathology. Clin Radiol. 2006;61(2):191-7. PMID: 16439225.

84. Liu WC, Lim JH, Park CK, et al. Poor sensitivity of sonography in detection of hepatocellular carcinoma in advanced liver cirrhosis: accuracy of pretransplantation sonography in 118 patients. Eur Radiol. 2003 Jul;13(7):1693-8. PMID: 12835987.

85. Luo BM, Wen YL, Yang HY, et al. Differentiation between malignant and benign nodules in the liver: use of contrast C3-MODE technology. World J Gastroenterol. 2005 Apr 28;11(16):2402-7. PMID: 15832408.

86. Luo W, Numata K, Kondo M, et al. Sonazoid-enhanced ultrasonography for evaluation of the enhancement patterns of focal liver tumors in the late phase by intermittent imaging with a high mechanical index. J Ultrasound Med. 2009 Apr;28(4):439-48. PMID: 19321671.

87. Luo W, Numata K, Morimoto M, et al. Focal liver tumors: characterization with 3D perflubutane microbubble contrast agent-enhanced US versus 3D contrast-enhanced multidetector CT. Radiology. 2009 Apr;251(1):287-95. PMID: 19221060.

88. Luo W, Numata K, Morimoto M, et al. Three-dimensional contrast-enhanced sonography of vascular patterns of focal liver tumors: pilot study of visualization methods. AJR Am J Roentgenol. 2009 Jan;192(1):165-73. PMID: 19098197.

89. Mita K, Kim SR, Kudo M, et al. Diagnostic sensitivity of imaging modalities for hepatocellular carcinoma smaller than 2 cm. World J Gastroenterol. 2010 Sep 7;16(33):4187-92. PMID: 20806437.

90. Mok TSK, Yu SCH, Lee C, et al. False-negative rate of abdominal sonography for detecting hepatocellular carcinoma in patients with hepatitis B and elevated serum alpha-fetoprotein levels. AJR Am J Roentgenol. 2004 Aug;183(2):453-8. PMID: 15269040.

91. Moriyasu F, Itoh K. Efficacy of perflubutane microbubble-enhanced ultrasound in the characterization and detection of focal liver lesions: phase 3 multicenter clinical trial. AJR Am J Roentgenol. 2009 Jul;193(1):86-95. PMID: 19542399.

92. Numata K, Fukuda H, Miwa H, et al. Contrast-enhanced ultrasonography findings using a perflubutane-based contrast agent in patients with early hepatocellular carcinoma. Eur J Radiol. 2014PMID: 24176532.

93. Ooi C-C, Low S-C, Schneider-Kolsky M, et al. Diagnostic accuracy of contrast-enhanced ultrasound in differentiating benign and malignant focal liver lesions: a retrospective study. J Med Imaging Radiat Oncol. 2010 Oct;54(5):421-30. PMID: 20958940.

94. Paul SB, Gulati MS, Sreenivas V, et al. Evaluating patients with cirrhosis for hepatocellular carcinoma: value of clinical symptomatology, imaging and alpha-fetoprotein. Oncology. 2007;72 Suppl 1:117-23. PMID: 18087192.

95. Pei XQ, Liu LZ, Xiong YH, et al. Quantitative analysis of contrast-enhanced ultrasonography: Differentiating focal nodular hyperplasia from hepatocellular carcinoma. Br J Radiol. 2013 Mar;86(1023):20120536 Epub 2013 Feb 7. PMID: 23392189.

96. Quaia E, Alaimo V, Baratella E, et al. The added diagnostic value of 64-row multidetector CT combined with contrast-enhanced US in the evaluation of hepatocellular nodule vascularity: implications in the diagnosis of malignancy in patients with liver cirrhosis. Eur Radiol. 2009 Mar;19(3):651-63. PMID: 18815790.

97. Quaia E, Bertolotto M, Calderan L, et al. US characterization of focal hepatic lesions with intermittent high-acoustic-power mode and contrast material. Acad Radiol. 2003 Jul;10(7):739-50. PMID: 12862283.

98. Rickes S, Schulze S, Neye H, et al. Improved diagnosing of small hepatocellular carcinomas by echo-enhanced power Doppler sonography in patients with cirrhosis. Eur J Gastroenterol Hepatol. 2003 Aug;15(8):893-900. PMID: 12867800.

99. Rode A, Bancel B, Douek P, et al. Small nodule detection in cirrhotic livers: evaluation with US, spiral CT, and MRI and correlation with pathologic examination of explanted liver. J Comput Assist Tomogr. 2001 May-Jun;25(3):327-36. PMID: 11351179.

100. Seitz K, Bernatik T, Strobel D, et al. Contrast-enhanced ultrasound (CEUS) for the characterization of focal liver lesions in clinical practice (DEGUM Multicenter Trial): CEUS vs. MRI--a prospective comparison in 269 patients. Ultraschall Med. 2010 Oct;31(5):492-9. PMID: 20652854.

101. Seitz K, Strobel D, Bernatik T, et al. Contrast-Enhanced Ultrasound (CEUS) for the characterization of focal liver lesions - prospective comparison in clinical practice: CEUS vs. CT (DEGUM multicenter trial). Parts of this manuscript were presented at the Ultrasound Dreilandertreffen 2008, Davos. Ultraschall Med. 2009 Aug;30(4):383-9. PMID: 19688670.

102. Shah SA, Tan JC, McGilvray ID, et al. Accuracy of staging as a predictor for recurrence after liver transplantation for hepatocellular carcinoma. Transplantation. 2006 Jun 27;81(12):1633-9. PMID: 16794527.

103. Singh P, Erickson RA, Mukhopadhyay P, et al. EUS for detection of the hepatocellular carcinoma: results of a prospective study. Gastrointest Endosc. 2007 Aug;66(2):265-73. PMID: 17543307.

104. Strobel D, Raeker S, Martus P, et al. Phase inversion harmonic imaging versus contrast-enhanced power Doppler sonography for the characterization of focal liver lesions. Int J Colorectal Dis. 2003 Jan;18(1):63-72. PMID: 12458384.

105. Sugimoto K, Moriyasu F, Saito K, et al. Comparison of Kupffer-phase Sonazoid-enhanced sonography and hepatobiliary-phase gadoxetic acid-enhanced magnetic resonance imaging of hepatocellular carcinoma and correlation with histologic grading. J Ultrasound Med. 2012 Apr;31(4):529-38. PMID: 22441909.

106. Sugimoto K, Moriyasu F, Shiraishi J, et al. Assessment of arterial hypervascularity of hepatocellular carcinoma: comparison of contrast-enhanced US and gadoxetate disodium-enhanced MR imaging. Eur Radiol. 2012 Jun;22(6):1205-13. PMID: 22270142.

107. Suzuki S, Iijima H, Moriyasu F, et al. Differential diagnosis of hepatic nodules using delayed parenchymal phase imaging of levovist contrast ultrasound: comparative study with SPIO-MRI. Hepatol Res. 2004 Jun;29(2):122-6. PMID: 15163434.

108. Takahashi M, Maruyama H, Shimada T, et al. Characterization of hepatic lesions (≤ 30 mm) with liver-specific contrast agents: a comparison between ultrasound and magnetic resonance imaging. Eur J Radiol. 2013;82(1):75-84. PMID: 23116806.

109. Tanaka S, Ioka T, Oshikawa O, et al. Dynamic sonography of hepatic tumors. AJR Am J Roentgenol. 2001 Oct;177(4):799-805. PMID: 11566675.

110. Teefey SA, Hildeboldt CC, Dehdashti F, et al. Detection of primary hepatic malignancy in liver transplant candidates: prospective comparison of CT, MR imaging, US, and PET. Radiology. 2003 Feb;226(2):533-42. PMID: 12563151.

111. Trojan J, Schroeder O, Raedle J, et al. Fluorine-18 FDG positron emission tomography for imaging of hepatocellular carcinoma. Am J Gastroenterol. 1999 Nov;94(11):3314-9. PMID: 10566736.

112. Van Thiel DH, Yong S, Li SD, et al. The development of de novo hepatocellular carcinoma in patients on a liver transplant list: frequency, size, and assessment of current screening methods. Liver Transpl. 2004 May;10(5):631-7. PMID: 15108254.

113. Wang J-H, Lu S-N, Hung C-H, et al. Small hepatic nodules (≤ 2 cm) in cirrhosis patients: characterization with contrast-enhanced ultrasonography. Liver Int. 2006 Oct;26(8):928-34. PMID: 16953832.

114. Wang ZL, Tang J, Weskott HP, et al. Undetermined focal liver lesions on gray-scale ultrasound in patients with fatty liver: characterization with contrast-enhanced ultrasound. J Gastroenterol Hepatol. 2008 Oct;23(10):1511-9. PMID: 18713302.

115. Xu HX, Lu MD, Liu LN, et al. Discrimination between neoplastic and non-neoplastic lesions in cirrhotic liver using contrast-enhanced ultrasound. Br J Radiol. 2012 Oct;85(1018):1376-84. PMID: 22553290.

116. Xu H-X, Xie X-Y, Lu M-D, et al. Contrast-enhanced sonography in the diagnosis of small hepatocellular carcinoma ≤ 2 cm. J Clin Ultrasound. 2008 Jun;36(5):257-66. PMID: 18088056.

117. Yamamoto K, Shiraki K, Deguchi M, et al. Diagnosis of hepatocellular carcinoma using digital subtraction imaging with the contrast agent, Levovist: comparison with helical CT, digital subtraction angiography, and US angiography. Oncol Rep. 2002 Jul-Aug;9(4):789-92. PMID: 12066210.

118. Yu NC, Chaudhari V, Raman SS, et al. CT and MRI improve detection of hepatocellular carcinoma, compared with ultrasound alone, in patients with cirrhosis. Clin Gastroenterol Hepatol. 2011 Feb;9(2):161-7. PMID: 20920597.

119. Zhou K-R, Yan F-H, Tu B-W. Arterial phase of biphase enhancement spiral CT in diagnosis of small hepatocellular carcinoma. Hepatobiliary Pancreat Dis Int. 2002 Feb;1(1):68-71. PMID: 14607626.

120. Addley HC, Griffin N, Shaw AS, et al. Accuracy of hepatocellular carcinoma detection on multidetector CT in a transplant liver population with explant liver correlation. Clin Radiol. 2011 Apr;66(4):349-56. PMID: 21295772.

121. Akai H, Kiryu S, Matsuda I, et al. Detection of hepatocellular carcinoma by Gd-EOB-DTPA-enhanced liver MRI: comparison with triple phase 64 detector row helical CT. Eur J Radiol. 2011 Nov;80(2):310-5. PMID: 20732773.

122. Baccarani U, Adani GL, Avellini C, et al. Comparison of clinical and pathological staging and long-term results of liver transplantation for hepatocellular carcinoma in a single transplant center. Transplant Proc. 2006 May;38(4):1111-3. PMID: 16757280.

123. Baek CK, Choi JY, Kim KA, et al. Hepatocellular carcinoma in patients with chronic liver disease: a comparison of gadoxetic acid-enhanced MRI and multiphasic MDCT. Clin Radiol. 2012 Feb;67(2):148-56. PMID: 21920517.

124. Bartolozzi C, Donati F, Cioni D, et al. MnDPDP-enhanced MRI vs dual-phase spiral CT in the detection of hepatocellular carcinoma in cirrhosis. Eur Radiol. 2000;10(11):1697-702. PMID: 11097390.

125. Bhattacharjya S, Bhattacharjya T, Quaglia A, et al. Liver transplantation in cirrhotic patients with small hepatocellular carcinoma: an analysis of pre-operative imaging, explant histology and prognostic histologic indicators. Dig Surg. 2004;21(2):152-9; discussion 9-60. PMID: 15166485.

126. Burrel M, Llovet JM, Ayuso C, et al. MRI angiography is superior to helical CT for detection of HCC prior to liver transplantation: an explant correlation. Hepatology. 2003 Oct;38(4):1034-42. PMID: 14512891.

127. Cheung TT, Ho CL, Lo CM, et al. 11C-acetate and 18F-FDG PET/CT for clinical staging and selection of patients with hepatocellular carcinoma for liver transplantation on the basis of milan criteria: Surgeon's perspective. J Nucl Med. 2013;54(2):192-200. PMID: 23321459.

128. Colagrande S, Fargnoli R, Dal Pozzo F, et al. Value of hepatic arterial phase CT versus lipiodol ultrafluid CT in the detection of hepatocellular carcinoma. J Comput Assist Tomogr. 2000 Nov-Dec;24(6):878-83. PMID: 11105704.

129. de Ledinghen V, Laharie D, Lecesne R, et al. Detection of nodules in liver cirrhosis: spiral computed tomography or magnetic resonance imaging? A prospective study of 88 nodules in 34 patients. Eur J Gastroenterol Hepatol. 2002 Feb;14(2):159-65. PMID: 11981340.

130. Denecke T, Grieser C, Froling V, et al. Multislice computed tomography using a triple-phase contrast protocol for preoperative assessment of hepatic tumor load in patients with hepatocellular carcinoma before liver transplantation. Transpl Int. 2009 Apr;22(4):395-402. PMID: 19000231.

131. Di Martino M, De Filippis G, De Santis A, et al. Hepatocellular carcinoma in cirrhotic patients: prospective comparison of US, CT and MR imaging. Eur Radiol. 2013;23:887-96. PMID: 23179521.

132. Doyle DJ, O'Malley ME, Jang H-J, et al. Value of the unenhanced phase for detection of hepatocellular carcinomas 3 cm or less when performing multiphase computed tomography in patients with cirrhosis. J Comput Assist Tomogr. 2007 Jan-Feb;31(1):86-92. PMID: 17259838.

133. Freeny PC, Grossholz M, Kaakaji K, et al. Significance of hyperattenuating and contrast-enhancing hepatic nodules detected in the cirrhotic liver during arterial phase helical CT in pre-liver transplant patients: radiologic-histopathologic correlation of explanted livers. Abdom Imaging. 2003 May-Jun;28(3):333-46. PMID: 12719903.

134. Golfieri R, Marini E, Bazzocchi A, et al. Small ($\leq$ 3 cm) hepatocellular carcinoma in cirrhosis: the role of double contrast agents in MR imaging vs. multidetector-row CT. Radiol Med (Torino). 2009 Dec;114(8):1239-66. PMID: 19697104.

135. Haradome H, Grazioli L, Tinti R, et al. Additional value of gadoxetic acid-DTPA-enhanced hepatobiliary phase MR imaging in the diagnosis of early-stage hepatocellular carcinoma: comparison with dynamic triple-phase multidetector CT imaging. J Magn Reson Imaging. 2011 Jul;34(1):69-78. PMID: 21598343.

136. Hidaka M, Takatsuki M, Okudaira S, et al. The expression of transporter OATP2/OATP8 decreases in undetectable hepatocellular carcinoma by Gd-EOB-MRI in the explanted cirrhotic liver. Hepatology International. 2012:1-7.

137. Higashihara H, Osuga K, Onishi H, et al. Diagnostic accuracy of C-arm CT during selective transcatheter angiography for hepatocellular carcinoma: comparison with intravenous contrast-enhanced, biphasic, dynamic MDCT. Eur Radiol. 2012 Apr;22(4):872-9. PMID: 22120061.

138. Hirakawa M, Yoshimitsu K, Irie H, et al. Performance of radiological methods in diagnosing hepatocellular carcinoma preoperatively in a recipient of living related liver transplantation: comparison with step section histopathology. Jpn J Radiol. 2011 Feb;29(2):129-37. PMID: 21359938.

139. Hori M, Murakami T, Kim T, et al. Detection of hypervascular hepatocellular carcinoma: comparison of SPIO-enhanced MRI with dynamic helical CT. J Comput Assist Tomogr. 2002 Sep-Oct;26(5):701-10. PMID: 12439302.

140. Hori M, Murakami T, Oi H, et al. Sensitivity in detection of hypervascular hepatocellular carcinoma by helical CT with intra-arterial injection of contrast medium, and by helical CT and MR imaging with intravenous injection of contrast medium. Acta Radiol. 1998 Mar;39(2):144-51. PMID: 9529444.

141. Hwang J, Kim SH, Lee MW, et al. Small ($\leq$ 2 cm) hepatocellular carcinoma in patients with chronic liver disease: comparison of gadoxetic acid-enhanced 3.0 T MRI and multiphasic 64-multirow detector CT. Br J Radiol. 2012 Jul;85(1015):e314-22. PMID: 22167508.

142. Iannaccone R, Laghi A, Catalano C, et al. Hepatocellular carcinoma: role of unenhanced and delayed phase multi-detector row helical CT in patients with cirrhosis. Radiology. 2005 Feb;234(2):460-7. PMID: 15671002.

143. Ichikawa T, Kitamura T, Nakajima H, et al. Hypervascular hepatocellular carcinoma: can double arterial phase imaging with multidetector CT improve tumor depiction in the cirrhotic liver? AJR Am J Roentgenol. 2002 Sep;179(3):751-8. PMID: 12185057.

144. Ichikawa T, Saito K, Yoshioka N, et al. Detection and characterization of focal liver lesions: a Japanese phase III, multicenter comparison between gadoxetic acid disodium-enhanced magnetic resonance imaging and contrast-enhanced computed tomography predominantly in patients with hepatocellular carcinoma and chronic liver disease. Invest Radiol. 2010 Mar;45(3):133-41. PMID: 20098330.

145. Inoue T, Kudo M, Komuta M, et al. Assessment of Gd-EOB-DTPA-enhanced MRI for HCC and dysplastic nodules and comparison of detection sensitivity versus MDCT. J Gastroenterol. 2012 Sep;47(9):1036-47. PMID: 22526270.

146. Iwazawa J, Ohue S, Hashimoto N, et al. Detection of hepatocellular carcinoma: comparison of angiographic C-arm CT and MDCT. AJR Am J Roentgenol. 2010 Oct;195(4):882-7. PMID: 20858813.

147. Jang HJ, Kim TK, Khalili K, et al. Characterization of 1- to 2-cm liver nodules detected on hcc surveillance ultrasound according to the criteria of the american association for the study of liver disease: Is quadriphasic CT necessary? AJR Am J Roentgenol. 2013;201(2):314-21. PMID: 23883211.

148. Jang HJ, Lim JH, Lee SJ, et al. Hepatocellular carcinoma: are combined CT during arterial portography and CT hepatic arteriography in addition to triple-phase helical CT all necessary for preoperative evaluation? Radiology. 2000 May;215(2):373-80. PMID: 10796910.

149. Jeng C-M, Kung C-H, Wang Y-C, et al. Spiral biphasic contrast-enhanced computerized tomography in the diagnosis of hepatocellular carcinoma. J Formos Med Assoc. 2002 Aug;101(8):588-92. PMID: 12440092.

150. Kakihara D, Nishie A, Harada N, et al. Performance of gadoxetic acid-enhanced MRI for detecting hepatocellular carcinoma in recipients of living-related-liver-transplantation: Comparison with dynamic multidetector row computed tomography and angiography-assisted computed tomography. J Magn Reson Imaging. 2013 Nov [Epub ahead of print]. PMID: 24259437.

151. Kang BK, Lim JH, Kim SH, et al. Preoperative depiction of hepatocellular carcinoma: ferumoxides-enhanced MR imaging versus triple-phase helical CT. Radiology. 2003 Jan;226(1):79-85. PMID: 12511672.

152. Kawaoka T, Aikata H, Takaki S, et al. FDG positron emission tomography/computed tomography for the detection of extrahepatic metastases from hepatocellular carcinoma. Hepatol Res. 2009;39(2):134-42. PMID: 19208034.

153. Kawata S, Murakami T, Kim T, et al. Multidetector CT: diagnostic impact of slice thickness on detection of hypervascular hepatocellular carcinoma. AJR Am J Roentgenol. 2002 Jul;179(1):61-6. PMID: 12076906.

154. Khan MA, Combs CS, Brunt EM, et al. Positron emission tomography scanning in the evaluation of hepatocellular carcinoma. J Hepatol. 2000 May;32(5):792-7. PMID: 10845666.

155. Kim KW, Lee JM, Klotz E, et al. Quantitative CT color mapping of the arterial enhancement fraction of the liver to detect hepatocellular carcinoma. Radiology. 2009 Feb;250(2):425-34. PMID: 19188314.

156. Kim SE, Lee HC, Shim JH, et al. Noninvasive diagnostic criteria for hepatocellular carcinoma in hepatic masses >2 cm in a hepatitis B virus-endemic area. Liver Int. 2011 Nov;31(10):1468-76. PMID: 21745284.

157. Kim SH, Choi D, Kim SH, et al. Ferucarbotran-enhanced MRI versus triple-phase MDCT for the preoperative detection of hepatocellular carcinoma. AJR Am J Roentgenol. 2005 Apr;184(4):1069-76. PMID: 15788575.

158. Kim SH, Kim SH, Lee J, et al. Gadoxetic acid-enhanced MRI versus triple-phase MDCT for the preoperative detection of hepatocellular carcinoma. AJR Am J Roentgenol. 2009 Jun;192(6):1675-81. PMID: 19457834.

159. Kim SJ, Kim SH, Lee J, et al. Ferucarbotran-enhanced 3.0-T magnetic resonance imaging using parallel imaging technique compared with triple-phase multidetector row computed tomography for the preoperative detection of hepatocellular carcinoma.[Erratum appears in J Comput Assist Tomogr. 2008 Jul-Aug;32(4):615]. J Comput Assist Tomogr. 2008 May-Jun;32(3):379-85. PMID: 18520541.

160. Kim SK, Lim JH, Lee WJ, et al. Detection of hepatocellular carcinoma: comparison of dynamic three-phase computed tomography images and four-phase computed tomography images using multidetector row helical computed tomography. J Comput Assist Tomogr. 2002 Sep-Oct;26(5):691-8. PMID: 12439300.

161. Kim T, Murakami T, Hori M, et al. Small hypervascular hepatocellular carcinoma revealed by double arterial phase CT performed with single breath-hold scanning and automatic bolus tracking. AJR Am J Roentgenol. 2002 Apr;178(4):899-904. PMID: 11906869.

162. Kim YK, Kim CS, Chung GH, et al. Comparison of gadobenate dimeglumine-enhanced dynamic MRI and 16-MDCT for the detection of hepatocellular carcinoma. AJR Am J Roentgenol. 2006 Jan;186(1):149-57. PMID: 16357395.

163. Kim YK, Kim CS, Han YM, et al. Detection of hepatocellular carcinoma: gadoxetic acid-enhanced 3-dimensional magnetic resonance imaging versus multi-detector row computed tomography. J Comput Assist Tomogr. 2009 Nov-Dec;33(6):844-50. PMID: 19940648.

164. Kim YK, Kwak HS, Kim CS, et al. Hepatocellular carcinoma in patients with chronic liver disease: comparison of SPIO-enhanced MR imaging and 16-detector row CT. Radiology. 2006 Feb;238(2):531-41. PMID: 16371577.

165. Kitamura T, Ichikawa T, Erturk SM, et al. Detection of hypervascular hepatocellular carcinoma with multidetector-row CT: single arterial-phase imaging with computer-assisted automatic bolus-tracking technique compared with double arterial-phase imaging. J Comput Assist Tomogr. 2008 Sep-Oct;32(5):724-9. PMID: 18830101.

166. Kumano S, Uemura M, Haraikawa T, et al. Efficacy of double arterial phase dynamic magnetic resonance imaging with the sensitivity encoding technique versus dynamic multidetector-row helical computed tomography for detecting hypervascular hepatocellular carcinoma. Jpn J Radiol. 2009 Jul;27(6):229-36. PMID: 19626408.

167. Laghi A, Iannaccone R, Rossi P, et al. Hepatocellular carcinoma: detection with triple-phase multi-detector row helical CT in patients with chronic hepatitis. Radiology. 2003 Feb;226(2):543-9. PMID: 12563152.

168. Lee CH, Kim KA, Lee J, et al. Using low tube voltage (80kVp) quadruple phase liver CT for the detection of hepatocellular carcinoma: two-year experience and comparison with Gd-EOB-DTPA enhanced liver MRI. Eur J Radiol. 2012 Apr;81(4):e605-11. PMID: 22297180.

169. Lee DH, Kim SH, Lee JM, et al. Diagnostic performance of multidetector row computed tomography, superparamagnetic iron oxide-enhanced magnetic resonance imaging, and dual-contrast magnetic resonance imaging in predicting the appropriateness of a transplant recipient based on milan criteria: correlation with histopathological findings. Invest Radiol. 2009 Jun;44(6):311-21. PMID: 19462486.

170. Lee J, Won JL, Hyo KL, et al. Early hepatocellular carcinoma: Three-phase helical CT features of 16 patients. Korean J Radiol. 2008;9(4):325-32. PMID: 18682670.

171. Lee JE, Jang JY, Jeong SW, et al. Diagnostic value for extrahepatic metastases of hepatocellular carcinoma in positron emission tomography/computed tomography scan. World J Gastroenterol. 2012 Jun 21;18(23):2979-87. PMID: 22736922.

172. Lee J-M, Kim I-H, Kwak H-S, et al. Detection of small hypervascular hepatocellular carcinomas in cirrhotic patients: comparison of superparamagnetic iron oxide-enhanced MR imaging with dual-phase spiral CT. Korean J Radiol. 2003 Jan-Mar;4(1):1-8. PMID: 12679628.

173. Li CS, Chen RC, Tu HY, et al. Imaging well-differentiated hepatocellular carcinoma with dynamic triple-phase helical computed tomography. Br J Radiol. 2006 Aug;79(944):659-65. PMID: 16641423.

174. Lim JH, Choi D, Kim SH, et al. Detection of hepatocellular carcinoma: value of adding delayed phase imaging to dual-phase helical CT. AJR Am J Roentgenol. 2002 Jul;179(1):67-73. PMID: 12076907.

175. Lim JH, Kim CK, Lee WJ, et al. Detection of hepatocellular carcinomas and dysplastic nodules in cirrhotic livers: accuracy of helical CT in transplant patients. AJR Am J Roentgenol. 2000 Sep;175(3):693-8. PMID: 10954452.

176. Lin M-T, Chen C-L, Wang C-C, et al. Diagnostic sensitivity of hepatocellular carcinoma imaging and its application to non-cirrhotic patients. J Gastroenterol Hepatol. 2011 Apr;26(4):745-50. PMID: 21418303.

177. Liu YI, Kamaya A, Jeffrey RB, et al. Multidetector computed tomography triphasic evaluation of the liver before transplantation: importance of equilibrium phase washout and morphology for characterizing hypervascular lesions. J Comput Assist Tomogr. 2012 Mar-Apr;36(2):213-9. PMID: 22446362.

178. Liu YI, Shin LK, Jeffrey RB, et al. Quantitatively defining washout in hepatocellular carcinoma. AJR Am J Roentgenol. 2013 Jan;200(1):84-9. PMID: 23255745.

179. Lu CH, Chen CL, Cheng YF, et al. Correlation between imaging and pathologic findings in explanted livers of hepatocellular carcinoma cases. Transplant Proc. 2010 Apr;42(3):830-3. PMID: 20430183.

180. Lv P, Lin XZ, Chen K, et al. Spectral CT in patients with small HCC: investigation of image quality and diagnostic accuracy. Eur Radiol. 2012 Oct;22(10):2117-24. PMID: 22618521.

181. Lv P, Lin XZ, Li J, et al. Differentiation of small hepatic hemangioma from small hepatocellular carcinoma: recently introduced spectral CT method. Radiology. 2011 Jun;259(3):720-9. PMID: 21357524.

182. Maetani YS, Ueda M, Haga H, et al. Hepatocellular carcinoma in patients undergoing living-donor liver transplantation. Accuracy of multidetector computed tomography by viewing images on digital monitors. Intervirology. 2008;51 Suppl 1:46-51. PMID: 18544948.

183. Marin D, Catalano C, De Filippis G, et al. Detection of hepatocellular carcinoma in patients with cirrhosis: added value of coronal reformations from isotropic voxels with 64-MDCT. AJR Am J Roentgenol. 2009 Jan;192(1):180-7. PMID: 19098199.

184. Marin D, Di Martino M, Guerrisi A, et al. Hepatocellular carcinoma in patients with cirrhosis: qualitative comparison of gadobenate dimeglumine-enhanced MR imaging and multiphasic 64-section CT. Radiology. 2009 Apr;251(1):85-95. PMID: 19332848.

185. Monzawa S, Ichikawa T, Nakajima H, et al. Dynamic CT for detecting small hepatocellular carcinoma: usefulness of delayed phase imaging. AJR Am J Roentgenol. 2007 Jan;188(1):147-53. PMID: 17179357.

186. Mortele KJ, De Keukeleire K, Praet M, et al. Malignant focal hepatic lesions complicating underlying liver disease: dual-phase contrast-enhanced spiral CT sensitivity and specificity in orthotopic liver transplant patients. Eur Radiol. 2001;11(9):1631-8. PMID: 11511882.

187. Murakami T, Kim T, Kawata S, et al. Evaluation of optimal timing of arterial phase imaging for the detection of hypervascular hepatocellular carcinoma by using triple arterial phase imaging with multidetector-row helical computed tomography. Invest Radiol. 2003 Aug;38(8):497-503. PMID: 12874516.

188. Murakami T, Kim T, Takamura M, et al. Hypervascular hepatocellular carcinoma: detection with double arterial phase multi-detector row helical CT. Radiology. 2001 Mar;218(3):763-7. PMID: 11230652.

189. Nagaoka S, Itano S, Ishibashi M, et al. Value of fusing PET plus CT images in hepatocellular carcinoma and combined hepatocellular and cholangiocarcinoma patients with extrahepatic metastases: preliminary findings. Liver Int. 2006 Sep;26(7):781-8. PMID: 16911459.

190. Nakamura H, Ito N, Kotake F, et al. Tumor-detecting capacity and clinical usefulness of SPIO-MRI in patients with hepatocellular carcinoma. J Gastroenterol. 2000;35(11):849-55. PMID: 11085494.

191. Nakamura Y, Tashiro H, Nambu J, et al. Detectability of hepatocellular carcinoma by gadoxetate disodium-enhanced hepatic MRI: Tumor-by-tumor analysis in explant livers. J Magn Reson Imaging. 2013;37(3):684-91. PMID: 23055436.

192. Nakayama A, Imamura H, Matsuyama Y, et al. Value of lipiodol computed tomography and digital subtraction angiography in the era of helical biphasic computed tomography as preoperative assessment of hepatocellular carcinoma. Ann Surg. 2001 Jul;234(1):56-62. PMID: 11420483.

193. Noguchi Y, Murakami T, Kim T, et al. Detection of hepatocellular carcinoma: comparison of dynamic MR imaging with dynamic double arterial phase helical CT. AJR Am J Roentgenol. 2003 Feb;180(2):455-60. PMID: 12540451.

194. Noguchi Y, Murakami T, Kim T, et al. Detection of hypervascular hepatocellular carcinoma by dynamic magnetic resonance imaging with double-echo chemical shift in-phase and opposed-phase gradient echo technique: comparison with dynamic helical computed tomography imaging with double arterial phase. J Comput Assist Tomogr. 2002 Nov-Dec;26(6):981-7. PMID: 12488747.

195. Onishi H, Kim T, Imai Y, et al. Hypervascular hepatocellular carcinomas: detection with gadoxetate disodium-enhanced MR imaging and multiphasic multidetector CT. Eur Radiol. 2012 Apr;22(4):845-54. PMID: 22057248.

196. Park JH, Kim SH, Park HS, et al. Added value of 80 kVp images to averaged 120 kVp images in the detection of hepatocellular carcinomas in liver transplantation candidates using dual-source dual-energy MDCT: results of JAFROC analysis. Eur J Radiol. 2011 Nov;80(2):e76-85. PMID: 20875937.

197. Peterson MS, Baron RL, Marsh JW, Jr., et al. Pretransplantation surveillance for possible hepatocellular carcinoma in patients with cirrhosis: epidemiology and CT-based tumor detection rate in 430 cases with surgical pathologic correlation. Radiology. 2000 Dec;217(3):743-9. PMID: 11110938.

198. Pitton MB, Kloeckner R, Herber S, et al. MRI versus 64-row MDCT for diagnosis of hepatocellular carcinoma. World J Gastroenterol. 2009 Dec 28;15(48):6044-51. PMID: 20027676.

199. Pozzi Mucelli RM, Como G, Del Frate C, et al. Multidetector CT with double arterial phase and high-iodine-concentration contrast agent in the detection of hepatocellular carcinoma. Radiol Med (Torino). 2006 Mar;111(2):181-91. PMID: 16671376.

200. Pugacheva O, Matsui O, Kozaka K, et al. Detection of small hypervascular hepatocellular carcinomas by EASL criteria: comparison with double-phase CT during hepatic arteriography. Eur J Radiol. 2011 Dec;80(3):e201-6. PMID: 20855175.

201. Rizvi S, Camci C, Yong Y, et al. Is post-Lipiodol CT better than i.v. contrast CT scan for early detection of HCC? A single liver transplant center experience. Transplant Proc. 2006 Nov;38(9):2993-5. PMID: 17112883.

202. Ronzoni A, Artioli D, Scardina R, et al. Role of MDCT in the diagnosis of hepatocellular carcinoma in patients with cirrhosis undergoing orthotopic liver transplantation. AJR Am J Roentgenol. 2007 Oct;189(4):792-8. PMID: 17885047.

203. Sano K, Ichikawa T, Motosugi U, et al. Imaging study of early hepatocellular carcinoma: usefulness of gadoxetic acid-enhanced MR imaging. Radiology. 2011 Dec;261(3):834-44. PMID: 21998047.

204. Schima W, Hammerstingl R, Catalano C, et al. Quadruple-phase MDCT of the liver in patients with suspected hepatocellular carcinoma: Effect of contrast material flow rate. AJR Am J Roentgenol. 2006;186(6):1571-9. PMID: 16714645.

205. Sofue K, Tsurusaki M, Kawasaki R, et al. Evaluation of hypervascular hepatocellular carcinoma in cirrhotic liver: comparison of different concentrations of contrast material with multi-detector row helical CT--a prospective randomized study. Eur J Radiol. 2011 Dec;80(3):e237-42. PMID: 21067880.

206. Sun HY, Lee JM, Shin CI, et al. Gadoxetic acid-enhanced magnetic resonance imaging for differentiating small hepatocellular carcinomas ($\leq$ 2 cm in diameter) from arterial enhancing pseudolesions: special emphasis on hepatobiliary phase imaging. Invest Radiol. 2010 Feb;45(2):96-103. PMID: 20057319.

207. Toyota N, Nakamura Y, Hieda M, et al. Diagnostic capability of gadoxetate disodium-enhanced liver MRI for diagnosis of hepatocellular carcinoma: Comparison with multi-detector CT. Hiroshima J Med Sci. 2013;62(3):55-61. PMID: 24279123.

208. Valls C, Cos M, Figueras J, et al. Pretransplantation diagnosis and staging of hepatocellular carcinoma in patients with cirrhosis: value of dual-phase helical CT. AJR Am J Roentgenol. 2004 Apr;182(4):1011-7. PMID: 15039179.

209. Wagnetz U, Atri M, Massey C, et al. Intraoperative ultrasound of the liver in primary and secondary hepatic malignancies: comparison with preoperative 1.5-T MRI and 64-MDCT. AJR Am J Roentgenol. 2011 Mar;196(3):562-8. PMID: 21343497.

210. Xiao X-g, Han X, Shan W-d, et al. Multi-slice CT angiography by triple-phase enhancement in preoperative evaluation of hepatocellular carcinoma. Chin Med J (Engl). 2005 May 20;118(10):844-9. PMID: 15989766.

211. Yan FH, Shen JZ, Li RC, et al. Enhancement patterns of small hepatocellular carcinoma shown by dynamic MRI and CT. Hepatobiliary Pancreat Dis Int. 2002 Aug;1(3):420-4. PMID: 14607719.

212. Yoo SH, Choi JY, Jang JW, et al. Gd-EOB-DTPA-enhanced MRI is better than MDCT in decision making of curative treatment for hepatocellular carcinoma. Ann Surg Oncol. 2013;20(9):2893-900. PMID: 23649931.

213. Yu Y, He N, Sun K, et al. Differentiating hepatocellular carcinoma from angiomyolipoma of the liver with CT spectral imaging: A preliminary study. Clin Radiol. 2013;68(9):e491-e7. PMID: 23702491.

214. Yu Y, Lin X, Chen K, et al. Hepatocellular carcinoma and focal nodular hyperplasia of the liver: differentiation with CT spectral imaging. Eur Radiol. 2013 Jun;23(6):1660-8 Epub 2013 Jan 10. PMID: 23306709.

215. Yukisawa S, Okugawa H, Masuya Y, et al. Multidetector helical CT plus superparamagnetic iron oxide-enhanced MR imaging for focal hepatic lesions in cirrhotic liver: a comparison with multi-phase CT during hepatic arteriography. Eur J Radiol. 2007 Feb;61(2):279-89. PMID: 17070663.

216. Zacherl J, Pokieser P, Wrba F, et al. Accuracy of multiphasic helical computed tomography and intraoperative sonography in patients undergoing orthotopic liver transplantation for hepatoma: what is the truth? Ann Surg. 2002 Apr;235(4):528-32. PMID: 11923609.

217. Zhao H, Yao JL, Han MJ, et al. Multiphase hepatic scans with multirow-detector helical CT in detection of hypervascular hepatocellular carcinoma. Hepatobiliary Pancreat Dis Int. 2004 May;3(2):204-8. PMID: 15138110.

218. Zhao H, Yao J-L, Wang Y, et al. Detection of small hepatocellular carcinoma: comparison of dynamic enhancement magnetic resonance imaging and multiphase multirow-detector helical CT scanning. World J Gastroenterol. 2007 Feb 28;13(8):1252-6. PMID: 17451209.

219. Zhao H, Zhou K-R, Yan F-H. Role of multiphase scans by multirow-detector helical CT in detecting small hepatocellular carcinoma. World J Gastroenterol. 2003 Oct;9(10):2198-201. PMID: 14562377.

220. Zheng X-H, Guan Y-S, Zhou X-P, et al. Detection of hypervascular hepatocellular carcinoma: Comparison of multi-detector CT with digital subtraction angiography and Lipiodol CT. World J Gastroenterol. 2005 Jan 14;11(2):200-3. PMID: 15633215.

221. Ahn SS, Kim M-J, Lim JS, et al. Added value of gadoxetic acid-enhanced hepatobiliary phase MR imaging in the diagnosis of hepatocellular carcinoma. Radiology. 2010 May;255(2):459-66. PMID: 20413759.

222. An C, Park MS, Kim D, et al. Added value of subtraction imaging in detecting arterial enhancement in small (<3 cm) hepatic nodules on dynamic contrast-enhanced MRI in patients at high risk of hepatocellular carcinoma. Eur Radiol. 2013;23:924-30. PMID: 23138382.

223. An C, Park M-S, Jeon H-M, et al. Prediction of the histopathological grade of hepatocellular carcinoma using qualitative diffusion-weighted, dynamic, and hepatobiliary phase MRI. Eur Radiol. 2012 Aug;22(8):1701-8. PMID: 22434421.

224. Baird AJ, Amos GJ, Saad NF, et al. Retrospective audit to determine the diagnostic accuracy of Primovist-enhanced MRI in the detection of hepatocellular carcinoma in cirrhosis with explant histopathology correlation. J Med Imaging Radiat Oncol. 2013;57(3):314-20. PMID: 23721140.

225. Cereser L, Furlan A, Bagatto D, et al. Comparison of portal venous and delayed phases of gadolinium-enhanced magnetic resonance imaging study of cirrhotic liver for the detection of contrast washout of hypervascular hepatocellular carcinoma. J Comput Assist Tomogr. 2010;34(5):706-11. PMID: 20861773.

226. Choi D, Kim SH, Lim JH, et al. Detection of hepatocellular carcinoma: combined T2-weighted and dynamic gadolinium-enhanced MRI versus combined CT during arterial portography and CT hepatic arteriography. J Comput Assist Tomogr. 2001 Sep-Oct;25(5):777-85. PMID: 11584240.

227. Choi SH, Lee JM, Yu NC, et al. Hepatocellular carcinoma in liver transplantation candidates: detection with gadobenate dimeglumine-enhanced MRI. AJR Am J Roentgenol. 2008 Aug;191(2):529-36. PMID: 18647927.

228. Chou C-T, Chen R-C, Chen W-T, et al. Characterization of hyperintense nodules on T1-weighted liver magnetic resonance imaging: comparison of Ferucarbotran-enhanced MRI with accumulation-phase FS-T1WI and gadolinium-enhanced MRI. J Chin Med Assoc. 2011 Feb;74(2):62-8. PMID: 21354082.

229. Chung J, Yu J-S, Kim DJ, et al. Hypervascular hepatocellular carcinoma in the cirrhotic liver: diffusion-weighted imaging versus superparamagnetic iron oxide-enhanced MRI. Magn Reson Imaging. 2011 Nov;29(9):1235-43. PMID: 21907517.

230. Chung S-H, Kim M-J, Choi J-Y, et al. Comparison of two different injection rates of gadoxetic acid for arterial phase MRI of the liver. J Magn Reson Imaging. 2010 Feb;31(2):365-72. PMID: 20099350.

231. Filippone A, Cianci R, Patriarca G, et al. The Value of Gadoxetic Acid-Enhanced Hepatospecific Phase MR Imaging for Characterization of Hepatocellular Nodules in the Cirrhotic Liver. European Journal of Clinical & Medical Oncology. 2010;2(4):1-8. PMID: 69823585.

232. Gatto A, De Gaetano AM, Giuga M, et al. Differentiating hepatocellular carcinoma from dysplastic nodules at gadobenate dimeglumine-enhanced hepatobiliary-phase magnetic resonance imaging. Abdom Imaging. 2013;38(4):736-44. PMID: 22986351.

233. Goshima S, Kanematsu M, Matsuo M, et al. Nodule-in-nodule appearance of hepatocellular carcinomas: comparison of gadolinium-enhanced and ferumoxides-enhanced magnetic resonance imaging. J Magn Reson Imaging. 2004 Aug;20(2):250-5. PMID: 15269950.

234. Guo L, Liang C, Yu T, et al. 3 T MRI of hepatocellular carcinomas in patients with cirrhosis: does T2-weighted imaging provide added value? Clin Radiol. 2012 Apr;67(4):319-28. PMID: 22099524.

235. Hardie AD, Kizziah MK, Boulter DJ. Diagnostic accuracy of diffusion-weighted MRI for identifying hepatocellular carcinoma with liver explant correlation. J Med Imaging Radiat Oncol. 2011 Aug;55(4):362-7. PMID: 21843170.

236. Hardie AD, Kizziah MK, Rissing MS. Can the patient with cirrhosis be imaged for hepatocellular carcinoma without gadolinium?: Comparison of combined T2-weighted, T2*-weighted, and diffusion-weighted MRI with gadolinium-enhanced MRI using liver explantation standard. J Comput Assist Tomogr. 2011 Nov-Dec;35(6):711-5. PMID: 22082541.

237. Hardie AD, Nance JW, Boulter DJ, et al. Assessment of the diagnostic accuracy of T2*-weighted MR imaging for identifying hepatocellular carcinoma with liver explant correlation. Eur J Radiol. 2011 Dec;80(3):e249-52. PMID: 21112710.

238. Hecht EM, Holland AE, Israel GM, et al. Hepatocellular carcinoma in the cirrhotic liver: gadolinium-enhanced 3D T1-weighted MR imaging as a stand-alone sequence for diagnosis. Radiology. 2006 May;239(2):438-47. PMID: 16641353.

239. Ito K, Fujita T, Shimizu A, et al. Multiarterial phase dynamic MRI of small early enhancing hepatic lesions in cirrhosis or chronic hepatitis: Differentiating between hypervascular hepatocellular carcinomas and pseudolesions. AJR Am J Roentgenol. 2004;183(3):699-705. PMID: 15333358.

240. Jeong MG, Yu JS, Kim KW, et al. Early homogeneously enhancing hemangioma versus hepatocellular carcinoma: differentiation using quantitative analysis of multiphasic dynamic magnetic resonance imaging. Yonsei Med J. 1999 Jun;40(3):248-55. PMID: 10412337.

241. Jeong WK, Byun JH, Lee SS, et al. Gadobenate dimeglumine-enhanced liver MR imaging in cirrhotic patients: quantitative and qualitative comparison of 1-hour and 3-hour delayed images. J Magn Reson Imaging. 2011 Apr;33(4):889-97. PMID: 21448954.

242. Jin Y, Nah S, Lee J, et al. Utility of Adding Primovist Magnetic Resonance Imaging to Analysis of Hepatocellular Carcinoma by Liver Dynamic Computed Tomography. Clin Gastroenterol Hepatol. 2013;11(2):187-92. PMID: 23142203.

243. Kamura T, Kimura M, Sakai K, et al. Small hypervascular hepatocellular carcinoma versus hypervascular pseudolesions: Differential diagnosis on MRI. Abdom Imaging. 2002;27(3):315-24. PMID: 12173363.

244. Kim AY, Kim YK, Lee MW, et al. Detection of hepatocellular carcinoma in gadoxetic acid-enhanced MRI and diffusion-weighted MRI with respect to the severity of liver cirrhosis. Acta Radiol. 2012 Oct 1;53(8):830-8. PMID: 22847903.

245. Kim DJ, Yu JS, Kim JH, et al. Small hypervascular hepatocellular carcinomas: value of diffusion-weighted imaging compared with "washout" appearance on dynamic MRI. Br J Radiol. 2012 Oct;85(1018):e879-86. PMID: 22573299.

246. Kim M-J, Lee M, Choi J-Y, et al. Imaging features of small hepatocellular carcinomas with microvascular invasion on gadoxetic acid-enhanced MR imaging. Eur J Radiol. 2012 Oct;81(10):2507-12. PMID: 22137613.

247. Kim TK, Lee KH, Jang H-J, et al. Analysis of gadobenate dimeglumine-enhanced MR findings for characterizing small (1-2-cm) hepatic nodules in patients at high risk for hepatocellular carcinoma. Radiology. 2011 Jun;259(3):730-8. PMID: 21364083.

248. Kim YK, Kim CS, Han YM, et al. Detection of liver malignancy with gadoxetic acid-enhanced MRI: is addition of diffusion-weighted MRI beneficial?.[Erratum appears in Clin Radiol. 2011 Oct;66(10):1006]. Clin Radiol. 2011 Jun;66(6):489-96. PMID: 21367403.

249. Kim YK, Kim CS, Han YM, et al. Detection of small hepatocellular carcinoma: can gadoxetic acid-enhanced magnetic resonance imaging replace combining gadopentetate dimeglumine-enhanced and superparamagnetic iron oxide-enhanced magnetic resonance imaging? Invest Radiol. 2010 Nov;45(11):740-6. PMID: 20644488.

250. Kim YK, Kim CS, Han YM, et al. Comparison of gadoxetic acid-enhanced MRI and superparamagnetic iron oxide-enhanced MRI for the detection of hepatocellular carcinoma. Clin Radiol. 2010 May;65(5):358-65. PMID: 20380933.

251. Kim YK, Kim CS, Han YM, et al. Detection of small hepatocellular carcinoma: intraindividual comparison of gadoxetic acid-enhanced MRI at 3.0 and 1.5 T.[Erratum appears in Invest Radiol. 2011 Sep;46(9):600]. Invest Radiol. 2011 Jun;46(6):383-9. PMID: 21467946.

252. Kim YK, Kim CS, Kwak HS, et al. Three-dimensional dynamic liver MR imaging using sensitivity encoding for detection of hepatocellular carcinomas: comparison with superparamagnetic iron oxide-enhanced mr imaging. J Magn Reson Imaging. 2004 Nov;20(5):826-37. PMID: 15503325.

253. Kim YK, Kim CS, Lee YH, et al. Comparison of superparamagnetic iron oxide-enhanced and gadobenate dimeglumine-enhanced dynamic MRI for detection of small hepatocellular carcinomas. AJR Am J Roentgenol. 2004 May;182(5):1217-23. PMID: 15100122.

254. Kim YK, Kwak HS, Han YM, et al. Usefulness of combining sequentially acquired gadobenate dimeglumine-enhanced magnetic resonance imaging and resovist-enhanced magnetic resonance imaging for the detection of hepatocellular carcinoma: comparison with computed tomography hepatic arteriography and computed tomography arterioportography using 16-slice multidetector computed tomography. J Comput Assist Tomogr. 2007 Sep-Oct;31(5):702-11. PMID: 17895780.

255. Kim YK, Lee YH, Kim CS, et al. Added diagnostic value of T2-weighted MR imaging to gadolinium-enhanced three-dimensional dynamic MR imaging for the detection of small hepatocellular carcinomas. Eur J Radiol. 2008 Aug;67(2):304-10. PMID: 17714904.

256. Kim YK, Lee YH, Kim CS, et al. Double-dose 1.0-M gadobutrol versus standard-dose 0.5-M gadopentetate dimeglumine in revealing small hypervascular hepatocellular carcinomas. Eur Radiol. 2008 Jan;18(1):70-7. PMID: 17404740.

257. Kondo H, Kanematsu M, Itoh K, et al. Does T2-weighted MR imaging improve preoperative detection of malignant hepatic tumors? Observer performance study in 49 surgically proven cases. Magn Reson Imaging. 2005 Jan;23(1):89-95. PMID: 15733793.

258. Koushima Y, Ebara M, Fukuda H, et al. Small hepatocellular carcinoma: assessment with T1-weighted spin-echo magnetic resonance imaging with and without fat suppression. Eur J Radiol. 2002 Jan;41(1):34-41. PMID: 11750150.

259. Krinsky GA, Lee VS, Theise ND, et al. Transplantation for hepatocellular carcinoma and cirrhosis: Sensitivity of magnetic resonance imaging. Liver Transpl. 2002;8(12):1156-64. PMID: 12474156.

260. Krinsky GA, Lee VS, Theise ND, et al. Hepatocellular carcinoma and dysplastic nodules in patients with cirrhosis: prospective diagnosis with MR imaging and explantation correlation. Radiology. 2001 May;219(2):445-54. PMID: 11323471.

261. Kwak H-S, Lee J-M, Kim C-S. Preoperative detection of hepatocellular carcinoma: comparison of combined contrast-enhanced MR imaging and combined CT during arterial portography and CT hepatic arteriography. Eur Radiol. 2004 Mar;14(3):447-57. PMID: 14531005.

262. Kwak H-S, Lee J-M, Kim Y-K, et al. Detection of hepatocellular carcinoma: comparison of ferumoxides-enhanced and gadolinium-enhanced dynamic three-dimensional volume interpolated breath-hold MR imaging. Eur Radiol. 2005 Jan;15(1):140-7. PMID: 15449000.

263. Lauenstein TC, Salman K, Morreira R, et al. Gadolinium-enhanced MRI for tumor surveillance before liver transplantation: center-based experience. AJR Am J Roentgenol. 2007 Sep;189(3):663-70. PMID: 17715115.

264. Lee JY, Kim SH, Jeon YH, et al. Ferucarbotran-enhanced magnetic resonance imaging versus gadoxetic acid-enhanced magnetic resonance imaging for the preoperative detection of hepatocellular carcinoma: initial experience. J Comput Assist Tomogr. 2010 Jan;34(1):127-34. PMID: 20118735.

265. Lee MH, Kim SH, Park MJ, et al. Gadoxetic acid-enhanced hepatobiliary phase MRI and high-b-value diffusion-weighted imaging to distinguish well-differentiated hepatocellular carcinomas from benign nodules in patients with chronic liver disease. AJR Am J Roentgenol. 2011 Nov;197(5):W868-75. PMID: 22021534.

266. Marrero JA, Hussain HK, Nghiem HV, et al. Improving the prediction of hepatocellular carcinoma in cirrhotic patients with an arterially-enhancing liver mass. Liver Transpl. 2005 Mar;11(3):281-9. PMID: 15719410.

267. Matsuo M, Kanematsu M, Itoh K, et al. Detection of malignant hepatic tumors: comparison of gadolinium-and ferumoxide-enhanced MR imaging. AJR Am J Roentgenol. 2001 Sep;177(3):637-43. PMID: 11517061.

268. Mori K, Yoshioka H, Takahashi N, et al. Triple arterial phase dynamic MRI with sensitivity encoding for hypervascular hepatocellular carcinoma: comparison of the diagnostic accuracy among the early, middle, late, and whole triple arterial phase imaging. AJR Am J Roentgenol. 2005 Jan;184(1):63-9. PMID: 15615952.

269. Motosugi U, Ichikawa T, Sou H, et al. Distinguishing hypervascular pseudolesions of the liver from hypervascular hepatocellular carcinomas with gadoxetic acid-enhanced MR imaging. Radiology. 2010 Jul;256(1):151-8. PMID: 20574092.

270. Ooka Y, Kanai F, Okabe S, et al. Gadoxetic acid-enhanced MRI compared with CT during angiography in the diagnosis of hepatocellular carcinoma. Magn Reson Imaging. 2013;31(5):748-54 Epub 2012 Dec 5. PMID: 23218794.

271. Park G, Kim YK, Kim CS, et al. Diagnostic efficacy of gadoxetic acid-enhanced MRI in the detection of hepatocellular carcinomas: comparison with gadopentetate dimeglumine. Br J Radiol. 2010 Dec;83(996):1010-6. PMID: 20682591.

272. Park MJ, Kim YK, Lee MH, et al. Validation of diagnostic criteria using gadoxetic acid-enhanced and diffusion-weighted MR imaging for small hepatocellular carcinoma (≤ 2.0 cm) in patients with hepatitis-induced liver cirrhosis. Acta Radiol. 2013;54(2):127-36. PMID: 23148300.

273. Park M-S, Kim S, Patel J, et al. Hepatocellular carcinoma: detection with diffusion-weighted versus contrast-enhanced magnetic resonance imaging in pretransplant patients. Hepatology. 2012 Jul;56(1):140-8. PMID: 22370974.

274. Park Y, Kim SH, Kim SH, et al. Gadoxetic acid (Gd-EOB-DTPA)-enhanced MRI versus gadobenate dimeglumine (Gd-BOPTA)-enhanced MRI for preoperatively detecting hepatocellular carcinoma: an initial experience. Korean J Radiol. 2010 Jul-Aug;11(4):433-40. PMID: 20592927.

275. Pauleit D, Textor J, Bachmann R, et al. Hepatocellular carcinoma: detection with gadolinium- and ferumoxides-enhanced MR imaging of the liver. Radiology. 2002 Jan;222(1):73-80. PMID: 11756708.

276. Petruzzi N, Mitchell D, Guglielmo F, et al. Hepatocellular carcinoma likelihood on MRI exams. Evaluation of a standardized categorization System. Acad Radiol. 2013 Jun;20(6):694-8 Epub 2013 Mar 28. PMID: 23541479.

277. Piana G, Trinquart L, Meskine N, et al. New MR imaging criteria with a diffusion-weighted sequence for the diagnosis of hepatocellular carcinoma in chronic liver diseases. J Hepatol. 2011 Jul;55(1):126-32. PMID: 21145857.

278. Rhee H, Kim MJ, Park MS, et al. Differentiation of early hepatocellular carcinoma from benign hepatocellular nodules on gadoxetic acid-enhanced MRI. Br J Radiol. 2012 Oct;85(1018):e837-44. PMID: 22553295.

279. Rimola J, Forner A, Tremosini S, et al. Non-invasive diagnosis of hepatocellular carcinoma ≤ 2 cm in cirrhosis. Diagnostic accuracy assessing fat, capsule and signal intensity at dynamic MRI. J Hepatol. 2012 Jun;56(6):1317-23. PMID: 22314420.

280. Secil M, Obuz F, Altay C, et al. The role of dynamic subtraction MRI in detection of hepatocellular carcinoma. Diagn Interv Radiol. 2008 Dec;14(4):200-4. PMID: 19061165.

281. Simon G, Link TM, Wortler K, et al. Detection of hepatocellular carcinoma: comparison of Gd-DTPA- and ferumoxides-enhanced MR imaging. Eur Radiol. 2005 May;15(5):895-903. PMID: 15800773.

282. Suh YJ, Kim M-J, Choi J-Y, et al. Differentiation of hepatic hyperintense lesions seen on gadoxetic acid-enhanced hepatobiliary phase MRI. AJR Am J Roentgenol. 2011 Jul;197(1):W44-52. PMID: 21700994.

283. Tanaka O, Ito H, Yamada K, et al. Higher lesion conspicuity for SENSE dynamic MRI in detecting hypervascular hepatocellular carcinoma: analysis through the measurements of liver SNR and lesion-liver CNR comparison with conventional dynamic MRI. Eur Radiol. 2005 Dec;15(12):2427-34. PMID: 16041592.

284. Tang Y, Yamashita Y, Arakawa A, et al. Detection of hepatocellular carcinoma arising in cirrhotic livers: comparison of gadolinium- and ferumoxides-enhanced MR imaging. AJR Am J Roentgenol. 1999 Jun;172(6):1547-54. PMID: 10350287.

285. Tanimoto A, Yuasa Y, Jinzaki M, et al. Routine MR imaging protocol with breath-hold fast scans: diagnostic efficacy for focal liver lesions. Radiat Med. 2002 Jul-Aug;20(4):169-79. PMID: 12296432.

286. Tsurusaki M, Semelka RC, Uotani K, et al. Prospective comparison of high- and low-spatial-resolution dynamic MR imaging with sensitivity encoding (SENSE) for hypervascular hepatocellular carcinoma. Eur Radiol. 2008 Oct;18(10):2206-12. PMID: 18446347.

287. Vandecaveye V, De Keyzer F, Verslype C, et al. Diffusion-weighted MRI provides additional value to conventional dynamic contrast-enhanced MRI for detection of hepatocellular carcinoma. Eur Radiol. 2009 Oct;19(10):2456-66. PMID: 19440718.

288. Xu P-J, Yan F-H, Wang J-H, et al. Added value of breathhold diffusion-weighted MRI in detection of small hepatocellular carcinoma lesions compared with dynamic contrast-enhanced MRI alone using receiver operating characteristic curve analysis. J Magn Reson Imaging. 2009 Feb;29(2):341-9. PMID: 19161186.

289. Xu P-J, Yan F-H, Wang J-H, et al. Contribution of diffusion-weighted magnetic resonance imaging in the characterization of hepatocellular carcinomas and dysplastic nodules in cirrhotic liver. J Comput Assist Tomogr. 2010 Jul;34(4):506-12. PMID: 20657216.

290. Yoshioka H, Takahashi N, Yamaguchi M, et al. Double arterial phase dynamic MRI with sensitivity encoding (SENSE) for hypervascular hepatocellular carcinomas. J Magn Reson Imaging. 2002 Sep;16(3):259-66. PMID: 12205581.

291. Youk JH, Lee JM, Kim CS. MRI for detection of hepatocellular carcinoma: comparison of mangafodipir trisodium and gadopentetate dimeglumine contrast agents. AJR Am J Roentgenol. 2004 Oct;183(4):1049-54. PMID: 15385303.

292. Yu JS, Chung JJ, Kim JH, et al. Small hypervascular hepatocellular carcinomas: value of "washout" on gadolinium-enhanced dynamic MR imaging compared to superparamagnetic iron oxide-enhanced imaging. Eur Radiol. 2009 Nov;19(11):2614-22. PMID: 19513719.

293. Yu JS, Kim KW, Park MS, et al. Transient peritumoral enhancement during dynamic MRI of the liver: Cavernous hemangioma versus hepatocellular carcinoma. J Comput Assist Tomogr. 2002 May-Jun;26(3):411-7. PMID: 12016371.

294. Yu JS, Lee JH, Chung JJ, et al. Small hypervascular hepatocellular carcinoma: limited value of portal and delayed phases on dynamic magnetic resonance imaging. Acta Radiol. 2008 Sep;49(7):735-43. PMID: 18608015.

295. Yu MH, Kim JH, Yoon JH, et al. Role of C-arm CT for transcatheter arterial chemoembolization of hepatocellular carcinoma: Diagnostic performance and predictive value for therapeutic response compared with gadoxetic acid-enhanced MRI. AJR Am J Roentgenol. 2013;201(3):675-83. PMID: 23971463.

296. Chen Y-K, Hsieh D-S, Liao C-S, et al. Utility of FDG-PET for investigating unexplained serum AFP elevation in patients with suspected hepatocellular carcinoma recurrence. Anticancer Res. 2005 Nov-Dec;25(6C):4719-25. PMID: 16334166.

297. Cheung TT, Chan SC, Ho CL, et al. Can positron emission tomography with the dual tracers [11 C]acetate and [18 F]fludeoxyglucose predict microvascular invasion in hepatocellular carcinoma? Liver Transpl. 2011 Oct;17(10):1218-25. PMID: 21688383.

298. Delbeke D, Martin WH, Sandler MP, et al. Evaluation of benign vs malignant hepatic lesions with positron emission tomography. Arch Surg. 1998 May;133(5):510-5; discussion 5-6. PMID: 9605913.

299. Eckel F, Herrmann K, Schmidt S, et al. Imaging of proliferation in hepatocellular carcinoma with the in vivo marker 18F-fluorothymidine. J Nucl Med. 2009 Sep;50(9):1441-7. PMID: 19690030.

300. Ho C-L, Chen S, Yeung DWC, et al. Dual-tracer PET/CT imaging in evaluation of metastatic hepatocellular carcinoma. J Nucl Med. 2007 Jun;48(6):902-9. PMID: 17504862.

301. Ho C-L, Yu SCH, Yeung DWC. 11C-acetate PET imaging in hepatocellular carcinoma and other liver masses. J Nucl Med. 2003 Feb;44(2):213-21. PMID: 12571212.

302. Hwang KH, Choi D-J, Lee S-Y, et al. Evaluation of patients with hepatocellular carcinomas using [(11)C]acetate and [(18)F]FDG PET/CT: A preliminary study. Appl Radiat Isot. 2009 Jul-Aug;67(7-8):1195-8. PMID: 19342249.

303. Ijichi H, Shirabe K, Taketomi A, et al. Clinical usefulness of 18F-fluorodeoxyglucose positron emission tomography/computed tomography for patients with primary liver cancer with special reference to rare histological types, hepatocellular carcinoma with sarcomatous change and combined hepatocellular and cholangiocarcinoma. Hepatol Res. 2013;43(5):481-7. PMID: 23145869.

304. Jeng L-B, Changlai S-P, Shen Y-Y, et al. Limited value of 18F-2-deoxyglucose positron emission tomography to detect hepatocellular carcinoma in hepatitis B virus carriers. Hepatogastroenterology. 2003 Nov-Dec;50(54):2154-6. PMID: 14696485.

305. Kim Y-K, Lee K-W, Cho SY, et al. Usefulness 18F-FDG positron emission tomography/computed tomography for detecting recurrence of hepatocellular carcinoma in posttransplant patients. Liver Transpl. 2010 Jun;16(6):767-72. PMID: 20517911.

306. Li S, Beheshti M, Peck-Radosavljevic M, et al. Comparison of (11)C-acetate positron emission tomography and (67)Gallium citrate scintigraphy in patients with hepatocellular carcinoma. Liver Int. 2006 Oct;26(8):920-7. PMID: 16953831.

307. Liangpunsakul S, Agarwal D, Horlander JC, et al. Positron emission tomography for detecting occult hepatocellular carcinoma in hepatitis C cirrhotics awaiting for liver transplantation. Transplant Proc. 2003 Dec;35(8):2995-7. PMID: 14697959.

308. Lin W-Y, Tsai S-C, Hung G-U. Value of delayed 18F-FDG-PET imaging in the detection of hepatocellular carcinoma. Nucl Med Commun. 2005 Apr;26(4):315-21. PMID: 15753790.

309. Park J-W, Kim JH, Kim SK, et al. A prospective evaluation of 18F-FDG and 11C-acetate PET/CT for detection of primary and metastatic hepatocellular carcinoma. J Nucl Med. 2008 Dec;49(12):1912-21. PMID: 18997056.

310. Sørensen M, Frisch K, Bender D, et al. The potential use of 2-[18F]fluoro-2-deoxy-D-galactose as a PET/CT tracer for detection of hepatocellular carcinoma. Eur J Nucl Med Mol Imaging. 2011;38(9):1723-31. PMID: 21553087.

311. Sugiyama M, Sakahara H, Torizuka T, et al. 18F-FDG PET in the detection of extrahepatic metastases from hepatocellular carcinoma. J Gastroenterol. 2004;39(10):961-8. PMID: 15549449.

312. Sun L, Guan YS, Pan WM, et al. Metabolic restaging of hepatocellular carcinoma using whole-body F-FDG PET/CT. World J Hepatol. 2009 Oct 31;1(1):90-7. PMID: 21160970.

313. Talbot J, Fartoux L, Balogova S, et al. Detection of hepatocellular carcinoma with PET/CT: a prospective comparison of 18F-fluorocholine and 18F-FDG in patients with cirrhosis or chronic liver disease. J Nucl Med. 2010 Nov;51(11):1699-706. PMID: 20956466.

314. Talbot J, Gutman F, Fartoux L, et al. PET/CT in patients with hepatocellular carcinoma using [(18)F]fluorocholine: preliminary comparison with [(18)F]FDG PET/CT. Eur J Nucl Med Mol Imaging. 2006 Nov;33(11):1285-9. PMID: 16802155.

315. Verhoef C, Valkema R, de Man RA, et al. Fluorine-18 FDG imaging in hepatocellular carcinoma using positron coincidence detection and single photon emission computed tomography. Liver. 2002 Feb;22(1):51-6. PMID: 11906619.

316. Wolfort RM, Papillion PW, Turnage RH, et al. Role of FDG-PET in the evaluation and staging of hepatocellular carcinoma with comparison of tumor size, AFP level, and histologic grade. Int Surg. 2010 Jan-Mar;95(1):67-75. PMID: 20480845.

317. Wu H-b, Wang Q-s, Li B-y, et al. F-18 FDG in conjunction with 11C-choline PET/CT in the diagnosis of hepatocellular carcinoma. Clin Nucl Med. 2011 Dec;36(12):1092-7. PMID: 22064078.

318. Wudel LJ, Jr., Delbeke D, Morris D, et al. The role of [18F]fluorodeoxyglucose positron emission tomography imaging in the evaluation of hepatocellular carcinoma. Am Surg. 2003 Feb;69(2):117-24; discussion 24-6. PMID: 12641351.

319. Yamamoto Y, Nishiyama Y, Kameyama R, et al. Detection of hepatocellular carcinoma using 11C-choline PET: Comparison with 18F-FDG PET. J Nucl Med. 2008 Aug;49(8):1245-8. PMID: 18632827.

320. Yoon KT, Kim JK, Kim DY, et al. Role of 18F-fluorodeoxyglucose positron emission tomography in detecting extrahepatic metastasis in pretreatment staging of hepatocellular carcinoma. Oncology. 2007;72 Suppl 1:104-10. PMID: 18087190.

321. Yoo HJ, Lee JM, Lee JY, et al. Additional value of SPIO-enhanced MR imaging for the noninvasive imaging diagnosis of hepatocellular carcinoma in cirrhotic liver. Invest Radiol. 2009 Dec;44(12):800-7. PMID: 19838119.

322. Pocha C, Dieperink E, McMaken KA, et al. Surveillance for hepatocellular cancer with ultrasonography vs. computed tomography - A randomised study. Aliment Pharmacol Ther. 2013;38(3):303-12. PMID: 23750991.

323. Chen JG, Parkin DM, Chen QG, et al. Screening for liver cancer: results of a randomised controlled trial in Qidong, China. J Med Screen. 2003;10(4):204-9. PMID: 14738659.

324. Naaktgeboren CA, de Groot JA, van Smeden M, et al. Evaluating diagnostic accuracy in the face of multiple reference standards. Ann Intern Med. 2013 Aug 6;159(3):195-202. PMID: 23922065.

325. Hunt CH, Hartman RP, Hesley GK. Frequency and severity of adverse effects of iodinated and gadolinium contrast materials: retrospective review of 456,930 doses. AJR Am J Roentgenol. 2009 Oct;193(4):1124-7. PMID: 19770337.

326. Nelson KL, Gifford LM, Lauber-Huber C, et al. Clinical safety of gadopentetate dimeglumine. Radiology. 1995 Aug;196(2):439-43. PMID: 7617858.

327. Niendorf HP, Haustein J, Cornelius I, et al. Safety of gadolinium-DTPA: extended clinical experience. Magn Reson Med. 1991 Dec;22(2):222-8; discussion 9-32. PMID: 1812350.

328. Katayama H, Yamaguchi K, Kozuka T, et al. Adverse reactions to ionic and nonionic contrast media. A report from the Japanese Committee on the Safety of Contrast Media. Radiology. 1990 Jun;175(3):621-8. PMID: 2343107.

329. Micro-bubble Contrast Agents (marketed as Definity (Perflutren Lipid Microsphere) Injectable Suspension and Optison (Perflutren Protein-Type A Microspheres for Injection). Silver Spring, MD: U.S. Food and Drug Administration; 2008. http://www.fda.gov/safety/medwatch/safetyinformation/safetyalertsforhumanmedicalproducts/ucm092270.htm. Accessed on November 12, 2013.

330. Piscaglia F, Bolondi L. The safety of Sonovue in abdominal applications: retrospective analysis of 23188 investigations. Ultrasound Med Biol. 2006 Sep;32(9):1369-75. PMID: 16965977.

331. Herzog CA. Incidence of adverse events associated with use of perflutren contrast agents for echocardiography. JAMA. 2008 May 7;299(17):2023-5. PMID: 18460662.

332. Patient Safety: Radiation Dose in X-Ray and CT Exams. Oak Brook, IL: Radiological Society of North America; 2013. http://www.radiologyinfo.org/en/safety/index.cfm?pg=sfty_xray. Accessed on November 13, 2013.

333. Colli A, Fraquelli M, Casazza G, et al. Accuracy of ultrasonography, spiral CT, magnetic resonance, and alpha-fetoprotein in diagnosing hepatocellular carcinoma: a systematic review. Am J Gastroenterol. 2006 Mar;101(3):513-23. PMID: 16542288.

334. Westwood M, Joore M, Grutters J, et al. Contrast-enhanced ultrasound using SonoVue(R) (sulphur hexafluoride microbubbles) compared with contrast-enhanced computed tomography and contrast-enhanced magnetic resonance imaging for the characterisation of focal liver lesions and detection of liver metastases: a systematic review and cost-effectiveness analysis. Health Technol Assess. 2013 Apr;17(16):1-243. PMID: 23611316.

335. Guang Y, Xie L, Ding H, et al. Diagnosis value of focal liver lesions with SonoVue-enhanced ultrasound compared with contrast-enhanced computed tomography and contrast-enhanced MRI: a meta-analysis. J Cancer Res Clin Oncol. 2011 Nov;137(11):1595-605. PMID: 21850382.

336. Xie L, Guang Y, Ding H, et al. Diagnostic value of contrast-enhanced ultrasound, computed tomography and magnetic resonance imaging for focal liver lesions: a meta-analysis. Ultrasound Med Biol. 2011 Jun;37(6):854-61. PMID: 21531500.

337. Chen L, Zhang L, Bao J, et al. Comparison of MRI with liver-specific contrast agents and multidetector row CT for the detection of hepatocellular carcinoma: a meta-analysis of 15 direct comparative studies. Gut. 2013 Oct;62(10):1520-1. PMID: 23929696.

338. Lin C-Y, Chen J-H, Liang J-A, et al. 18F-FDG PET or PET/CT for detecting extrahepatic metastases or recurrent hepatocellular carcinoma: a systematic review and meta-analysis. Eur J Radiol. 2012 Sep;81(9):2417-22. PMID: 21899970.

339. Aghoram R, Cai P, Dickinson JA. Alpha-foetoprotein and/or liver ultrasonography for screening of hepatocellular carcinoma in patients with chronic hepatitis B. Cochrane Database Syst Rev. 2012;9. PMID: 22972059.

340. Lachs MS, Nachamkin I, Edelstein PH, et al. Spectrum bias in the evaluation of diagnostic tests: lessons from the rapid dipstick test for urinary tract infection. Ann Intern Med. 1992 Jul 15;117(2):135-40. PMID: 1605428.

341. Morana G, Salviato E, Guarise A. Contrast agents for hepatic MRI. Cancer Imaging. 2007;7 Spec No A:S24-7. PMID: 17921081.

342. Lijmer JG, Bossuyt PM, Heisterkamp SH. Exploring sources of heterogeneity in systematic reviews of diagnostic tests. Stat Med. 2002 Jun 15;21(11):1525-37. PMID: 12111918.

343. Gatsonis C, Paliwato P. Meta-analysis of diagnostic and screening test accuracy evaluations: methodologic primer. AJR Am J Roentgenol. 2006 Aug;187(2):271-81. PMID: 16861527.

344. Macaskill P, Gatsonis C, Deeks J, et al. Chapter 10. Analysing and Presenting Results. In: Deeks JJ, Bossuyt PM, Gatsonis C, eds. Cochrane Handbook for Systematic Reviews of Diagnostic Test Accuracy. Version 1.0 ed. Oxford: The Cochrane Collaboration; 2010. Available from: http://srdta.cochrane.org/.

345. Deeks JJ, Macaskill P, Irwig L. The performance of tests of publication bias and other sample size effects in systematic reviews of diagnostic test accuracy was assessed. J Clin Epidemiol. 2005 Sep;58(9):882-93. PMID: 16085191.

346. Song F, Khan KS, Dinnes J, et al. Asymmetric funnel plots and publication bias in meta-analyses of diagnostic accuracy. Int J Epidemiol. 2002 Feb;31(1):88-95. PMID: 11914301.

347. Liver Imaging Reporting and Data System version 2013.1. American College of Radiology. http://www.acr.org/Quality-Safety/Resources/LIRADS/. Accessed on April 2014.

Abbreviations and Acronyms

AASLD	American Association for the Study of Liver Diseases
AFP	Alpha-fetoprotein
AFROC	alternate free response operating characteristic
AHRQ	Agency for Healthcare Research and Quality
AUROC	area under the receiver operating characteristic
BCLC	Barcelona Clinic Liver Cancer
CER	Comparative effectiveness review
CT	Computed tomography
EASL	European Association for the Study of the Liver
EPC	Evidence-based Practice Center
FDA	U.S. Food and Drug Administration
FDG	^{18}F-fluorodeoxyglucose
FLT	^{18}F-fluorothymidine
HBV	Hepatitis B virus
HCC	Hepatocellular carcinoma
HCV	Hepatitis C virus
KQ	Key Question
LR	Likelihood ratio
MRI	Magnetic resonance imaging
PET	Positron emission tomography
PICOTS	Populations, interventions, comparators, outcomes, timing, setting
QUADAS	Quality Assessment of Diagnostic Accuracy Studies
SIP	Scientific information packet
TEP	Technical expert panel
UCSF	University of California, San Francisco
US	Ultrasound

Appendix A. Included Studies

1. Addley HC, Griffin N, Shaw AS, et al. Accuracy of hepatocellular carcinoma detection on multidetector CT in a transplant liver population with explant liver correlation. Clin Radiol. 2011 Apr;66(4):349-56. PMID: 21295772.

2. Ahn SS, Kim M-J, Lim JS, et al. Added value of gadoxetic acid-enhanced hepatobiliary phase MR imaging in the diagnosis of hepatocellular carcinoma. Radiology. 2010 May;255(2):459-66. PMID: 20413759.

3. Akai H, Kiryu S, Matsuda I, et al. Detection of hepatocellular carcinoma by Gd-EOB-DTPA-enhanced liver MRI: comparison with triple phase 64 detector row helical CT. Eur J Radiol. 2011 Nov;80(2):310-5. PMID: 20732773.

4. Alaboudy A, Inoue T, Hatanaka K, et al. Usefulness of combination of imaging modalities in the diagnosis of hepatocellular carcinoma using Sonazoid(R)-enhanced ultrasound, gadolinium diethylene-triamine-pentaacetic acid-enhanced magnetic resonance imaging, and contrast-enhanced computed tomography. Oncology. 2011;81 Suppl 1:66-72. PMID: 22212939.

5. An C, Park MS, Kim D, et al. Added value of subtraction imaging in detecting arterial enhancement in small (<3 cm) hepatic nodules on dynamic contrast-enhanced MRI in patients at high risk of hepatocellular carcinoma. Eur Radiol. 2013;23:924-30. PMID: 23138382.

6. An C, Park M-S, Jeon H-M, et al. Prediction of the histopathological grade of hepatocellular carcinoma using qualitative diffusion-weighted, dynamic, and hepatobiliary phase MRI. Eur Radiol. 2012 Aug;22(8):1701-8. PMID: 22434421.

7. Baccarani U, Adani GL, Avellini C, et al. Comparison of clinical and pathological staging and long-term results of liver transplantation for hepatocellular carcinoma in a single transplant center. Transplant Proc. 2006 May;38(4):1111-3. PMID: 16757280.

8. Baek CK, Choi JY, Kim KA, et al. Hepatocellular carcinoma in patients with chronic liver disease: a comparison of gadoxetic acid-enhanced MRI and multiphasic MDCT. Clin Radiol. 2012 Feb;67(2):148-56. PMID: 21920517.

9. Baird AJ, Amos GJ, Saad NF, et al. Retrospective audit to determine the diagnostic accuracy of Primovist-enhanced MRI in the detection of hepatocellular carcinoma in cirrhosis with explant histopathology correlation. J Med Imaging Radiat Oncol. 2013;57(3):314-20. PMID: 23721140.

10. Bartolozzi C, Donati F, Cioni D, et al. MnDPDP-enhanced MRI vs dual-phase spiral CT in the detection of hepatocellular carcinoma in cirrhosis. Eur Radiol. 2000;10(11):1697-702. PMID: 11097390.

11. Bennett GL, Krinsky GA, Abitbol RJ, et al. Sonographic detection of hepatocellular carcinoma and dysplastic nodules in cirrhosis: correlation of pretransplantation sonography and liver explant pathology in 200 patients. AJR Am J Roentgenol. 2002 Jul;179(1):75-80. PMID: 12076908.

12. Bhattacharjya S, Bhattacharjya T, Quaglia A, et al. Liver transplantation in cirrhotic patients with small hepatocellular carcinoma: an analysis of pre-operative imaging, explant histology and prognostic histologic indicators. Dig Surg. 2004;21(2):152-9; discussion 9-60. PMID: 15166485.

13. Burrel M, Llovet JM, Ayuso C, et al. MRI angiography is superior to helical CT for detection of HCC prior to liver transplantation: an explant correlation. Hepatology. 2003 Oct;38(4):1034-42. PMID: 14512891.

14. Catala V, Nicolau C, Vilana R, et al. Characterization of focal liver lesions: comparative study of contrast-enhanced ultrasound versus spiral computed tomography. Eur Radiol. 2007 Apr;17(4):1066-73. PMID: 17072617.

15. Cereser L, Furlan A, Bagatto D, et al. Comparison of portal venous and delayed phases of gadolinium-enhanced magnetic

resonance imaging study of cirrhotic liver for the detection of contrast washout of hypervascular hepatocellular carcinoma. J Comput Assist Tomogr. 2010;34(5):706-11. PMID: 20861773.

16. Chalasani N, Horlander JC, Sr., Said A, et al. Screening for hepatocellular carcinoma in patients with advanced cirrhosis. Am J Gastroenterol. 1999 Oct;94(10):2988-93. PMID: 10520857.

17. Chen MH, Wu W, Yang W, et al. The use of contrast-enhanced ultrasonography in the selection of patients with hepatocellular carcinoma for radio frequency ablation therapy. J Ultrasound Med. 2007;26(8):1055-63. PMID: 17646367.

18. Chen MH, Yang W, Yan K, et al. The role of contrast-enhanced ultrasound in planning treatment protocols for hepatocellular carcinoma before radiofrequency ablation. Clin Radiol. 2007 Aug;62(8):752-60. PMID: 17604763.

19. Chen Y-K, Hsieh D-S, Liao C-S, et al. Utility of FDG-PET for investigating unexplained serum AFP elevation in patients with suspected hepatocellular carcinoma recurrence. Anticancer Res. 2005 Nov-Dec;25(6C):4719-25. PMID: 16334166.

20. Cheung TT, Chan SC, Ho CL, et al. Can positron emission tomography with the dual tracers [11 C]acetate and [18 F]fludeoxyglucose predict microvascular invasion in hepatocellular carcinoma? Liver Transpl. 2011 Oct;17(10):1218-25. PMID: 21688383.

21. Cheung TT, Ho CL, Lo CM, et al. 11C-acetate and 18F-FDG PET/CT for clinical staging and selection of patients with hepatocellular carcinoma for liver transplantation on the basis of milan criteria: Surgeon's perspective. J Nucl Med. 2013;54(2):192-200. PMID: 23321459.

22. Choi D, Kim SH, Lim JH, et al. Detection of hepatocellular carcinoma: combined T2-weighted and dynamic gadolinium-enhanced MRI versus combined CT during arterial portography and CT hepatic arteriography. J Comput Assist Tomogr. 2001 Sep-Oct;25(5):777-85. PMID: 11584240.

23. Choi SH, Lee JM, Yu NC, et al. Hepatocellular carcinoma in liver transplantation candidates: detection with gadobenate dimeglumine-enhanced MRI. AJR Am J Roentgenol. 2008 Aug;191(2):529-36. PMID: 18647927.

24. Chou C-T, Chen R-C, Chen W-T, et al. Characterization of hyperintense nodules on T1-weighted liver magnetic resonance imaging: comparison of Ferucarbotran-enhanced MRI with accumulation-phase FS-T1WI and gadolinium-enhanced MRI. J Chin Med Assoc. 2011 Feb;74(2):62-8. PMID: 21354082.

25. Chung J, Yu J-S, Kim DJ, et al. Hypervascular hepatocellular carcinoma in the cirrhotic liver: diffusion-weighted imaging versus superparamagnetic iron oxide-enhanced MRI. Magn Reson Imaging. 2011 Nov;29(9):1235-43. PMID: 21907517.

26. Chung S-H, Kim M-J, Choi J-Y, et al. Comparison of two different injection rates of gadoxetic acid for arterial phase MRI of the liver. J Magn Reson Imaging. 2010 Feb;31(2):365-72. PMID: 20099350.

27. Colagrande S, Fargnoli R, Dal Pozzo F, et al. Value of hepatic arterial phase CT versus lipiodol ultrafluid CT in the detection of hepatocellular carcinoma. J Comput Assist Tomogr. 2000 Nov-Dec;24(6):878-83. PMID: 11105704.

28. Dai Y, Chen MH, Fan ZH, et al. Diagnosis of small hepatic nodules detected by surveillance ultrasound in patients with cirrhosis: Comparison between contrast-enhanced ultrasound and contrast-enhanced helical computed tomography. Hepatol Res. 2008 Mar;38(3):281-90. PMID: 17908168.

29. de Ledinghen V, Laharie D, Lecesne R, et al. Detection of nodules in liver cirrhosis: spiral computed tomography or magnetic resonance imaging? A prospective study of 88 nodules in 34 patients. Eur J Gastroenterol Hepatol. 2002 Feb;14(2):159-65. PMID: 11981340.

30. Delbeke D, Martin WH, Sandler MP, et al. Evaluation of benign vs malignant hepatic lesions with positron emission tomography. Arch Surg. 1998 May;133(5):510-5; discussion 5-6. PMID: 9605913.

31. Denecke T, Grieser C, Froling V, et al. Multislice computed tomography using a triple-phase contrast protocol for preoperative assessment of hepatic tumor load in patients with hepatocellular

carcinoma before liver transplantation. Transpl Int. 2009 Apr;22(4):395-402. PMID: 19000231.

32. Di Martino M, De Filippis G, De Santis A, et al. Hepatocellular carcinoma in cirrhotic patients: prospective comparison of US, CT and MR imaging. Eur Radiol. 2013;23:887-96. PMID: 23179521.

33. Di Martino M, Marin D, Guerrisi A, et al. Intraindividual comparison of gadoxetate disodium-enhanced MR imaging and 64-section multidetector CT in the Detection of hepatocellular carcinoma in patients with cirrhosis. Radiology. 2010 Sep;256(3):806-16. PMID: 20720069.

34. D'Onofrio M, Rozzanigo U, Masinielli BM, et al. Hypoechoic focal liver lesions: characterization with contrast enhanced ultrasonography. J Clin Ultrasound. 2005 May;33(4):164-72. PMID: 15856516.

35. Doyle DJ, O'Malley ME, Jang H-J, et al. Value of the unenhanced phase for detection of hepatocellular carcinomas 3 cm or less when performing multiphase computed tomography in patients with cirrhosis. J Comput Assist Tomogr. 2007 Jan-Feb;31(1):86-92. PMID: 17259838.

36. Eckel F, Herrmann K, Schmidt S, et al. Imaging of proliferation in hepatocellular carcinoma with the in vivo marker 18F-fluorothymidine. J Nucl Med. 2009 Sep;50(9):1441-7. PMID: 19690030.

37. Egger C, Goertz RS, Strobel D, et al. Dynamic contrast-enhanced ultrasound (DCE-US) for easy and rapid evaluation of hepatocellular carcinoma compared to dynamic contrast-enhanced computed tomography (DCE-CT)--a pilot study. Ultraschall Med. 2012;33(6):587-92. PMID: 23154871.

38. Filippone A, Cianci R, Patriarca G, et al. The Value of Gadoxetic Acid-Enhanced Hepatospecific Phase MR Imaging for Characterization of Hepatocellular Nodules in the Cirrhotic Liver. European Journal of Clinical & Medical Oncology. 2010;2(4):1-8. PMID: 69823585.

39. Forner A, Vilana R, Ayuso C, et al. Diagnosis of hepatic nodules 20 mm or smaller in cirrhosis: Prospective validation of the noninvasive diagnostic criteria for hepatocellular carcinoma.[Erratum appears in Hepatology. 2008 Feb;47(2):769]. Hepatology. 2008 Jan;47(1):97-104. PMID: 18069697.

40. Fowler KJ, Karimova EJ, Arauz AR, et al. Validation of organ procurement and transplant network (OPTN)/united network for organ sharing (UNOS) criteria for imaging diagnosis of hepatocellular carcinoma. Transplantation. 2013;95(12):1506-11. PMID: 23778569.

41. Fracanzani AL, Burdick L, Borzio M, et al. Contrast-enhanced Doppler ultrasonography in the diagnosis of hepatocellular carcinoma and premalignant lesions in patients with cirrhosis. Hepatology. 2001 Dec;34(6):1109-12. PMID: 11731999.

42. Freeman RB, Mithoefer A, Ruthazer R, et al. Optimizing staging for hepatocellular carcinoma before liver transplantation: A retrospective analysis of the UNOS/OPTN database. Liver Transpl. 2006 Oct;12(10):1504-11. PMID: 16952174.

43. Freeny PC, Grossholz M, Kaakaji K, et al. Significance of hyperattenuating and contrast-enhancing hepatic nodules detected in the cirrhotic liver during arterial phase helical CT in pre-liver transplant patients: radiologic-histopathologic correlation of explanted livers. Abdom Imaging. 2003 May-Jun;28(3):333-46. PMID: 12719903.

44. Furuse J, Maru Y, Yoshino M, et al. Assessment of arterial tumor vascularity in small hepatocellular carcinoma. Comparison between color doppler ultrasonography and radiographic imagings with contrast medium: dynamic CT, angiography, and CT hepatic arteriography. Eur J Radiol. 2000 Oct;36(1):20-7. PMID: 10996754.

45. Gaiani S, Celli N, Piscaglia F, et al. Usefulness of contrast-enhanced perfusional sonography in the assessment of hepatocellular carcinoma hypervascular at spiral computed tomography. J Hepatol. 2004 Sep;41(3):421-6. PMID: 15336445.

46. Gambarin-Gelwan M, Wolf DC, Shapiro R, et al. Sensitivity of commonly available screening tests in detecting hepatocellular carcinoma in cirrhotic patients undergoing liver transplantation. Am J Gastroenterol. 2000 Jun;95(6):1535-8. PMID: 10894592.

47. Gatto A, De Gaetano AM, Giuga M, et al. Differentiating hepatocellular carcinoma

48. Giorgio A, De Stefano G, Coppola C, et al. Contrast-enhanced sonography in the characterization of small hepatocellular carcinomas in cirrhotic patients: comparison with contrast-enhanced ultrafast magnetic resonance imaging. Anticancer Res. 2007 Nov-Dec;27(6C):4263-9. PMID: 18214030.

49. Giorgio A, Ferraioli G, Tarantino L, et al. Contrast-enhanced sonographic appearance of hepatocellular carcinoma in patients with cirrhosis: Comparison with contrast-enhanced helical CT appearance. AJR Am J Roentgenol. 2004;183(5):1319-26. PMID: 15505297.

50. Golfieri R, Marini E, Bazzocchi A, et al. Small (≤ 3 cm) hepatocellular carcinoma in cirrhosis: the role of double contrast agents in MR imaging vs. multidetector-row CT. Radiol Med (Torino). 2009 Dec;114(8):1239-66. PMID: 19697104.

51. Goshima S, Kanematsu M, Matsuo M, et al. Nodule-in-nodule appearance of hepatocellular carcinomas: comparison of gadolinium-enhanced and ferumoxides-enhanced magnetic resonance imaging. J Magn Reson Imaging. 2004 Aug;20(2):250-5. PMID: 15269950.

52. Goto E, Masuzaki R, Tateishi R, et al. Value of post-vascular phase (Kupffer imaging) by contrast-enhanced ultrasonography using Sonazoid in the detection of hepatocellular carcinoma. J Gastroenterol. 2012;47(4):477-85. PMID: 22200940.

53. Guo L, Liang C, Yu T, et al. 3 T MRI of hepatocellular carcinomas in patients with cirrhosis: does T2-weighted imaging provide added value? Clin Radiol. 2012 Apr;67(4):319-28. PMID: 22099524.

54. Haradome H, Grazioli L, Tinti R, et al. Additional value of gadoxetic acid-DTPA-enhanced hepatobiliary phase MR imaging in the diagnosis of early-stage hepatocellular carcinoma: comparison with dynamic triple-phase multidetector CT imaging. J Magn Reson Imaging. 2011 Jul;34(1):69-78. PMID: 21598343.

55. Hardie AD, Kizziah MK, Boulter DJ. Diagnostic accuracy of diffusion-weighted MRI for identifying hepatocellular carcinoma with liver explant correlation. J Med Imaging Radiat Oncol. 2011 Aug;55(4):362-7. PMID: 21843170.

56. Hardie AD, Kizziah MK, Rissing MS. Can the patient with cirrhosis be imaged for hepatocellular carcinoma without gadolinium?: Comparison of combined T2-weighted, T2*-weighted, and diffusion-weighted MRI with gadolinium-enhanced MRI using liver explantation standard. J Comput Assist Tomogr. 2011 Nov-Dec;35(6):711-5. PMID: 22082541.

57. Hardie AD, Nance JW, Boulter DJ, et al. Assessment of the diagnostic accuracy of T2*-weighted MR imaging for identifying hepatocellular carcinoma with liver explant correlation. Eur J Radiol. 2011 Dec;80(3):e249-52. PMID: 21112710.

58. Hatanaka K, Kudo M, Minami Y, et al. Differential diagnosis of hepatic tumors: value of contrast-enhanced harmonic sonography using the newly developed contrast agent, Sonazoid. Intervirology. 2008;51 Suppl 1:61-9. PMID: 18544950.

59. Hecht EM, Holland AE, Israel GM, et al. Hepatocellular carcinoma in the cirrhotic liver: gadolinium-enhanced 3D T1-weighted MR imaging as a stand-alone sequence for diagnosis. Radiology. 2006 May;239(2):438-47. PMID: 16641353.

60. Hidaka M, Takatsuki M, Okudaira S, et al. The expression of transporter OATP2/OATP8 decreases in undetectable hepatocellular carcinoma by Gd-EOB-MRI in the explanted cirrhotic liver. Hepatology International. 2012:1-7.

61. Higashihara H, Osuga K, Onishi H, et al. Diagnostic accuracy of C-arm CT during selective transcatheter angiography for hepatocellular carcinoma: comparison with intravenous contrast-enhanced, biphasic, dynamic MDCT. Eur Radiol. 2012 Apr;22(4):872-9. PMID: 22120061.

62. Hirakawa M, Yoshimitsu K, Irie H, et al. Performance of radiological methods in diagnosing hepatocellular carcinoma preoperatively in a recipient of living related liver transplantation: comparison with step section histopathology. Jpn J Radiol. 2011 Feb;29(2):129-37. PMID: 21359938.

63. Ho C-l, Chen S, Yeung DWC, et al. Dual-

tracer PET/CT imaging in evaluation of metastatic hepatocellular carcinoma. J Nucl Med. 2007 Jun;48(6):902-9. PMID: 17504862.

64. Ho C-L, Yu SCH, Yeung DWC. 11C-acetate PET imaging in hepatocellular carcinoma and other liver masses. J Nucl Med. 2003 Feb;44(2):213-21. PMID: 12571212.

65. Hori M, Murakami T, Kim T, et al. Detection of hypervascular hepatocellular carcinoma: comparison of SPIO-enhanced MRI with dynamic helical CT. J Comput Assist Tomogr. 2002 Sep-Oct;26(5):701-10. PMID: 12439302.

66. Hori M, Murakami T, Oi H, et al. Sensitivity in detection of hypervascular hepatocellular carcinoma by helical CT with intra-arterial injection of contrast medium, and by helical CT and MR imaging with intravenous injection of contrast medium. Acta Radiol. 1998 Mar;39(2):144-51. PMID: 9529444.

67. Hwang J, Kim SH, Lee MW, et al. Small (≤ 2 cm) hepatocellular carcinoma in patients with chronic liver disease: comparison of gadoxetic acid-enhanced 3.0 T MRI and multiphasic 64-multirow detector CT. Br J Radiol. 2012 Jul;85(1015):e314-22. PMID: 22167508.

68. Hwang KH, Choi D-J, Lee S-Y, et al. Evaluation of patients with hepatocellular carcinomas using [(11)C]acetate and [(18)F]FDG PET/CT: A preliminary study. Appl Radiat Isot. 2009 Jul-Aug;67(7-8):1195-8. PMID: 19342249.

69. Iannaccone R, Laghi A, Catalano C, et al. Hepatocellular carcinoma: role of unenhanced and delayed phase multi-detector row helical CT in patients with cirrhosis. Radiology. 2005 Feb;234(2):460-7. PMID: 15671002.

70. Iavarone M, Sangiovanni A, Forzenigo LV, et al. Diagnosis of hepatocellular carcinoma in cirrhosis by dynamic contrast imaging: the importance of tumor cell differentiation. Hepatology. 2010 Nov;52(5):1723-30. PMID: 20842697.

71. Ichikawa T, Kitamura T, Nakajima H, et al. Hypervascular hepatocellular carcinoma: can double arterial phase imaging with multidetector CT improve tumor depiction in the cirrhotic liver? AJR Am J Roentgenol. 2002 Sep;179(3):751-8. PMID: 12185057.

72. Ichikawa T, Saito K, Yoshioka N, et al. Detection and characterization of focal liver lesions: a Japanese phase III, multicenter comparison between gadoxetic acid disodium-enhanced magnetic resonance imaging and contrast-enhanced computed tomography predominantly in patients with hepatocellular carcinoma and chronic liver disease. Invest Radiol. 2010 Mar;45(3):133-41. PMID: 20098330.

73. Ijichi H, Shirabe K, Taketomi A, et al. Clinical usefulness of 18F-fluorodeoxyglucose positron emission tomography/computed tomography for patients with primary liver cancer with special reference to rare histological types, hepatocellular carcinoma with sarcomatous change and combined hepatocellular and cholangiocarcinoma. Hepatol Res. 2013;43(5):481-7. PMID: 23145869.

74. Imamura M, Shiratori Y, Shiina S, et al. Power Doppler sonography for hepatocellular carcinoma: factors affecting the power Doppler signals of the tumors. Liver. 1998 Dec;18(6):427-33. PMID: 9869398.

75. Inoue T, Kudo M, Hatanaka K, et al. Imaging of hepatocellular carcinoma: Qualitative and quantitative analysis of postvascular phase contrast-enhanced ultrasonography with sonazoid. Oncology. 2008;75(SUPPL. 1):48-54. PMID: 19092272.

76. Inoue T, Kudo M, Komuta M, et al. Assessment of Gd-EOB-DTPA-enhanced MRI for HCC and dysplastic nodules and comparison of detection sensitivity versus MDCT. J Gastroenterol. 2012 Sep;47(9):1036-47. PMID: 22526270.

77. Inoue T, Kudo M, Maenishi O, et al. Value of liver parenchymal phase contrast-enhanced sonography to diagnose premalignant and borderline lesions and overt hepatocellular carcinoma. AJR Am J Roentgenol. 2009 Mar;192(3):698-705. PMID: 19234266.

78. Ito K, Fujita T, Shimizu A, et al. Multiarterial phase dynamic MRI of small early enhancing hepatic lesions in cirrhosis or chronic hepatitis: Differentiating between hypervascular hepatocellular carcinomas

and pseudolesions. AJR Am J Roentgenol. 2004;183(3):699-705. PMID: 15333358.

79. Iwazawa J, Ohue S, Hashimoto N, et al. Detection of hepatocellular carcinoma: comparison of angiographic C-arm CT and MDCT. AJR Am J Roentgenol. 2010 Oct;195(4):882-7. PMID: 20858813.

80. Jang HJ, Kim TK, Khalili K, et al. Characterization of 1- to 2-cm liver nodules detected on hcc surveillance ultrasound according to the criteria of the american association for the study of liver disease: Is quadriphasic CT necessary? AJR Am J Roentgenol. 2013;201(2):314-21. PMID: 23883211.

81. Jang HJ, Kim TK, Wilson SR. Small nodules (1-2 cm) in liver cirrhosis: characterization with contrast-enhanced ultrasound. Eur J Radiol. 2009 Dec;72(3):418-24. PMID: 18834687.

82. Jang HJ, Lim JH, Lee SJ, et al. Hepatocellular carcinoma: are combined CT during arterial portography and CT hepatic arteriography in addition to triple-phase helical CT all necessary for preoperative evaluation? Radiology. 2000 May;215(2):373-80. PMID: 10796910.

83. Jeng C-M, Kung C-H, Wang Y-C, et al. Spiral biphasic contrast-enhanced computerized tomography in the diagnosis of hepatocellular carcinoma. J Formos Med Assoc. 2002 Aug;101(8):588-92. PMID: 12440092.

84. Jeng L-B, Changlai S-P, Shen Y-Y, et al. Limited value of 18F-2-deoxyglucose positron emission tomography to detect hepatocellular carcinoma in hepatitis B virus carriers. Hepatogastroenterology. 2003 Nov-Dec;50(54):2154-6. PMID: 14696485.

85. Jeong MG, Yu JS, Kim KW, et al. Early homogeneously enhancing hemangioma versus hepatocellular carcinoma: differentiation using quantitative analysis of multiphasic dynamic magnetic resonance imaging. Yonsei Med J. 1999 Jun;40(3):248-55. PMID: 10412337.

86. Jeong WK, Byun JH, Lee SS, et al. Gadobenate dimeglumine-enhanced liver MR imaging in cirrhotic patients: quantitative and qualitative comparison of 1-hour and 3-hour delayed images. J Magn Reson Imaging. 2011 Apr;33(4):889-97. PMID: 21448954.

87. Jin Y, Nah S, Lee J, et al. Utility of Adding Primovist Magnetic Resonance Imaging to Analysis of Hepatocellular Carcinoma by Liver Dynamic Computed Tomography. Clin Gastroenterol Hepatol. 2013;11(2):187-92. PMID: 23142203.

88. Kakihara D, Nishie A, Harada N, et al. Performance of gadoxetic acid-enhanced MRI for detecting hepatocellular carcinoma in recipients of living-related-liver-transplantation: Comparison with dynamic multidetector row computed tomography and angiography-assisted computed tomography. J Magn Reson Imaging. 2013PMID: 24259437.

89. Kamura T, Kimura M, Sakai K, et al. Small hypervascular hepatocellular carcinoma versus hypervascular pseudolesions: Differential diagnosis on MRI. Abdom Imaging. 2002;27(3):315-24. PMID: 12173363.

90. Kang BK, Lim JH, Kim SH, et al. Preoperative depiction of hepatocellular carcinoma: ferumoxides-enhanced MR imaging versus triple-phase helical CT. Radiology. 2003 Jan;226(1):79-85. PMID: 12511672.

91. Kawada N, Ohkawa K, Tanaka S, et al. Improved diagnosis of well-differentiated hepatocellular carcinoma with gadolinium ethoxybenzyl diethylene triamine pentaacetic acid-enhanced magnetic resonance imaging and Sonazoid contrast-enhanced ultrasonography. Hepatol Res. 2010;40(9):930-6. PMID: 20887598.

92. Kawaoka T, Aikata H, Takaki S, et al. FDG positron emission tomography/computed tomography for the detection of extrahepatic metastases from hepatocellular carcinoma. Hepatol Res. 2009;39(2):134-42. PMID: 19208034.

93. Kawata S, Murakami T, Kim T, et al. Multidetector CT: diagnostic impact of slice thickness on detection of hypervascular hepatocellular carcinoma. AJR Am J Roentgenol. 2002 Jul;179(1):61-6. PMID: 12076906.

94. Khalili K, Kim TK, Jang H-J, et al. Optimization of imaging diagnosis of 1-2 cm hepatocellular carcinoma: an analysis of diagnostic performance and resource

utilization. J Hepatol. 2011 Apr;54(4):723-8. PMID: 21156219.

95. Khan MA, Combs CS, Brunt EM, et al. Positron emission tomography scanning in the evaluation of hepatocellular carcinoma. J Hepatol. 2000 May;32(5):792-7. PMID: 10845666.

96. Kim AY, Kim YK, Lee MW, et al. Detection of hepatocellular carcinoma in gadoxetic acid-enhanced MRI and diffusion-weighted MRI with respect to the severity of liver cirrhosis. Acta Radiol. 2012 Oct 1;53(8):830-8. PMID: 22847903.

97. Kim CK, Lim JH, Lee WJ. Detection of hepatocellular carcinomas and dysplastic nodules in cirrhotic liver: accuracy of ultrasonography in transplant patients. J Ultrasound Med. 2001 Feb;20(2):99-104. PMID: 11211142.

98. Kim DJ, Yu JS, Kim JH, et al. Small hypervascular hepatocellular carcinomas: value of diffusion-weighted imaging compared with "washout" appearance on dynamic MRI. Br J Radiol. 2012 Oct;85(1018):e879-86. PMID: 22573299.

99. Kim KW, Lee JM, Klotz E, et al. Quantitative CT color mapping of the arterial enhancement fraction of the liver to detect hepatocellular carcinoma. Radiology. 2009 Feb;250(2):425-34. PMID: 19188314.

100. Kim M-J, Lee M, Choi J-Y, et al. Imaging features of small hepatocellular carcinomas with microvascular invasion on gadoxetic acid-enhanced MR imaging. Eur J Radiol. 2012 Oct;81(10):2507-12. PMID: 22137613.

101. Kim PN, Choi D, Rhim H, et al. Planning ultrasound for percutaneous radiofrequency ablation to treat small (≤ 3 cm) hepatocellular carcinomas detected on computed tomography or magnetic resonance imaging: a multicenter prospective study to assess factors affecting ultrasound visibility. J Vasc Interv Radiol. 2012 May;23(5):627-34. PMID: 22387030.

102. Kim SE, Lee HC, Shim JH, et al. Noninvasive diagnostic criteria for hepatocellular carcinoma in hepatic masses >2 cm in a hepatitis B virus-endemic area. Liver Int. 2011 Nov;31(10):1468-76. PMID: 21745284.

103. Kim SH, Choi D, Kim SH, et al. Ferucarbotran-enhanced MRI versus triple-phase MDCT for the preoperative detection of hepatocellular carcinoma. AJR Am J Roentgenol. 2005 Apr;184(4):1069-76. PMID: 15788575.

104. Kim SH, Kim SH, Lee J, et al. Gadoxetic acid-enhanced MRI versus triple-phase MDCT for the preoperative detection of hepatocellular carcinoma. AJR Am J Roentgenol. 2009 Jun;192(6):1675-81. PMID: 19457834.

105. Kim SJ, Kim SH, Lee J, et al. Ferucarbotran-enhanced 3.0-T magnetic resonance imaging using parallel imaging technique compared with triple-phase multidetector row computed tomography for the preoperative detection of hepatocellular carcinoma.[Erratum appears in J Comput Assist Tomogr. 2008 Jul-Aug;32(4):615]. J Comput Assist Tomogr. 2008 May-Jun;32(3):379-85. PMID: 18520541.

106. Kim SK, Lim JH, Lee WJ, et al. Detection of hepatocellular carcinoma: comparison of dynamic three-phase computed tomography images and four-phase computed tomography images using multidetector row helical computed tomography. J Comput Assist Tomogr. 2002 Sep-Oct;26(5):691-8. PMID: 12439300.

107. Kim T, Murakami T, Hori M, et al. Small hypervascular hepatocellular carcinoma revealed by double arterial phase CT performed with single breath-hold scanning and automatic bolus tracking. AJR Am J Roentgenol. 2002 Apr;178(4):899-904. PMID: 11906869.

108. Kim TK, Lee KH, Jang H-J, et al. Analysis of gadobenate dimeglumine-enhanced MR findings for characterizing small (1-2-cm) hepatic nodules in patients at high risk for hepatocellular carcinoma. Radiology. 2011 Jun;259(3):730-8. PMID: 21364083.

109. Kim YK, Kim CS, Chung GH, et al. Comparison of gadobenate dimeglumine-enhanced dynamic MRI and 16-MDCT for the detection of hepatocellular carcinoma. AJR Am J Roentgenol. 2006 Jan;186(1):149-57. PMID: 16357395.

110. Kim YK, Kim CS, Han YM, et al. Detection of hepatocellular carcinoma: gadoxetic acid-enhanced 3-dimensional magnetic resonance

imaging versus multi-detector row computed tomography. J Comput Assist Tomogr. 2009 Nov-Dec;33(6):844-50. PMID: 19940648.

111. Kim YK, Kim CS, Han YM, et al. Detection of liver malignancy with gadoxetic acid-enhanced MRI: is addition of diffusion-weighted MRI beneficial?.[Erratum appears in Clin Radiol. 2011 Oct;66(10):1006]. Clin Radiol. 2011 Jun;66(6):489-96. PMID: 21367403.

112. Kim YK, Kim CS, Han YM, et al. Detection of small hepatocellular carcinoma: can gadoxetic acid-enhanced magnetic resonance imaging replace combining gadopentetate dimeglumine-enhanced and superparamagnetic iron oxide-enhanced magnetic resonance imaging? Invest Radiol. 2010 Nov;45(11):740-6. PMID: 20644488.

113. Kim YK, Kim CS, Han YM, et al. Comparison of gadoxetic acid-enhanced MRI and superparamagnetic iron oxide-enhanced MRI for the detection of hepatocellular carcinoma. Clin Radiol. 2010 May;65(5):358-65. PMID: 20380933.

114. Kim YK, Kim CS, Han YM, et al. Detection of small hepatocellular carcinoma: intraindividual comparison of gadoxetic acid-enhanced MRI at 3.0 and 1.5 T.[Erratum appears in Invest Radiol. 2011 Sep;46(9):600]. Invest Radiol. 2011 Jun;46(6):383-9. PMID: 21467946.

115. Kim YK, Kim CS, Kwak HS, et al. Three-dimensional dynamic liver MR imaging using sensitivity encoding for detection of hepatocellular carcinomas: comparison with superparamagnetic iron oxide-enhanced mr imaging. J Magn Reson Imaging. 2004 Nov;20(5):826-37. PMID: 15503325.

116. Kim YK, Kim CS, Lee YH, et al. Comparison of superparamagnetic iron oxide-enhanced and gadobenate dimeglumine-enhanced dynamic MRI for detection of small hepatocellular carcinomas. AJR Am J Roentgenol. 2004 May;182(5):1217-23. PMID: 15100122.

117. Kim YK, Kwak HS, Han YM, et al. Usefulness of combining sequentially acquired gadobenate dimeglumine-enhanced magnetic resonance imaging and resovist-enhanced magnetic resonance imaging for the detection of hepatocellular carcinoma: comparison with computed tomography hepatic arteriography and computed tomography arterioportography using 16-slice multidetector computed tomography. J Comput Assist Tomogr. 2007 Sep-Oct;31(5):702-11. PMID: 17895780.

118. Kim YK, Kwak HS, Kim CS, et al. Hepatocellular carcinoma in patients with chronic liver disease: comparison of SPIO-enhanced MR imaging and 16-detector row CT. Radiology. 2006 Feb;238(2):531-41. PMID: 16371577.

119. Kim YK, Lee YH, Kim CS, et al. Added diagnostic value of T2-weighted MR imaging to gadolinium-enhanced three-dimensional dynamic MR imaging for the detection of small hepatocellular carcinomas. Eur J Radiol. 2008 Aug;67(2):304-10. PMID: 17714904.

120. Kim YK, Lee YH, Kim CS, et al. Double-dose 1.0-M gadobutrol versus standard-dose 0.5-M gadopentetate dimeglumine in revealing small hypervascular hepatocellular carcinomas. Eur Radiol. 2008 Jan;18(1):70-7. PMID: 17404740.

121. Kim Y-K, Lee K-W, Cho SY, et al. Usefulness 18F-FDG positron emission tomography/computed tomography for detecting recurrence of hepatocellular carcinoma in posttransplant patients. Liver Transpl. 2010 Jun;16(6):767-72. PMID: 20517911.

122. Kitamura T, Ichikawa T, Erturk SM, et al. Detection of hypervascular hepatocellular carcinoma with multidetector-row CT: single arterial-phase imaging with computer-assisted automatic bolus-tracking technique compared with double arterial-phase imaging. J Comput Assist Tomogr. 2008 Sep-Oct;32(5):724-9. PMID: 18830101.

123. Kondo H, Kanematsu M, Itoh K, et al. Does T2-weighted MR imaging improve preoperative detection of malignant hepatic tumors? Observer performance study in 49 surgically proven cases. Magn Reson Imaging. 2005 Jan;23(1):89-95. PMID: 15733793.

124. Korenaga K, Korenaga M, Furukawa M, et al. Usefulness of Sonazoid contrast-enhanced ultrasonography for hepatocellular carcinoma: Comparison with pathological diagnosis and superparamagnetic iron oxide magnetic resonance images. J Gastroenterol.

2009;44(7):733-41. PMID: 19387532.

125. Koushima Y, Ebara M, Fukuda H, et al. Small hepatocellular carcinoma: assessment with T1-weighted spin-echo magnetic resonance imaging with and without fat suppression. Eur J Radiol. 2002 Jan;41(1):34-41. PMID: 11750150.

126. Krinsky GA, Lee VS, Theise ND, et al. Transplantation for hepatocellular carcinoma and cirrhosis: Sensitivity of magnetic resonance imaging. Liver Transpl. 2002;8(12):1156-64. PMID: 12474156.

127. Krinsky GA, Lee VS, Theise ND, et al. Hepatocellular carcinoma and dysplastic nodules in patients with cirrhosis: prospective diagnosis with MR imaging and explantation correlation. Radiology. 2001 May;219(2):445-54. PMID: 11323471.

128. Kumano S, Uemura M, Haraikawa T, et al. Efficacy of double arterial phase dynamic magnetic resonance imaging with the sensitivity encoding technique versus dynamic multidetector-row helical computed tomography for detecting hypervascular hepatocellular carcinoma. Jpn J Radiol. 2009 Jul;27(6):229-36. PMID: 19626408.

129. Kunishi Y, Numata K, Morimoto M, et al. Efficacy of fusion imaging combining sonography and hepatobiliary phase MRI with Gd-EOB-DTPA to detect small hepatocellular carcinoma. AJR Am J Roentgenol. 2012 Jan;198(1):106-14. PMID: 22194485.

130. Kwak H-S, Lee J-M, Kim C-S. Preoperative detection of hepatocellular carcinoma: comparison of combined contrast-enhanced MR imaging and combined CT during arterial portography and CT hepatic arteriography. Eur Radiol. 2004 Mar;14(3):447-57. PMID: 14531005.

131. Kwak H-S, Lee J-M, Kim Y-K, et al. Detection of hepatocellular carcinoma: comparison of ferumoxides-enhanced and gadolinium-enhanced dynamic three-dimensional volume interpolated breath-hold MR imaging. Eur Radiol. 2005 Jan;15(1):140-7. PMID: 15449000.

132. Laghi A, Iannaccone R, Rossi P, et al. Hepatocellular carcinoma: detection with triple-phase multi-detector row helical CT in patients with chronic hepatitis. Radiology. 2003 Feb;226(2):543-9. PMID: 12563152.

133. Lauenstein TC, Salman K, Morreira R, et al. Gadolinium-enhanced MRI for tumor surveillance before liver transplantation: center-based experience. AJR Am J Roentgenol. 2007 Sep;189(3):663-70. PMID: 17715115.

134. Lee CH, Kim KA, Lee J, et al. Using low tube voltage (80kVp) quadruple phase liver CT for the detection of hepatocellular carcinoma: two-year experience and comparison with Gd-EOB-DTPA enhanced liver MRI. Eur J Radiol. 2012 Apr;81(4):e605-11. PMID: 22297180.

135. Lee DH, Kim SH, Lee JM, et al. Diagnostic performance of multidetector row computed tomography, superparamagnetic iron oxide-enhanced magnetic resonance imaging, and dual-contrast magnetic resonance imaging in predicting the appropriateness of a transplant recipient based on milan criteria: correlation with histopathological findings. Invest Radiol. 2009 Jun;44(6):311-21. PMID: 19462486.

136. Lee J, Won JL, Hyo KL, et al. Early hepatocellular carcinoma: Three-phase helical CT features of 16 patients. Korean J Radiol. 2008;9(4):325-32. PMID: 18682670.

137. Lee JE, Jang JY, Jeong SW, et al. Diagnostic value for extrahepatic metastases of hepatocellular carcinoma in positron emission tomography/computed tomography scan. World J Gastroenterol. 2012 Jun 21;18(23):2979-87. PMID: 22736922.

138. Lee J-M, Kim I-H, Kwak H-S, et al. Detection of small hypervascular hepatocellular carcinomas in cirrhotic patients: comparison of superparamagnetic iron oxide-enhanced MR imaging with dual-phase spiral CT. Korean J Radiol. 2003 Jan-Mar;4(1):1-8. PMID: 12679628.

139. Lee JY, Kim SH, Jeon YH, et al. Ferucarbotran-enhanced magnetic resonance imaging versus gadoxetic acid-enhanced magnetic resonance imaging for the preoperative detection of hepatocellular carcinoma: initial experience. J Comput Assist Tomogr. 2010 Jan;34(1):127-34. PMID: 20118735.

140. Lee MH, Kim SH, Park MJ, et al. Gadoxetic acid-enhanced hepatobiliary phase MRI and high-b-value diffusion-weighted imaging to

distinguish well-differentiated hepatocellular carcinomas from benign nodules in patients with chronic liver disease. AJR Am J Roentgenol. 2011 Nov;197(5):W868-75. PMID: 22021534.

141. Lee MW, Kim YJ, Park HS, et al. Targeted sonography for small hepatocellular carcinoma discovered by CT or MRI: factors affecting sonographic detection. AJR Am J Roentgenol. 2010 May;194(5):W396-400. PMID: 20410384.

142. Li CS, Chen RC, Tu HY, et al. Imaging well-differentiated hepatocellular carcinoma with dynamic triple-phase helical computed tomography. Br J Radiol. 2006 Aug;79(944):659-65. PMID: 16641423.

143. Li R, Guo Y, Hua X, et al. Characterization of focal liver lesions: comparison of pulse-inversion harmonic contrast-enhanced sonography with contrast-enhanced CT. J Clin Ultrasound. 2007 Mar-Apr;35(3):109-17. PMID: 17295272.

144. Li S, Beheshti M, Peck-Radosavljevic M, et al. Comparison of (11)C-acetate positron emission tomography and (67)Gallium citrate scintigraphy in patients with hepatocellular carcinoma. Liver Int. 2006 Oct;26(8):920-7. PMID: 16953831.

145. Liangpunsakul S, Agarwal D, Horlander JC, et al. Positron emission tomography for detecting occult hepatocellular carcinoma in hepatitis C cirrhotics awaiting for liver transplantation. Transplant Proc. 2003 Dec;35(8):2995-7. PMID: 14697959.

146. Libbrecht L, Bielen D, Verslype C, et al. Focal lesions in cirrhotic explant livers: pathological evaluation and accuracy of pretransplantation imaging examinations. Liver Transpl. 2002 Sep;8(9):749-61. PMID: 12200773.

147. Lim JH, Choi D, Kim SH, et al. Detection of hepatocellular carcinoma: value of adding delayed phase imaging to dual-phase helical CT. AJR Am J Roentgenol. 2002 Jul;179(1):67-73. PMID: 12076907.

148. Lim JH, Kim CK, Lee WJ, et al. Detection of hepatocellular carcinomas and dysplastic nodules in cirrhotic livers: accuracy of helical CT in transplant patients. AJR Am J Roentgenol. 2000 Sep;175(3):693-8. PMID: 10954452.

149. Lim JH, Kim SH, Lee WJ, et al. Ultrasonographic detection of hepatocellular carcinoma: Correlation of preoperative ultrasonography and resected liver pathology. Clin Radiol. 2006;61(2):191-7. PMID: 16439225.

150. Lin M-T, Chen C-L, Wang C-C, et al. Diagnostic sensitivity of hepatocellular carcinoma imaging and its application to non-cirrhotic patients. J Gastroenterol Hepatol. 2011 Apr;26(4):745-50. PMID: 21418303.

151. Lin W-Y, Tsai S-C, Hung G-U. Value of delayed 18F-FDG-PET imaging in the detection of hepatocellular carcinoma. Nuclear Medicine Communications. 2005 Apr;26(4):315-21. PMID: 15753790.

152. Liu WC, Lim JH, Park CK, et al. Poor sensitivity of sonography in detection of hepatocellular carcinoma in advanced liver cirrhosis: accuracy of pretransplantation sonography in 118 patients. Eur Radiol. 2003 Jul;13(7):1693-8. PMID: 12835987.

153. Liu YI, Kamaya A, Jeffrey RB, et al. Multidetector computed tomography triphasic evaluation of the liver before transplantation: importance of equilibrium phase washout and morphology for characterizing hypervascular lesions. J Comput Assist Tomogr. 2012 Mar-Apr;36(2):213-9. PMID: 22446362.

154. Liu YI, Shin LK, Jeffrey RB, et al. Quantitatively defining washout in hepatocellular carcinoma. AJR Am J Roentgenol. 2013 Jan;200(1):84-9. PMID: 23255745.

155. Lu CH, Chen CL, Cheng YF, et al. Correlation between imaging and pathologic findings in explanted livers of hepatocellular carcinoma cases. Transplant Proc. 2010 Apr;42(3):830-3. PMID: 20430183.

156. Luca A, Caruso S, Milazzo M, et al. Multidetector-row computed tomography (MDCT) for the diagnosis of hepatocellular carcinoma in cirrhotic candidates for liver transplantation: prevalence of radiological vascular patterns and histological correlation with liver explants.[Erratum appears in Eur Radiol. 2011 Jul;21(7):1574 Note: Grutttadauria, Salvatore [corrected to Gruttadauria, Salvatore]]. Eur Radiol. 2010 Apr;20(4):898-907. PMID: 19802612.

157. Luo BM, Wen YL, Yang HY, et al. Differentiation between malignant and benign nodules in the liver: use of contrast C3-MODE technology. World J Gastroenterol. 2005 Apr 28;11(16):2402-7. PMID: 15832408.

158. Luo W, Numata K, Kondo M, et al. Sonazoid-enhanced ultrasonography for evaluation of the enhancement patterns of focal liver tumors in the late phase by intermittent imaging with a high mechanical index. J Ultrasound Med. 2009 Apr;28(4):439-48. PMID: 19321671.

159. Luo W, Numata K, Morimoto M, et al. Focal liver tumors: characterization with 3D perflubutane microbubble contrast agent-enhanced US versus 3D contrast-enhanced multidetector CT. Radiology. 2009 Apr;251(1):287-95. PMID: 19221060.

160. Luo W, Numata K, Morimoto M, et al. Three-dimensional contrast-enhanced sonography of vascular patterns of focal liver tumors: pilot study of visualization methods. AJR Am J Roentgenol. 2009 Jan;192(1):165-73. PMID: 19098197.

161. Lv P, Lin XZ, Chen K, et al. Spectral CT in patients with small HCC: investigation of image quality and diagnostic accuracy. Eur Radiol. 2012 Oct;22(10):2117-24. PMID: 22618521.

162. Lv P, Lin XZ, Li J, et al. Differentiation of small hepatic hemangioma from small hepatocellular carcinoma: recently introduced spectral CT method. Radiology. 2011 Jun;259(3):720-9. PMID: 21357524.

163. Maetani YS, Ueda M, Haga H, et al. Hepatocellular carcinoma in patients undergoing living-donor liver transplantation. Accuracy of multidetector computed tomography by viewing images on digital monitors. Intervirology. 2008;51 Suppl 1:46-51. PMID: 18544948.

164. Marin D, Catalano C, De Filippis G, et al. Detection of hepatocellular carcinoma in patients with cirrhosis: added value of coronal reformations from isotropic voxels with 64-MDCT. AJR Am J Roentgenol. 2009 Jan;192(1):180-7. PMID: 19098199.

165. Marin D, Di Martino M, Guerrisi A, et al. Hepatocellular carcinoma in patients with cirrhosis: qualitative comparison of gadobenate dimeglumine-enhanced MR imaging and multiphasic 64-section CT. Radiology. 2009 Apr;251(1):85-95. PMID: 19332848.

166. Marrero JA, Hussain HK, Nghiem HV, et al. Improving the prediction of hepatocellular carcinoma in cirrhotic patients with an arterially-enhancing liver mass. Liver Transpl. 2005 Mar;11(3):281-9. PMID: 15719410.

167. Matsuo M, Kanematsu M, Itoh K, et al. Detection of malignant hepatic tumors: comparison of gadolinium-and ferumoxide-enhanced MR imaging. AJR Am J Roentgenol. 2001 Sep;177(3):637-43. PMID: 11517061.

168. Mita K, Kim SR, Kudo M, et al. Diagnostic sensitivity of imaging modalities for hepatocellular carcinoma smaller than 2 cm. World J Gastroenterol. 2010 Sep 7;16(33):4187-92. PMID: 20806437.

169. Mok TSK, Yu SCH, Lee C, et al. False-negative rate of abdominal sonography for detecting hepatocellular carcinoma in patients with hepatitis B and elevated serum alpha-fetoprotein levels. AJR Am J Roentgenol. 2004 Aug;183(2):453-8. PMID: 15269040.

170. Monzawa S, Ichikawa T, Nakajima H, et al. Dynamic CT for detecting small hepatocellular carcinoma: usefulness of delayed phase imaging. AJR Am J Roentgenol. 2007 Jan;188(1):147-53. PMID: 17179357.

171. Mori K, Yoshioka H, Takahashi N, et al. Triple arterial phase dynamic MRI with sensitivity encoding for hypervascular hepatocellular carcinoma: comparison of the diagnostic accuracy among the early, middle, late, and whole triple arterial phase imaging. AJR Am J Roentgenol. 2005 Jan;184(1):63-9. PMID: 15615952.

172. Moriyasu F, Itoh K. Efficacy of perflubutane microbubble-enhanced ultrasound in the characterization and detection of focal liver lesions: phase 3 multicenter clinical trial. AJR Am J Roentgenol. 2009 Jul;193(1):86-95. PMID: 19542399.

173. Mortele KJ, De Keukeleire K, Praet M, et al. Malignant focal hepatic lesions complicating underlying liver disease: dual-phase contrast-enhanced spiral CT sensitivity and specificity in orthotopic liver transplant

patients. Eur Radiol. 2001;11(9):1631-8. PMID: 11511882.

174. Motosugi U, Ichikawa T, Sou H, et al. Distinguishing hypervascular pseudolesions of the liver from hypervascular hepatocellular carcinomas with gadoxetic acid-enhanced MR imaging. Radiology. 2010 Jul;256(1):151-8. PMID: 20574092.

175. Murakami T, Kim T, Kawata S, et al. Evaluation of optimal timing of arterial phase imaging for the detection of hypervascular hepatocellular carcinoma by using triple arterial phase imaging with multidetector-row helical computed tomography. Invest Radiol. 2003 Aug;38(8):497-503. PMID: 12874516.

176. Murakami T, Kim T, Takamura M, et al. Hypervascular hepatocellular carcinoma: detection with double arterial phase multi-detector row helical CT. Radiology. 2001 Mar;218(3):763-7. PMID: 11230652.

177. Nagaoka S, Itano S, Ishibashi M, et al. Value of fusing PET plus CT images in hepatocellular carcinoma and combined hepatocellular and cholangiocarcinoma patients with extrahepatic metastases: preliminary findings. Liver Int. 2006 Sep;26(7):781-8. PMID: 16911459.

178. Nakamura H, Ito N, Kotake F, et al. Tumor-detecting capacity and clinical usefulness of SPIO-MRI in patients with hepatocellular carcinoma. J Gastroenterol. 2000;35(11):849-55. PMID: 11085494.

179. Nakamura Y, Tashiro H, Nambu J, et al. Detectability of hepatocellular carcinoma by gadoxetate disodium-enhanced hepatic MRI: Tumor-by-tumor analysis in explant livers. J Magn Reson Imaging. 2013;37(3):684-91. PMID: 23055436.

180. Nakayama A, Imamura H, Matsuyama Y, et al. Value of lipiodol computed tomography and digital subtraction angiography in the era of helical biphasic computed tomography as preoperative assessment of hepatocellular carcinoma. Ann Surg. 2001 Jul;234(1):56-62. PMID: 11420483.

181. Noguchi Y, Murakami T, Kim T, et al. Detection of hepatocellular carcinoma: comparison of dynamic MR imaging with dynamic double arterial phase helical CT. AJR Am J Roentgenol. 2003 Feb;180(2):455-60. PMID: 12540451.

182. Noguchi Y, Murakami T, Kim T, et al. Detection of hypervascular hepatocellular carcinoma by dynamic magnetic resonance imaging with double-echo chemical shift in-phase and opposed-phase gradient echo technique: comparison with dynamic helical computed tomography imaging with double arterial phase. J Comput Assist Tomogr. 2002 Nov-Dec;26(6):981-7. PMID: 12488747.

183. Numata K, Fukuda H, Miwa H, et al. Contrast-enhanced ultrasonography findings using a perflubutane-based contrast agent in patients with early hepatocellular carcinoma. Eur J Radiol. 2014 PMID: 24176532.

184. Onishi H, Kim T, Imai Y, et al. Hypervascular hepatocellular carcinomas: detection with gadoxetate disodium-enhanced MR imaging and multiphasic multidetector CT. Eur Radiol. 2012 Apr;22(4):845-54. PMID: 22057248.

185. Ooi C-C, Low S-C, Schneider-Kolsky M, et al. Diagnostic accuracy of contrast-enhanced ultrasound in differentiating benign and malignant focal liver lesions: a retrospective study. J Med Imaging Radiat Oncol. 2010 Oct;54(5):421-30. PMID: 20958940.

186. Ooka Y, Kanai F, Okabe S, et al. Gadoxetic acid-enhanced MRI compared with CT during angiography in the diagnosis of hepatocellular carcinoma. Magn Reson Imaging. 2013;31(5):748-54 Epub 2012 Dec 5. PMID: 23218794.

187. Park G, Kim YK, Kim CS, et al. Diagnostic efficacy of gadoxetic acid-enhanced MRI in the detection of hepatocellular carcinomas: comparison with gadopentetate dimeglumine. Br J Radiol. 2010 Dec;83(996):1010-6. PMID: 20682591.

188. Park JH, Kim SH, Park HS, et al. Added value of 80 kVp images to averaged 120 kVp images in the detection of hepatocellular carcinomas in liver transplantation candidates using dual-source dual-energy MDCT: results of JAFROC analysis. Eur J Radiol. 2011 Nov;80(2):e76-85. PMID: 20875937.

189. Park J-W, Kim JH, Kim SK, et al. A prospective evaluation of 18F-FDG and 11C-acetate PET/CT for detection of primary and metastatic hepatocellular carcinoma. J Nucl Med. 2008

Dec;49(12):1912-21. PMID: 18997056.

190. Park MJ, Kim YK, Lee MH, et al. Validation of diagnostic criteria using gadoxetic acid-enhanced and diffusion-weighted MR imaging for small hepatocellular carcinoma (≤ 2.0 cm) in patients with hepatitis-induced liver cirrhosis. Acta Radiol. 2013;54(2):127-36. PMID: 23148300.

191. Park M-S, Kim S, Patel J, et al. Hepatocellular carcinoma: detection with diffusion-weighted versus contrast-enhanced magnetic resonance imaging in pretransplant patients. Hepatology. 2012 Jul;56(1):140-8. PMID: 22370974.

192. Park Y, Kim SH, Kim SH, et al. Gadoxetic acid (Gd-EOB-DTPA)-enhanced MRI versus gadobenate dimeglumine (Gd-BOPTA)-enhanced MRI for preoperatively detecting hepatocellular carcinoma: an initial experience. Korean J Radiol. 2010 Jul-Aug;11(4):433-40. PMID: 20592927.

193. Paul SB, Gulati MS, Sreenivas V, et al. Evaluating patients with cirrhosis for hepatocellular carcinoma: value of clinical symptomatology, imaging and alpha-fetoprotein. Oncology. 2007;72 Suppl 1:117-23. PMID: 18087192.

194. Pauleit D, Textor J, Bachmann R, et al. Hepatocellular carcinoma: detection with gadolinium- and ferumoxides-enhanced MR imaging of the liver. Radiology. 2002 Jan;222(1):73-80. PMID: 11756708.

195. Pei XQ, Liu LZ, Xiong YH, et al. Quantitative analysis of contrast-enhanced ultrasonography: Differentiating focal nodular hyperplasia from hepatocellular carcinoma. Br J Radiol. 2013 Mar;86(1023):20120536 Epub 2013 Feb 7. PMID: 23392189.

196. Peterson MS, Baron RL, Marsh JW, Jr., et al. Pretransplantation surveillance for possible hepatocellular carcinoma in patients with cirrhosis: epidemiology and CT-based tumor detection rate in 430 cases with surgical pathologic correlation. Radiology. 2000 Dec;217(3):743-9. PMID: 11110938.

197. Petruzzi N, Mitchell D, Guglielmo F, et al. Hepatocellular carcinoma likelihood on MRI exams. Evaluation of a standardized categorization System. Acad Radiol. 2013 Jun;20(6):694-8 Epub 2013 Mar 28. PMID: 23541479.

198. Piana G, Trinquart L, Meskine N, et al. New MR imaging criteria with a diffusion-weighted sequence for the diagnosis of hepatocellular carcinoma in chronic liver diseases. J Hepatol. 2011 Jul;55(1):126-32. PMID: 21145857.

199. Pitton MB, Kloeckner R, Herber S, et al. MRI versus 64-row MDCT for diagnosis of hepatocellular carcinoma. World J Gastroenterol. 2009 Dec 28;15(48):6044-51. PMID: 20027676.

200. Pocha C, Dieperink E, McMaken KA, et al. Surveillance for hepatocellular cancer with ultrasonography vs. computed tomography - A randomised study. Alimentary Pharmacology and Therapeutics. 2013;38(3):303-12. PMID: 23750991.

201. Pozzi Mucelli RM, Como G, Del Frate C, et al. Multidetector CT with double arterial phase and high-iodine-concentration contrast agent in the detection of hepatocellular carcinoma. Radiol Med (Torino). 2006 Mar;111(2):181-91. PMID: 16671376.

202. Pugacheva O, Matsui O, Kozaka K, et al. Detection of small hypervascular hepatocellular carcinomas by EASL criteria: comparison with double-phase CT during hepatic arteriography. Eur J Radiol. 2011 Dec;80(3):e201-6. PMID: 20855175.

203. Quaia E, Alaimo V, Baratella E, et al. The added diagnostic value of 64-row multidetector CT combined with contrast-enhanced US in the evaluation of hepatocellular nodule vascularity: implications in the diagnosis of malignancy in patients with liver cirrhosis. Eur Radiol. 2009 Mar;19(3):651-63. PMID: 18815790.

204. Quaia E, Bertolotto M, Calderan L, et al. US characterization of focal hepatic lesions with intermittent high-acoustic-power mode and contrast material. Acad Radiol. 2003 Jul;10(7):739-50. PMID: 12862283.

205. Rhee H, Kim MJ, Park MS, et al. Differentiation of early hepatocellular carcinoma from benign hepatocellular nodules on gadoxetic acid-enhanced MRI. Br J Radiol. 2012 Oct;85(1018):e837-44. PMID: 22553295.

206. Rickes S, Schulze S, Neye H, et al.

Improved diagnosing of small hepatocellular carcinomas by echo-enhanced power Doppler sonography in patients with cirrhosis. Eur J Gastroenterol Hepatol. 2003 Aug;15(8):893-900. PMID: 12867800.

207. Rimola J, Forner A, Tremosini S, et al. Non-invasive diagnosis of hepatocellular carcinoma ≤ 2 cm in cirrhosis. Diagnostic accuracy assessing fat, capsule and signal intensity at dynamic MRI. J Hepatol. 2012 Jun;56(6):1317-23. PMID: 22314420.

208. Rizvi S, Camci C, Yong Y, et al. Is post-Lipiodol CT better than i.v. contrast CT scan for early detection of HCC? A single liver transplant center experience. Transplant Proc. 2006 Nov;38(9):2993-5. PMID: 17112883.

209. Rode A, Bancel B, Douek P, et al. Small nodule detection in cirrhotic livers: evaluation with US, spiral CT, and MRI and correlation with pathologic examination of explanted liver. J Comput Assist Tomogr. 2001 May-Jun;25(3):327-36. PMID: 11351179.

210. Ronzoni A, Artioli D, Scardina R, et al. Role of MDCT in the diagnosis of hepatocellular carcinoma in patients with cirrhosis undergoing orthotopic liver transplantation. AJR Am J Roentgenol. 2007 Oct;189(4):792-8. PMID: 17885047.

211. Sangiovanni A, Manini MA, Iavarone M, et al. The diagnostic and economic impact of contrast imaging techniques in the diagnosis of small hepatocellular carcinoma in cirrhosis. Gut. 2010 May;59(5):638-44. PMID: 19951909.

212. Sano K, Ichikawa T, Motosugi U, et al. Imaging study of early hepatocellular carcinoma: usefulness of gadoxetic acid-enhanced MR imaging. Radiology. 2011 Dec;261(3):834-44. PMID: 21998047.

213. Schima W, Hammerstingl R, Catalano C, et al. Quadruple-phase MDCT of the liver in patients with suspected hepatocellular carcinoma: Effect of contrast material flow rate. AJR Am J Roentgenol. 2006;186(6):1571-9. PMID: 16714645.

214. Secil M, Obuz F, Altay C, et al. The role of dynamic subtraction MRI in detection of hepatocellular carcinoma. Diagn Interv Radiol. 2008 Dec;14(4):200-4. PMID: 19061165.

215. Seitz K, Bernatik T, Strobel D, et al. Contrast-enhanced ultrasound (CEUS) for the characterization of focal liver lesions in clinical practice (DEGUM Multicenter Trial): CEUS vs. MRI--a prospective comparison in 269 patients. Ultraschall Med. 2010 Oct;31(5):492-9. PMID: 20652854.

216. Seitz K, Strobel D, Bernatik T, et al. Contrast-Enhanced Ultrasound (CEUS) for the characterization of focal liver lesions - prospective comparison in clinical practice: CEUS vs. CT (DEGUM multicenter trial). Parts of this manuscript were presented at the Ultrasound Dreilandertreffen 2008, Davos. Ultraschall Med. 2009 Aug;30(4):383-9. PMID: 19688670.

217. Serste T, Barrau V, Ozenne V, et al. Accuracy and disagreement of computed tomography and magnetic resonance imaging for the diagnosis of small hepatocellular carcinoma and dysplastic nodules: role of biopsy. Hepatology. 2012 Mar;55(3):800-6. PMID: 22006503.

218. Shah SA, Tan JC, McGilvray ID, et al. Accuracy of staging as a predictor for recurrence after liver transplantation for hepatocellular carcinoma. Transplantation. 2006 Jun 27;81(12):1633-9. PMID: 16794527.

219. Simon G, Link TM, Wortler K, et al. Detection of hepatocellular carcinoma: comparison of Gd-DTPA- and ferumoxides-enhanced MR imaging. Eur Radiol. 2005 May;15(5):895-903. PMID: 15800773.

220. Singh P, Erickson RA, Mukhopadhyay P, et al. EUS for detection of the hepatocellular carcinoma: results of a prospective study. Gastrointest Endosc. 2007 Aug;66(2):265-73. PMID: 17543307.

221. Sofue K, Tsurusaki M, Kawasaki R, et al. Evaluation of hypervascular hepatocellular carcinoma in cirrhotic liver: comparison of different concentrations of contrast material with multi-detector row helical CT--a prospective randomized study. Eur J Radiol. 2011 Dec;80(3):e237-42. PMID: 21067880.

222. Sørensen M, Frisch K, Bender D, et al. The potential use of 2-[18F]fluoro-2-deoxy-D-galactose as a PET/CT tracer for detection of hepatocellular carcinoma. Eur J Nucl Med Mol Imaging. 2011;38(9):1723-31.

PMID: 21553087.

223. Strobel D, Raeker S, Martus P, et al. Phase inversion harmonic imaging versus contrast-enhanced power Doppler sonography for the characterization of focal liver lesions. Int J Colorectal Dis. 2003 Jan;18(1):63-72. PMID: 12458384.

224. Sugimoto K, Moriyasu F, Saito K, et al. Comparison of Kupffer-phase Sonazoid-enhanced sonography and hepatobiliary-phase gadoxetic acid-enhanced magnetic resonance imaging of hepatocellular carcinoma and correlation with histologic grading. J Ultrasound Med. 2012 Apr;31(4):529-38. PMID: 22441909.

225. Sugimoto K, Moriyasu F, Shiraishi J, et al. Assessment of arterial hypervascularity of hepatocellular carcinoma: comparison of contrast-enhanced US and gadoxetate disodium-enhanced MR imaging. Eur Radiol. 2012 Jun;22(6):1205-13. PMID: 22270142.

226. Sugiyama M, Sakahara H, Torizuka T, et al. 18F-FDG PET in the detection of extrahepatic metastases from hepatocellular carcinoma. J Gastroenterol. 2004;39(10):961-8. PMID: 15549449.

227. Suh YJ, Kim M-J, Choi J-Y, et al. Differentiation of hepatic hyperintense lesions seen on gadoxetic acid-enhanced hepatobiliary phase MRI. AJR Am J Roentgenol. 2011 Jul;197(1):W44-52. PMID: 21700994.

228. Sun HY, Lee JM, Shin CI, et al. Gadoxetic acid-enhanced magnetic resonance imaging for differentiating small hepatocellular carcinomas (≤ 2 cm in diameter) from arterial enhancing pseudolesions: special emphasis on hepatobiliary phase imaging. Invest Radiol. 2010 Feb;45(2):96-103. PMID: 20057319.

229. Sun L, Guan YS, Pan WM, et al. Metabolic restaging of hepatocellular carcinoma using whole-body F-FDG PET/CT. World J Hepatol. 2009 Oct 31;1(1):90-7. PMID: 21160970.

230. Suzuki S, Iijima H, Moriyasu F, et al. Differential diagnosis of hepatic nodules using delayed parenchymal phase imaging of levovist contrast ultrasound: comparative study with SPIO-MRI. Hepatol Res. 2004 Jun;29(2):122-6. PMID: 15163434.

231. Takahashi M, Maruyama H, Shimada T, et al. Characterization of hepatic lesions (≤ 30 mm) with liver-specific contrast agents: a comparison between ultrasound and magnetic resonance imaging. Eur J Radiol. 2013;82(1):75-84. PMID: 23116806.

232. Talbot J, Fartoux L, Balogova S, et al. Detection of hepatocellular carcinoma with PET/CT: a prospective comparison of 18F-fluorocholine and 18F-FDG in patients with cirrhosis or chronic liver disease. J Nucl Med. 2010 Nov;51(11):1699-706. PMID: 20956466.

233. Talbot J, Gutman F, Fartoux L, et al. PET/CT in patients with hepatocellular carcinoma using [(18)F]fluorocholine: preliminary comparison with [(18)F]FDG PET/CT. Eur J Nucl Med Mol Imaging. 2006 Nov;33(11):1285-9. PMID: 16802155.

234. Tanaka O, Ito H, Yamada K, et al. Higher lesion conspicuity for SENSE dynamic MRI in detecting hypervascular hepatocellular carcinoma: analysis through the measurements of liver SNR and lesion-liver CNR comparison with conventional dynamic MRI. Eur Radiol. 2005 Dec;15(12):2427-34. PMID: 16041592.

235. Tanaka S, Ioka T, Oshikawa O, et al. Dynamic sonography of hepatic tumors. AJR Am J Roentgenol. 2001 Oct;177(4):799-805. PMID: 11566675.

236. Tang Y, Yamashita Y, Arakawa A, et al. Detection of hepatocellular carcinoma arising in cirrhotic livers: comparison of gadolinium- and ferumoxides-enhanced MR imaging. AJR Am J Roentgenol. 1999 Jun;172(6):1547-54. PMID: 10350287.

237. Tanimoto A, Yuasa Y, Jinzaki M, et al. Routine MR imaging protocol with breath-hold fast scans: diagnostic efficacy for focal liver lesions. Radiat Med. 2002 Jul-Aug;20(4):169-79. PMID: 12296432.

238. Teefey SA, Hildeboldt CC, Dehdashti F, et al. Detection of primary hepatic malignancy in liver transplant candidates: prospective comparison of CT, MR imaging, US, and PET. Radiology. 2003 Feb;226(2):533-42. PMID: 12563151.

239. Toyota N, Nakamura Y, Hieda M, et al. Diagnostic capability of gadoxetate disodium-enhanced liver MRI for diagnosis of hepatocellular carcinoma: Comparison

with multi-detector CT. Hiroshima Journal of Medical Sciences. 2013;62(3):55-61. PMID: 24279123.

240. Trinchet JC, Chaffaut C, Bourcier V, et al. Ultrasonographic surveillance of hepatocellular carcinoma in cirrhosis: a randomized trial comparing 3- and 6-month periodicities. Hepatology. 2011 Dec;54(6):1987-97. PMID: 22144108.

241. Trojan J, Schroeder O, Raedle J, et al. Fluorine-18 FDG positron emission tomography for imaging of hepatocellular carcinoma. Am J Gastroenterol. 1999 Nov;94(11):3314-9. PMID: 10566736.

242. Tsurusaki M, Semelka RC, Uotani K, et al. Prospective comparison of high- and low-spatial-resolution dynamic MR imaging with sensitivity encoding (SENSE) for hypervascular hepatocellular carcinoma. Eur Radiol. 2008 Oct;18(10):2206-12. PMID: 18446347.

243. Valls C, Cos M, Figueras J, et al. Pretransplantation diagnosis and staging of hepatocellular carcinoma in patients with cirrhosis: value of dual-phase helical CT. AJR Am J Roentgenol. 2004 Apr;182(4):1011-7. PMID: 15039179.

244. Van Thiel DH, Yong S, Li SD, et al. The development of de novo hepatocellular carcinoma in patients on a liver transplant list: frequency, size, and assessment of current screening methods. Liver Transpl. 2004 May;10(5):631-7. PMID: 15108254.

245. Vandecaveye V, De Keyzer F, Verslype C, et al. Diffusion-weighted MRI provides additional value to conventional dynamic contrast-enhanced MRI for detection of hepatocellular carcinoma. Eur Radiol. 2009 Oct;19(10):2456-66. PMID: 19440718.

246. Verhoef C, Valkema R, de Man RA, et al. Fluorine-18 FDG imaging in hepatocellular carcinoma using positron coincidence detection and single photon emission computed tomography. Liver. 2002 Feb;22(1):51-6. PMID: 11906619.

247. Wagnetz U, Atri M, Massey C, et al. Intraoperative ultrasound of the liver in primary and secondary hepatic malignancies: comparison with preoperative 1.5-T MRI and 64-MDCT. AJR Am J Roentgenol. 2011 Mar;196(3):562-8. PMID: 21343497.

248. Wang JH, Chang KC, Kee KM, et al. Hepatocellular carcinoma surveillance at 4- vs. 12-month intervals for patients with chronic viral hepatitis: a randomized study in community. Am J Gastroenterol. 2013 Mar;108(3):416-24. PMID: 23318478.

249. Wang J-H, Lu S-N, Hung C-H, et al. Small hepatic nodules (≤ 2 cm) in cirrhosis patients: characterization with contrast-enhanced ultrasonography. Liver Int. 2006 Oct;26(8):928-34. PMID: 16953832.

250. Wang ZL, Tang J, Weskott HP, et al. Undetermined focal liver lesions on gray-scale ultrasound in patients with fatty liver: characterization with contrast-enhanced ultrasound. J Gastroenterol Hepatol. 2008 Oct;23(10):1511-9. PMID: 18713302.

251. Wolfort RM, Papillion PW, Turnage RH, et al. Role of FDG-PET in the evaluation and staging of hepatocellular carcinoma with comparison of tumor size, AFP level, and histologic grade. Int Surg. 2010 Jan-Mar;95(1):67-75. PMID: 20480845.

252. Wu H-b, Wang Q-s, Li B-y, et al. F-18 FDG in conjunction with 11C-choline PET/CT in the diagnosis of hepatocellular carcinoma. Clin Nucl Med. 2011 Dec;36(12):1092-7. PMID: 22064078.

253. Wudel LJ, Jr., Delbeke D, Morris D, et al. The role of [18F]fluorodeoxyglucose positron emission tomography imaging in the evaluation of hepatocellular carcinoma. Am Surg. 2003 Feb;69(2):117-24; discussion 24-6. PMID: 12641351.

254. Xiao X-g, Han X, Shan W-d, et al. Multi-slice CT angiography by triple-phase enhancement in preoperative evaluation of hepatocellular carcinoma. Chin Med J (Engl). 2005 May 20;118(10):844-9. PMID: 15989766.

255. Xu HX, Lu MD, Liu LN, et al. Discrimination between neoplastic and non-neoplastic lesions in cirrhotic liver using contrast-enhanced ultrasound. Br J Radiol. 2012 Oct;85(1018):1376-84. PMID: 22553290.

256. Xu H-X, Xie X-Y, Lu M-D, et al. Contrast-enhanced sonography in the diagnosis of small hepatocellular carcinoma ≤ 2 cm. J Clin Ultrasound. 2008 Jun;36(5):257-66. PMID: 18088056.

257. Xu P-J, Yan F-H, Wang J-H, et al. Added value of breathhold diffusion-weighted MRI in detection of small hepatocellular carcinoma lesions compared with dynamic contrast-enhanced MRI alone using receiver operating characteristic curve analysis. J Magn Reson Imaging. 2009 Feb;29(2):341-9. PMID: 19161186.

258. Xu P-J, Yan F-H, Wang J-H, et al. Contribution of diffusion-weighted magnetic resonance imaging in the characterization of hepatocellular carcinomas and dysplastic nodules in cirrhotic liver. J Comput Assist Tomogr. 2010 Jul;34(4):506-12. PMID: 20657216.

259. Yamamoto K, Shiraki K, Deguchi M, et al. Diagnosis of hepatocellular carcinoma using digital subtraction imaging with the contrast agent, Levovist: comparison with helical CT, digital subtraction angiography, and US angiography. Oncol Rep. 2002 Jul-Aug;9(4):789-92. PMID: 12066210.

260. Yamamoto Y, Nishiyama Y, Kameyama R, et al. Detection of hepatocellular carcinoma using 11C-choline PET: Comparison with 18F-FDG PET. J Nucl Med. 2008 Aug;49(8):1245-8. PMID: 18632827.

261. Yan FH, Shen JZ, Li RC, et al. Enhancement patterns of small hepatocellular carcinoma shown by dynamic MRI and CT. Hepatobiliary Pancreat Dis Int. 2002 Aug;1(3):420-4. PMID: 14607719.

262. Yoo HJ, Lee JM, Lee JY, et al. Additional value of SPIO-enhanced MR imaging for the noninvasive imaging diagnosis of hepatocellular carcinoma in cirrhotic liver. Invest Radiol. 2009 Dec;44(12):800-7. PMID: 19838119.

263. Yoo SH, Choi JY, Jang JW, et al. Gd-EOB-DTPA-enhanced MRI is better than MDCT in decision making of curative treatment for hepatocellular carcinoma. Ann Surg Oncol. 2013;20(9):2893-900. PMID: 23649931.

264. Yoon KT, Kim JK, Kim DY, et al. Role of 18F-fluorodeoxyglucose positron emission tomography in detecting extrahepatic metastasis in pretreatment staging of hepatocellular carcinoma. Oncology. 2007;72 Suppl 1:104-10. PMID: 18087190.

265. Yoshioka H, Takahashi N, Yamaguchi M, et al. Double arterial phase dynamic MRI with sensitivity encoding (SENSE) for hypervascular hepatocellular carcinomas. J Magn Reson Imaging. 2002 Sep;16(3):259-66. PMID: 12205581.

266. Youk JH, Lee JM, Kim CS. MRI for detection of hepatocellular carcinoma: comparison of mangafodipir trisodium and gadopentetate dimeglumine contrast agents. AJR Am J Roentgenol. 2004 Oct;183(4):1049-54. PMID: 15385303.

267. Yu JS, Chung JJ, Kim JH, et al. Small hypervascular hepatocellular carcinomas: value of "washout" on gadolinium-enhanced dynamic MR imaging compared to superparamagnetic iron oxide-enhanced imaging. Eur Radiol. 2009 Nov;19(11):2614-22. PMID: 19513719.

268. Yu JS, Kim KW, Park MS, et al. Transient peritumoral enhancement during dynamic MRI of the liver: Cavernous hemangioma versus hepatocellular carcinoma. J Comput Assist Tomogr. 2002 May-Jun;26(3):411-7. PMID: 12016371.

269. Yu JS, Lee JH, Chung JJ, et al. Small hypervascular hepatocellular carcinoma: limited value of portal and delayed phases on dynamic magnetic resonance imaging. Acta Radiol. 2008 Sep;49(7):735-43. PMID: 18608015.

270. Yu MH, Kim JH, Yoon JH, et al. Role of C-arm CT for transcatheter arterial chemoembolization of hepatocellular carcinoma: Diagnostic performance and predictive value for therapeutic response compared with gadoxetic acid-enhanced MRI. AJR Am J Roentgenol. 2013;201(3):675-83. PMID: 23971463.

271. Yu NC, Chaudhari V, Raman SS, et al. CT and MRI improve detection of hepatocellular carcinoma, compared with ultrasound alone, in patients with cirrhosis. Clin Gastroenterol Hepatol. 2011 Feb;9(2):161-7. PMID: 20920597.

272. Yu Y, He N, Sun K, et al. Differentiating hepatocellular carcinoma from angiomyolipoma of the liver with CT spectral imaging: A preliminary study. Clin Radiol. 2013;68(9):e491-e7. PMID: 23702491.

273. Yu Y, Lin X, Chen K, et al. Hepatocellular carcinoma and focal nodular hyperplasia of the liver: differentiation with CT spectral imaging. Eur Radiol. 2013 Jun;23(6):1660-8

Epub 2013 Jan 10. PMID: 23306709.

274. Yukisawa S, Okugawa H, Masuya Y, et al. Multidetector helical CT plus superparamagnetic iron oxide-enhanced MR imaging for focal hepatic lesions in cirrhotic liver: a comparison with multi-phase CT during hepatic arteriography. Eur J Radiol. 2007 Feb;61(2):279-89. PMID: 17070663.

275. Zacherl J, Pokieser P, Wrba F, et al. Accuracy of multiphasic helical computed tomography and intraoperative sonography in patients undergoing orthotopic liver transplantation for hepatoma: what is the truth? Ann Surg. 2002 Apr;235(4):528-32. PMID: 11923609.

276. Zhang BH, Yang BH, Tang ZY. Randomized controlled trial of screening for hepatocellular carcinoma. J Cancer Res Clin Oncol. 2004 Jul;130(7):417-22. PMID: 15042359.

277. Zhao H, Yao JL, Han MJ, et al. Multiphase hepatic scans with multirow-detector helical CT in detection of hypervascular hepatocellular carcinoma. Hepatobiliary Pancreat Dis Int. 2004 May;3(2):204-8. PMID: 15138110.

278. Zhao H, Yao J-L, Wang Y, et al. Detection of small hepatocellular carcinoma: comparison of dynamic enhancement magnetic resonance imaging and multiphase multirow-detector helical CT scanning. World J Gastroenterol. 2007 Feb 28;13(8):1252-6. PMID: 17451209.

279. Zhao H, Zhou K-R, Yan F-H. Role of multiphase scans by multirow-detector helical CT in detecting small hepatocellular carcinoma. World J Gastroenterol. 2003 Oct;9(10):2198-201. PMID: 14562377.

280. Zheng X-H, Guan Y-S, Zhou X-P, et al. Detection of hypervascular hepatocellular carcinoma: Comparison of multi-detector CT with digital subtraction angiography and Lipiodol CT. World J Gastroenterol. 2005 Jan 14;11(2):200-3. PMID: 15633215.

281. Zhou K-R, Yan F-H, Tu B-W. Arterial phase of biphase enhancement spiral CT in diagnosis of small hepatocellular carcinoma. Hepatobiliary Pancreat Dis Int. 2002 Feb;1(1):68-71. PMID: 14607626.

Appendix B. Excluded Studies

Abe Y, Yamashita Y, Tang Y, Namimoto T, Takahashi M. Calculation of T2 relaxation time from ultrafast single shot sequences for differentiation of liver tumors: comparison of echo-planar, HASTE, and spin-echo sequences. Radiat Med. 2000;18(1):7-14, PMID: 10852650. *Excluded: Wrong outcome/Did not report diagnostic accuracy measures*

Achkar JP, Araya V, Baron RL, Marsh JW, Dvorchik I, Rakela J. Undetected hepatocellular carcinoma: clinical features and outcome after liver transplantation. Liver Transpl Surg. 1998;4(6):477-482, PMID: 9791158. *Excluded: Wrong outcome/Did not report diagnostic accuracy measures*

Ahn SJ, Kim M-J, Hong H-S, Kim KA, Song H-T. Distinguishing hemangiomas from malignant solid hepatic lesions: a comparison of heavily T2-weighted images obtained before and after administration of gadoxetic acid. J Magn Reson Imaging. 2011;34(2):310-317, PMID: 21598345. *Excluded: Wrong population*

Ainsworth AP, Pless T, Nielsen HO. Potential impact of adding endoscopic ultrasound to standard imaging procedures in the preoperative assessment of resectability in patients with liver tumors. Scand J Gastroenterol. 2011;46(7-8):1020-1023, PMID: 21504382. *Excluded: Wrong intervention*

Akai H, Matsuda I, Kiryu S, et al. Fate of hypointense lesions on Gd-EOB-DTPA-enhanced magnetic resonance imaging. Eur J Radiol. 2012;81(11):2973-2977, PMID: 22280873. *Excluded: Wrong outcome/Did not report diagnostic accuracy measures*

Altenbernd J, Heusner TA, Ringelstein A, Ladd SC, Forsting M, Antoch G. Dual-energy-CT of hypervascular liver lesions in patients with HCC: investigation of image quality and sensitivity. Eur Radiol. 2011;21(4):738-743, PMID: 20936520. *Excluded: Wrong outcome/Did not report diagnostic accuracy measures*

Andersson KL, Salomon JA, Goldie SJ, Chung RT. Cost effectiveness of alternative surveillance strategies for hepatocellular carcinoma in patients with cirrhosis. Clin Gastroenterol Hepatol. 2008;6(12):1418-1424, PMID: 18848905. *Excluded: Background*

Ando E, Tanaka M, Yamashita F, et al. Diagnostic clues for recurrent hepatocellular carcinoma: comparison of tumour markers and imaging studies. Eur J Gastroenterol Hepatol. 2003;15(6):641-648, PMID: 12840676. *Excluded: Imaging before 1995*

Ansari D, Keussen I, Andersson R. Positron emission tomography in malignancies of the liver, pancreas and biliary tract - indications and potential pitfalls. [Review]. Scandinavian Journal of Gastroenterology. Vol 482013:259-265. *Excluded: Wrong publication type*

Barone C, Koeberle D, Metselaar H, Parisi G, Sansonno D, Spinzi G. Multidisciplinary approach for HCC patients: hepatology for the oncologists. [Review]. Annals of Oncology. Vol 242013. *Excluded: Wrong publication type*

Bartolotta TV, Taibbi A, Galia M, et al. Characterization of hypoechoic focal hepatic lesions in patients with fatty liver: diagnostic performance and confidence of contrast-enhanced ultrasound. Eur Radiol. 2007;17(3):650-661, PMID: 17180328. *Excluded: Wrong population*

Bartolotta TV, Taibbi A, Midiri M, La Grutta L, De Maria M, Lagalla R. Characterisation of focal liver lesions undetermined at grey-scale US: contrast-enhanced US versus 64-row MDCT and MRI with liver-specific contrast agent. Radiol Med. 2010;115(5):714-731, PMID: 20082225. *Excluded: Inadequate reference standard*

Bartolozzi C, Battaglia V, Bargellini I, et al. Contrast-enhanced magnetic resonance imaging of 102 nodules in cirrhosis: correlation with histological findings on explanted livers. Abdom Imaging. 2013;38(2):290-296. *Excluded: Wrong outcome/Did not report diagnostic accuracy measures*

Bashir MR, Gupta RT, Davenport MS, et al. Hepatocellular carcinoma in a North American population: does hepatobiliary MR imaging with Gd-EOB-DTPA improve sensitivity and confidence for diagnosis? J Magn Reson Imaging. 2013;37(2):398-406. *Excluded: Inadequate reference standard*

Ba-Ssalamah A, Heinz-Peer G, Schima W, et al. Detection of focal hepatic lesions: comparison of unenhanced and SHU 555 A-enhanced MR imaging versus biphasic helical CTAP. J Magn Reson Imaging. 2000;11(6):665-672, PMID:

10862066. *Excluded: Wrong population*

Beaton C, Cochlin D, Kumar N. Contrast enhanced ultrasound should be the initial radiological investigation to characterise focal liver lesions. Eur J Surg Oncol. 2010;36(1):43-46, PMID: 19709846. *Excluded: Wrong outcome/Did not report diagnostic accuracy measures*

Beissert M, Delorme S, Mutze S, et al. Comparison of B-mode and conventional colour/power Doppler ultrasound, contrast-enhanced Doppler ultrasound and spiral CT in the diagnosis of focal lesions of the liver: Results of a multicentre study. Ultraschall Med. 2002;23(4):245-250, PMID: 12226762. *Excluded: Wrong population*

Bharat A, Brown DB, Crippin JS, et al. Pre-liver transplantation locoregional adjuvant therapy for hepatocellular carcinoma as a strategy to improve longterm survival. J Am Coll Surg. 2006;203(4):411-420, PMID: 17000383. *Excluded: Wrong intervention*

Bhartia B, Ward J, Guthrie JA, Robinson PJ. Hepatocellular carcinoma in cirrhotic livers: double-contrast thin-section MR imaging with pathologic correlation of explanted tissue. AJR Am J Roentgenol. 2003;180(3):577-584, PMID: 12591657. *Excluded: Wrong intervention*

Bieze M, Bennink RJ, El-Massoudi Y, et al. The use of 18F-fluoromethylcholine PET/CT in differentiating focal nodular hyperplasia from hepatocellular adenoma: A prospective study of diagnostic accuracy. Nuclear Medicine Communications. 2013;34(2):146-154. *Excluded: Wrong population*

Bieze M, van den Esschert JW, Nio CY, et al. Diagnostic accuracy of MRI in differentiating hepatocellular adenoma from focal nodular hyperplasia: prospective study of the additional value of gadoxetate disodium. AJR Am J Roentgenol. 2012;199(1):26-34, PMID: 22733890. *Excluded: Wrong population*

Bleuzen A, Huang C, Olar M, Tchuenbou J, Tranquart F. Diagnostic accuracy of contrast-enhanced ultrasound in focal lesions of the liver using cadence contrast pulse sequencing. Ultraschall Med. 2006;27(1):40-48, PMID: 16470478. *Excluded: Wrong population*

Bluemke DA, Paulson EK, Choti MA, DeSena S, Clavien PA. Detection of hepatic lesions in candidates for surgery: comparison of ferumoxides-enhanced MR imaging and dual-phase helical CT. AJR Am J Roentgenol. 2000;175(6):1653-1658, PMID: 11090399. *Excluded: Wrong population*

Bluemke DA, Weber TM, Rubin D, et al. Hepatic MR imaging with ferumoxides: multicenter study of safety and effectiveness of direct injection protocol. Radiology. 2003;228(2):457-464, PMID: 12893904. *Excluded: Wrong population*

Boeve WJ, Kok T, Haagsma EB, Slooff MJ, Sluiter WJ, Kamman RL. Superior diagnostic strength of combined contrast enhanced MR-angiography and MR-imaging compared to intra-arterial DSA in liver transplantation candidates. Magn Reson Imaging. 2001;19(5):609-622, PMID: 11672618. *Excluded: Wrong outcome/Did not report diagnostic accuracy measures*

Boin IFSF, Pracucho EM, Rique MC, et al. Expanded Milan criteria on pathological examination after liver transplantation: analysis of preoperative data. Transplant Proc. 2008;40(3):777-779, PMID: 18455014. *Excluded: Inadequate reference standard*

Bruegel M, Gaa J, Waldt S, et al. Diagnosis of hepatic metastasis: comparison of respiration-triggered diffusion-weighted echo-planar MRI and five t2-weighted turbo spin-echo sequences. AJR Am J Roentgenol. 2008;191(5):1421-1429, PMID: 18941080. *Excluded: Wrong population*

Bryant TH, Blomley MJ, Albrecht T, et al. Improved characterization of liver lesions with liver-phase uptake of liver-specific microbubbles: prospective multicenter study. Radiology. 2004;232(3):799-809, PMID: 15284434. *Excluded: Wrong outcome/Did not report diagnostic accuracy measures*

Carlos RC, Kim HM, Hussain HK, Francis IR, Nghiem HV, Fendrick AM. Developing a prediction rule to assess hepatic malignancy in patients with cirrhosis. AJR Am J Roentgenol. 2003;180(4):893-900, PMID: 12646426. *Excluded: Wrong outcome/Did not report diagnostic accuracy measures*

Caturelli E, Bartolucci F, Biasini E, et al. Diagnosis of liver nodules observed in chronic liver disease patients during ultrasound screening for early detection of hepatocellular carcinoma. Am J Gastroenterol. 2002;97(2):397-405, PMID: 11866279. *Excluded: Wrong outcome/Did not report diagnostic accuracy measures*

Cedrone A, Pompili M, Sallustio G, Lorenzelli GP, Gasbarrini G, Rapaccini GL. Comparison between color power Doppler ultrasound with echo-enhancer and spiral computed tomography in the evaluation of hepatocellular carcinoma vascularization before and after ablation procedures. Am J Gastroenterol. 2001;96(6):1854-1859, PMID: 11419839. *Excluded: Wrong population*

Cha DI, Lee MW, Kim YK, et al. Assessing patients with hepatocellular carcinoma meeting the milan criteria: Is liver 3 tesla MR with gadoxetic acid necessary in addition to liver CT? J Magn Reson Imaging. 2013. *Excluded: Wrong outcome/Did not report diagnostic accuracy measures*

Cha MJ, Lee MW, Cha DI, et al. Size discrepancy between sonographic and computed tomographic/magnetic resonance imaging measurement of hepatocellular carcinoma : the necessity of tumor size measurement standardization. J Ultrasound Med. 2013;32(10):1703-1709. *Excluded: Wrong outcome/Did not report diagnostic accuracy measures*

Chami L, Lassau N, Malka D, et al. Benefits of contrast-enhanced sonography for the detection of liver lesions: comparison with histologic findings.[Erratum appears in AJR Am J Roentgenol. 2008 May;190(5):1152]. AJR Am J Roentgenol. 2008;190(3):683-690, PMID: 18287439. *Excluded: Wrong population*

Chang JM, Lee JM, Lee MW, et al. Superparamagnetic iron oxide-enhanced liver magnetic resonance imaging: comparison of 1.5 T and 3.0 T imaging for detection of focal malignant liver lesions. Invest Radiol. 2006;41(2):168-174, PMID: 16428988. *Excluded: Wrong population*

Chen HY, Ma XM, Ye M, Hou YL, Hu B, Bai YR. CT-pathologic correlation in primary hepatocellular carcinoma: An implication for target delineation. J Radiat Res (Tokyo). 2013;54(5):938-942. *Excluded: Wrong outcome/Did not report diagnostic accuracy measures*

Chen JG, Parkin DM, Chen QG, et al. Screening for liver cancer: results of a randomised controlled trial in Qidong, China. J Med Screen. 2003;10(4):204-209, PMID: 14738659. *Excluded: Wrong intervention*

Chen MM, Yang W, Dai Y, Wu W. High mechanical index post-contrast ultrasonography improves tissue structural display of hepatocellular carcinoma. Chin Med J (Engl). 2005;118(24):2046-2051. *Excluded: Wrong outcome/Did not report diagnostic accuracy measures*

Chen R-C, Lii J-M, Chou C-T, et al. T2-weighted and T1-weighted dynamic superparamagnetic iron oxide (ferucarbotran) enhanced MRI of hepatocellular carcinoma and hyperplastic nodules. J Formos Med Assoc. 2008;107(10):798-805, PMID: 18926947. *Excluded: Wrong outcome/Did not report diagnostic accuracy measures*

Chen TH-H, Chen C-J, Yen M-F, et al. Ultrasound screening and risk factors for death from hepatocellular carcinoma in a high risk group in Taiwan. Int J Cancer. 2002;98(2):257-261, PMID: 11857416. *Excluded: Wrong intervention*

Chen Z, Liang H, Zhang X, et al. [Value of (18)F-FDG PET/CT and CECT in detecting postoperative recurrence and extrahepatic metastasis of hepatocellular carcinoma in patients with elevated serum alpha-fetoprotein]. [Chinese]. Nan Fang Yi Ke Da Xue Xue Bao. 2012;32(11):1615-1619. *Excluded: Not English language*

Cheung TT, Ho CL, Chen S, et al. Reply: Underestimated role of 18F-FDG PET for HCC evaluation and promise of 18F-FDG PET/MR imaging in this setting. J Nucl Med. 2013;54(8):1511-1512. *Excluded: Wrong publication type*

Cho CS, Curran S, Schwartz LH, et al. Preoperative radiographic assessment of hepatic steatosis with histologic correlation. J Am Coll Surg. 2008;206(3):480-488, PMID: 18308219. *Excluded: Wrong population*

Choi D, Kim S, Lim J, et al. Preoperative detection of hepatocellular carcinoma: ferumoxides-enhanced mr imaging versus combined helical CT during arterial portography and CT hepatic arteriography. AJR Am J Roentgenol. 2001;176(2):475-482, PMID: 11159099. *Excluded: Wrong intervention*

Choi JS, Kim MJ, Kim JH, et al. Comparison of multi-echo and single-echo gradient-recalled echo sequences for SPIO-enhanced liver MRI at 3 T. Clin Radiol. 2010;65(11):916-923, PMID: 20933647. *Excluded: Wrong population*

Chou CT, Chen RC, Chen WT, Lii JM. Detection of hepatocellular carcinoma by ferucarbotran-enhanced magnetic resonance imaging: the efficacy of accumulation phase fat-suppressed T1-weighted imaging. Clin Radiol. 2009;64(1):22-29. *Excluded: Wrong intervention*

Chou CT, Chen RC, Chen WT, Lii JM. Percentage of signal intensity loss for characterisation of focal liver lesions in patients with chronic liver disease using ferucarbotran-enhanced MRI. Br J Radiol. 2010;83(996):1023-1028, PMID: 20413445. *Excluded: Wrong population*

Chung YE, Kim M-J, Park M-S, et al. The impact of CT follow-up interval on stages of hepatocellular carcinomas detected during the surveillance of patients with liver cirrhosis. AJR Am J Roentgenol. 2012;199(4):816-821, PMID: 22997373. *Excluded: Wrong outcome/Did not report diagnostic accuracy measures*

Cieszanowski A, Anysz-Grodzicka A, Szeszkowski W, et al. Characterization of focal liver lesions using quantitative techniques: comparison of apparent diffusion coefficient values and T2 relaxation times. Eur Radiol. 2012;22(11):2514-2524. *Excluded: Wrong population*

Coates GG, Borrello JA, McFarland EG, Mirowitz SA, Brown JJ. Hepatic T2-weighted MRI: a prospective comparison of sequences, including breath-hold, half-Fourier turbo spin echo (HASTE). J Magn Reson Imaging. 1998;8(3):642-649, PMID: 9626880. *Excluded: Wrong population*

Colagrande S, La Villa G, Bartolucci M, Lanini F, Barletta G, Villari N. Spiral computed tomography versus ultrasound in the follow-up of cirrhotic patients previously treated for hepatocellular carcinoma: a prospective study. J Hepatol. 2003;39(1):93-98, PMID: 12821049. *Excluded: Wrong outcome/Did not report diagnostic accuracy measures*

Colli A, Fraquelli M, Casazza G, et al. Accuracy of ultrasonography, spiral CT, magnetic resonance, and alpha-fetoprotein in diagnosing hepatocellular carcinoma: a systematic review. Am J Gastroenterol. 2006;101(3):513-523, PMID: 16542288. *Excluded: Systematic review; studies checked for inclusion*

Cruite I, Tang A, Sirlin CB. Imaging-based diagnostic systems for hepatocellular carcinoma. [Review]. AJR Am J Roentgenol. 2013;201(1):41-55. *Excluded: Wrong publication type*

Davarpanah AH, Weinreb JC. The role of imaging in hepatocellular carcinoma: the present and future. J Clin Gastroenterol. 2013;47(10). *Excluded: Wrong publication type*

De Cecco CN, Buffa V, Fedeli S, et al. Dual energy CT (DECT) of the liver: conventional versus virtual unenhanced images. Eur Radiol. 2010;20(12):2870-2875, PMID: 20623126. *Excluded: Wrong outcome/Did not report diagnostic accuracy measures*

Di Tommaso L, Sangiovanni A, Borzio M, Park YN, Farinati F, Roncalli M. Advanced precancerous lesions in the liver. [Review]. Baillieres Best Pract Res Clin Gastroenterol. 2013;27(2):269-284. *Excluded: Wrong publication type*

Dietrich CF, Ignee A, Trojan J, Fellbaum C, Schuessler G. Improved characterisation of histologically proven liver tumours by contrast enhanced ultrasonography during the portal venous and specific late phase of SHU 508A. Gut. 2004;53(3):401-405, PMID: 14960524. *Excluded: Wrong outcome/Did not report diagnostic accuracy measures*

D'Onofrio M, Faccioli N, Zamboni G, et al. Focal liver lesions in cirrhosis: value of contrast-enhanced ultrasonography compared with Doppler ultrasound and alpha-fetoprotein levels. Radiol Med (Torino). 2008;113(7):978-991, PMID: 18779929. *Excluded: Wrong population*

D'Onofrio M, Martone E, Faccioli N, Zamboni G, Malago R, Mucelli RP. Focal liver lesions: sinusoidal phase of CEUS. Abdom Imaging. Vol 31. 2006/06/28 ed2006:529-536. *Excluded: Wrong population*

Dumitrescu CI, Gheonea IA, Săndulescu L, Surlin V, Săftoiu A, Dumitrescu D. Contrast enhanced ultrasound and magnetic resonance imaging in hepatocellular carcinoma diagnosis. Med. 2013;15(4):261-267. *Excluded: Inadequate reference standard*

Earls JP. Comparison studies of CT and MRI in patients with hepatic metastases. Oncology (Williston). 2000;14(6 Suppl 3):21-28, PMID: 10887648. *Excluded: Background*

Earls JP, Rofsky NM, DeCorato DR, Krinsky GA, Weinreb JC. Echo-train STIR MRI of the liver: comparison of breath-hold and non-breath-hold imaging strategies. J Magn Reson Imaging. 1999;9(1):87-92, PMID: 10030655. *Excluded: Wrong population*

Efremidis SC, Hytiroglou P, Matsui O. Enhancement patterns and signal-intensity characteristics of small hepatocellular carcinoma in cirrhosis: pathologic basis and diagnostic challenges. Eur Radiol. 2007;17(11):2969-2982, PMID: 17618439. *Excluded: Background*

Efremidis SC, Vougiouklis N, Zafiriadou E, et al.

Pathways of lymph node involvement in upper abdominal malignancies: evaluation with high-resolution CT. Eur Radiol. 1999;9(5):868-874, PMID: 10369981. *Excluded: Wrong outcome/Did not report diagnostic accuracy measures*

Eisele RM, Schumacher G, Lopez-Hanninen E, Neuhaus P. Role of B-mode ultrasound screening in detection of local tumor recurrence in the first year after radiofrequency ablation in the liver. Cancer Detect Prev. 2007;31(4):316-322, PMID: 17935909. *Excluded: Inadequate reference standard*

el-Desouki M, Mohamadiyeh M, al-Rashed R, Othman S, al-Mofleh I. Features of hepatic cavernous hemangioma on planar and SPECT Tc-99m-labeled red blood cell scintigraphy. Clin Nucl Med. 1999;24(8):583-589, PMID: 10439179. *Excluded: Wrong population*

El-Serag HB, Marrero JA, Rudolph L, Reddy KR. Diagnosis and treatment of hepatocellular carcinoma. Gastroenterology. 2008;134(6):1752-1763, PMID: 18471552. *Excluded: Background*

Erturk SM, Ichikawa T, Sano K, Motosugi U, Sou H, Araki T. Diffusion-weighted magnetic resonance imaging for characterization of focal liver masses: impact of parallel imaging (SENSE) and b value. J Comput Assist Tomogr. 2008;32(6):865-871, PMID: 19204445. *Excluded: Wrong population*

Ewertsen C, Henriksen BM, Torp-Pedersen S, Bachmann Nielsen M. Characterization by biopsy or CEUS of liver lesions guided by image fusion between ultrasonography and CT, PET/CT or MRI. Ultraschall Med. 2011;32(2):191-197, PMID: 21225564. *Excluded: Wrong outcome/Did not report diagnostic accuracy measures*

Fasani P, Sangiovanni A, De Fazio C, et al. High prevalence of multinodular hepatocellular carcinoma in patients with cirrhosis attributable to multiple risk factors. Hepatology. 1999;29(6):1704-1707, PMID: 10347111. *Excluded: Wrong outcome/Did not report diagnostic accuracy measures*

Federle M, Chezmar J, Rubin DL, et al. Efficacy and safety of mangafodipir trisodium (MnDPDP) injection for hepatic MRI in adults: results of the U.S. Multicenter phase III clinical trials. Efficacy of early imaging. J Magn Reson Imaging. 2000;12(5):689-701, PMID: 11050638. *Excluded: Wrong intervention*

Fedorov VD, Karmazanovskii GG, Kubyshkin VA, et al. [Spiral computer tomography in diagnosis of hepatic diseases]. Khirurgiia (Mosk). 1998(5):9-14, PMID: 9642951. *Excluded: Background*

Fenlon HM, Tello R, deCarvalho VL, Yucel EK. Signal characteristics of focal liver lesions on double echo T2-weighted conventional spin echo MRI: observer performance versus quantitative measurements of T2 relaxation times. J Comput Assist Tomogr. 2000;24(2):204-211, PMID: 10752879. *Excluded: Wrong population*

Foroutani A, Garland AM, Berber E, et al. Laparoscopic ultrasound vs triphasic computed tomography for detecting liver tumors. Arch Surg. 2000;135(8):933-938, PMID: 10922255. *Excluded: Wrong population*

Friedrich-Rust M, Klopffleisch T, Nierhoff J, et al. Contrast-Enhanced Ultrasound for the differentiation of benign and malignant focal liver lesions: a meta-analysis. [Review]. Liver Int. 2013;33(5):739-755. *Excluded: Systematic review; studies checked for inclusion*

Fu G-L, Du Y, Zee C-S, et al. Gadobenate dimeglumine-enhanced liver magnetic resonance imaging: value of hepatobiliary phase for the detection of focal liver lesions. J Comput Assist Tomogr. 2012;36(1):14-19, PMID: 22261765. *Excluded: Wrong outcome/Did not report diagnostic accuracy measures*

Fujinaga Y, Kadoya M, Kozaka K, et al. Prediction of macroscopic findings of hepatocellular carcinoma on hepatobiliary phase of gadolinium-ethoxybenzyl-diethylenetriamine pentaacetic acid-enhanced magnetic resonance imaging: Correlation with pathology. Hepatol Res. 2013;43(5):488-494. *Excluded: Wrong outcome/Did not report diagnostic accuracy measures*

Fujita T, Ito K, Honjo K, Okazaki H, Matsumoto T, Matsunaga N. Detection of hepatocellular carcinoma: comparison of T2-weighted breath-hold fast spin-echo sequences and high-resolution dynamic MR imaging with a phased-array body coil. J Magn Reson Imaging. 1999;9(2):274-279, PMID: 10077024. *Excluded: Inadequate reference standard*

Fukuda H, Ito R, Ohto M, et al. US-CT 3D dual imaging by mutual display of the same sections for depicting minor changes in hepatocellular carcinoma. Eur J Radiol. 2012;81(9):2014-2019, PMID: 21676568. *Excluded: Wrong outcome/Did not report diagnostic accuracy measures*

Fukukura Y, Kamiyama T, Takumi K, Shindo T, Higashi R, Nakajo M. Comparison of ferucarbotran-enhanced fluid-attenuated inversion-recovery echo-planar, T2-weighted turbo spin-echo, T2*-weighted gradient-echo, and diffusion-weighted echo-planar imaging for detection of malignant liver lesions. J Magn Reson Imaging. 2010;31(3):607-616, PMID: 20187203. *Excluded: Wrong population*

Fung KTT, Li FTW, Raimondo ML, et al. Systematic review of radiological imaging for hepatocellular carcinoma in cirrhotic patients. Br J Radiol. 2004;77(920):633-640, PMID: 15326039. *Excluded: Background*

Furlan A, Marin D, Cabassa P, et al. Enhancement pattern of small hepatocellular carcinoma (HCC) at contrast-enhanced US (CEUS), MDCT, and MRI: intermodality agreement and comparison of diagnostic sensitivity between 2005 and 2010 American Association for the Study of Liver Diseases (AASLD) guidelines. Eur J Radiol. 2012;81(9):2099-2105, PMID: 21906896. *Excluded: Inadequate reference standard*

Furuichi K, Furukawa A, Takahashi M, Murata K. Role of combined CT hepatic angiography and CT during arterial portography in the management of patients with hepatocellular carcinomas and liver metastases. Hepatol Res. 2004;28(4):191-197. *Excluded: Wrong intervention*

Gabata T, Matsui O, Kadoya M, et al. Delayed MR imaging of the liver: correlation of delayed enhancement of hepatic tumors and pathologic appearance. Abdom Imaging. 1998;23(3):309-313, PMID: 9569304. *Excluded: Wrong outcome/Did not report diagnostic accuracy measures*

Gehl HB, Bourne M, Grazioli L, Moller A, Lodemann KP. Off-site evaluation of liver lesion detection by Gd-BOPTA-enhanced MR imaging. Eur Radiol. 2001;11(2):187-192, PMID: 11218012. *Excluded: Wrong population*

Geng L, Lin C, Huang B, et al. Solitary necrotic nodule of the liver: MR findings in 33 pathologically proved lesions. Eur J Radiol. 2012;81(4):623-629, PMID: 21354738. *Excluded: Wrong population*

Goetti R, Reiner CS, Knuth A, et al. Quantitative perfusion analysis of malignant liver tumors: dynamic computed tomography and contrast-enhanced ultrasound. Invest Radiol. 2012;47(1):18-24, PMID: 21788906. *Excluded: Wrong population*

Golfieri R, Grazioli L, Orlando E, et al. Which is the best MRI marker of malignancy for atypical cirrhotic nodules: hypointensity in hepatobiliary phase alone or combined with other features? Classification after Gd-EOB-DTPA administration. J Magn Reson Imaging. 2012;36(3):648-657, PMID: 22592930. *Excluded: Wrong outcome/Did not report diagnostic accuracy measures*

Golfieri R, Renzulli M, Lucidi V, Corcioni B, Trevisani F, Bolondi L. Contribution of the hepatobiliary phase of Gd-EOB-DTPA-enhanced MRI to Dynamic MRI in the detection of hypovascular small (<= 2 cm) HCC in cirrhosis. Eur Radiol. 2011;21(6):1233-1242, PMID: 21293864. *Excluded: Wrong outcome/Did not report diagnostic accuracy measures*

Goshima S, Kanematsu M, Kondo H, et al. Diffusion-weighted imaging of the liver: optimizing b value for the detection and characterization of benign and malignant hepatic lesions. J Magn Reson Imaging. 2008;28(3):691-697, PMID: 18777553. *Excluded: Wrong population*

Gourtsoyianni S, Papanikolaou N, Yarmenitis S, Maris T, Karantanas A, Gourtsoyiannis N. Respiratory gated diffusion-weighted imaging of the liver: value of apparent diffusion coefficient measurements in the differentiation between most commonly encountered benign and malignant focal liver lesions. Eur Radiol. 2008;18(3):486-492, PMID: 17994317. *Excluded: Wrong population*

Granito A, Galassi M, Piscaglia F, et al. Impact of gadoxetic acid (Gd-EOB-DTPA)-enhanced magnetic resonance on the non-invasive diagnosis of small hepatocellular carcinoma: a prospective study. Aliment Pharmacol Ther. 2013;37(3):355-363. *Excluded: Inadequate reference standard*

Grazioli L, Morana G, Kirchin MA, Schneider G. Accurate differentiation of focal nodular hyperplasia from hepatic adenoma at gadobenate dimeglumine-enhanced MR imaging: prospective study. Radiology. 2005;236(1):166-177, PMID: 15955857. *Excluded: Wrong population*

Grazioli L, Olivetti L, Fugazzola C, et al. The pseudocapsule in hepatocellular carcinoma: correlation between dynamic MR imaging and pathology. Eur Radiol. 1999;9(1):62-67, PMID: 9933382. *Excluded: Wrong outcome/Did not report diagnostic accuracy measures*

Guang Y, Xie L, Ding H, Cai A, Huang Y. Diagnosis value of focal liver lesions with SonoVue-enhanced ultrasound compared with contrast-enhanced computed tomography and contrast-enhanced MRI: a meta-analysis. J Cancer Res Clin Oncol. 2011;137(11):1595-1605, PMID: 21850382. *Excluded: Systematic review; studies checked for inclusion*

Guimaraes CM, Correia MM, Baldisserotto M, de Queiroz Aires EP, Coelho JF. Intraoperative ultrasonography of the liver in patients with abdominal tumors: a new approach. J Ultrasound Med. 2004;23(12):1549-1555, PMID: 15557298. *Excluded: Wrong population*

Guiu B, Loffroy R, Ben Salem D, et al. Combined SPIO-gadolinium magnetic resonance imaging in cirrhotic patients: negative predictive value and role in screening for hepatocellular carcinoma. Abdom Imaging. 2008;33(5):520-528, PMID: 17912584. *Excluded: Wrong intervention*

Hafeez S, Alam MS, Sajjad Z, Khan ZA, Akhter W, Mubarak F. Triphasic computed tomography (CT) scan in focal tumoral liver lesions. JPMA J Pak Med Assoc. 2011;61(6):571-575, PMID: 22204213. *Excluded: Wrong population*

Haider MA, Amitai MM, Rappaport DC, et al. Multi-detector row helical CT in preoperative assessment of small (< or = 1.5 cm) liver metastases: is thinner collimation better? Radiology. 2002;225(1):137-142, PMID: 12354997. *Excluded: Wrong population*

Hammerstingl R, Adam G, Ayuso J-R, et al. Comparison of 1.0 M gadobutrol and 0.5 M gadopentetate dimeglumine-enhanced magnetic resonance imaging in five hundred seventy-two patients with known or suspected liver lesions: results of a multicenter, double-blind, interindividual, randomized clinical phase-III trial. Invest Radiol. 2009;44(3):168-176, PMID: 19169143. *Excluded: Wrong population*

Hammerstingl R, Huppertz A, Breuer J, et al. Diagnostic efficacy of gadoxetic acid (Primovist)-enhanced MRI and spiral CT for a therapeutic strategy: comparison with intraoperative and histopathologic findings in focal liver lesions. Eur Radiol. 2008;18(3):457-467, PMID: 18058107. *Excluded: Wrong population*

Hann LE, Schwartz LH, Panicek DM, Bach AM, Fong Y, Blumgart LH. Tumor involvement in hepatic veins: comparison of MR imaging and US for preoperative assessment. Radiology. 1998;206(3):651-656, PMID: 9494482. *Excluded: Wrong population*

Hanna RF, Kased N, Kwan SW, et al. Double-contrast MRI for accurate staging of hepatocellular carcinoma in patients with cirrhosis. AJR Am J Roentgenol. 2008;190(1):47-57, PMID: 18094293. *Excluded: Wrong intervention*

Hara K, Numata K, FJSUM, et al. Diagnosis of advanced hepatocellular carcinoma using contrast-enhanced harmonic gray-scale imaging with enhancement agents (Levovist): Correlation with helical CT and US angiography. Journal of Medical Ultrasonics. 2001;28(AUTUMN):127-133. *Excluded: Wrong comparator/Wrong reference standard*

Haradome H, Grazioli L, Morone M, et al. T2-weighted and diffusion-weighted MRI for discriminating benign from malignant focal liver lesions: diagnostic abilities of single versus combined interpretations. J Magn Reson Imaging. 2012;35(6):1388-1396, PMID: 22246647. *Excluded: Wrong population*

Hardie AD, Romano PB. The use of T2*-weighted multi-echo GRE imaging as a novel method to diagnose hepatocellular carcinoma compared with gadolinium-enhanced MRI: a feasibility study. Magn Reson Imaging. 2010;28(2):281-285, PMID: 20071122. *Excluded: Inadequate reference standard*

Harms J, Feussner H, Baumgartner M, Schneider A, Donhauser M, Wessels G. Three-dimensional navigated laparoscopic ultrasonography: first experiences with a new minimally invasive diagnostic device. Surg Endosc. 2001;15(12):1459-1462, PMID: 11965466. *Excluded: Background*

Hatanaka K, Chung H, Kudo M, et al. Usefulness of the post-vascular phase of contrast-enhanced ultrasonography with sonazoid in the evaluation of gross types of hepatocellular carcinoma. Oncology. 2010;78(SUPPL. 1):53-59. *Excluded: Wrong outcome/Did not report diagnostic accuracy measures*

Hatanaka K, Kudo M, Minami Y, Maekawa K. Sonazoid-enhanced ultrasonography for diagnosis of hepatic malignancies: comparison with contrast-enhanced CT. Oncology. 2008;75 Suppl 1:42-47, PMID: 19092271. *Excluded:*

Wrong population

Hayashi M, Matsui O, Ueda K, Kawamori Y, Gabata T, Kadoya M. Progression to hypervascular hepatocellular carcinoma: Correlation with intranodular blood supply evaluated with CT during intraarterial injection of contrast material. Radiology. 2002;225(1):143-149. *Excluded: Wrong outcome/Did not report diagnostic accuracy measures*

Hayashida M, Ito K, Fujita T, et al. Small hepatocellular carcinomas in cirrhosis: differences in contrast enhancement effects between helical CT and MR imaging during multiphasic dynamic imaging. Magn Reson Imaging. 2008;26(1):65-71. *Excluded: Wrong outcome/Did not report diagnostic accuracy measures*

Helmberger TK, Laubenberger J, Rummeny E, et al. MRI characteristics in focal hepatic disease before and after administration of MnDPDP: discriminant analysis as a diagnostic tool. Eur Radiol. 2002;12(1):62-70, PMID: 11868075. *Excluded: Wrong intervention*

Hennedige T, Venkatesh SK. Imaging of hepatocellular carcinoma: diagnosis, staging and treatment monitoring. [Review]. Cancer Imaging. 2013;12:530-547. *Excluded: Background*

Henrion J, Libon E, De Maeght S, et al. Surveillance for hepatocellular carcinoma: compliance and results according to the aetiology of cirrhosis in a cohort of 141 patients. Acta Gastroenterol Belg. 2000;63(1):5-9, PMID: 10907311. *Excluded: Wrong outcome/Did not report diagnostic accuracy measures*

Herman P, Pugliese V, Machado MA, et al. Hepatic adenoma and focal nodular hyperplasia: differential diagnosis and treatment. World J Surg. 2000;24(3):372-376, PMID: 10658075. *Excluded: Wrong population*

Higashihara H, Murakami T, Kim T, et al. Differential diagnosis between metastatic tumors and nonsolid benign lesions of the liver using ferucarbotran-enhanced MR imaging. Eur J Radiol. 2010;73(1):125-130, PMID: 19019608. *Excluded: Wrong population*

Hiraoka A, Hirooka M, Ochi H, et al. Importance of screening for synchronous malignant neoplasms in patients with hepatocellular carcinoma: Impact of FDG PET/CT. Liver Int. 2013;33(7):1085-1091. *Excluded: Wrong population*

Hohmann J, Skrok J, Basilico R, et al. Characterisation of focal liver lesions with unenhanced and contrast enhanced low MI real time ultrasound: on-site unblinded versus off-site blinded reading. Eur J Radiol. 2012;81(3):e317-324, PMID: 22100374. *Excluded: Wrong population*

Holalkere N-S, Sahani DV, Blake MA, Halpern EF, Hahn PF, Mueller PR. Characterization of small liver lesions: Added role of MR after MDCT. J Comput Assist Tomogr. 2006;30(4):591-596, PMID: 16845289. *Excluded: Wrong population*

Holzapfel K, Eiber MJ, Fingerle AA, Bruegel M, Rummeny EJ, Gaa J. Detection, classification, and characterization of focal liver lesions: Value of diffusion-weighted MR imaging, gadoxetic acid-enhanced MR imaging and the combination of both methods. Abdom Imaging. 2012;37(1):74-82, PMID: 21597893. *Excluded: Wrong population*

Honda T, Kumada T, Kiriyama S, et al. Comparison of contrast-enhanced harmonic ultrasonography and power Doppler ultrasonography for depicting vascularity of hepatocellular carcinoma identified by angiography-assisted CT. Hepatol Res. 2003;27(4):314-321. *Excluded: Wrong outcome/Did not report diagnostic accuracy measures*

Hori M, Murakami T, Kim T, et al. Sensitivity of double-phase helical CT during arterial portography for detection of hypervascular hepatocellular carcinoma. J Comput Assist Tomogr. 1998;22(6):861-867, PMID: 9843222. *Excluded: Wrong intervention*

Huang JS, Pan HB, Chou CP, et al. Optimizing scanning phases in detecting small (<2 cm) hepatocellular carcinoma: Whole-liver dynamic study with multidetector row CT. J Comput Assist Tomogr. 2008;32(3):341-346. *Excluded: Wrong outcome/Did not report diagnostic accuracy measures*

Huang Y-L, Chen J-H, Shen W-C. Diagnosis of hepatic tumors with texture analysis in nonenhanced computed tomography images. Acad Radiol. 2006;13(6):713-720, PMID: 16679273. *Excluded: Wrong population*

Hussain SM, van den Bos IC, Dwarkasing RS, Kuiper JW, den Hollander J. Hepatocellular adenoma: Findings at state-of-the-art magnetic resonance imaging, ultrasound, computed tomography and pathologic analysis. Eur Radiol. 2006;16(9):1873-1886. *Excluded: Background*

Hustinx R, Paulus P, Jacquet N, Jerusalem G, Bury T, Rigo P. Clinical evaluation of whole-body 18F-fluorodeoxyglucose positron emission tomography in the detection of liver metastases. Ann Oncol. 1998;9(4):397-401, PMID: 9636830. *Excluded: Wrong population*

Hwang J, Kim SH, Kim YS, et al. Gadoxetic acid-enhanced MRI versus multiphase multidetector row computed tomography for evaluating the viable tumor of hepatocellular carcinomas treated with image-guided tumor therapy. J Magn Reson Imaging. 2010;32(3):629-638, PMID: 20815061. *Excluded: Wrong population*

Iannaccone R, Piacentini F, Murakami T, et al. Hepatocellular carcinoma in patients with nonalcoholic fatty liver disease: Helical CT and MR imaging findings with clinical-pathologic comparison. Radiology. 2007;243(2):422-430. *Excluded: Wrong outcome/Did not report diagnostic accuracy measures*

Iannicelli E, Di Pietropaolo M, Marignani M, et al. Gadoxetic acid-enhanced MRI for hepatocellular carcinoma and hypointense nodule observed in the hepatobiliary phase. Radiol Med (Torino). 2013:1-10. *Excluded: Wrong outcome/Did not report diagnostic accuracy measures*

Iavarone M, Manini MA, Sangiovanni A, et al. Contrast-enhanced computed tomography and ultrasound-guided liver biopsy to diagnose dysplastic liver nodules in cirrhosis. Dig Liver Dis. 2013;45(1):43-49. *Excluded: Wrong outcome/Did not report diagnostic accuracy measures*

Ichikawa T, Federle MP, Grazioli L, Nalesnik M. Hepatocellular adenoma: Multiphasic CT and histopathologic findings in 25 patients. Radiology. 2000;214(3):861-868. *Excluded: Wrong population*

Ichikawa T, Haradome H, Hachiya J, Nitatori T, Araki T. Diffusion-weighted MR imaging with a single-shot echoplanar sequence: detection and characterization of focal hepatic lesions. AJR Am J Roentgenol. 1998;170(2):397-402, PMID: 9456953. *Excluded: Wrong population*

Ichikawa T, Motosugi U, Morisaka H, Sano K, Ali M, Araki T. Volumetric low-tube-voltage CT imaging for evaluating hypervascular hepatocellular carcinoma; Effects on radiation exposure, image quality, and diagnostic performance. Jpn J Radiol. 2013;31(8):521-529. *Excluded: Wrong outcome/Did not report diagnostic accuracy measures*

Ichikawa T, Okada M, Kondo H, et al. Recommended iodine dose for multiphasic contrast-enhanced mutidetector-row computed tomography imaging of liver for assessing hypervascular hepatocellular carcinoma: multicenter prospective study in 77 general hospitals in Japan. Acad Radiol. 2013;20(9):1130-1136. *Excluded: Wrong outcome/Did not report diagnostic accuracy measures*

Imai Y, Murakami T, Hori M, et al. Hypervascular hepatocellular carcinoma: Combined dynamic MDCT and SPIO-enhanced MRI versus combined CTHA and CTAP. Hepatol Res. 2008;38(2):147-158. *Excluded: Wrong intervention*

Inoue E, Fujita M, Hosomi N, et al. Double phase CT arteriography of the whole liver in the evaluation of hepatic tumors. J Comput Assist Tomogr. 1998;22(1):64-68, PMID: 9448763. *Excluded: Wrong intervention*

Ishigami K, Tajima T, Fujita N, et al. Hepatocellular carcinoma with marginal superparamagnetic iron oxide uptake on T2*-weighted magnetic resonance imaging: histopathologic correlation. Eur J Radiol. 2011;80(3):e293-298, PMID: 21288675. *Excluded: Wrong outcome/Did not report diagnostic accuracy measures*

Ishigami K, Yoshimitsu K, Nishihara Y, et al. Hepatocellular carcinoma with a pseudocapsule on gadolinium-enhanced MR images: correlation with histopathologic findings. Radiology. 2009;250(2):435-443, PMID: 19095782. *Excluded: Wrong population*

Ishikawa M, Yogita S, Miyake H, et al. Differential diagnosis of small hepatocellular carcinoma and borderline lesions and therapeutic strategy. Hepatogastroenterology. 2002;49(48):1591-1596, PMID: 12397743. *Excluded: Imaging before 1995*

Itoh S, Ikeda M, Achiwa M, Satake H, Iwano S, Ishigaki T. Late-arterial and portal-venous phase imaging of the liver with a multislice CT scanner in patients without circulatory disturbances: automatic bolus tracking or empirical scan delay? Eur Radiol. 2004;14(9):1665-1673, PMID: 15067427. *Excluded: Wrong outcome/Did not report diagnostic accuracy measures*

Iwamoto S, Sanefuji H, Okuda K. Computed tomography angiographic findings in hepatocellular carcinoma less than 2 cm detected during follow-up in 29 patients. J Gastroenterol Hepatol. 2003;18(9):1076-1080, PMID: 12911666. *Excluded: Wrong outcome/Did not report diagnostic accuracy measures*

Iwata Y, Shiomi S, Sasaki N, et al. Clinical usefulness of positron emission tomography with fluorine-18-fluorodeoxyglucose in the diagnosis of liver tumors. Ann Nucl Med. 2000;14(2):121-126, PMID: 10830530. *Excluded: Wrong outcome/Did not report diagnostic accuracy measures*

Iwazawa J, Nishida N, Yamamoto A, et al. Detection of portal perfusion abnormalities: comparison of 3 ferucarbotran-enhanced magnetic resonance imaging sequences. J Comput Assist Tomogr. 2006;30(2):165-172, PMID: 16628027. *Excluded: Wrong outcome/Did not report diagnostic accuracy measures*

Izumi N. Diagnostic and treatment algorithm of the Japanese society of hepatology: a consensus-based practice guideline. Oncology. 2010;78 Suppl 1:78-86, PMID: 20616588. *Excluded: Background*

Jadvar H. Hepatocellular carcinoma and gastroenteropancreatic neuroendocrine tumors: Potential role of other positron emission tomography radiotracers. Semin Nucl Med. 2012;42(4):247-254. *Excluded: Background*

Jakab Z. [Investigation of the blood supply of liver tumors--ultrasonography with contrast agents]. Orv Hetil. 2004;145(7 Suppl 1):378-381, PMID: 15049055. *Excluded: Background*

Jeon UB, Lee JW, Choo KS, et al. Iodized oil uptake assessment with cone-beam CT in chemoembolization of small hepatocellular carcinomas. World J Gastroenterol. 2009;15(46):5833-5837, PMID: 19998505. *Excluded: Wrong population*

Jeong HT, Kim MJ, Kim YE, Park YN, Choi GH, Choi JS. MRI features of hepatocellular carcinoma expressing progenitor cell markers. Liver Int. 2012;32(3):430-440. *Excluded: Wrong outcome/Did not report diagnostic accuracy measures*

Jeong YY, Mitchell DG, Kamishima T. Small (<20 mm) enhancing hepatic nodules seen on arterial phase MR imaging of the cirrhotic liver: clinical implications. AJR Am J Roentgenol. 2002;178(6):1327-1334, PMID: 12034592. *Excluded: Wrong intervention*

Jeong YY, Yim NY, Kang HK. Hepatocellular carcinoma in the cirrhotic liver with helical CT and MRI: Imaging spectrum and pitfalls of cirrhosis-related nodules. AJR Am J Roentgenol. 2005;185(4):1024-1032. *Excluded: Background*

Jin Y-J, Lee HC, Lee D, et al. Role of the routine use of chest computed tomography and bone scan in staging workup of hepatocellular carcinoma. J Hepatol. 2012;56(6):1324-1329, PMID: 22322236. *Excluded: Wrong comparator/Wrong reference standard*

Joo I, Kim SH, Lee JY, Lee JM, Han JK, Choi BI. Comparison of semiautomated and manual measurements for simulated hypo- and hyper-attenuating hepatic tumors on MDCT: effect of slice thickness and reconstruction increment on their accuracy. Acad Radiol. 2011;18(5):626-633, PMID: 21393028. *Excluded: Wrong outcome/Did not report diagnostic accuracy measures*

Jou JH, Chen P-H, Jazwinski A, Bouneva I, Smith AD, Muir AJ. Rates of surveillance and management of hepatocellular carcinoma in patients evaluated at a liver transplant center. Dig Dis Sci. 2010;55(12):3591-3596, PMID: 20683659. *Excluded: Wrong outcome/Did not report diagnostic accuracy measures*

Jung G, Breuer J, Poll LW, et al. Imaging characteristics of hepatocellular carcinoma using the hepatobiliary contrast agent Gd-EOB-DTPA. Acta Radiol. 2006;47(1):15-23, PMID: 16498928. *Excluded: Wrong intervention*

Junqiang L, Yinzhong W, Li Z, et al. Gadoxetic acid disodium (Gd-EOB-DTPA)-enhanced magnetic resonance imaging for the detection of hepatocellular carcinoma: A meta-analysis. J Magn Reson Imaging. 2013. *Excluded: Systematic review; studies checked for inclusion*

Kaihara S, Kiuchi T, Ueda M, et al. Living-donor liver transplantation for hepatocellular carcinoma. Transplantation. 2003;75(3 Suppl):S37-40, PMID: 12589138. *Excluded: Wrong outcome/Did not report diagnostic accuracy measures*

Kakeda S, Korogi Y, Ohnari N, et al. Usefulness of cone-beam volume CT with flat panel detectors in conjunction with catheter angiography for transcatheter arterial embolization. J Vasc Interv Radiol. 2007;18(12):1508-1516, PMID: 18057285. *Excluded: Wrong intervention*

Kamel IR, Choti MA, Horton KM, et al. Surgically staged focal liver lesions: accuracy and reproducibility of dual-phase helical CT for detection and characterization. Radiology. 2003;227(3):752-757, PMID: 12773679. *Excluded: Wrong population*

Kamel IR, Liapi E, Fishman EK. Multidetector CT of hepatocellular carcinoma. Baillieres Best Pract Res Clin Gastroenterol. 2005;19(1):63-89, PMID: 15757805. *Excluded: Background*

Kan M, Hiraoka A, Uehara T, et al. Evaluation of contrast-enhanced ultrasonography using perfluorobutane (sonazoid®) in patients with small hepatocellular carcinoma: Comparison with dynamic computed tomography. Oncol Lett. 2010;1(3):485-488. *Excluded: Inadequate reference standard*

Kanata N, Yoshikawa T, Ohno Y, et al. HCC-to-liver contrast on arterial-dominant phase images of EOB-enhanced MRI: Comparison with dynamic CT. Magn Reson Imaging. 2013;31(1):17-22. *Excluded: Wrong outcome/Did not report diagnostic accuracy measures*

Kane SV, Ganger DR. Management of hepatocellular carcinoma: staging and treatment. Am J Ther. 1997;4(1):39-45, PMID: 10423590. *Excluded: Background*

Kanematsu M, Goshima S, Kondo H, et al. Optimizing scan delays of fixed duration contrast injection in contrast-enhanced biphasic multidetector-row CT for the liver and the detection of hypervascular hepatocellular carcinoma. J Comput Assist Tomogr. 2005;29(2):195-201, PMID: 15772536. *Excluded: Background*

Kanematsu M, Hoshi H, Murakami T, et al. Fat-suppressed T2-weighted MR imaging of hepatocellular carcinoma and metastases: comparison of conventional spin-echo, fast spin-echo, and echoplanar pulse sequences. J Magn Reson Imaging. 1999;10(1):25-32, PMID: 10398974. *Excluded: Wrong population*

Kanematsu M, Hoshi H, Murakami T, et al. Detection of hepatocellular carcinoma: comparison of low- and high-spatial-resolution dynamic MR images. AJR Am J Roentgenol. 1999;173(5):1207-1212, PMID: 10541090. *Excluded: Background*

Kanematsu M, Itoh K, Matsuo M, et al. Malignant hepatic tumor detection with ferumoxides-enhanced MR imaging with a 1.5-T system: comparison of four imaging pulse sequences. J Magn Reson Imaging. 2001;13(2):249-257, PMID: 11169831. *Excluded: Wrong population*

Karadeniz-Bilgili MY, Braga L, Birchard KR, et al. Hepatocellular carcinoma missed on gadolinium enhanced MR imaging, discovered in liver explants: retrospective evaluation. J Magn Reson Imaging. 2006;23(2):210-215, PMID: 16416439. *Excluded: Wrong outcome/Did not report diagnostic accuracy measures*

Karahan OI, Yikilmaz A, Artis T, Canoz O, Coskun A, Torun E. Contrast-enhanced dynamic magnetic resonance imaging findings of hepatocellular carcinoma and their correlation with histopathologic findings. Eur J Radiol. 2006;57(3):445-452. *Excluded: Background*

Karahan OI, Yikilmaz A, Isin S, Orhan S. Characterization of hepatocellular carcinomas with triphasic CT and correlation with histopathologic findings. Acta Radiol. 2003;44(6):566-571. *Excluded: Background*

Kaseb AO, Abaza YM, Roses RE. Multidisciplinary management of hepatocellular carcinoma. Recent Results Cancer Res. 2013;190:247-259, PMID: 22941025. *Excluded: Background*

Kashiwagi T. FDG-PET and hepatocellular carcinoma. J Gastroenterol. 2004;39(10):1017-1018. *Excluded: Background*

Katyal S, Oliver JH, 3rd, Peterson MS, Ferris JV, Carr BS, Baron RL. Extrahepatic metastases of hepatocellular carcinoma. Radiology. 2000;216(3):698-703, PMID: 10966697. *Excluded: Wrong outcome/Did not report diagnostic accuracy measures*

Kawada T. Receiver operating characteristic curve analysis, sensitivity comparison and individual difference. Clin Radiol. 2012;67(9):940, PMID: 22608247. *Excluded: Wrong outcome/Did not report diagnostic accuracy measures*

Kawamura E, Habu D, Ohfuji S, et al. Clinical role of FDG-PET for HCC: relationship of glucose metabolic indicator to Japan Integrated Staging (JIS) score. Hepatogastroenterology. 2008;55(82-83):582-586, PMID: 18613412. *Excluded: Wrong outcome/Did not report diagnostic accuracy measures*

Kawamura Y, Ikeda K, Seko Y, et al. Heterogeneous type 4 enhancement of hepatocellular carcinoma on dynamic CT is associated with tumor recurrence after radiofrequency ablation. AJR Am J Roentgenol. 2011;197(4):W665-673, PMID: 21940538. *Excluded: Background*

Kchaou-Ouakaa A, Belhadjbrik N, Elloumi H, et al. [Surveillance for hepatocellular carcinoma: does it work?]. Tunis Med. 2007;85(10):866-870, PMID: 18236810. *Excluded: Background*

Ke S, Zhang F, Wang W, et al. Multiple target-specific molecular imaging agents detect liver cancer in a preclinical model. Curr Mol Med. 2012;12(8):944-951, PMID: 22779431. *Excluded: Background*

Kehagias D, Metafa A, Hatziioannou A, et al. Comparison of CT, MRI and CT during arterial portography in the detection of malignant hepatic lesions. Hepatogastroenterology. 2000;47(35):1399-1403, PMID: 11100361. *Excluded: Wrong population*

Khalili K, Kim TK, Jang H-J, Yazdi LK, Guindi M, Sherman M. Indeterminate 1-2-cm nodules found on hepatocellular carcinoma surveillance: biopsy for all, some, or none? Hepatology. 2011;54(6):2048-2054, PMID: 22057624. *Excluded: Background*

Khan AS, Hussain HK, Johnson TD, Weadock WJ, Pelletier SJ, Marrero JA. Value of delayed hypointensity and delayed enhancing rim in magnetic resonance imaging diagnosis of small hepatocellular carcinoma in the cirrhotic liver. J Magn Reson Imaging. 2010;32(2):360-366, PMID: 20677263. *Excluded: Background*

Kilickesmez O, Bayramoglu S, Inci E, Cimilli T. Value of apparent diffusion coefficient measurement for discrimination of focal benign and malignant hepatic masses. J Med Imaging Radiat Oncol. 2009;53(1):50-55, PMID: 19453528. *Excluded: Wrong outcome/Did not report diagnostic accuracy measures*

Kim AY, Lee MW, Rhim H, et al. Pretreatment evaluation with contrast-enhanced ultrasonography for percutaneous radiofrequency ablation of hepatocellular carcinomas with poor conspicuity on conventional ultrasonography. Korean J Radiol. 2013;14(5):754-763. *Excluded: Wrong outcome/Did not report diagnostic accuracy measures*

Kim BK, Han KH, Park YN, et al. Prediction of microvascular invasion before curative resection of hepatocellular carcinoma. J Surg Oncol. 2008;97(3):246-252, PMID: 18095300. *Excluded: Wrong outcome/Did not report diagnostic accuracy measures*

Kim BK, Kang WJ, Kim JK, et al. 18F-fluorodeoxyglucose uptake on positron emission tomography as a prognostic predictor in locally advanced hepatocellular carcinoma. Cancer. 2011;117(20):4779-4787, PMID: 21469082. *Excluded: Wrong outcome/Did not report diagnostic accuracy measures*

Kim CK, Lim JH, Lee WJ. Detection of hepatocellular carcinoma and dysplastic nodule in cirrhotic liver: Accuracy of ultrasonography. Ultrasound Med Biol. 2000;26(SUPPL. 2). *Excluded: Wrong publication type*

Kim H, Park M-S, Choi JY, et al. Can microvessel invasion of hepatocellular carcinoma be predicted by pre-operative MRI? Eur Radiol. 2009;19(7):1744-1751, PMID: 19247666. *Excluded: Wrong outcome/Did not report diagnostic accuracy measures*

Kim H-C, Kim AY, Han JK, et al. Hepatic arterial and portal venous phase helical CT in patients treated with transcatheter arterial chemoembolization for hepatocellular carcinoma: added value of unenhanced images. Radiology. 2002;225(3):773-780, PMID: 12461260. *Excluded: Wrong population*

Kim HJ, Kim TK, Kim PN, et al. Assessment of the therapeutic response of hepatocellular carcinoma treated with transcatheter arterial chemoembolization: comparison of contrast-enhanced sonography and 3-phase computed tomography. J Ultrasound Med. 2006;25(4):477-486, PMID: 16567437. *Excluded: Wrong population*

Kim HO, Kim JS, Shin YM, Ryu J-S, Lee YS, Lee SG. Evaluation of metabolic characteristics and viability of lipiodolized hepatocellular carcinomas using 18F-FDG PET/CT. J Nucl Med. 2010;51(12):1849-1856, PMID: 21098794. *Excluded: Wrong population*

Kim HY, Choi JY, Kim CW, et al. Gadolinium ethoxybenzyl diethylenetriamine pentaacetic acid-enhanced magnetic resonance imaging predicts the histological grade of hepatocellular carcinoma only in patients with Child-Pugh class A cirrhosis. Liver Transpl. 2012;18(7):850-857, PMID: 22407909. *Excluded: Wrong outcome/Did not report diagnostic accuracy measures*

Kim I, Kim MJ. Histologic characteristics of hepatocellular carcinomas showing atypical enhancement patterns on 4-phase MDCT examination. Korean J Radiol. 2012;13(5):586-593. *Excluded: Wrong outcome/Did not report diagnostic accuracy measures*

Kim J-E, Kim SH, Lee SJ, Rhim H. Hypervascular hepatocellular carcinoma 1 cm or smaller in patients with chronic liver disease:

characterization with gadoxetic acid-enhanced MRI that includes diffusion-weighted imaging. AJR Am J Roentgenol. 2011;196(6):W758-765, PMID: 21606265. *Excluded: Wrong outcome/Did not report diagnostic accuracy measures*

Kim JH, Kim MJ, Park YN, et al. Mangafodipir trisodium-enhanced MRI of hepatocellular carcinoma: correlation with histological characteristics. Clin Radiol. 2008;63(11):1195-1204. *Excluded: Wrong outcome/Did not report diagnostic accuracy measures*

Kim JY, Kim MJ, Kim KA, Jeong HT, Park YN. Hyperintense HCC on hepatobiliary phase images of gadoxetic acid-enhanced MRI: Correlation with clinical and pathological features. Eur J Radiol. 2012;81(12):3877-3882. *Excluded: Background*

Kim K-B, Kim CW, Kim GH. Area extraction of the liver and hepatocellular carcinoma in CT scans. J Digit Imaging. 2008;21 Suppl 1:S89-103, PMID: 17846836. *Excluded: Background*

Kim MJ, Jin YC, Joon SL, et al. Optimal scan window for detection of hypervascular hepatocellular carcinomas during MDCT examination. AJR Am J Roentgenol. 2006;187(1):198-206. *Excluded: Background*

Kim MJ, Lim HK, Choi D, Lee WJ, Rhim HC, Kim S. Sonography guided percutaneous radiofrequency ablation of hepatocellular carcinoma: effect of cooperative training on the pretreatment assessment of the operation's feasibility. Korean J Radiol. 2008;9(1):29-37, PMID: 18253073. *Excluded: Wrong outcome/Did not report diagnostic accuracy measures*

Kim M-J, Choi J-Y, Chung YE, Choi SY. Magnetic resonance imaging of hepatocellular carcinoma using contrast media. Oncology. 2008;75 Suppl 1:72-82, PMID: 19092275. *Excluded: Background*

Kim M-J, Kim JH, Chung J-J, Park MS, Lim JS, Oh YT. Focal hepatic lesions: detection and characterization with combination gadolinium- and superparamagnetic iron oxide-enhanced MR imaging. Radiology. 2003;228(3):719-726, PMID: 12881583. *Excluded: Wrong population*

Kim M-J, Kim JH, Lim JS, et al. Detection and characterization of focal hepatic lesions: mangafodipir vs. superparamagnetic iron oxide-enhanced magnetic resonance imaging. J Magn Reson Imaging. 2004;20(4):612-621, PMID: 15390224. *Excluded: Wrong intervention*

Kim S, Mannelli L, Hajdu CH, et al. Hepatocellular carcinoma: assessment of response to transarterial chemoembolization with image subtraction. J Magn Reson Imaging. 2010;31(2):348-355, PMID: 20099348. *Excluded: Wrong population*

Kim SH, Choi BI, Lee JY, et al. Diagnostic accuracy of multi-/single-detector row CT and contrast-enhanced MRI in the detection of hepatocellular carcinomas meeting the milan criteria before liver transplantation. Intervirology. 2008;51 Suppl 1:52-60, PMID: 18544949. *Excluded: Systematic review; studies checked for inclusion*

Kim SH, Choi D, Lim JH, et al. Optimal pulse sequence for ferumoxides-enhanced MR imaging used in the detection of hepatocellular carcinoma: a comparative study using seven pulse sequences. Korean J Radiol. 2002;3(2):87-97, PMID: 12087198. *Excluded: Wrong outcome/Did not report diagnostic accuracy measures*

Kim SH, Lee JM, Lee JY, et al. Value of contrast-enhanced sonography for the characterization of focal hepatic lesions in patients with diffuse liver disease: receiver operating characteristic analysis. AJR Am J Roentgenol. 2005;184(4):1077-1084, PMID: 15788576. *Excluded: Wrong outcome/Did not report diagnostic accuracy measures*

Kim SH, Lee WJ, Lim HK, Park CK. SPIO-enhanced mri findings of well-differentiated hepatocellular carcinomas: correlation with MDCT findings. Korean J Radiol. 2009;10(2):112-120. *Excluded: Inadequate reference standard*

Kim SK, Kim SH, Lee WJ, et al. Preoperative detection of hepatocellular carcinoma: ferumoxides-enhanced versus mangafodipir trisodium-enhanced MR imaging. AJR Am J Roentgenol. 2002;179(3):741-750, PMID: 12185056. *Excluded: Wrong intervention*

Kim T, Murakami T, Takahashi S, Hori M, Tsuda K, Nakamura H. Diffusion-weighted single-shot echoplanar MR imaging for liver disease. AJR Am J Roentgenol. 1999;173(2):393-398, PMID: 10430143. *Excluded: Wrong population*

Kim T, Murakami T, Takahashi S, et al. Optimal phases of dynamic CT for detecting hepatocellular carcinoma: Evaluation of unenhanced and triple-phase images. Abdom Imaging. 1999;24(5):473-480. *Excluded: Wrong intervention*

Kim TK, Jang H-J, Wilson SR. Imaging diagnosis of hepatocellular carcinoma with differentiation from other pathology. Clin Liver Dis. 2005;9(2):253-279, PMID: 15831272. *Excluded: Background*

Kim TK, Lee KH, Khalili K, Jang H-J. Hepatocellular nodules in liver cirrhosis: contrast-enhanced ultrasound. Abdom Imaging. 2011;36(3):244-263, PMID: 21253723. *Excluded: Background*

Kim YJ, Yun M, Lee WJ, Kim KS, Lee JD. Usefulness of 18F-FDG PET in intrahepatic cholangiocarcinoma. Eur J Nucl Med Mol Imaging. 2003;30(11):1467-1472, PMID: 14579085. *Excluded: Wrong population*

Kim YK, Kim CS, Han YM. Detection of small hepatocellular carcinoma: Comparison of conventional gadolinium-enhanced MRI with gadoliniumenhanced MRI after the administration of ferucarbotran. Br J Radiol. 2009;82(978):468-474. *Excluded: Inadequate reference standard*

Kim YK, Kwak HS, Kim CS, Han YM. Detection and characterization of focal hepatic tumors: a comparison of T2-weighted MR images before and after the administration of gadoxetic acid. J Magn Reson Imaging. 2009;30(2):437-443, PMID: 19629973. *Excluded: Wrong intervention*

Kim YK, Lee YH, Kwak HS, Kim CS, Han YM. Small malignant hepatic tumor detection in gadolinium- and ferucarbotran-enhanced magnetic resonance imaging: does combining ferucarbotran-enhanced T2*-weighted gradient echo and T2-weighted turbo spin echo images have additive efficacy? Korean J Radiol. 2008;9(6):510-519, PMID: 19039267. *Excluded: Wrong intervention*

Klein D, Jenett M, Gassel HJ, Sandstede J, Hahn D. Quantitative dynamic contrast-enhanced sonography of hepatic tumors. Eur Radiol. 2004;14(6):1082-1091, PMID: 15108017. *Excluded: Wrong outcome/Did not report diagnostic accuracy measures*

Kluge R, Schmidt F, Caca K, et al. Positron emission tomography with [(18)F]fluoro-2-deoxy-D-glucose for diagnosis and staging of bile duct cancer. Hepatology. 2001;33(5):1029-1035, PMID: 11343227. *Excluded: Wrong population*

Kneteman N, Livraghi T, Madoff D, de Santibanez E, Kew M. Tools for monitoring patients with hepatocellular carcinoma on the waiting list and after liver transplantation. Liver Transpl. 2011;17 Suppl 2:S117-127, PMID: 21584926. *Excluded: Background*

Kondo H, Kanematsu M, Hoshi H, et al. Preoperative detection of malignant hepatic tumors: comparison of combined methods of MR imaging with combined methods of CT. AJR Am J Roentgenol. 2000;174(4):947-954, PMID: 10749228. *Excluded: Wrong population*

Konopke R, Bunk A, Kersting S. The role of contrast-enhanced ultrasound for focal liver lesion detection: an overview. Ultrasound Med Biol. 2007;33(10):1515-1526, PMID: 17618038. *Excluded: Background*

Korpraphong P, Leyendecker JR, Hildebolt CF, Narra V, Bae KT, Brown JJ. Serial MR imaging of small arterially-enhancing liver lesions in patients with chronic liver disease. J Med Assoc Thai. 2009;92(4):548-555, PMID: 19374308. *Excluded: Wrong outcome/Did not report diagnostic accuracy measures*

Kosari K, Gomes M, Hunter D, Hess DJ, Greeno E, Sielaff TD. Local, intrahepatic, and systemic recurrence patterns after radiofrequency ablation of hepatic malignancies. J Gastrointest Surg. 2002;6(2):255-263, PMID: 11992812. *Excluded: Wrong population*

Koyama K, Okamura T, Kawabe J, et al. The usefulness of 18F-FDG PET images obtained 2 hours after intravenous injection in liver tumor. Ann Nucl Med. 2002;16(3):169-176, PMID: 12126041. *Excluded: Wrong outcome/Did not report diagnostic accuracy measures*

Krinsky G. Imaging of dysplastic nodules and small hepatocellular carcinomas: experience with explanted livers. Intervirology. 2004;47(3-5):191-198, PMID: 15383729. *Excluded: Background*

Krinsky GA, Lee VS. MR imaging of cirrhotic nodules. Abdom Imaging. 2000;25(5):471-482, PMID: 10931980. *Excluded: Background*

Krinsky GA, Lee VS, Theise ND. Focal lesions in the cirrhotic liver: high resolution ex vivo MRI with pathologic correlation. J Comput Assist Tomogr. 2000;24(2):189-196, PMID: 10752877. *Excluded: Background*

Kubota K, Ina H, Okada Y, Irie T. Growth rate of primary single hepatocellular carcinoma: determining optimal screening interval with contrast enhanced computed tomography. Dig Dis Sci. 2003;48(3):581-586, PMID: 12757173. *Excluded: Wrong outcome/Did not report*

Kudo M. Hepatocellular carcinoma 2009 and beyond: from the surveillance to molecular targeted therapy. Oncology. 2008;75 Suppl 1:1-12, PMID: 19092266. *Excluded: Background*

Kudo M. Real practice of hepatocellular carcinoma in Japan: conclusions of the Japan Society of Hepatology 2009 Kobe Congress. Oncology. 2010;78 Suppl 1:180-188, PMID: 20616602. *Excluded: Background*

Kudo M, Hatanaka K, Maekawa K. Newly developed novel ultrasound technique, defect reperfusion ultrasound imaging, using sonazoid in the management of hepatocellular carcinoma. Oncology. 2010;78 Suppl 1:40-45, PMID: 20616583. *Excluded: Inadequate reference standard*

Kudo M, Matsui O, Sakamoto M, et al. Role of gadolinium-ethoxybenzyl-diethylenetriamine pentaacetic acid-enhanced magnetic resonance imaging in the management of hepatocellular carcinoma: Consensus at the symposium of the 48th annual meeting of the liver cancer study group of Japan. Oncology (Switzerland). 2013;84(SUPPL.1):21-27. *Excluded: Background*

Kudo M, Zheng RQ, Kim SR, et al. Diagnostic accuracy of imaging for liver cirrhosis compared to histologically proven liver cirrhosis. A multicenter collaborative study. Intervirology. 2008;51 Suppl 1:17-26, PMID: 18544944. *Excluded: Wrong population*

Kuehl H, Antoch G, Stergar H, et al. Comparison of FDG-PET, PET/CT and MRI for follow-up of colorectal liver metastases treated with radiofrequency ablation: initial results. Eur J Radiol. 2008;67(2):362-371, PMID: 18155866. *Excluded: Wrong population*

Kuehl H, Rosenbaum-Krumme S, Veit-Haibach P, et al. Impact of whole-body imaging on treatment decision to radio-frequency ablation in patients with malignant liver tumors: comparison of [18F]fluorodeoxyglucose-PET/computed tomography, PET and computed tomography. Nuclear Medicine Communications. 2008;29(7):599-606, PMID: 18528181. *Excluded: Wrong population*

Kulemann V, Schima W, Tamandl D, et al. Preoperative detection of colorectal liver metastases in fatty liver: MDCT or MRI? Eur J Radiol. 2011;79(2):e1-6, PMID: 20392584. *Excluded: Wrong population*

Kumada T, Toyoda H, Tada T, et al. Evolution of hypointense hepatocellular nodules observed only in the hepatobiliary phase of gadoxetate disodium-enhanced MRI. AJR Am J Roentgenol. 2011;197(1):58-63, PMID: 21701011. *Excluded: Wrong outcome/Did not report diagnostic accuracy measures*

Lai ECH, Tang CN, Ha JPY, Tsui DKK, Li MKW. The evolving influence of laparoscopy and laparoscopic ultrasonography on patients with hepatocellular carcinoma. Am J Surg. 2008;196(5):736-740. *Excluded: Wrong intervention*

Lam MG, Kwee TC, Basu S, Alavi A. Underestimated role of 18F-FDG PET for HCC evaluation and promise of 18F-FDG PET/MR imaging in this setting. J Nucl Med. 2013;54(8):1510-1511. *Excluded: Wrong publication type*

Lamerz R, Runge M, Stieber P, Meissner E. Use of serum PIVKA-II (DCP) determination for differentiation between benign and malignant liver diseases. Anticancer Res. 1999;19(4A):2489-2493, PMID: 10470180. *Excluded: Wrong intervention*

Lanka B, Jang H-J, Kim TK, Burns PN, Wilson SR. Impact of contrast-enhanced ultrasonography in a tertiary clinical practice. J Ultrasound Med. 2007;26(12):1703-1714, PMID: 18029922. *Excluded: Wrong population*

Larcos G, Sorokopud H, Berry G, Farrell GC. Sonographic screening for hepatocellular carcinoma in patients with chronic hepatitis or cirrhosis: an evaluation. AJR Am J Roentgenol. 1998;171(2):433-435, PMID: 9694470. *Excluded: Wrong outcome/Did not report diagnostic accuracy measures*

Lee DH, Lee JM, Klotz E, et al. Detection of recurrent hepatocellular carcinoma in cirrhotic liver after transcatheter arterial chemoembolization: value of quantitative color mapping of the arterial enhancement fraction of the liver. Korean J Radiol. 2013;14(1):51-60. *Excluded: Inadequate reference standard*

Lee JA, Jeong WK, Kim Y, et al. Dual-energy CT to detect recurrent HCC after TACE: initial experience of color-coded iodine CT imaging. Eur J Radiol. 2013;82(4):569-576. *Excluded: Wrong outcome/Did not report diagnostic accuracy measures*

Lee JK, Chung Y-H, Song B-C, et al. Recurrences of hepatocellular carcinoma following initial remission by transcatheter arterial chemoembolization. J Gastroenterol Hepatol. 2002;17(1):52-58, PMID: 11895553. *Excluded: Wrong outcome/Did not report diagnostic accuracy measures*

Lee JM, Trevisani F, Vilgrain V, Wald C. Imaging diagnosis and staging of hepatocellular carcinoma. Liver Transpl. 2011;17 Suppl 2:S34-43, PMID: 21739567. *Excluded: Background*

Lee JM, Yoon J-H, Kim KW. Diagnosis of hepatocellular carcinoma: newer radiological tools. Semin Oncol. 2012;39(4):399-409, PMID: 22846858. *Excluded: Background*

Lee JY, Choi BI, Han JK, Lee JM, Kim SH. State-of-the-art ultrasonography of hepatocellular carcinoma. Eur J Radiol. 2006;58(2):177-185. *Excluded: Background*

Lee KHY, O'Malley ME, Haider MA, Hanbidge A. Triple-Phase MDCT of Hepatocellular Carcinoma. AJR Am J Roentgenol. 2004;182(3):643-649. *Excluded: Wrong outcome/Did not report diagnostic accuracy measures*

Lee MH, Kim YK, Park MJ, et al. Gadoxetic acid-enhanced fat suppressed three-dimensional T1-weighted MRI using a multiecho dixon technique at 3 tesla: Emphasis on image quality and hepatocellular carcinoma detection. J Magn Reson Imaging. 2013;38(2):401-410. *Excluded: Wrong outcome/Did not report diagnostic accuracy measures*

Lee MW, Rhim H, Ik Cha D, Jun Kim Y, Lim HK. Planning US for percutaneous radiofrequency ablation of small hepatocellular carcinomas (1-3 cm): Value of fusion imaging with conventional US and CT/MR Images. Journal of Vascular and Interventional Radiology. 2013;24(7):958-965. *Excluded: Inadequate reference standard*

Lee SD, Kim SH, Kim YK, et al. 18F-FDG-PET/CT predicts early tumor recurrence in living donor liver transplantation for hepatocellular carcinoma. Transpl Int. 2013;26(1):50-60. *Excluded: Wrong outcome/Did not report diagnostic accuracy measures*

Lee SW, Kim HJ, Park JH, et al. Clinical usefulness of 18F-FDG PET-CT for patients with gallbladder cancer and cholangiocarcinoma. J Gastroenterol. 2010;45(5):560-566, PMID: 20035356. *Excluded: Wrong population*

Leen E, Ceccotti P, Kalogeropoulou C, Angerson WJ, Moug SJ, Horgan PG. Prospective multicenter trial evaluating a novel method of characterizing focal liver lesions using contrast-enhanced sonography. AJR Am J Roentgenol. 2006;186(6):1551-1559, PMID: 16714643. *Excluded: Wrong population*

Lencioni R. Surveillance and early diagnosis of hepatocellular carcinoma. Dig Liver Dis. 2010;42 Suppl 3:S223-227, PMID: 20547307. *Excluded: Background*

Lencioni R, Della Pina C, Bruix J, et al. Clinical management of hepatic malignancies: ferucarbotran-enhanced magnetic resonance imaging versus contrast-enhanced spiral computed tomography. Dig Dis Sci. 2005;50(3):533-537, PMID: 15810637. *Excluded: Wrong population*

Lencioni R, Della Pina C, Crocetti L, Bozzi E, Cioni D. Clinical management of focal liver lesions: the key role of real-time contrast-enhanced US. Eur Radiol. 2007;17 Suppl 6:F73-79, PMID: 18376460. *Excluded: Background*

Lencioni R, Piscaglia F, Bolondi L. Contrast-enhanced ultrasound in the diagnosis of hepatocellular carcinoma. J Hepatol. 2008;48(5):848-857, PMID: 18328590. *Excluded: Background*

Leoni S, Piscaglia F, Golfieri R, et al. The impact of vascular and nonvascular findings on the noninvasive diagnosis of small hepatocellular carcinoma based on the EASL and AASLD criteria. Am J Gastroenterol. 2010;105(3):599-609, PMID: 19935786. *Excluded: Background*

Leoni S, Piscaglia F, Righini R, Bolondi L. Management of small hepatocellular carcinoma. Acta Gastroenterol Belg. 2006;69(2):230-235, PMID: 16929622. *Excluded: Background*

Li CS, Chen RC, Lii JM, et al. Magnetic resonance imaging appearance of well-differentiated hepatocellular carcinoma. J Comput Assist Tomogr. 2006;30(4):597-603. *Excluded: Wrong outcome/Did not report diagnostic accuracy measures*

Li X-D, Li Z-G, Song X-X, Liu C-F. A variant in microRNA-196a2 is associated with susceptibility to hepatocellular carcinoma in Chinese patients with cirrhosis. Pathology. 2010;42(7):669-673, PMID: 21080878. *Excluded: Wrong intervention*

Li Y-Y, Sha W-H, Zhou Y-J, Nie Y-Q. Short and long term efficacy of high intensity focused ultrasound therapy for advanced hepatocellular carcinoma. J Gastroenterol Hepatol. 2007;22(12):2148-2154, PMID: 18031373. *Excluded: Wrong intervention*

Liang P-C, Ch'ang H-J, Hsu C, Tseng SS, Shih TTF, Wu Liu T. Dynamic MRI signals in the second week of radiotherapy relate to treatment outcomes of hepatocellular carcinoma: a preliminary result. Liver Int. 2007;27(4):516-528, PMID: 17403192. *Excluded: Wrong population*

Lim JH, Cho JM, Kim EY, Park CK. Dysplastic nodules in liver cirrhosis: evaluation of hemodynamics with CT during arterial portography and CT hepatic arteriography. Radiology. 2000;214(3):869-874, PMID: 10715060. *Excluded: Wrong intervention*

Lim JH, Choi D, Park CK, Lee WJ, Lim HK. Encapsulated hepatocellular carcinoma: CT-pathologic correlations. Eur Radiol. 2006;16(10):2326-2333. *Excluded: Wrong outcome/Did not report diagnostic accuracy measures*

Lim JH, Jang HJ, Kim EY, Park CK, Joh JW, Kim YI. Early recurring hepatocellular carcinoma after partial hepatic resection: preoperative CT findings. Korean J Radiol. 2000;1(1):38-42, PMID: 11752927. *Excluded: Wrong outcome/Did not report diagnostic accuracy measures*

Lim KS. Diffusion-weighted MRI of hepatocellular carcinoma in cirrhosis. Clin Radiol. 2013. *Excluded: Wrong publication type*

Limanond P, Raman SS, Sayre J, Lu DSK. Comparison of dynamic gadolinium-enhanced and ferumoxides-enhanced MRI of the liver on high- and low-field scanners. J Magn Reson Imaging. 2004;20(4):640-647, PMID: 15390231. *Excluded: Wrong population*

Lin C-Y, Chen J-H, Liang J-A, Lin C-C, Jeng L-B, Kao C-H. 18F-FDG PET or PET/CT for detecting extrahepatic metastases or recurrent hepatocellular carcinoma: a systematic review and meta-analysis. Eur J Radiol. 2012;81(9):2417-2422, PMID: 21899970. *Excluded: Systematic review; studies checked for inclusion*

Liu G-J, Xu H-X, Xie X-Y, et al. Does the echogenicity of focal liver lesions on baseline gray-scale ultrasound interfere with the diagnostic performance of contrast-enhanced ultrasound? Eur Radiol. 2009;19(5):1214-1222, PMID: 19137313. *Excluded: Wrong population*

Liu J, Wang J-Z, Zhao J-D, Xu Z-Y, Jiang G-L. Use of combined maximum and minimum intensity projections to determine internal target volume in 4-dimensional CT scans for hepatic malignancies. Radiat. 2012;7:11, PMID: 22284745. *Excluded: Wrong outcome/Did not report diagnostic accuracy measures*

Liu Q, Chen J, Li H, Liang B, Zhang L, Hu T. Hepatocellular carcinoma with bile duct tumor thrombi: correlation of magnetic resonance imaging features to histopathologic manifestations. Eur J Radiol. 2010;76(1):103-109, PMID: 19501994. *Excluded: Wrong outcome/Did not report diagnostic accuracy measures*

Liu QY, Huang SQ, Chen JY, et al. Small hepatocellular carcinoma with bile duct tumor thrombi: CT and MRI findings. Abdom Imaging. 2010;35(5):537-542. *Excluded: Wrong outcome/Did not report diagnostic accuracy measures*

Liu Q-Y, Zhang W-D, Chen J-Y, Li H-G, Liu C, Liang B-L. Hepatocellular carcinoma with bile duct tumor thrombus: dynamic computed tomography findings and histopathologic correlation. J Comput Assist Tomogr. 2011;35(2):187-194, PMID: 21412088. *Excluded: Wrong outcome/Did not report diagnostic accuracy measures*

Liu W-Y, Jin Y, Rong R-H, Ta X, Zhu X-S. Multi-phase helical CT in diagnosis of early hepatocellular carcinoma. Hepatobiliary Pancreat Dis Int. 2003;2(1):73-76, PMID: 14607651. *Excluded: Wrong outcome/Did not report diagnostic accuracy measures*

Liu X, Zou L, Liu F, Zhou Y, Song B. Gadoxetic Acid Disodium-Enhanced Magnetic Resonance Imaging for the Detection of Hepatocellular Carcinoma: A Meta-Analysis. PLoS ONE. 2013;8(8). *Excluded: Systematic review; studies checked for inclusion*

Liu Y, Chen Z, Liu C, Yu D, Lu Z, Zhang N. Gadolinium-loaded polymeric nanoparticles modified with Anti-VEGF as multifunctional MRI contrast agents for the diagnosis of liver cancer. Biomaterials. 2011;32(22):5167-5176, PMID: 21521627. *Excluded: Wrong outcome/Did not report diagnostic accuracy measures*

Lo CM, Fan ST, Liu CL, et al. Determining resectability for hepatocellular carcinoma: the role of laparoscopy and laparoscopic ultrasonography. J Hepatobiliary Pancreat Surg. 2000;7(3):260-264, PMID: 10982624. *Excluded: Background*

Loffroy R, Lin M, Rao P, et al. Comparing the detectability of hepatocellular carcinoma by C-arm dual-phase cone-beam computed tomography during hepatic arteriography with conventional contrast-enhanced magnetic resonance imaging. Cardiovasc Intervent Radiol. 2012;35(1):97-104, PMID: 21328023. *Excluded: Wrong outcome/Did not report diagnostic accuracy measures*

Lok AS, Sterling RK, Everhart JE, et al. Des-gamma-carboxy prothrombin and alpha-fetoprotein as biomarkers for the early detection of hepatocellular carcinoma. Gastroenterology. 2010;138(2):493-502, PMID: 19852963. *Excluded: Wrong population*

Lopez Hanninen E, Vogl TJ, Bechstein WO, et al. Biphasic spiral computed tomography for detection of hepatocellular carcinoma before resection or orthotopic liver transplantation. Invest Radiol. 1998;33(4):216-221, PMID: 9556746. *Excluded: Imaging before 1995*

Low RN. Abdominal MRI advances in the detection of liver tumours and characterisation. Lancet Oncol. 2007;8(6):525-535, PMID: 17540304. *Excluded: Background*

Loyer EM, Chin H, DuBrow RA, David CL, Eftekhari F, Charnsangavej C. Hepatocellular carcinoma and intrahepatic peripheral cholangiocarcinoma: Enhancement patterns with quadruple phase helical CT - A comparative study. Radiology. 1999;212(3):866-875. *Excluded: Wrong outcome/Did not report diagnostic accuracy measures*

Lu DS, Siripongsakun S, Kyong Lee J, et al. Complete tumor encapsulation on magnetic resonance imaging: A potentially useful imaging biomarker for better survival in solitary large hepatocellular carcinoma. Liver Transpl. 2013;19(3):283-291. *Excluded: Wrong outcome/Did not report diagnostic accuracy measures*

Lu Q, Luo Y, Yuan C-X, et al. Value of contrast-enhanced intraoperative ultrasound for cirrhotic patients with hepatocellular carcinoma: a report of 20 cases. World J Gastroenterol. 2008;14(25):4005-4010, PMID: 18609684. *Excluded: Wrong intervention*

Lu X, Zhao H, Yang H, et al. A prospective clinical study on early recurrence of hepatocellular carcinoma after hepatectomy. J Surg Oncol. 2009;100(6):488-493, PMID: 19653238. *Excluded: Wrong outcome/Did not report diagnostic accuracy measures*

Luciani A, Baranes L, Decaens T, et al. Non-invasive diagnostic imaging of hepatocellular carcinoma: Targeting cellular characterization? J Hepatol. 2011;55(1):224-226. *Excluded: Background*

Luke FE, Allen BC, Moshiri ST, et al. Multiphase multi-detector row computed tomography in the setting of chronic liver disease and orthotopic liver transplantation: can a series be eliminated in order to reduce radiation dose? J Comput Assist Tomogr. 2013;37(3):408-414. *Excluded: Background*

Luo MY, Shan H, Jiang ZB, Li LF, Huang HQ. Study on hepatocellular carcinoma-associated hepatic arteriovenous shunt using multidetector CT. World J Gastroenterol. 2003;9(11):2455-2459. *Excluded: Wrong outcome/Did not report diagnostic accuracy measures*

Luo MY, Shan H, Jiang ZB, Liang WW, Zhang JS, Li LF. Capability of multidetector CT to diagnose hepatocellular carcinoma-associated arterioportal shunt. World J Gastroenterol. 2005;11(17):2666-2669. *Excluded: Wrong outcome/Did not report diagnostic accuracy measures*

Luo W, Numata K, Morimoto M, et al. Clinical utility of contrast-enhanced three-dimensional ultrasound imaging with Sonazoid: findings on hepatocellular carcinoma lesions. Eur J Radiol. 2009;72(3):425-431, PMID: 18930616. *Excluded: Wrong outcome/Did not report diagnostic accuracy measures*

Ma H, Liu J, Liu F. CT-guided single high-dose percutaneous acetic acid injection for small hepatocellular carcinoma: A long-term follow-up study. Eur J Radiol. 2012;81(6):1184-1186. *Excluded: Wrong population*

Ma X, Samir AE, Holalkere N-S, Sahani DV. Optimal arterial phase imaging for detection of hypervascular hepatocellular carcinoma determined by continuous image capture on 16-MDCT. AJR Am J Roentgenol. 2008;191(3):772-777, PMID: 18716108. *Excluded: Wrong outcome/Did not report diagnostic accuracy measures*

Macarini L, Milillo P, Cascavilla A, et al. MR characterisation of dysplastic nodules and hepatocarcinoma in the cirrhotic liver with hepatospecific superparamagnetic contrast agents: pathological correlation in explanted livers. Radiol Med (Torino). 2009;114(8):1267-1282, PMID: 19902328. *Excluded: Wrong intervention*

Macdonald GA, Peduto AJ. Magnetic resonance imaging (MRI) and diseases of the liver and biliary tract. Part 1. Basic principles, MRI in the assessment of diffuse and focal hepatic disease. J Gastroenterol Hepatol. 2000;15(9):980-991, PMID: 11059926. *Excluded: Background*

Maciel AC, Cerski CT, Moreira RK, Resende VL, Zanotelli ML, Matiotti SB. Hepatocellular carcinoma in patients undergoing orthotopic liver transplantation: radiological findings with anatomopathological correlation in Brazil. Arq Gastroenterol. 2006;43(1):24-29, PMID: 16699614. *Excluded: Imaging before 1995*

Magini G, Farsad M, Frigerio M, et al. C-11 acetate does not enhance usefulness of F-18 FDG PET/CT in differentiating between focal nodular hyperplasia and hepatic adenoma. Clin Nucl Med. 2009;34(10):659-665, PMID: 19893396. *Excluded: Wrong population*

Makita O, Yamashita Y, Arakawa A, et al. Diffuse perfusion abnormality of the liver parenchyma on angiography-assisted helical CT in relation to cirrhosis and previous treatments: a potential diagnostic pitfall for detecting hepatocellular carcinoma. Clin Imaging. 2000;24(5):292-297, PMID: 11331160. *Excluded: Wrong intervention*

Makita O, Yamashita Y, Arakawa A, et al. Diagnostic accuracy of helical CT arterial portography and CT hepatic arteriography for hypervascular hepatocellular carcinoma in chronic liver damage. An ROC analysis. Acta Radiol. 2000;41(5):464-469, PMID: 11016767. *Excluded: Wrong intervention*

Malagari K, Koskinas J, Brountzos E, et al. CT portography and post-lipiodol CT in the preinterventional work-up of primary and secondary liver tumors. A single center experience. Hepatogastroenterology. 1999;46(29):2901-2908, PMID: 10576370. *Excluded: Wrong intervention*

Mallikarjuna Swamy CM, Arathi CA, Kodandaswamy CR. Value of ultrasonography-guided fine needle aspiration cytology in the investigative sequence of hepatic lesions with an emphasis on hepatocellular carcinoma. J Cytol. 2011;28(4):178-184. *Excluded: Wrong intervention*

Mandai M, Koda M, Matono T, et al. Assessment of hepatocellular carcinoma by contrast-enhanced ultrasound with perfluorobutane microbubbles: comparison with dynamic CT. Br J Radiol. 2011;84(1002):499-507, PMID: 20959373. *Excluded: Inadequate reference standard*

Manichon AF, Bancel B, Durieux-Millon M, et al. Hepatocellular adenoma: Evaluation with contrast-enhanced ultrasound and MRI and correlation with pathologic and phenotypic classification in 26 lesions. HPB Surgery. 2012;2012. *Excluded: Wrong population*

Mann GN, Marx HF, Lai LL, Wagman LD. Clinical and cost effectiveness of a new hepatocellular MRI contrast agent, mangafodipir trisodium, in the preoperative assessment of liver resectability. Ann Surg Oncol. 2001;8(7):573-579, PMID: 11508618. *Excluded: Wrong population*

Marchianò A, Spreafico C, Lanocita R, et al. Does iodine concentration affect the diagnostic efficacy of biphasic spiral CT in patients with hepatocellular carcinoma? Abdom Imaging. 2005;30(3):274-280. *Excluded: Wrong outcome/Did not report diagnostic accuracy measures*

Marrero JA, Welling T. Modern diagnosis and management of hepatocellular carcinoma. Clin Liver Dis. 2009;13(2):233-247, PMID: 19442916. *Excluded: Background*

Martie A, Sporea I, Popescu A, et al. Contrast enhanced ultrasound for the characterization of hepatocellular carcinoma. Med Ultrason. 2011;13(2):108-113, PMID: 21655536. *Excluded: Inadequate reference standard*

Maruyama H, Takahashi M, Ishibashi H, et al. Ultrasound-guided treatments under low acoustic power contrast harmonic imaging for hepatocellular carcinomas undetected by B-mode ultrasonography. Liver Int. 2009;29(5):708-714. *Excluded: Wrong intervention*

Massarweh NN, Park JO, Bruix J, et al. Diagnostic imaging and biopsy use among elderly medicare beneficiaries with hepatocellular carcinoma. J Oncol Pract. 2011;7(3):155-160. *Excluded: Wrong intervention*

Matoba M, Kitadate M, Kondou T, Yokota H, Tonami H. Depiction of hypervascular hepatocellular carcinoma with 64-MDCT: Comparison of moderate- and high-concentration contrast material with and without saline flush. AJR Am J Roentgenol. 2009;193(3):738-744. *Excluded: Wrong outcome/Did not report diagnostic accuracy measures*

Matsui O, Kobayashi S, Sanada J, et al. Hepatocellular nodules in liver cirrhosis: hemodynamic evaluation (angiography-assisted CT) with special reference to multi-step hepatocarcinogenesis. Abdom Imaging. 2011;36(3):264-272, PMID: 21267562. *Excluded: Wrong intervention*

Matsui O, Ueda K, Kobayashi S, et al. Intra- and perinodular hemodynamics of hepatocellular carcinoma: CT observation during intra-arterial contrast injection. Abdom Imaging. 2002;27(2):147-156. *Excluded: Background*

Matsuo M, Kanematsu M, Inaba Y, et al. Pre-operative detection of malignant hepatic tumours: value of combined helical CT during arterial portography and biphasic CT during hepatic arteriography. Clin Radiol. 2001;56(2):138-145, PMID: 11222073. *Excluded: Wrong intervention*

Matsushima M, Naganawa S, Ikeda M, et al. Diagnostic value of SPIO-mediated breath-hold, black-blood, fluid-attenuated, inversion recovery (BH-BB-FLAIR) imaging in patients with hepatocellular carcinomas. Magn. 2010;9(2):49-58, PMID: 20585194. *Excluded: Inadequate reference standard*

Mejia GA, Gomez MA, Serrano J, et al. Correlation between the radiologic and histologic size of hepatocellular carcinoma in patients eligible for liver transplantation. Transplant Proc. 2006;38(5):1394-1395, PMID: 16797313. *Excluded: Background*

Mi B, Wan W, Yu C, You X, Xu Q. Sarcomatoid hepatocellular carcinoma diagnosed by FDG PET/CT. Clin Nucl Med. 2011;36(10):925-927. *Excluded: Background*

Mikami S, Kubo S, Hirohashi K, et al. Computed tomography during arteriography and arterial portography in small hepatocellular carcinoma and dysplastic nodule: a prospective study. Jpn J Cancer Res. 2000;91(8):859-863, PMID: 10965029. *Excluded: Wrong intervention*

Mikami S, Tateishi R, Akahane M, et al. Computed tomography follow-up for the detection of hepatocellular carcinoma recurrence after initial radiofrequency ablation: a single-center experience. J Vasc Interv Radiol. 2012;23(10):1269-1275. *Excluded: Wrong outcome/Did not report diagnostic accuracy measures*

Miller FH, Hammond N, Siddiqi AJ, et al. Utility of diffusion-weighted MRI in distinguishing benign and malignant hepatic lesions. J Magn Reson Imaging. 2010;32(1):138-147, PMID: 20578020. *Excluded: Wrong population*

Min YW, Gwak G-Y, Lee MW, et al. Clinical course of sub-centimeter-sized nodules detected during surveillance for hepatocellular carcinoma. World J Gastroenterol. 2012;18(21):2654-2660, PMID: 22690074. *Excluded: Wrong outcome/Did not report diagnostic accuracy measures*

Miyamoto N, Sakurai Y, Nishimori H, Tsuji K, Kang J-H, Maguchi H. Optimal scan timing for coronal enhancement of hypervascular hepatocellular carcinomas and correlation with tumor size: evaluation with four-phase CT hepatic arteriography. Radiat Med. 2005;23(6):456-462, PMID: 16389992. *Excluded: Wrong intervention*

Miyayama S, Matsui O, Yamashiro M, et al. Detection of hepatocellular carcinoma by CT during arterial portography using a cone-beam CT technology: Comparison with conventional CTAP. Abdom Imaging. 2009;34(4):502-506. *Excluded: Wrong intervention*

Miyayama S, Yamashiro M, Okuda M, et al. Detection of corona enhancement of hypervascular hepatocellular carcinoma by C-arm dual-phase cone-beam CT during hepatic arteriography. Cardiovasc Intervent Radiol. 2011;34(1):81-86, PMID: 20333382. *Excluded: Wrong intervention*

Mochizuki T, Tsuda T, Sugawara Y, et al. Tc-99m PMT hepatobiliary scintigraphy in the differential diagnosis of extrahepatic metastases and hepatocellular carcinoma. Clin Nucl Med. 2000;25(12):991-995, PMID: 11129165. *Excluded: Wrong intervention*

Mody RJ, Pohlen JA, Malde S, Strouse PJ, Shulkin BL. FDG PET for the study of primary hepatic malignancies in children. Pediatr Blood Cancer. 2006;47(1):51-55, PMID: 16078228. *Excluded: Wrong population*

Mok TSK, Yeo W, Yu S, et al. An intensive surveillance program detected a high incidence of hepatocellular carcinoma among hepatitis B virus carriers with abnormal alpha-fetoprotein levels or abdominal ultrasonography results. J Clin Oncol. 2005;23(31):8041-8047. *Excluded: Inadequate reference standard*

Montorsi M, Santambrogio R, Bianchi P, et al. Laparoscopy with laparoscopic ultrasound for pretreatment staging of hepatocellular carcinoma: a prospective study. J Gastrointest

Surg. 2001;5(3):312-315, PMID: 11360055. *Excluded: Wrong intervention*

Monzawa S, Omata K, Shimazu N, Yagawa A, Hosoda K, Araki T. Well-differentiated hepatocellular carcinoma: Findings of US, CT, and MR imaging. Abdom Imaging. 1999;24(4):392-397. *Excluded: Wrong outcome/Did not report diagnostic accuracy measures*

Morana G, Grazioli L, Kirchin MA, et al. Solid hypervascular liver lesions: accurate identification of true benign lesions on enhanced dynamic and hepatobiliary phase magnetic resonance imaging after gadobenate dimeglumine administration. Invest Radiol. 2011;46(4):225-239, PMID: 21102346. *Excluded: Wrong population*

Morana G, Grazioli L, Schneider G, et al. Hypervascular hepatic lesions: dynamic and late enhancement pattern with Gd-BOPTA. Acad Radiol. 2002;9 Suppl 2:S476-479, PMID: 12188313. *Excluded: Background*

Mori K, Scheidler J, Helmberger T, et al. Detection of malignant hepatic lesions before orthotopic liver transplantation: accuracy of ferumoxides-enhanced MR imaging. AJR Am J Roentgenol. 2002;179(4):1045-1051, PMID: 12239063. *Excluded: Wrong intervention*

Moribata K, Tamai H, Shingaki N, et al. Assessment of malignant potential of small hypervascular hepatocellular carcinoma using B-mode ultrasonography. Hepatol Res. 2011;41(3):233-239. *Excluded: Wrong outcome/Did not report diagnostic accuracy measures*

Muhi A, Ichikawa T, Motosugi U, et al. High-b-value diffusion-weighted MR imaging of hepatocellular lesions: estimation of grade of malignancy of hepatocellular carcinoma. J Magn Reson Imaging. 2009;30(5):1005-1011, PMID: 19856432. *Excluded: Wrong outcome/Did not report diagnostic accuracy measures*

Murakami T, Imai Y, Okada M, et al. Ultrasonography, computed tomography and magnetic resonance imaging of hepatocellular carcinoma: toward improved treatment decisions. Oncology. 2011;81 Suppl 1:86-99, PMID: 22212941. *Excluded: Background*

Murakami T, Kim T, Hori M, Federle MP. Double Arterial Phase Multi-Detector Row Helical CT for Detection of Hypervascular Hepatocellular Carcinoma [3]. Radiology. 2003;229(3):931-932. *Excluded: Background*

Murakami T, Okada M, Hyodo T. CT versus MR imaging of hepatocellular carcinoma: toward improved treatment decisions. Magn. 2012;11(2):75-81, PMID: 22790293. *Excluded: Background*

Murakami T, Takamura M, Kim T, et al. Double phase CT during hepatic arteriography for diagnosis of hepatocellular carcinoma. Eur J Radiol. 2005;54(2):246-252, PMID: 15837405. *Excluded: Wrong intervention*

Nakagawara H, Ogawa M, Matsumoto N, et al. Evaluation of malignancy of hepatocellular carcinoma using the ultrasonic B-mode method: Clinical significance of extracapsular invasion of hepatocellular carcinoma using ultrasonography. Journal of Medical Ultrasonics. 2007;34(2):83-91. *Excluded: Wrong outcome/Did not report diagnostic accuracy measures*

Nakai M, Sato M, Ikoma A, et al. Triple-phase computed tomography during arterial portography with bolus tracking for hepatic tumors. Jpn J Radiol. 2010;28(2):149-156, PMID: 20182850. *Excluded: Wrong intervention*

Nakamura Y, Toyota N, Shuji D, et al. Clinical significance of the transitional phase at gadoxetate disodium-enhanced hepatic MRI for the diagnosis of hepatocellular carcinoma: Preliminary results. J Comput Assist Tomogr. 2011;35(6):723-727. *Excluded: Wrong outcome/Did not report diagnostic accuracy measures*

Nakanishi M, Chuma M, Hige S, et al. Relationship between diffusion-weighted magnetic resonance imaging and histological tumor grading of hepatocellular carcinoma. Ann Surg Oncol. 2012;19(4):1302-1309. *Excluded: Wrong outcome/Did not report diagnostic accuracy measures*

Nakaura T, Awai K, Yanaga Y, et al. Detection of early enhancement of hypervascular hepatocellular carcinoma using single breath-hold 3D pixel shift dynamic subtraction MDCT. AJR Am J Roentgenol. 2008;190(1):W13-18, PMID: 18094267. *Excluded: Wrong outcome/Did not report diagnostic accuracy measures*

Nakayama M, Kamura T, Kimura M, Seki H, Tsukada K, Sakai K. Quantitative MRI of hepatocellular carcinoma in cirrhotic and noncirrhotic livers. Clin Imaging. 1998;22(4):280-283. *Excluded: Wrong outcome/Did not report diagnostic accuracy measures*

Nakayama M, Yamashita Y, Mitsuzaki K, et al. Improved tissue characterization of focal liver lesions with ferumoxide-enhanced T1 and T2-weighted MR imaging. J Magn Reson Imaging. 2000;11(6):647-654, PMID: 10862064. *Excluded: Wrong outcome/Did not report diagnostic accuracy measures*

Namkung S, Zech CJ, Helmberger T, Reiser MF, Schoenberg SO. Superparamagnetic iron oxide (SPIO)-enhanced liver MRI with ferucarbotran: efficacy for characterization of focal liver lesions. J Magn Reson Imaging. 2007;25(4):755-765, PMID: 17335040. *Excluded: Wrong population*

Nanashima A, Abo T, Sakamoto I, et al. Three-dimensional fusion images of hepatic vasculature and bile duct used for preoperative simulation before hepatic surgery. Hepatogastroenterology. 2012;59(118):1748-1757, PMID: 22369745. *Excluded: Wrong outcome/Did not report diagnostic accuracy measures*

Negi N, Yoshikawa T, Ohno Y, et al. Hepatic CT perfusion measurements: a feasibility study for radiation dose reduction using new image reconstruction method. Eur J Radiol. 2012;81(11):3048-3054, PMID: 22613507. *Excluded: Wrong intervention*

Ng CS, Chandler AG, Wei W, et al. Effect of dual vascular input functions on CT perfusion parameter values and reproducibility in liver tumors and normal liver. J Comput Assist Tomogr. 2012;36(4):388-393, PMID: 22805665. *Excluded: Wrong outcome/Did not report diagnostic accuracy measures*

Ng CS, Chandler AG, Wei W, et al. Reproducibility of CT perfusion parameters in liver tumors and normal liver. Radiology. 2011;260(3):762-770, PMID: 21788525. *Excluded: Wrong outcome/Did not report diagnostic accuracy measures*

Ng CS, Raunig DL, Jackson EF, et al. Reproducibility of perfusion parameters in dynamic contrast-enhanced MRI of lung and liver tumors: effect on estimates of patient sample size in clinical trials and on individual patient responses. AJR Am J Roentgenol. 2010;194(2):W134-140, PMID: 20093564. *Excluded: Wrong outcome/Did not report diagnostic accuracy measures*

Nguyen P, Feng JC, Chang KJ. Endoscopic ultrasound (EUS) and EUS-guided fine-needle aspiration (FNA) of liver lesions. Gastrointest Endosc. 1999;50(3):357-361, PMID: 10462656. *Excluded: Wrong intervention*

Nicolau C, Vilana R, Catala V, et al. Importance of evaluating all vascular phases on contrast-enhanced sonography in the differentiation of benign from malignant focal liver lesions. AJR Am J Roentgenol. 2006;186(1):158-167, PMID: 16357396. *Excluded: Wrong population*

Niizawa G, Ikegami T, Matsuzaki Y, et al. Monitoring of hepatocellular carcinoma, following proton radiotherapy, with contrast-enhanced color Doppler ultrasonography. J Gastroenterol. 2005;40(3):283-290, PMID: 15830288. *Excluded: Wrong population*

Nishie A, Tajima T, Asayama Y, et al. Diagnostic performance of apparent diffusion coefficient for predicting histological grade of hepatocellular carcinoma. Eur J Radiol. 2011;80(2):e29-33, PMID: 20619566. *Excluded: Wrong outcome/Did not report diagnostic accuracy measures*

Nishie A, Tajima T, Ishigami K, et al. Detection of hepatocellular carcinoma (HCC) using super paramagnetic iron oxide (SPIO)-enhanced MRI: Added value of diffusion-weighted imaging (DWI). J Magn Reson Imaging. 2010;31(2):373-382, PMID: 20099351. *Excluded: Wrong intervention*

Nishie A, Yoshimitsu K, Asayama Y, et al. Detection of combined hepatocellular and cholangiocarcinomas on enhanced CT: Comparison with histologic findings. AJR Am J Roentgenol. 2005;184(4):1157-1162. *Excluded: Wrong outcome/Did not report diagnostic accuracy measures*

Nishie A, Yoshimitsu K, Asayama Y, et al. Radiologic detectability of minute portal venous invasion in hepatocellular carcinoma. AJR Am J Roentgenol. 2008;190(1):81-87, PMID: 18094297. *Excluded: Wrong outcome/Did not report diagnostic accuracy measures*

Niu Y, Huang T, Lian F, Li F. Contrast-enhanced ultrasonography for the diagnosis of small hepatocellular carcinoma: a meta-analysis and meta-regression analysis. Tumor Biology. 2013:1-8. *Excluded: Systematic review; studies checked for inclusion*

Nouso K, Tanaka H, Uematsu S, et al. Cost-effectiveness of the surveillance program of hepatocellular carcinoma depends on the medical circumstances. J Gastroenterol Hepatol.

2008;23(3):437-444, PMID: 17683496. *Excluded: Wrong outcome/Did not report diagnostic accuracy measures*

Numminen K, Halavaara J, Isoniemi H, et al. Magnetic resonance imaging of the liver: true fast imaging with steady state free precession sequence facilitates rapid and reliable distinction between hepatic hemangiomas and liver malignancies. J Comput Assist Tomogr. 2003;27(4):571-576, PMID: 12886146. *Excluded: Wrong population*

Numminen K, Halavaara J, Tervahartiala P, et al. Liver tumour MRI: what do we need for lesion characterization? Scand J Gastroenterol. 2004;39(1):67-73, PMID: 14992564. *Excluded: Wrong population*

Numminen K, Isoniemi H, Halavaara J, et al. Preoperative assessment of focal liver lesions: multidetector computed tomography challenges magnetic resonance imaging. Acta Radiol. 2005;46(1):9-15, PMID: 15841734. *Excluded: Wrong population*

Obuz F, Oksuzler M, Secil M, Sagol O, Karademir S, Astarcioglu H. Efficiency of MR imaging in the detection of malignant liver lesions. Diagn Interv Radiol. 2006;12(1):17-21, PMID: 16538579. *Excluded: Wrong outcome/Did not report diagnostic accuracy measures*

Ogata R, Majima Y, Tateishi Y, et al. Bright loop appearance; a characteristic ultrasonography sign of early hepatocellular carcinoma. Oncol Rep. 2000;7(6):1293-1298, PMID: 11032932. *Excluded: Wrong outcome/Did not report diagnostic accuracy measures*

Ogawa S, Kumada T, Toyoda H, et al. Evaluation of pathological features of hepatocellular carcinoma by contrast-enhanced ultrasonography: Comparison with pathology on resected specimen. Eur J Radiol. 2006;59(1):74-81. *Excluded: Wrong outcome/Did not report diagnostic accuracy measures*

Ohto M, Ito R, Soma N, et al. Contrast-enhanced 3D ultrasonography in minute hepatocellular carcinoma. Journal of Medical Ultrasonics. 2011;38(1):3-12. *Excluded: Wrong study design for Key Question*

Okada M, Imai Y, Kim T, et al. Comparison of enhancement patterns of histologically confirmed hepatocellular carcinoma between gadoxetate- and ferucarbotran-enhanced magnetic resonance imaging. J Magn Reson Imaging. 2010;32(4):903-913, PMID: 20882621. *Excluded: Wrong outcome/Did not report diagnostic accuracy measures*

Okamoto E, Sato S, Sanchez-Siles AA, et al. Evaluation of virtual CT sonography for enhanced detection of small hepatic nodules: a prospective pilot study. AJR Am J Roentgenol. 2010;194(5):1272-1278, PMID: 20410414. *Excluded: Wrong outcome/Did not report diagnostic accuracy measures*

Okumura E, Sanada S, Suzuki M, Matsui O. A computer-aided temporal and dynamic subtraction technique of the liver for detection of small hepatocellular carcinomas on abdominal CT images. Phys Med Biol. 2006;51(19):4759-4771, PMID: 16985269. *Excluded: Wrong outcome/Did not report diagnostic accuracy measures*

Okumura E, Sanada S, Suzuki M, Takemura A, Matsui O. Effectiveness of temporal and dynamic subtraction images of the liver for detection of small HCC on abdominal CT images: comparison of 3D nonlinear image-warping and 3D global-matching techniques. Radiol Phys Technol. 2011;4(2):109-120, PMID: 21229338. *Excluded: Wrong outcome/Did not report diagnostic accuracy measures*

Onaya H, Itai Y, Satake M, et al. Highly enhanced hepatic masses seen on CT during arterial portography: Early hepatocellular carcinoma and adenomatous hyperplasia. Jpn J Clin Oncol. 2000;30(10):440-445. *Excluded: Wrong intervention*

Onur MR, Cicekci M, Kayali A, Poyraz AK, Kocakoc E. The role of ADC measurement in differential diagnosis of focal hepatic lesions. Eur J Radiol. 2012;81(3):e171-176, PMID: 21353418. *Excluded: Wrong outcome/Did not report diagnostic accuracy measures*

Ouedraogo W, Tran-Van Nhieu J, Baranes L, et al. [Evaluation of noninvasive diagnostic criteria for hepatocellular carcinoma on pretransplant MRI (2010): correlation between MR imaging features and histological features on liver specimen]. J Radiol. 2011;92(7-8):688-700, PMID: 21819911. *Excluded: Not English language*

Ozsunar Y, Skjoldbye B, Court-Payen M, Karstrup S, Burcharth F. Impact of intraoperative ultrasonography on surgical treatment of liver tumours. Acta Radiol. 2000;41(1):97-101, PMID: 10665881. *Excluded: Wrong intervention*

Parikh A, Taouli B. Imaging of hepatocellular

carcinoma: current concepts. Recent Results Cancer Res. 2013;190:33-55, PMID: 22941012. *Excluded: Background*

Park HS, Lee J-M, Kim SH, et al. Differentiation of well-differentiated hepatocellular carcinomas from other hepatocellular nodules in cirrhotic liver: value of SPIO-enhanced MR imaging at 3.0 Tesla. J Magn Reson Imaging. 2009;29(2):328-335, PMID: 19161184. *Excluded: Wrong intervention*

Patel D, Terrault NA, Yao FY, Bass NM, Ladabaum U. Cost-effectiveness of hepatocellular carcinoma surveillance in patients with hepatitis C virus-related cirrhosis. Clin Gastroenterol Hepatol. 2005;3(1):75-84, PMID: 15645408. *Excluded: Background*

Patel M, Shariff MIF, Ladep NG, et al. Hepatocellular carcinoma: diagnostics and screening. J Eval Clin Pract. 2012;18(2):335-342, PMID: 21114800. *Excluded: Background*

Paudyal B, Oriuchi N, Paudyal P, et al. Early diagnosis of recurrent hepatocellular carcinoma with 18F-FDG PET after radiofrequency ablation therapy. Oncol Rep. 2007;18(6):1469-1473. *Excluded: Wrong outcome/Did not report diagnostic accuracy measures*

Pauleit D, Textor J, Bachmann R, et al. Improving the detectability of focal liver lesions on T2-weighted MR images: ultrafast breath-hold or respiratory-triggered thin-section MRI? J Magn Reson Imaging. 2001;14(2):128-133, PMID: 11477670. *Excluded: Wrong population*

Pawluk RS, Tummala S, Brown JJ, Borrello JA. A retrospective analysis of the accuracy of T2-weighted images and dynamic gadolinium-enhanced sequences in the detection and characterization of focal hepatic lesions. J Magn Reson Imaging. 1999;9(2):266-273, PMID: 10077023. *Excluded: Imaging before 1995*

Peck-Radosavljevic M. Imaging and early diagnosis of hepatocellular carcinoma. Minerva Gastroenterol Dietol. 2011;57(3):273-286, PMID: 21769077. *Excluded: Background*

Pei XQ, Liu LZ, Liu M, et al. Contrast-enhanced ultrasonography of hepatocellular carcinoma: correlation between quantitative parameters and histological grading. Br J Radiol. 2012;85(1017):e740-747, PMID: 22096225. *Excluded: Wrong outcome/Did not report diagnostic accuracy measures*

Peschl R, Werle A, Mathis G. Differential diagnosis of focal liver lesions in signal-enhanced ultrasound using BR 1, a second-generation ultrasound signal enhancer. Dig Dis. 2004;22(1):73-80, PMID: 15292698. *Excluded: Inadequate reference standard*

Petersein J, Spinazzi A, Giovagnoni A, et al. Focal liver lesions: evaluation of the efficacy of gadobenate dimeglumine in MR imaging--a multicenter phase III clinical study. Radiology. 2000;215(3):727-736, PMID: 10831691. *Excluded: Wrong population*

Phongkitkarun S, Srianujata T, Jatchavala J. Supplement value of magnetic resonance imaging in small hepatic lesion (< or = 20 mm) detected on routine computed tomography. J Med Assoc Thai. 2009;92(5):677-686, PMID: 19459531. *Excluded: Wrong outcome/Did not report diagnostic accuracy measures*

Pirovano G, Vanzulli A, Marti-Bonmati L, et al. Evaluation of the accuracy of gadobenate dimeglumine-enhanced MR imaging in the detection and characterization of focal liver lesions. AJR Am J Roentgenol. 2000;175(4):1111-1120, PMID: 11000175. *Excluded: Wrong population*

Piscaglia F, Lencioni R, Sagrini E, et al. Characterization of focal liver lesions with contrast-enhanced ultrasound. Ultrasound Med Biol. 2010;36(4):531-550, PMID: 20350680. *Excluded: Wrong publication type*

Pleguezuelo M, Germani G, Marelli L, et al. Evidence-based diagnosis and locoregional therapy for hepatocellular carcinoma. Expert Rev Gastroenterol Hepatol. 2008;2(6):761-784, PMID: 19090737. *Excluded: Background*

Poeckler-Schoeniger C, Koepke J, Gueckel F, Sturm J, Georgi M. MRI with superparamagnetic iron oxide: efficacy in the detection and characterization of focal hepatic lesions. Magn Reson Imaging. 1999;17(3):383-392, PMID: 10195581. *Excluded: Wrong population*

Preis O, Blake MA, Scott JA. Neural network evaluation of PET scans of the liver: a potentially useful adjunct in clinical interpretation. Radiology. 2011;258(3):714-721, PMID: 21339347. *Excluded: Inadequate reference standard*

Purysko AS, Remer EM, Coppa CP, Leao Filho HM, Thupili CR, Veniero JC. LI-RADS: a case-based review of the new categorization of liver findings in patients with end-stage liver disease. Radiographics. 2012;32(7):1977-1995.

Excluded: Wrong outcome/Did not report diagnostic accuracy measures

Purysko AS, Remer EM, Coppa CP, Obuchowski NA, Schneider E, Veniero JC. Characteristics and distinguishing features of hepatocellular adenoma and focal nodular hyperplasia on gadoxetate disodium-enhanced MRI. AJR Am J Roentgenol. 2012;198(1):115-123, PMID: 22194486. *Excluded: Wrong population*

Qayyum A, Thoeni RF, Coakley FV, Lu Y, Guay JP, Ferrell LD. Detection of hepatocellular carcinoma by ferumoxides-enhanced MR imaging in cirrhosis: Incremental value of dynamic gadolinium-enhancement. J Magn Reson Imaging. 2006;23(1):17-22, PMID: 16315209. *Excluded: Wrong intervention*

Qian MYY, Yuwei J R, Angus P, Schelleman T, Johnson L, Gow P. Efficacy and cost of a hepatocellular carcinoma screening program at an Australian teaching hospital. J Gastroenterol Hepatol. 2010;25(5):951-956, PMID: 20546449. *Excluded: Wrong publication type*

Quaia E, Alaimo V, Baratella E, et al. Effect of observer experience in the differentiation between benign and malignant liver tumors after ultrasound contrast agent injection. J Ultrasound Med. 2010;29(1):25-36, PMID: 20040772. *Excluded: Wrong population*

Quaia E, Calliada F, Bertolotto M, et al. Characterization of focal liver lesions with contrast-specific US modes and a sulfur hexafluoride-filled microbubble contrast agent: diagnostic performance and confidence. Radiology. 2004;232(2):420-430, PMID: 15286314. *Excluded: Wrong population*

Quaia E, De Paoli L, Pizzolato R, et al. Predictors of dysplastic nodule diagnosis in patients with liver cirrhosis on unenhanced and gadobenate dimeglumine-enhanced MRI with dynamic and hepatobiliary phase. AJR Am J Roentgenol. 2013;200(3):553-562. *Excluded: Wrong outcome/Did not report diagnostic accuracy measures*

Quaia E, Lorusso A, Grisi G, Stacul F, Cova MA. The role of CEUS in the characterization of hepatocellular nodules detected during the US surveillance program--current practices in Europe. Ultraschall Med. 2012;33 Suppl 1:S48-56, PMID: 22723029. *Excluded: Background*

Quaia E, Pizzolato R, De Paoli L, Angileri R, Ukmar M, Cova MA. Arterial enhancing-only nodules less than 2 cm in diameter in patients with liver cirrhosis: predictors of hepatocellular carcinoma diagnosis on gadobenate dimeglumine-enhanced MR imaging. J Magn Reson Imaging. 2013;37(4):892-902. *Excluded: Wrong outcome/Did not report diagnostic accuracy measures*

Quaia E, Stacul F, Gaiani S, et al. Comparison of diagnostic performance of unenhanced vs SonoVue - enhanced ultrasonography in focal liver lesions characterization. The experience of three Italian centers. Radiol Med (Torino). 2004;108(1-2):71-81, PMID: 15269691. *Excluded: Wrong population*

Rabenandrasana HA, Furukawa A, Furuichi K, Yamasaki M, Takahashi M, Murata K. Comparison between tissue harmonic imaging and liver-specific late-phase contrast-enhanced pulse-inversion imaging in the detection of hepatocellular carcinoma and liver metastasis. Radiat Med. 2004;22(2):90-97, PMID: 15176603. *Excluded: Inadequate reference standard*

Raman SS, Lu DS, Chen SC, Sayre J, Eilber F, Economou J. Hepatic MR imaging using ferumoxides: prospective evaluation with surgical and intraoperative sonographic confirmation in 25 cases. AJR Am J Roentgenol. 2001;177(4):807-812, PMID: 11566677. *Excluded: Wrong population*

Reimer P, Jahnke N, Fiebich M, et al. Hepatic lesion detection and characterization: value of nonenhanced MR imaging, superparamagnetic iron oxide-enhanced MR imaging, and spiral CT-ROC analysis. Radiology. 2000;217(1):152-158, PMID: 11012438. *Excluded: Wrong population*

Ren FY, Piao XX, Jin AL. Efficacy of ultrasonography and alpha-fetoprotein on early detection of hepatocellular carcinoma. World J Gastroenterol. 2006;12(29):4656-4659. *Excluded: Wrong outcome/Did not report diagnostic accuracy measures*

Rennert J, Jung E-M, Schreyer AG, et al. MR-arterioportography: a new technical approach for detection of liver lesions. World J Gastroenterol. 2011;17(13):1739-1745, PMID: 21483635. *Excluded: Background*

Robinson PJ, Arnold P, Wilson D. Small "indeterminate" lesions on CT of the liver: a follow-up study of stability. Br J Radiol. 2003;76(912):866-874, PMID: 14711773. *Excluded: Wrong outcome/Did not report diagnostic accuracy measures*

Ronot M, Bahrami S, Calderaro J, et al. Hepatocellular adenomas: Accuracy of magnetic resonance imaging and liver biopsy in subtype classification. Hepatology. 2011;53(4):1182-1191. *Excluded: Wrong population*

Rosenkrantz AB, Mannelli L, Mossa D, Babb JS. Breath-hold T2-weighted MRI of the liver at 3T using the BLADE technique: impact upon image quality and lesion detection. Clin Radiol. 2011;66(5):426-433, PMID: 21300326. *Excluded: Inadequate reference standard*

Ruelas-Villavicencio AL, Vargas-Vorackova F. In whom, how and how often is surveillance for hepatocellular carcinoma cost-effective? Ann Hepatol. 2004;3(4):152-159, PMID: 15657557. *Excluded: Background*

Rydberg JN, Tervonen OA, Rydberg DB, Lomas DJ, Ehman RL, Riederer SJ. Dual-echo breathhold T(2)-weighted fast spin echo MR imaging of liver lesions. Magn Reson Imaging. 2000;18(2):117-124, PMID: 10722970. *Excluded: Inadequate reference standard*

Saab S, Ly D, Nieto J, et al. Hepatocellular carcinoma screening in patients waiting for liver transplantation: a decision analytic model. Liver Transpl. 2003;9(7):672-681, PMID: 12827551. *Excluded: Background*

Sacks A, Peller PJ, Surasi DS, Chatburn L, Mercier G, Subramaniam RM. Value of PET/CT in the management of primary hepatobiliary tumors, part 2. AJR Am J Roentgenol. 2011;197(2):W260-265, PMID: 21785051. *Excluded: Background*

Saito K, Moriyasu F, Sugimoto K, et al. Histological grade of differentiation of hepatocellular carcinoma: Comparison of the efficacy of diffusion-weighted MRI with T2-weighted imaging and angiography-assisted CT. J Med Imaging Radiat Oncol. 2012;56(3):261-269. *Excluded: Background*

Saito K, Moriyasu F, Sugimoto K, et al. Diagnostic efficacy of gadoxetic acid-enhanced MRI for hepatocellular carcinoma and dysplastic nodule. World J Gastroenterol. 2011;17(30):3503-3509. *Excluded: Wrong outcome/Did not report diagnostic accuracy measures*

Sandrasegaran K, Akisik FM, Lin C, Tahir B, Rajan J, Aisen AM. The value of diffusion-weighted imaging in characterizing focal liver masses. Acad Radiol. 2009;16(10):1208-1214, PMID: 19608435. *Excluded: Wrong population*

Sandrasegaran K, Ramaswamy R, Ghosh S, et al. Diffusion-weighted MRI of the transplanted liver. Clin Radiol. 2011;66(9):820-825, PMID: 21621199. *Excluded: Wrong outcome/Did not report diagnostic accuracy measures*

Sangiovanni A, Del Ninno E, Fasani P, et al. Increased survival of cirrhotic patients with a hepatocellular carcinoma detected during surveillance. Gastroenterology. 2004;126(4):1005-1014, PMID: 15057740. *Excluded: Wrong outcome/Did not report diagnostic accuracy measures*

Sangiovanni A, Prati GM, Fasani P, et al. The natural history of compensated cirrhosis due to hepatitis C virus: A 17-year cohort study of 214 patients. Hepatology. 2006;43(6):1303-1310, PMID: 16729298. *Excluded: Wrong outcome/Did not report diagnostic accuracy measures*

Santagostino E, Colombo M, Rivi M, et al. A 6-month versus a 12-month surveillance for hepatocellular carcinoma in 559 hemophiliacs infected with the hepatitis C virus. Blood. 2003;102(1):78-82, PMID: 12649165. *Excluded: Wrong outcome/Did not report diagnostic accuracy measures*

Santi V, Trevisani F, Gramenzi A, et al. Semiannual surveillance is superior to annual surveillance for the detection of early hepatocellular carcinoma and patient survival. J Hepatol. 2010;53(2):291-297, PMID: 20483497. *Excluded: Wrong outcome/Did not report diagnostic accuracy measures*

Savranoglu P, Obuz F, Karasu S, et al. The role of SPIO-enhanced MRI in the detection of malignant liver lesions. Clin Imaging. 2006;30(6):377-381, PMID: 17101405. *Excluded: Wrong population*

Schindera ST, Diedrichsen L, Muller HC, et al. Iterative reconstruction algorithm for abdominal multidetector CT at different tube voltages: assessment of diagnostic accuracy, image quality, and radiation dose in a phantom study. Radiology. 2011;260(2):454-462, PMID: 21493795. *Excluded: Wrong population*

Schindera ST, Hareter LF, Raible S, et al. Effect of tumor size and tumor-to-liver contrast of hypovascular liver tumors on the diagnostic performance of hepatic CT imaging. Invest Radiol. 2012;47(3):197-201, PMID: 22233758. *Excluded: Wrong population*

Schultz JF, Bell JD, Goldstein RM, Kuhn JA, McCarty TM. Hepatic tumor imaging using iron oxide MRI: comparison with computed tomography, clinical impact, and cost analysis. Ann Surg Oncol. 1999;6(7):691-698, PMID: 10560856. *Excluded: Wrong population*

Seltzer SE, Getty DJ, Pickett RM, et al. Multimodality diagnosis of liver tumors: feature analysis with CT, liver-specific and contrast-enhanced MR, and a computer model. Acad Radiol. 2002;9(3):256-269, PMID: 11887942. *Excluded: Wrong population*

Semelka RC, Lee JK, Worawattanakul S, Noone TC, Patt RH, Ascher SM. Sequential use of ferumoxide particles and gadolinium chelate for the evaluation of focal liver lesions on MRI. J Magn Reson Imaging. 1998;8(3):670-674, PMID: 9626884. *Excluded: Wrong population*

Semelka RC, Martin DR, Balci C, Lance T. Focal liver lesions: comparison of dual-phase CT and multisequence multiplanar MR imaging including dynamic gadolinium enhancement. J Magn Reson Imaging. 2001;13(3):397-401, PMID: 11241813. *Excluded: Wrong population*

Seo JW, Lim JH, Choi D, Jang HJ, Lee WJ, Lim HK. Indeterminate small, low-attenuating hepatocellular nodules on helical CT in patients with chronic liver disease: 2-Year follow-up. Clin Imaging. 2005;29(4):266-272. *Excluded: Wrong outcome/Did not report diagnostic accuracy measures*

Shah AJ, Parsons B, Pope I, Callaway M, Finch-Jones MD, Thomas MG. The clinical impact of magnetic resonance imaging in diagnosing focal hepatic lesions and suspected cancer. Clin Imaging. 2009;33(3):209-212, PMID: 19411027. *Excluded: Wrong population*

Shah TU, Semelka RC, Pamuklar E, et al. The risk of hepatocellular carcinoma in cirrhotic patients with small liver nodules on MRI. Am J Gastroenterol. 2006;101(3):533-540, PMID: 16542290. *Excluded: Wrong setting*

Sharma P, Saini SD, Kuhn LB, et al. Knowledge of hepatocellular carcinoma screening guidelines and clinical practices among gastroenterologists. Dig Dis Sci. 2011;56(2):569-577, PMID: 20978844. *Excluded: Background*

Sherman M. The radiological diagnosis of hepatocellular carcinoma. Am J Gastroenterol. 2010;105(3):610-612, PMID: 20203642. *Excluded: Background*

Shimizu A, Ito K, Sasaki K, et al. Small hyperintense hepatic lesions on T1-weighted images in patients with cirrhosis: evaluation with serial MRI and imaging features for clinical benignity. Magn Reson Imaging. 2007;25(10):1430-1436, PMID: 17524587. *Excluded: Inadequate reference standard*

Shiraishi J, Sugimoto K, Moriyasu F, Kamiyama N, Doi K. Computer-aided diagnosis for the classification of focal liver lesions by use of contrast-enhanced ultrasonography. Med Phys. 2008;35(5):1734-1746, PMID: 18561648. *Excluded: Wrong outcome/Did not report diagnostic accuracy measures*

Shokry A. Value of dynamic multidetector CT in different grades of hepatocellular carcinoma. Egyptian Journal of Radiology and Nuclear Medicine. 2012;43(3):361-368. *Excluded: Wrong outcome/Did not report diagnostic accuracy measures*

Smith JT, Hawkins RM, Guthrie JA, et al. Effect of slice thickness on liver lesion detection and characterisation by multidetector CT. J Med Imaging Radiat Oncol. 2010;54(3):188-193, PMID: 20598005. *Excluded: Wrong outcome/Did not report diagnostic accuracy measures*

Snowberger N, Chinnakotla S, Lepe RM, et al. Alpha fetoprotein, ultrasound, computerized tomography and magnetic resonance imaging for detection of hepatocellular carcinoma in patients with advanced cirrhosis. Aliment Pharmacol Ther. 2007;26(9):1187-1194, PMID: 17944733. *Excluded: Imaging before 1995*

Song Z-Z. Diagnosis of hepatic nodules 20 mm or smaller in cirrhosis: prospective validation of the noninvasive diagnostic criteria for hepatocellular carcinoma. Hepatology. 2008;47(6):2145-2146; author reply 2146-2147, PMID: 18508292. *Excluded: Wrong outcome/Did not report diagnostic accuracy measures*

Soresi M, Magliarisi C, Campagna P, et al. Usefulness of alpha-fetoprotein in the diagnosis of hepatocellular carcinoma. Anticancer Res. 2003;23(2C):1747-1753, PMID: 12820452. *Excluded: Background*

Soussan M, Aube C, Bahrami S, Boursier J, Valla DC, Vilgrain V. Incidental focal solid liver lesions: diagnostic performance of contrast-enhanced ultrasound and MR imaging. Eur Radiol. 2010;20(7):1715-1725, PMID: 20069427. *Excluded: Wrong population*

Soye JA, Mullan CP, Porter S, Beattie H, Barltrop AH, Nelson WM. The use of contrast-enhanced ultrasound in the characterisation of focal liver lesions. Ulster Med J. 2007;76(1):22-25, PMID: 17288301. *Excluded: Wrong outcome/Did not report diagnostic accuracy measures*

Soyer P, Corno L, Boudiaf M, et al. Differentiation between cavernous hemangiomas and untreated malignant neoplasms of the liver with free-breathing diffusion-weighted MR imaging: comparison with T2-weighted fast spin-echo MR imaging. Eur J Radiol. 2011;80(2):316-324, PMID: 20800983. *Excluded: Wrong population*

Soyer P, Dufresne AC, Somveille E, Lenormand S, Scherrer A, Rymer R. Differentiation between hepatic cavernous hemangioma and malignant tumor with T2-weighted MRI: comparison of fast spin-echo and breathhold fast spin-echo pulse sequences. Clin Imaging. 1998;22(3):200-210, PMID: 9559233. *Excluded: Wrong population*

Sporea I, Badea R, Martie A, et al. Contrast Enhanced Ultrasound for the evaluation of focal liver lesions in daily practice. A multicentre study. Med. 2012;14(2):95-100, PMID: 22675708. *Excluded: Wrong population*

Sporea I, Sirli R, Martie A, Popescu A, Danila M. How useful is contrast enhanced ultrasonography for the characterization of focal liver lesions? J Gastrontest Liver Dis. 2010;19(4):393-398, PMID: 21188330. *Excluded: Wrong population*

Steingruber IE, Mallouhi A, Czermak BV, et al. Pretransplantation evaluation of the cirrhotic liver with explantation correlation: accuracy of CT arterioportography and digital subtraction hepatic angiography in revealing hepatocellular carcinoma. AJR Am J Roentgenol. 2003;181(1):99-108, PMID: 12818838. *Excluded: Background*

Stoker J, Romijn MG, de Man RA, et al. Prospective comparative study of spiral computer tomography and magnetic resonance imaging for detection of hepatocellular carcinoma. Gut. 2002;51(1):105-107, PMID: 12077101. *Excluded: Inadequate reference standard*

Strobel D, Bernatik T, Blank W, et al. Diagnostic accuracy of CEUS in the differential diagnosis of small (<=20 mm) and subcentimetric (<=10 mm) focal liver lesions in comparison with histology. Results of the DEGUM multicenter trial. Ultraschall Med. 2011;32(6):593-597, PMID: 22161556. *Excluded: Wrong population*

Strobel D, Seitz K, Blank W, et al. Contrast-enhanced ultrasound for the characterization of focal liver lesions--diagnostic accuracy in clinical practice (DEGUM multicenter trial). Ultraschall Med. 2008;29(5):499-505, PMID: 19241506. *Excluded: Wrong population*

Sugihara S, Suto Y, Kamba M, Ogawa T. Comparison of various techniques of iron oxide-enhanced breath-hold MR imaging of hepatocellular carcinoma. Clin Imaging. 2001;25(2):104-109, PMID: 11483419. *Excluded: Wrong outcome/Did not report diagnostic accuracy measures*

Suzuki K, Yamamoto M, Shirahata N, et al. Evaluation of contrast-enhanced ultrasonography in the diagnosis of hepatocellular carcinoma. Act Hepato. 2001;42(10):528-535. *Excluded: Not English language*

Szklaruk J, Silverman PM, Charnsangavej C. Imaging in the diagnosis, staging, treatment, and surveillance of hepatocellular carcinoma. AJR Am J Roentgenol. 2003;180(2):441-454, PMID: 12540450. *Excluded: Background*

Tada T, Kumada T, Toyoda H, et al. Diagnosis of hepatocellular carcinoma by contrast-enhanced ultrasound with perflurobutane and enhanced magnetic resonance imaging with Gd-EOB-DTPA. Act Hepato. 2010;51(3):99-106. *Excluded: Not English language*

Tahir B, Sandrasegaran K, Ramaswamy R, et al. Does the hepatocellular phase of gadobenate dimeglumine help to differentiate hepatocellular carcinoma in cirrhotic patients according to histological grade? Clin Radiol. 2011;66(9):845-852, PMID: 21771548. *Excluded: Wrong outcome/Did not report diagnostic accuracy measures*

Tajima T, Zhang X, Kitagawa T, et al. Computer-aided detection (CAD) of hepatocellular carcinoma on multiphase CT images. Progress in Biomedical Optics and Imaging - Proceedings of SPIE. 2007;6514. *Excluded: Inadequate reference standard*

Takahashi M, Maruyama H, Ishibashi H, Yoshikawa M, Yokosuka O. Contrast-enhanced ultrasound with perflubutane microbubble agent: evaluation of differentiation of hepatocellular carcinoma. AJR Am J Roentgenol. 2011;196(2):W123-131, PMID: 21257852. *Excluded: Wrong outcome/Did not report diagnostic accuracy measures*

Takayasu K, Arii S, Ikai I, et al. Overall survival

after transarterial lipiodol infusion chemotherapy with or without embolization for unresectable hepatocellular carcinoma: propensity score analysis. AJR Am J Roentgenol. 2010;194(3):830-837, PMID: 20173167. *Excluded: Background*

Takayasu K, Maeda T, Iwata R. Sensitivity of superselective arteriography for small hepatocellular carcinoma compared with proximal arteriography and computed tomography during superselective arteriography. Jpn J Clin Oncol. 2002;32(6):191-195, PMID: 12110634. *Excluded: Wrong population*

Takayasu K, Muramatsu Y, Mizuguchi Y, Ojima H. CT Imaging of early hepatocellular carcinoma and the natural outcome of hypoattenuating nodular lesions in chronic liver disease. Oncology. 2007;72 Suppl 1:83-91, PMID: 18087187. *Excluded: Wrong publication type*

Takayasu K, Yoshie K, Muramatsu Y, et al. Haemodynamic changes in non-alcoholic (viral) liver cirrhosis studied by computed tomography (CT) arterial portography and CT arteriography. J Gastroenterol Hepatol. 1999;14(9):908-914, PMID: 10535474. *Excluded: Wrong intervention*

Takeshita K, Nagashima I, Frui S, et al. Effect of superparamagnetic iron oxide-enhanced MRI of the liver with hepatocellular carcinoma and hyperplastic nodule. J Comput Assist Tomogr. 2002;26(3):451-455. *Excluded: Wrong population*

Takumi K, Fukukura Y, Shindo T, et al. Feasibility of a fixed scan delay technique using a previous bolus tracking technique data for dynamic hepatic CT. Eur J Radiol. 2012;81(11):2996-3001, PMID: 22749800. *Excluded: Wrong outcome/Did not report diagnostic accuracy measures*

Tamada T, Ito K, Ueki A, et al. Peripheral low intensity sign in hepatic hemangioma: diagnostic pitfall in hepatobiliary phase of Gd-EOB-DTPA-enhanced MRI of the liver. J Magn Reson Imaging. 2012;35(4):852-858, PMID: 22127980. *Excluded: Wrong population*

Tan C, Thng C, Low A, et al. Wash-out of hepatocellular carcinoma: quantitative region of interest analysis on CT. Ann Acad Med Singapore. 2011;40(6):269-275, PMID: 21779615. *Excluded: Wrong comparator/Wrong reference standard*

Tanabe N, Ito K, Shimizu A, et al. Hepatocellular lesions with increased iron uptake on superparamagnetic iron oxide-enhanced magnetic resonance imaging in cirrhosis or chronic hepatitis: comparison of four magnetic resonance sequences for lesion conspicuity. Magn Reson Imaging. 2009;27(6):801-806, PMID: 19144487. *Excluded: Wrong outcome/Did not report diagnostic accuracy measures*

Tanaka H, Iijima H, Higashiura A, et al. New malignant grading system for hepatocellular carcinoma using the Sonazoid contrast agent for ultrasonography. J Gastroenterol. 2013:1-9. *Excluded: Wrong outcome/Did not report diagnostic accuracy measures*

Tanaka H, Iijima H, Nouso K, et al. Cost-effectiveness analysis on the surveillance for hepatocellular carcinoma in liver cirrhosis patients using contrast-enhanced ultrasonography. Hepatol Res. 2012;42(4):376-384. *Excluded: Wrong study design for Key Question*

Tanaka S, Oshikawa O, Sasaki T, Ioka T, Tsukuma H. Evaluation of tissue harmonic imaging for the diagnosis of focal liver lesions. Ultrasound Med Biol. 2000;26(2):183-187, PMID: 10722906. *Excluded: Wrong population*

Tanaka Y, Sasaki Y, Katayama K, et al. Probability of hepatocellular carcinoma of small hepatocellular nodules undetectable by computed tomography during arterial portography. Hepatology. 2000;31(4):890-898, PMID: 10733545. *Excluded: Wrong population*

Tang A, Cruite I, Sirlin CB. Toward a standardized system for hepatocellular carcinoma diagnosis using computed tomography and MRI. [Review]. Expert Rev Gastroenterol Hepatol. 2013;7(3):269-279. *Excluded: Wrong outcome/Did not report diagnostic accuracy measures*

Tanimoto A, Wakabayashi G, Shinmoto H, Nakatsuka S, Okuda S, Kuribayashi S. Superparamagnetic iron oxide-enhanced MR imaging for focal hepatic lesions: a comparison with CT during arterioportography plus CT during hepatic arteriography. J Gastroenterol. 2005;40(4):371-380, PMID: 15870974. *Excluded: Wrong intervention*

Tanimoto A, Wakabayashi G, Shinmoto H, Okuda S, Kuribayashi S, Mukai M. The mechanism of ring enhancement in hepatocellular carcinoma on superparamagnetic iron oxide-enhanced T1-weighted images: an investigation into peritumoral Kupffer cells. J Magn Reson Imaging. 2005;21(3):230-236, PMID: 15723373. *Excluded: Wrong outcome/Did not report diagnostic accuracy measures*

Tao R, Zhang J, Dai Y, et al. Characterizing hepatocellular carcinoma using multi-breath-hold two-dimensional susceptibility-weighted imaging: Comparison to conventional liver MRI. Clin Radiol. 2012;67(12):e91-e97. *Excluded: Wrong outcome/Did not report diagnostic accuracy measures*

Taouli B, Goh JSK, Lu Y, et al. Growth rate of hepatocellular carcinoma: Evaluation with serial computed tomography or magnetic resonance imaging. J Comput Assist Tomogr. 2005;29(4):425-429. *Excluded: Wrong outcome/Did not report diagnostic accuracy measures*

Taouli B, Vilgrain V, Dumont E, Daire JL, Fan B, Menu Y. Evaluation of liver diffusion isotropy and characterization of focal hepatic lesions with two single-shot echo-planar MR imaging sequences: prospective study in 66 patients. Radiology. 2003;226(1):71-78, PMID: 12511671. *Excluded: Wrong population*

Tatsumi M, Clark PA, Nakamoto Y, Wahl RL. Impact of body habitus on quantitative and qualitative image quality in whole-body FDG-PET. Eur J Nucl Med Mol Imaging. 2003;30(1):40-45, PMID: 12483408. *Excluded: Wrong outcome/Did not report diagnostic accuracy measures*

Tello R, Fenlon HM, Gagliano T, deCarvalho VL, Yucel EK. Prediction rule for characterization of hepatic lesions revealed on MR imaging: estimation of malignancy. AJR Am J Roentgenol. 2001;176(4):879-884, PMID: 11264070. *Excluded: Wrong population*

Thompson Coon J, Rogers G, Hewson P, et al. Surveillance of cirrhosis for hepatocellular carcinoma: a cost-utility analysis. Br J Cancer. 2008;98(7):1166-1175, PMID: 18382459. *Excluded: Wrong study design for Key Question*

Tonan T, Fujimoto K, Azuma S, et al. Evaluation of small (<or=2 cm) dysplastic nodules and well-differentiated hepatocellular carcinomas with ferucarbotran-enhanced MRI in a 1.0-T MRI unit: utility of T2*-weighted gradient echo sequences with an intermediate-echo time. Eur J Radiol. 2007;64(1):133-139, PMID: 17408900. *Excluded: Wrong intervention*

Toyoda H, Kumada T, Sone Y. Impact of a unified CT angiography system on outcome of patients with hepatocellular carcinoma. AJR Am J Roentgenol. 2009;192(3):766-774, PMID: 19234276. *Excluded: Wrong population*

Toyoda H, Kumada T, Tada T, et al. Non-hypervascular hypointense nodules detected by Gd-EOB-DTPA-enhanced MRI are a risk factor for recurrence of HCC after hepatectomy. J Hepatol. 2013. *Excluded: Wrong outcome/Did not report diagnostic accuracy measures*

Tradati F, Colombo M, Mannucci PM, et al. A prospective multicenter study of hepatocellular carcinoma in italian hemophiliacs with chronic hepatitis C. The Study Group of the Association of Italian Hemophilia Centers. Blood. 1998;91(4):1173-1177, PMID: 9454746. *Excluded: Wrong outcome/Did not report diagnostic accuracy measures*

Treglia G, Giovannini E, Di Franco D, et al. The role of positron emission tomography using carbon-11 and fluorine-18 choline in tumors other than prostate cancer: a systematic review. Ann Nucl Med. 2012;26(6):451-461, PMID: 22566040. *Excluded: Wrong population*

Trevisani F, Cantarini MC, Labate AMM, et al. Surveillance for hepatocellular carcinoma in elderly Italian patients with cirrhosis: effects on cancer staging and patient survival.[Erratum appears in Am J Gastroenterol. 2004 Oct;99(10):2074]. Am J Gastroenterol. 2004;99(8):1470-1476, PMID: 15307862. *Excluded: Wrong study design for Key Question*

Trillaud H, Bruel J-M, Valette P-J, et al. Characterization of focal liver lesions with SonoVue-enhanced sonography: international multicenter-study in comparison to CT and MRI. World J Gastroenterol. 2009;15(30):3748-3756, PMID: 19673015. *Excluded: Wrong population*

Tsai C-C, Yen T-C, Tzen K-Y. The value of Tc-99m red blood cell SPECT in differentiating giant cavernous hemangioma of the liver from other liver solid masses. Clin Nucl Med. 2002;27(8):578-581, PMID: 12170003. *Excluded: Wrong population*

Tsurusaki M, Sugimoto K, Fujii M, Fukuda T, Matsumoto S, Sugimura K. Combination of CT during arterial portography and double-phase CT hepatic arteriography with multi-detector row helical CT for evaluation of hypervascular hepatocellular carcinoma. Clin Radiol. 2007;62(12):1189-1197, PMID: 17981167. *Excluded: Wrong intervention*

Tzen KY, Yen TC, Lin WY, Tsai CC, Lin KJ. Diagnostic value of 99mTc-labeled red blood cell SPET for a solitary solid liver mass in HBV carrier patients with different echogenicities. Hepatogastroenterology. 2000;47(35):1375-1378, PMID: 11100355. *Excluded: Wrong population*

Vajragupta L, Kittisatra K, Sasiwimonphan K. Magnetic resonance imaging findings of hepatocellular carcinoma: Typical and atypical findings. Asian Biomedicine. 2010;4(1):113-124. *Excluded: Wrong outcome/Did not report diagnostic accuracy measures*

Valls C, Lopez E, Guma A, et al. Helical CT versus CT arterial portography in the detection of hepatic metastasis of colorectal carcinoma. AJR Am J Roentgenol. 1998;170(5):1341-1347, PMID: 9574613. *Excluded: Wrong population*

van den Esschert JW, Bieze M, Beuers UH, van Gulik TM, Bennink RJ. Differentiation of hepatocellular adenoma and focal nodular hyperplasia using 18F-fluorocholine PET/CT. Eur J Nucl Med Mol Imaging. 2011;38(3):436-440, PMID: 20717825. *Excluded: Wrong population*

Vilana R, Bianchi L, Varela M, et al. Is microbubble-enhanced ultrasonography sufficient for assessment of response to percutaneous treatment in patients with early hepatocellular carcinoma? Eur Radiol. 2006;16(11):2454-2462, PMID: 16710666. *Excluded: Wrong population*

Vogel WV, van Dalen JA, Wiering B, et al. Evaluation of image registration in PET/CT of the liver and recommendations for optimized imaging. J Nucl Med. 2007;48(6):910-919, PMID: 17504865. *Excluded: Wrong outcome/Did not report diagnostic accuracy measures*

Vogl TJ, Schwarz W, Blume S, et al. Preoperative evaluation of malignant liver tumors: comparison of unenhanced and SPIO (Resovist)-enhanced MR imaging with biphasic CTAP and intraoperative US. Eur Radiol. 2003;13(2):262-272, PMID: 12598989. *Excluded: Wrong intervention*

von Herbay A, Vogt C, Haussinger D. Late-phase pulse-inversion sonography using the contrast agent levovist: differentiation between benign and malignant focal lesions of the liver. AJR Am J Roentgenol. 2002;179(5):1273-1279, PMID: 12388513. *Excluded: Wrong population*

von Herbay A, Vogt C, Haussinger D. Pulse inversion sonography in the early phase of the sonographic contrast agent Levovist: differentiation between benign and malignant focal liver lesions. J Ultrasound Med. 2002;21(11):1191-1200, PMID: 12418760. *Excluded: Wrong outcome/Did not report diagnostic accuracy measures*

von Herbay A, Vogt C, Willers R, Haussinger D. Real-time imaging with the sonographic contrast agent SonoVue: differentiation between benign and malignant hepatic lesions. J Ultrasound Med. 2004;23(12):1557-1568, PMID: 15557299. *Excluded: Wrong outcome/Did not report diagnostic accuracy measures*

von Herbay A, Westendorff J, Gregor M. Contrast-enhanced ultrasound with SonoVue: differentiation between benign and malignant focal liver lesions in 317 patients. J Clin Ultrasound. 2010;38(1):1-9, PMID: 19790253. *Excluded: Wrong population*

Vossen JA, Buijs M, Liapi E, Eng J, Bluemke DA, Kamel IR. Receiver operating characteristic analysis of diffusion-weighted magnetic resonance imaging in differentiating hepatic hemangioma from other hypervascular liver lesions. J Comput Assist Tomogr. 2008;32(5):750-756, PMID: 18830105. *Excluded: Wrong population*

Wang B, Gao ZQ, Yan X. Correlative study of angiogenesis and dynamic contrast-enhanced magnetic resonance imaging features of hepatocellular carcinoma. Acta Radiol. 2005;46(4):353-358. *Excluded: Wrong outcome/Did not report diagnostic accuracy measures*

Wang DB, Zhou KR, Zeng MS, Chen KM, Wang YXJ. Mn-DPDP-enhanced 24-h delayed-scan MRI of hepatocellular carcinoma is correlated with histology [1]. Eur Radiol. 2004;14(4):743-745. *Excluded: Wrong intervention*

Wang H, Mu XT, Zhong X. Comparative study of dynamic MRI and MSCT in hepatocellular carcinoma with cirrhosis. Chinese Journal of Medical Imaging Technology. 2007;23(7):1046-1048. *Excluded: Not English language*

Wang J-H, Lu S-N, Tung H-D, et al. Flash-echo contrast sonography in the evaluation of response of small hepatocellular carcinoma to percutaneous ablation. J Clin Ultrasound. 2006;34(4):161-168, PMID: 16615047. *Excluded: Wrong population*

Wang WP, Ding H, Qi Q, Mao F, Xu ZZ, Kudo M.

Characterization of focal hepatic lesions with contrast-enhanced C-cube gray scale ultrasonography. World J Gastroenterol. 2003;9(8):1667-1674, PMID: 12918098. *Excluded: Wrong outcome/Did not report diagnostic accuracy measures*

Wang W-P, Wu Y, Luo Y, et al. Clinical value of contrast-enhanced ultrasonography in the characterization of focal liver lesions: a prospective multicenter trial. Hepatobiliary Pancreat Dis Int. 2009;8(4):370-376, PMID: 19666405. *Excluded: Wrong population*

Wang XY, Chen D, Zhang XS, Chen ZF, Hu AB. Value of 18F-FDG-PET/CT in the detection of recurrent hepatocellular carcinoma after hepatectomy or radiofrequency ablation: A comparative study with contrast-enhanced ultrasound. Journal of Digestive Diseases. 2013;14(8):433-438. *Excluded: Inadequate reference standard*

Wang Z, Tang J, An L, et al. Contrast-enhanced ultrasonography for assessment of tumor vascularity in hepatocellular carcinoma. J Ultrasound Med. 2007;26(6):757-762. *Excluded: Wrong outcome/Did not report diagnostic accuracy measures*

Ward J, Chen F, Guthrie JA, et al. Hepatic lesion detection after superparamagnetic iron oxide enhancement: comparison of five T2-weighted sequences at 1.0 T by using alternative-free response receiver operating characteristic analysis. Radiology. 2000;214(1):159-166, PMID: 10644117. *Excluded: Wrong population*

Ward J, Guthrie JA, Scott DJ, et al. Hepatocellular carcinoma in the cirrhotic liver: double-contrast MR imaging for diagnosis. Radiology. 2000;216(1):154-162, PMID: 10887242. *Excluded: Wrong population*

Watanabe H, Kanematsu M, Goshima S, et al. Detection of focal hepatic lesions with 3-T MRI: comparison of two-dimensional and three-dimensional T2-weighted sequences. Jpn J Radiol. 2012;30(9):721-728. *Excluded: Wrong outcome/Did not report diagnostic accuracy measures*

Watanabe S, Katada Y, Gohkyu M, Nakajima M, Kawabata H, Nozaki M. Liver perfusion CT during hepatic arteriography for the hepatocellular carcinoma: Dose reduction and quantitative evaluation for normal- and ultralow-dose protocol. Eur J Radiol. 2012;81(12):3993-3997. *Excluded: Wrong intervention*

Willkomm P, Bender H, Bangard M, Decker P, Grunwald F, Biersack HJ. FDG PET and immunoscintigraphy with 99mTc-labeled antibody fragments for detection of the recurrence of colorectal carcinoma. J Nucl Med. 2000;41(10):1657-1663, PMID: 11037995. *Excluded: Wrong population*

Wilson SR, Burns PN, Muradali D, Wilson JA, Lai X. Harmonic hepatic US with microbubble contrast agent: initial experience showing improved characterization of hemangioma, hepatocellular carcinoma, and metastasis. Radiology. 2000;215(1):153-161, PMID: 10751481. *Excluded: Wrong outcome/Did not report diagnostic accuracy measures*

Wilson SR, Kim TK, Jang H-J, Burns PN. Enhancement patterns of focal liver masses: discordance between contrast-enhanced sonography and contrast-enhanced CT and MRI. AJR Am J Roentgenol. 2007;189(1):W7-W12, PMID: 17579140. *Excluded: Wrong outcome/Did not report diagnostic accuracy measures*

Winters SD, Jackson S, Armstrong GA, Birchall IW, Lee KHY, Low G. Value of subtraction MRI in assessing treatment response following image-guided loco-regional therapies for hepatocellular carcinoma. Clin Radiol. 2012;67(7):649-655. *Excluded: Wrong population*

Witjes CDM, Willemssen FEJA, Verheij J, et al. Histological differentiation grade and microvascular invasion of hepatocellular carcinoma predicted by dynamic contrast-enhanced MRI. J Magn Reson Imaging. 2012;36(3):641-647, PMID: 22532493. *Excluded: Wrong outcome/Did not report diagnostic accuracy measures*

Wolf GK, Lang H, Prokop M, Schreiber M, Zoller W. Volume measurements of localized hepatic lesions using three-dimensional sonography in comparison with three-dimensional computed tomography. Eur J Med Res. 1998;3(3):157-164, PMID: 9502756. *Excluded: Wrong outcome/Did not report diagnostic accuracy measures*

Wong K, Paulson EK, Nelson RC. Breath-hold three-dimensional CT of the liver with multi-detector row helical CT. Radiology. 2001;219(1):75-79, PMID: 11274537. *Excluded: Wrong population*

Woodall CE, Scoggins CR, Loehle J, Ravindra KV, McMasters KM, Martin RCG. Hepatic imaging characteristics predict overall survival in hepatocellular carcinoma. Ann Surg Oncol.

2007;14(10):2824-2830, PMID: 17690939. *Excluded: Wrong outcome/Did not report diagnostic accuracy measures*

Wu LM, Xu JR, Gu HY, et al. Is Liver-Specific Gadoxetic Acid-Enhanced Magnetic Resonance Imaging a Reliable Tool for Detection of Hepatocellular Carcinoma in Patients with Chronic Liver Disease? Dig Dis Sci. 2013:1-13. *Excluded: Systematic review; studies checked for inclusion*

Wu LM, Xu JR, Lu Q, Hua J, Chen J, Hu J. A pooled analysis of diffusion-weighted imaging in the diagnosis of hepatocellular carcinoma in chronic liver diseases. [Review]. J Gastroenterol Hepatol. 2013;28(2):227-234. *Excluded: Systematic review; studies checked for inclusion*

Wu W, Chen M-H, Yin S-S, et al. The role of contrast-enhanced sonography of focal liver lesions before percutaneous biopsy. AJR Am J Roentgenol. 2006;187(3):752-761, PMID: 16928941. *Excluded: Wrong population*

Xia D, Jing J, Shen H, Wu J. Value of diffusion-weighted magnetic resonance images for discrimination of focal benign and malignant hepatic lesions: a meta-analysis. J Magn Reson Imaging. 2010;32(1):130-137, PMID: 20578019. *Excluded: Wrong study design for Key Question*

Xie L, Guang Y, Ding H, Cai A, Huang Y. Diagnostic value of contrast-enhanced ultrasound, computed tomography and magnetic resonance imaging for focal liver lesions: a meta-analysis. Ultrasound Med Biol. 2011;37(6):854-861, PMID: 21531500. *Excluded: Systematic review; studies checked for inclusion*

Xing GS, Wang S, Ouyang H, Ma XH, Zhou CW. Comparison of CT and dynamic-enhancement MRI for the diagnosis of hepatocellular carcinoma. Chinese Journal of Medical Imaging Technology. 2010;26(1):1-4. *Excluded: Not English language*

Xu HX, Liu GJ, Lu MD, et al. Characterization of focal liver lesions using contrast-enhanced sonography with a low mechanical index mode and a sulfur hexafluoride-filled microbubble contrast agent. J Clin Ultrasound. 2006;34(6):261-272, PMID: 16788957. *Excluded: Inadequate reference standard*

Xu HX, Liu GJ, Lu MD, et al. Characterization of small focal liver lesions using real-time contrast-enhanced sonography: diagnostic performance analysis in 200 patients. J Ultrasound Med. 2006;25(3):349-361, PMID: 16495496. *Excluded: Inadequate reference standard*

Xu H-X, Lu M-D, Xie X-H, et al. Three-dimensional contrast-enhanced ultrasound of the liver: experience of 92 cases. Ultrasonics. 2009;49(3):377-385, PMID: 19041996. *Excluded: Wrong outcome/Did not report diagnostic accuracy measures*

Xu J, Wu Y, Dong F. Clinical value of contrast-enhanced ultrasound in differentiating benign and malignant focal liver lesions. J Huazhong Univ Sci Technolog Med Sci. 2007;27(6):703-705, PMID: 18231748. *Excluded: Wrong outcome/Did not report diagnostic accuracy measures*

Yan FH, Zeng MS, Zhou KR. Role and pitfalls of hepatic helical multi-phase CT scanning in differential diagnosis of small hemangioma and small hepatocellular carcinoma. World Journal of Gastroenterology. Vol 41998:343-347. *Excluded: Wrong outcome/Did not report diagnostic accuracy measures*

Yanaga Y, Awai K, Nakaura T, et al. Hepatocellular carcinoma in patients weighing 70 kg or less: Initial trial of compact-bolus dynamic CT with low-dose contrast material at 80 kVp. AJR Am J Roentgenol. 2011;196(6):1324-1331. *Excluded: Wrong outcome/Did not report diagnostic accuracy measures*

Yang DM, Jahng GH, Kim HC, et al. The detection and discrimination of malignant and benign focal hepatic lesions: T2 weighted vs diffusion-weighted MRI. Br J Radiol. 2011;84(1000):319-326, PMID: 20959371. *Excluded: Wrong population*

Yao QJ, Hu HT, Li HL, Guo CY, Meng YL, Li YN. Xper CT in diagnosis and treatment of micro hepatocellular carcinoma. Chinese Journal of Medical Imaging Technology. 2012;28(7):1363-1366. *Excluded: Wrong population*

Yaqoob J, Bari V, Usman MU, Munir K, Mosharaf F, Akhtar W. The Evaluation of Hepatocellular Carcinoma with Biphasic Contrast enhanced Helical CT Scan. Journal of the Pakistan Medical Association. 2004;54(3):123-127. *Excluded: Wrong outcome/Did not report diagnostic accuracy measures*

Yen Y-H, Wang J-H, Lu S-N, et al. Contrast-enhanced ultrasonographic spoke-wheel sign in hepatic focal nodular hyperplasia. Eur J Radiol. 2006;60(3):439-444, PMID: 16916591. *Excluded: Wrong population*

Yi J, Gwak GY, Sinn DH, et al. Screening for extrahepatic metastases by additional staging modalities is required for hepatocellular carcinoma patients beyond modified UICC stage T1. Hepato Gastroenterology. 2013;60(122):328-332. *Excluded: Wrong outcome/Did not report diagnostic accuracy measures*

Yoo HJ, Lee JM, Lee MW, et al. Hepatocellular carcinoma in cirrhotic liver: double-contrast-enhanced, high-resolution 3.0T-MR imaging with pathologic correlation. Invest Radiol. 2008;43(7):538-546, PMID: 18580337. *Excluded: Wrong intervention*

Yoon J-H, Lee E-J, Cha S-S, et al. Comparison of gadoxetic acid-enhanced MR imaging versus four-phase multi-detector row computed tomography in assessing tumor regression after radiofrequency ablation in subjects with hepatocellular carcinomas. J Vasc Interv Radiol. 2010;21(3):348-356, PMID: 20116285. *Excluded: Wrong population*

Yoon MA, Kim SH, Park HS, et al. Value of dual contrast liver MRI at 3.0 T in differentiating well-differentiated hepatocellular carcinomas from dysplastic nodules: preliminary results of multivariate analysis. Invest Radiol. 2009;44(10):641-649, PMID: 19724237. *Excluded: Wrong outcome/Did not report diagnostic accuracy measures*

Yoon SH, Lee JM, So YH, et al. Multiphasic MDCT enhancement pattern of hepatocellular carcinoma smaller than 3 cm in diameter: Tumor size and cellular differentiation. AJR Am J Roentgenol. 2009;193(6):W482-W489. *Excluded: Wrong outcome/Did not report diagnostic accuracy measures*

Yoshioka H, Sato J, Takahashi N, et al. Dual double arterial phase dynamic MR imaging with sensitivity encoding (SENSE): which is better for diagnosing hypervascular hepatocellular carcinomas, in-phase or opposed-phase imaging? Magn Reson Imaging. 2004;22(3):361-367, PMID: 15062931. *Excluded: Wrong outcome/Did not report diagnostic accuracy measures*

Yu DX, Ma XX, Wei HG, Zhang XM, Wang Q, Li CF. Angiogenesis and its maturation of hepatocellular carcinoma and its correlation with the deoxyhemoglobin parameters R2 * and T2 * values by using noninvasive magnetic resonance imaging. Acta Academiae Medicinae Sinicae. 2009;31(5):589-593. *Excluded: Wrong outcome/Did not report diagnostic accuracy measures*

Yu EWR, Chie WC, Chen THH. Does screening or surveillance for primary hepatocellular carcinoma with ultrasonography improve the prognosis of patients? Cancer J. 2004;10(5):317-325. *Excluded: Wrong study design for Key Question*

Yu JS, Kim KW, Kim YH, Jeong EK, Chien D. Comparison of multishot turbo spin echo and HASTE sequences for T2-weighted MRI of liver lesions. J Magn Reson Imaging. 1998;8(5):1079-1084, PMID: 9786145. *Excluded: Wrong outcome/Did not report diagnostic accuracy measures*

Yu JS, Kim KW, Lee JT, Yoo HS. MR imaging during arterial portography for assessment of hepatocellular carcinoma: comparison with CT during arterial portography. AJR Am J Roentgenol. 1998;170(6):1501-1506, PMID: 9609162. *Excluded: Wrong intervention*

Yu JS, Kim KW, Lee JT, Yoo HS. Focal lesions in cirrhotic liver: comparing MR imaging during arterial portography with Gd-enhanced dynamic MR imaging. Yonsei Med J. 2000;41(5):546-555, PMID: 11079613. *Excluded: Wrong population*

Yu MH, Lee JM, Yoon JH, et al. Low tube voltage intermediate tube current liver MDCT: Sinogram-affirmed iterative reconstruction algorithm for detection of hypervascular hepatocellular carcinoma. AJR Am J Roentgenol. 2013;201(1):23-32. *Excluded: Wrong intervention*

Yucel C, Ozdemir H, Gurel S, Ozer S, Arac M. Detection and differential diagnosis of hepatic masses using pulse inversion harmonic imaging during the liver-specific late phase of contrast enhancement with Levovist. J Clin Ultrasound. 2002;30(4):203-212, PMID: 11981929. *Excluded: Wrong population*

Zacherl J, Scheuba C, Imhof M, et al. Current value of intraoperative sonography during surgery for hepatic neoplasms. World J Surg. 2002;26(5):550-554, PMID: 12098044. *Excluded: Wrong intervention*

Zandrino F, Curone P, Benzi L, Musante F. Value of an early arteriographic acquisition for evaluating the splanchnic vessels as an adjunct to biphasic CT using a multislice scanner. Eur Radiol. 2003;13(5):1072-1079, PMID: 12695830. *Excluded: Wrong intervention*

Zech CJ, Grazioli L, Breuer J, Reiser MF, Schoenberg SO. Diagnostic performance and description of morphological features of focal nodular hyperplasia in Gd-EOB-DTPA-enhanced liver magnetic resonance imaging: results of a multicenter trial. Invest Radiol. 2008;43(7):504-511, PMID: 18580333. *Excluded: Wrong population*

Zhang B, Yang B. Combined alpha fetoprotein testing and ultrasonography as a screening test for primary liver cancer. J Med Screen. 1999;6(2):108-110, PMID: 10444731. *Excluded: Wrong population*

Zhang HP, Du LF, Li F, He YQ. Differential diagnosis of isolated hepatocellular carcinoma and metastatic hepatic carcinoma with contrast-enhanced ultrasonography. Chinese Journal of Medical Imaging Technology. 2009;25(11):2053-2056. *Excluded: Wrong outcome/Did not report diagnostic accuracy measures*

Zhang J-W, Feng X-Y, Liu H-Q, et al. CT volume measurement for prognostic evaluation of unresectable hepatocellular carcinoma after TACE. World J Gastroenterol. 2010;16(16):2038-2045, PMID: 20419843. *Excluded: Wrong population*

Zhang K, Kokudo N, Hasegawa K, et al. Detection of new tumors by intraoperative ultrasonography during repeated hepatic resections for hepatocellular carcinoma. Arch Surg. 2007;142(12):1170-1175. *Excluded: Wrong intervention*

Zhang L-J, Peng J, Wu S-Y, et al. Liver virtual non-enhanced CT with dual-source, dual-energy CT: a preliminary study. Eur Radiol. 2010;20(9):2257-2264, PMID: 20393717. *Excluded: Wrong outcome/Did not report diagnostic accuracy measures*

Zhang M-G, Huang X-J, Zhu Q, Geng J, Zhang A-J. Relationship between CT grouping and complications of liver cirrhosis. Hepatobiliary Pancreat Dis Int. 2006;5(2):219-223, PMID: 16698579. *Excluded: Wrong outcome/Did not report diagnostic accuracy measures*

Zhang P, Zhou P, Tian SM, Qian Y, Deng J, Zhang L. Application of acoustic radiation force impulse imaging for the evaluation of focal liver lesion elasticity. Hepatobiliary Pancreat Dis Int. 2013;12(2):165-170. *Excluded: Inadequate reference standard*

Zhang R, Qin S, Zhou Y, Song Y, Sun L. Comparison of imaging characteristics between hepatic benign regenerative nodules and hepatocellular carcinomas associated with Budd-Chiari syndrome by contrast enhanced ultrasound. Eur J Radiol. 2012;81(11):2984-2989, PMID: 22341409. *Excluded: Wrong population*

Zhang X, Kanematsu M, Fujita H, et al. Application of an artificial neural network to the computer-aided differentiation of focal liver disease in MR imaging. Radiol Phys Technol. 2009;2(2):175-182, PMID: 20821117. *Excluded: Wrong outcome/Did not report diagnostic accuracy measures*

Zheng J, Li J, Cui X, Ye H, Ye L. Comparison of diagnostic sensitivity of C-arm CT, DSA and CT in detecting small HCC. Hepatogastroenterology. 2013;60(126):1509-1512. *Excluded: Inadequate reference standard*

Zhong-Zhen S, Kai L, Rong-Qin Z, et al. A feasibility study for determining ablative margin with 3D-CEUS-CT/MR image fusion after radiofrequency ablation of hepatocellular carcinoma. Ultraschall Med. 2012;33(7):E250-E255. *Excluded: Wrong population*

Zhou JS, Huan Y, Wei MG. Quantitative analysis of hepatocellular adenomas with triphasic contrast enhanced multislice spiral computed tomography (MSCT). Afr J Biotechnol. 2010;9(23):3448-3457. *Excluded: Wrong setting*

Zhou JS, Huan Y, Wei MQ, Jiang XQ. Detection of hepatocellular carcinoma with multi-slice spiral CT by using double-arterial phase and portal venous phase enhanced scanning: Effect of iodine concentration of contrast material. Afr J Biotechnol. 2010;9(23):3443-3447. *Excluded: Wrong population*

Zhou J-Y, Wong DWK, Ding F, et al. Liver tumour segmentation using contrast-enhanced multi-detector CT data: performance benchmarking of three semiautomated methods. Eur Radiol. 2010;20(7):1738-1748, PMID: 20157817. *Excluded: Wrong outcome/Did not report diagnostic accuracy measures*

Zhu GY, Teng GJ, Guo JH, et al. Application of PET-CT in monitoring residual and extrahepatic metastatic lesions for hepatocellular carcinoma with positive alpha fetoproteins after interventional therapy. Chinese Journal of Radiology. 2010;44(7):726-730. *Excluded: Not English language*

Zhuang H, Sinha P, Pourdehnad M, Duarte PS,

Yamamoto AJ, Alavi A. The role of positron emission tomography with fluorine-18-deoxyglucose in identifying colorectal cancer metastases to liver. Nuclear Medicine Communications. 2000;21(9):793-798, PMID: 11065150. *Excluded: Wrong population*

Zimmerman P, Lu DS, Yang LY, Chen S, Sayre J, Kadell B. Hepatic metastases from breast carcinoma: comparison of noncontrast, arterial-dominant, and portal-dominant phase spiral CT. J Comput Assist Tomogr. 2000;24(2):197-203, PMID: 10752878. *Excluded: Wrong population*

Zorger N, Jung E-M, Schreyer AG, et al. Ultrasound-arterioportography (US-AP): A new technical approach to perform detection of liver lesions. Clin Hemorheol Microcirc. 2010;46(2-3):117-126, PMID: 21135487. *Excluded: Wrong intervention*

Zuber-Jerger I, Schacherer D, Woenckhaus M, Jung EM, Scholmerich J, Klebl F. Contrast-enhanced ultrasound in diagnosing liver malignancy. Clin Hemorheol Microcirc. 2009;43(1-2):109-118, PMID: 19713605. *Excluded: Wrong population*

Appendix C. Risk of Bias

Table C1. Risk of bias: Diagnostic studies

Author, Year	Random or Consecutive Sample	Avoidance of Case-control Design	Avoidance of Inappropriate Exclusions	Index Test Results Interpreted Without Knowledge of Reference Standard	Use of Pre-specified Threshold or Definition for a Positive Test	Credible Reference Standard	Reference Standard Interpreted Independently From the Test Under Evaluation	Appropriate Interval Between Index Test and Reference Standard	Same Reference Standard Applied to All Patients	Were All Patients Included in the Analysis?	Overall Risk of Bias (Low, Moderate, High)
Addley, 2011[1]	Yes	Yes	Yes	Yes	Yes	Yes (explant)	Yes	Unclear (up to 5 months but the study did not report a mean length of time)	Yes	Yes	Moderate
Ahn, 2010[2]	Yes	Yes	Yes	Yes	Yes	Yes (varied)	Unclear	Unclear	No	Yes	High
Akai, 2011[3]	Yes	Yes	Yes	Yes	Yes	Yes (explant)	Unclear	Unclear	Yes	Yes	Moderate
Alaboudy, 2011[4]	Unclear	No (all cases)	Yes	Yes	Yes	Yes	Unclear	Unclear	Yes	Yes	Moderate
An, 2013[5]	Yes	No (all cases)	Yes	Yes	No	Yes	Unclear	Yes	Yes	No	Moderate
An, 2012[6]	Unclear	No (all cases)	No	Unclear	Yes	Yes	Unclear	Unclear	Yes	No	High
Baccarani U, 2006[7]	Unclear	Yes	Yes	Yes; imaging done prior to transplant; its interpretation is part of qualifier for transplant	Yes	Yes	Unclear	Unclear	Yes	Yes	Moderate
Baek, 2012[8]	Yes	No (all cases)	Unclear	Yes	Yes	Yes	Unclear	Unclear	No	No	High
Baird, 2013[9]	Unclear	Yes	Yes	Yes	Unclear	Yes	Unclear	Unclear	Yes	Yes	Moderate
Bartolozzi, 2000[10]	Unclear	No (all cases)	Yes	Yes	Unclear	Yes	Unclear	Unclear	No	Unclear	High
Bennett, 2002[11]	Unclear	Yes	Yes	Unclear	Yes	Yes (explant)	Unclear	Yes	Yes	Yes	Moderate
Bhattacharjya, 2004[12]	Unclear	No (all cases)	Yes	Unclear	Unclear	Yes (explant)	Unclear	Yes	Yes	Yes	High

Author, Year	Random or Consecutive Sample	Avoidance of Case-control Design	Avoidance of Inappropriate Exclusions	Index Test Results Interpreted Without Knowledge of Reference Standard	Use of Pre-specified Threshold or Definition for a Positive Test	Credible Reference Standard	Reference Standard Interpreted Independently From the Test Under Evaluation	Appropriate Interval Between Index Test and Reference Standard	Same Reference Standard Applied to All Patients	Were All Patients Included in the Analysis?	Overall Risk of Bias (Low, Moderate, High)
Burrel, 2003[13]	Unclear	No (all cases)	Yes	Yes	Yes	Yes (explant)	Yes	Yes (mean 46 or 53 days)	Yes	No (3/29 excluded for CT)	High
Catala, 2007[14]	Unclear	Yes	Yes	Yes	Unclear	Yes	Unclear	Unclear	No	Yes	High
Cereser, 2010[15]	Yes	No (all cases)	Yes	Yes	Yes	Yes	Unclear	Unclear	No	Yes	Moderate
Chalasani, 1999[16]	Yes	Yes	Yes	Unclear	Yes	Yes	Unclear	Unclear	No	Yes	Moderate
Chen, 2005[17]	Unclear	No (25/26 cases)	Yes	Unclear	Yes	Yes (biopsy or clinical f/u)	Unclear	Unclear	No	Yes	High
Cheung, 2013[18]	Unclear	No (all cases)	Yes	Unclear	Yes	Yes	Unclear	Yes	No	Yes	High
Cheung, 2011[19]	Unclear	No (all cases)	Yes	Unclear	Yes	Unclear	Unclear	Unclear	Unclear	Yes	High
Choi, 2008[20]	Yes	Yes	Yes	Yes	Yesd	Yes	Unclear	Yes	Yes	Yes	Moderate
Choi, 2001[21]	Yes	No (all cases)	Yes	Yes	Yes	Yes	Unclear	Unclear	Yes	Yes	Moderate
Chou, 2011[22]	Unclear	Yes	Yes	Yes	Yes	Yes	Unclear	Yes	Yes	No (excluded nodules without histological diagnosis)	Moderate
Chung, 2011[23]	Unclear	Yes	Yes	Yes	Yes	Yes	Unclear	Unclear	No	Yes	Moderate
Chung, 2010[24]	Yes	Yes	Yes	Unclear	Unclear	Yes	Unclear	Unclear	No	Yes	Moderate
Colagrande, 2000[25]	Unclear	No (22/24 cases)	Yes	Yes	Yes	Unclear	Unclear	Unclear	No	No (patients who did not undergo lipiodol CT excluded)	High
Dai, 2008[26]	Yes	Yes	Yes	Yes	Yes	Yes	Unclear	Unclear	Yes	Yes	High
de Ledinghen, 2002[27]	Unclear	Yes	Yes	Yes	Yes	Yes (explant)	No	Yes (mean 44 days)	Yes	Yes	Moderate
Delbeke, 1998[28]	Yes	Yes	Yes	Yes	Yes	Yes (pathology)	Unclear	Yes (<2 months)	Yes	Yes	Moderate
Denecke, 2009[29]	Yes	No (all cases)	Yes	Unclear	Yes	Yes	Unclear	Yes	Yes	Yes	Moderate

Author, Year	Random or Consecutive Sample	Avoidance of Case-control Design	Avoidance of Inappropriate Exclusions	Index Test Results Interpreted Without Knowledge of Reference Standard	Use of Pre-specified Threshold or Definition for a Positive Test	Credible Reference Standard	Reference Standard Interpreted Independently From the Test Under Evaluation	Appropriate Interval Between Index Test and Reference Standard	Same Reference Standard Applied to All Patients	Were All Patients Included in the Analysis?	Overall Risk of Bias (Low, Moderate, High)
Di Martino, 2013[30]	Yes	Yes	Yes	Yes	Yes	Yes	Unclear	Unclear	No	No (34 excluded due to loss to f/u or insufficient proof of tumor burden; 140 excluded due to >1 month between CT and MRI)	Moderate
Di Martino, 2010[31]	Yes	Yes	Yes	Yes	Yes	Yes	Unclear	Unclear	No	No (37 excluded due to incomplete imaging or follow-up)	Moderate
D'Onofrio, 2005[32]	Yes	Yes	Yes	Yes	Yes	Unclear	Unclear	Unclear	No	Yes	Moderate
Doyle, 2007[33]	Unclear	No (case-control)	Yes	Unclear	Yes	Yes	Unclear	Unclear	No	Yes	High
Eckel, 2009[34]	Unclear	No (cases only)	Yes	Unclear	Yes	Yes	Unclear	Unclear	No	Yes	High
Egger, 2012[35]	Unclear	No (all cases)	Yes	Unclear	Yes	Yes	Unclear	Unclear	Yes	Yes	Moderate
Filippone, 2010[36]	Unclear	No (all cases)	Yes	Yes	Yes	Yes	Unclear	Unclear	No	Yes	Moderate
Forner, 2008[37]	Unclear	Yes	Yes	Unclear	Yes	Yes	Unclear	Unclear	Yes	Yes	Moderate
Fowler, 2013[38]	Yes	No (all cases)	Yes	Unclear	Yes	Yes	Unclear	Unclear	Yes	Yes	Moderate
Fracanzani, 2001[39]	Yes	Yes	Yes	Unclear	Unclear	Yes	Unclear	Unclear	Yes	Yes	Moderate
Freeman, 2006[40]	Yes	Yes	Yes	No	Yes	Yes	Unclear	Unclear	Yes	Yes	Moderate
Freeny, 2003[41]	Yes	Yes	Yes	Yes	Yes	Yes (explant)	Unclear	No (mean 249 or 168 days)	Yes	Yes	High
Furuse, 2000[42]	Yes	No (all cases)	Yes	Unclear	Unclear	Yes	Unclear	Unclear	Yes	Yes	Moderate

Author, Year	Random or Consecutive Sample	Avoidance of Case-control Design	Avoidance of Inappropriate Exclusions	Index Test Results Interpreted Without Knowledge of Reference Standard	Use of Pre-specified Threshold or Definition for a Positive Test	Credible Reference Standard	Reference Standard Interpreted Independently From the Test Under Evaluation	Appropriate Interval Between Index Test and Reference Standard	Same Reference Standard Applied to All Patients	Were All Patients Included in the Analysis?	Overall Risk of Bias (Low, Moderate, High)
Gaiani, 2004[43]	Yes	No (all cases)	Yes	Unclear	Yes	Unclear (US evaluated and Doppler US used as part of reference standard)	Unclear	Unclear	Yes	Yes	High
Gambarin-Gelwan, 2000[44]	Yes	Yes	Yes	Unclear	Yes	Yes (explant)	Unclear	Unclear (within 6 months)	Yes	Yes	Moderate
Gatto, 2013[45]	Unclear	Yes	Yes	Unclear	Yes	Yes	Unclear	Unclear	Yes	Yes	Moderate
Giorgio, 2007[46]	Yes	Yes	Yes	Yes	Yes	Unclear	Unclear	Unclear	No	Yes	Moderate
Giorgio, 2004[47]	Yes	No (all cases)	Yes	Unclear	Yes	Yes	Unclear	Yes	Yes	Yes	Moderate
Golfieri, 2009[48]	Yes	Yes	Yes	Unclear	Yes	Yes	Unclear	Unclear	No	Yes	Moderate
Goshima, 2004[49]	Yes	No (all cases)	Yes	Unclear	Yes	Unclear	Unclear	Unclear	No	Yes	Moderate
Goto, 2012[50]	Yes	No (all cases)	Yes	Yes	Yes	Unclear (CT only including lesions <2 cm)	Yes	Yes	Yes	Yes	Moderate
Guo, 2012[51]	Unclear	No (all cases)	No (excluded difficult to dx patients)	Yes	Yes	Yes	Unclear	Unclear	No	Yes	Moderate
Haradome, 2011[52]	Yes	Yes	Yes	Unclear	Yes	Yes	Unclear	Unclear	Yes	Yes	Moderate
Hardie, 2011[53]	Yes	Yes	Yes	Yes	Unclear	Yes	Unclear	Yes	Yes	Yes	High
Hardie, 2011 (2)[54]	Unclear	Yes	Yes	Unclear	Unclear	Yes	Unclear	Yes	Yes	Yes	High
Hardie, 2011 (3)[55]	Yes	Yes	Yes	Yes	Unclear	Yes (explant)	Unclear	Yes	Yes	Yes	Moderate
Hatanaka, 2008[56]	Yes	Yes	Yes	Yes	Yes	Yes	Unclear	Unclear	No	Yes	Moderate
Hecht, 2006[57]	Yes	Yes	Yes	Unclear	Yes	Yes (explant)	Yes	Yes	Yes	Yes	Moderate

Author, Year	Random or Consecutive Sample	Avoidance of Case-control Design	Avoidance of Inappropriate Exclusions	Index Test Results Interpreted Without Knowledge of Reference Standard	Use of Pre-specified Threshold or Definition for a Positive Test	Credible Reference Standard	Reference Standard Interpreted Independently From the Test Under Evaluation	Appropriate Interval Between Index Test and Reference Standard	Same Reference Standard Applied to All Patients	Were All Patients Included in the Analysis?	Overall Risk of Bias (Low, Moderate, High)
Hidaka, 2013[58]	Unclear	No (all cases)	Unclear	Yes	Yes	Yes	Unclear	Unclear	Yes	Yes	High
Higashihara, 2012[59]	Unclear	No (all cases)	Yes	Unclear	Yes	Unclear	Unclear	Yes	No	Yes	High
Hirawaka, 2011[60]	Unclear	No	Yes	Unclear	Yes	Yes	Unclear	Yes	Yes	Yes	Moderate
Ho, 2003[61]	Unclear	Yes	Yes	Yes	Yes	Yes	Unclear	Unclear	Yes	No (7/39 patients with HCC excluded)	Moderate
Ho, 2007[62]	Yes	Yes	Yes	Unclear	Yes	Yes (multiple criteria)	Unclear	Unclear	No	Yes	Moderate
Hori, 2002[63]	Unclear	No (90% had HCC)	Yes	Unclear	Yes	Unclear	Unclear	Unclear	No	No (16 patients excluded due to no reference standard)	High
Hori, 1998[64]	Unclear	No (all cases)	Yes	Yes	Unclear	Unclear	Unclear	Yes	No	Yes	High
Hwang, 2012[65]	Yes	No (all cases)	Yes	Unclear	Yes	Yes	Unclear	Unclear	No	Yes	Moderate
Hwang, 2009[66]	Unclear	No (90% had HCC)	Yes	Unclear	Unclear	Unclear	Unclear	Unclear	No	No	High
Iannaccone, 2005[67]	Unclear	Yes	Yes	Yes	Yes	Yes	Unclear	Unclear	Yes	Yes	Moderate
Iavarone, 2010[68]	Yes	No (all cases)	Yes	Yes	Yes	Yes	Unclear	Unclear	Yes	Yes	Moderate
Ichikawa, 2010[69]	Unclear	Yes	Yes	Yes (for blinded readers)	Unclear	Unclear	Unclear	Yes	No	No (denominators varied)	Moderate
Ichikawa, 2002[70]	Unclear	No (all cases)	Yes	Yes	Yes	Yes	Unclear	Unclear	Unclear	Yes	Moderate
Ijichi, 2013[71]	Unclear	No (all cases)	Yes	Unclear	Unclear	Yes	Unclear	Unclear	Yes	Yes	Moderate

Author, Year	Random or Consecutive Sample	Avoidance of Case-control Design	Avoidance of Inappropriate Exclusions	Index Test Results Interpreted Without Knowledge of Reference Standard	Use of Pre-specified Threshold or Definition for a Positive Test	Credible Reference Standard	Reference Standard Interpreted Independently From the Test Under Evaluation	Appropriate Interval Between Index Test and Reference Standard	Same Reference Standard Applied to All Patients	Were All Patients Included in the Analysis?	Overall Risk of Bias (Low, Moderate, High)
Imamura, 1998[72]	Yes	No (all cases)	Yes	Yes	Yes	Yes	Unclear	Unclear	Yes	Yes	Moderate
Inoue, 2012[73]	Unclear	Unclear	Yes	Unclear	Yes	Yes	Unclear	Unclear	Yes	Yes	Moderate
Inoue, 2009[74]	Yes	Yes	Yes	Yes	Yes	Yes	Unclear	Unclear	Yes	Yes	Moderate
Inoue, 2008[75]	Unclear	No (all cases)	Yes	Yes	Unclear	Yes	Unclear	Unclear	No	Yes	High
Ito, 2004[76]	Unclear	No (all cases)	Yes	Unclear	Unclear	Unclear	Unclear	Unclear	No	Yes	Moderate
Iwazawa, 2010[77]	Yes	No (all cases)	Yes	Yes	Yes	Unclear	Unclear	Unclear	No	Yes	Moderate
Jang, 2000[78]	Yes	No (all cases)	Yes	Yes	Yes	Yes	Unclear	Unclear	Yes	No (7/59 excluded due to no pathologic proof and 18 excluded due to follow-up with spiral CT <12 months)	Moderate
Jang, 2013[79]	Unclear	Yes	Yes	Unclear	Yes	Unclear	Unclear	Unclear	No	Yes	Moderate
Jang, 2009[80]	Unclear	Yes	Yes	Unclear	Yes	Yes	Unclear	Unclear	No	Yes	Moderate
Jeong, 2003[81]	Unclear	Yes	Yes	Yes	Yes	Yes	Unclear	Unclear	Yes	Yes	Moderate
Jeong, 2002[82]	Unclear	No (all cases)	Yes	Unclear	Unclear	Unclear	Unclear	Unclear	Yes	Yes	High
Jeong, 2011[83]	Unclear	No (all cases)	Yes	Unclear	Yes	Unclear	Unclear	Unclear	No	No	High
Jeong, 1999[84]	Unclear	No (cases and controls)	Yes	Yes	No (post-hoc)	Yes	Unclear	Unclear	No	Yes	High
Jin, 2013[85]	Yes	Yes	Yes	Unclear	Yes	Unclear	Unclear	Unclear	No	Yes	Moderate
Kakihara, 2013[86]	Yes	No (all cases)	Yes	Yes	Yes	Yes	Unclear	Unclear	Yes	Yes	Moderate
Kamura, 2002[87]	Unclear	No (case-control)	Unclear	Unclear	Yes	Unclear	Unclear	Unclear	No	Yes	High

Author, Year	Random or Consecutive Sample	Avoidance of Case-control Design	Avoidance of Inappropriate Exclusions	Index Test Results Interpreted Without Knowledge of Reference Standard	Use of Pre-specified Threshold or Definition for a Positive Test	Credible Reference Standard	Reference Standard Interpreted Independently From the Test Under Evaluation	Appropriate Interval Between Index Test and Reference Standard	Same Reference Standard Applied to All Patients	Were All Patients Included in the Analysis?	Overall Risk of Bias (Low, Moderate, High)
Kang, 2003[88]	Yes	No (all cases)	Yes	Unclear	Yes	Yes	Unclear	Unclear	Yes	Yes	Moderate
Kawada, 2010[89]	Unclear	No (all cases)	Yes	Unclear	Yes	Yes	Unclear	Unclear	Yes	Yes	High
Kawaoka, 2009[90]	Yes	Yes	Yes	Unclear	No	Unclear	Unclear	Unclear	No	Yes	High
Kawata, 2002[91]	Yes	No (only analyzed cases)	Yes	Yes	Yes	Yes	Unclear	Unclear	No	Yes	Moderate
Khalili, 2011[92]	Yes	Yes	Yes	Yes	Yes	Yes	Unclear	Unclear	No	Yes	Moderate
Khan, 2000[93]	Yes	No (all cases)	Yes	Yes	Yes	Yes (histology or cytology)	Yes	Unclear	No	Yes	High
Kim AY, 2012[94]	Unclear	No (all cases)	Yes	Unclear (for PET)	Yes	Yes	Unclear	Unclear	No	Yes	Moderate
Kim CK, 2001[95]	Yes	Yes	Yes	Yes	Yes	Yes (explant)	Unclear	Yes	Yes	Yes	Moderate
Kim DJ, 2012[96]	Yes	Yes	Yes	Unclear	Yes	Yes	Unclear	Unclear	No	Yes	Moderate
Kim KW, 2009[97]	Yes	No (case-control)	Yes	Yes	Yes	Yes	Unclear	Unclear	No	Yes	Moderate
Kim MJ, 2012[98]	Unclear	No (all cases)	Yes	Yes	Yes	Yes	Unclear	Yes	Yes	Yes	Moderate
Kim PN, 2012[99]	Unclear	No (all cases)	Yes	Yes	Unclear	Yes	Yes	Yes	Yes	Yes	Moderate
Kim SE, 2011[100]	Yes	Yes	Yes	No	Yes	Yes	Unclear	Unclear	Yes	Yes	Moderate
Kim SH, 2009[101]	Yes	No (all cases)	Yes	Yes	Yes	Yes	Unclear	Unclear	Yes	Yes	Moderate
Kim SH, 2005[102]	Yes	No (all cases)	Yes	Yes	Yes	Yes	Unclear	Unclear	Yes	Yes	Moderate
Kim SJ, 2008[103]	Unclear	No (all cases)	Yes	Yes	Yes	Yes	Unclear	Yes	Yes	Yes	High

Author, Year	Random or Consecutive Sample	Avoidance of Case-control Design	Avoidance of Inappropriate Exclusions	Index Test Results Interpreted Without Knowledge of Reference Standard	Use of Pre-specified Threshold or Definition for a Positive Test	Credible Reference Standard	Reference Standard Interpreted Independently From the Test Under Evaluation	Appropriate Interval Between Index Test and Reference Standard	Same Reference Standard Applied to All Patients	Were All Patients Included in the Analysis?	Overall Risk of Bias (Low, Moderate, High)
Kim SK, 2002 (2)[104]	Yes	No (all cases)	Unclear (excluded 25 patients with HCC with unresectable distribution)	Unclear	Yes	Yes	Unclear	Unclear	Yes	Yes	Moderate
Kim T, 2002[105]	Yes	Yes	Yes	Yes	Yes	Yes	Unclear	Unclear	No	Yes	Moderate
Kim TK, 2011[106]	Yes	Yes	Yes	Yes	No	Yes	Unclear	Unclear	No	Yes	Moderate
Kim YK, 2011[107]	Unclear	No (all cases)	Yes	Yes	Yes	Yes	Unclear	Unclear	No	Yes	Moderate
Kim YK, 2011 (2)[108]	Unclear	No (all cases)	Yes	Yes	Yes	Yes	Unclear	Unclear	No	Yes	Moderate
Kim YK, 2010[109]	Unclear	No (all cases)	Yes	Yes	Yes	Unclear	Unclear	Unclear	No	Yes	High
Kim YK, 2010 (2)[110]	Unclear	No (all cases)	Yes	Yes	Yes	Unclear	Unclear	Unclear	No	Yes	High
Kim YK, 2010 (3)[111]	Yes	No (all cases)	Yes	Yes	Yes	Unclear	Unclear	Unclear	Unclear	Yes	High
Kim YK, 2009 (2)[112]	Unclear	No (all cases)	Yes	Yes	Yes	Unclear	Unclear	Unclear	No	Yes	High
Kim YK, 2008[113]	Unclear	No (all cases)	Unclear	Yes	Yes	Yes	Unclear	Unclear	No	Yes	Moderate
Kim YK, 2008 (2)[114]	Unclear	No (all cases)	Yes	Yes	Yes	Yes	Unclear	Unclear	No	Yes	High
Kim YK, 2007[115]	Unclear	No (all cases)	Yes	Yes	Yes	Yes	Unclear	Unclear	No	No (excluded 8 patients without reference exam diagnosis)	Moderate
Kim YK, 2006[116]	Unclear	No (all cases)	Yes	Yes	Yes	Yes	Unclear	Unclear	No	Yes	Moderate

Author, Year	Random or Consecutive Sample	Avoidance of Case-control Design	Avoidance of Inappropriate Exclusions	Index Test Results Interpreted Without Knowledge of Reference Standard	Use of Pre-specified Threshold or Definition for a Positive Test	Credible Reference Standard	Reference Standard Interpreted Independently From the Test Under Evaluation	Appropriate Interval Between Index Test and Reference Standard	Same Reference Standard Applied to All Patients	Were All Patients Included in the Analysis?	Overall Risk of Bias (Low, Moderate, High)
Kim YK, 2006[117]	Unclear	No (all cases)	Yes	Yes	Yes	Unclear (for lesions after the first HCC in each patient)	Unclear	Unclear	No	Yes	High
Kim YK, 2004[118]	Yes	No (all cases)	Yes	Yes	Yes	Unclear	Unclear	Unclear	No	No (excluded 20 patients without reference exam diagnosis)	High
Kim YK, 2004 (2)[119]	Yes	No (all cases)	Yes	Yes	Yes	Yes	Unclear	Unclear	No	Yes	Moderate
Kitamura, 2008[120]	Unclear	No (all cases)	Yes	Yes	Yes	Unclear	Unclear	Unclear	No	Yes	Moderate
Kondo, 2005[121]	Yes	No (all cases)	Yes	Yes	Yes	Yes	Unclear	Unclear	Yes	Yes	Moderate
Korenaga, 2009[122]	Yes	No (all cases)	Yes	Yes	Only AUROC reported	Yes	Unclear	Unclear	Yes	Yes	Moderate
Koushima, 2002[123]	Unclear	No (case-control)	Yes	Unclear	Only AUROC reported	Yes	Unclear	Unclear	Yes	No	High
Krinsky, 2002[124]	Yes	No (all cases)	Yes	Yes	Yes	Yes	Unclear	Yes	Yes	Yes	Moderate
Krinsky, 2001[125]	Unclear	Yes	Yes	Unclear	Yes	Yes (explant)	Unclear	Yes	Yes	Yes	Moderate
Kumano, 2009[126]	Yes	No (all cases)	Yes	Unclear	Yes	Yes	Unclear	Unclear	No	Yes	Moderate
Kunishi, 2012[127]	Unclear	No (all cases)	Yes	Yes	Yes	Yes	Yes	Unclear	No	Yes	Moderate
Kwak, 2005[128]	Yes	No (all cases)	Yes	Unclear	Yes	Unclear	Unclear	Unclear	Yes	Yes	Moderate
Kwak, 2004[129]	Unclear	No (all cases)	Yes	Yes	Yes	Unclear	Unclear	Unclear	Unclear	Yes	Moderate
Laghi, 2003[130]	Yes	Yes	Yes	Yes	Yes	Yes	Unclear	Unclear	Yes	Yes	Moderate

Author, Year	Random or Consecutive Sample	Avoidance of Case-control Design	Avoidance of Inappropriate Exclusions	Index Test Results Interpreted Without Knowledge of Reference Standard	Use of Pre-specified Threshold or Definition for a Positive Test	Credible Reference Standard	Reference Standard Interpreted Independently From the Test Under Evaluation	Appropriate Interval Between Index Test and Reference Standard	Same Reference Standard Applied to All Patients	Were All Patients Included in the Analysis?	Overall Risk of Bias (Low, Moderate, High)
Lauenstein, 2007[131]	Yes	Yes	Yes	Yes	Yes	Yes	Unclear	Yes	Yes	Yes	Moderate
Lee CH, 2012[132]	Yes	No (all cases)	Yes	Yes	Yes	Unclear	Unclear	Unclear	No	Yes	Moderate
Lee DH, 2009[133]	Yes	Yes	Yes	Yes	Yes	Yes	Unclear	Yes	Yes	Yes	Moderate
Lee J, 2008[134]	Yes	No (all cases)	Yes	No	Unclear	Yes	Unclear	Yes	Yes	Yes	Moderate
Lee JE, 2012[135]	Yes	Yes	Yes	Yes	Yes	Yes	Unclear	Unclear	Yes	Yes	Moderate
Lee JM, 2003[136]	Unclear	No (all cases)	Yes	Yes	Yes	Unclear	Unclear	No	Yes	Yes	Moderate
Lee JY, 2010[137]	Yes	No (all cases)	Yes	Yes	Yes	Yes	Unclear	Yes	Yes	Yes	Moderate
Lee MH, 2011[138]	Yes	No (case-control)	Yes	Yes	Yes	Yes	Unclear	Yes	Yes	Yes	Moderate
Lee MW, 2010[139]	Yes	No (all cases)	Yes	Unclear	Yes	Yes	Yes (reference studies performed prior to test)	Unclear	Yes	Yes	Moderate
Li, 2007[140]	Unclear	Yes	Yes	Unclear	Unclear	Yes	Unclear	Unclear	Yes	Yes	Moderate
Li, 2006[141]	Yes	No (all cases)	Yes	No	Yes	Yes	Unclear	Unclear	Yes	Yes	Moderate
Li CS, 2006[142]	Yes	No (all cases)	Yes	Unclear	Yes	Yes	Unclear	Unclear	Yes	Yes	Moderate
Liangpunsakul, 2003[143]	Unclear	Yes	Yes	Unclear	Yes	Unclear	Unclear	Unclear	Unclear	Yes	High
Libbrecht, 2002[144]	Yes	Yes	Yes	Unclear	Yes	Yes (explant)	Yes	Yes	Yes	No	High
Lim JH 2006[145]	Yes	No (all cases)	Yes	Unclear	Yes	Yes	Unclear	Unclear	Yes	Yes	Moderate

Author, Year	Random or Consecutive Sample	Avoidance of Case-control Design	Avoidance of Inappropriate Exclusions	Index Test Results Interpreted Without Knowledge of Reference Standard	Use of Pre-specified Threshold or Definition for a Positive Test	Credible Reference Standard	Reference Standard Interpreted Independently From the Test Under Evaluation	Appropriate Interval Between Index Test and Reference Standard	Same Reference Standard Applied to All Patients	Were All Patients Included in the Analysis?	Overall Risk of Bias (Low, Moderate, High)
Lim JH 2002[146]	Yes	No (all cases)	Unclear (excluded 115 patients with multiple HCC with unresectable distribution or main portal vein obstruction)	Unclear	Yes	Yes	Unclear	Yes	Yes	Yes	Moderate
Lim JH 2000[147]	Yes	Yes	Yes	Yes	Yes	Yes (explant)	Unclear	Yes	Yes	Yes	Moderate
Lin MT, 2011[148]	Unclear	No (all cases)	Unclear	Unclear	Unclear	Yes	Unclear	Unclear	Yes	Yes	High
Lin WY, 2005[149]	Unclear	No (all cases)	Yes	Unclear	Yes	Yes	Unclear	Unclear	No	Yes	High
Liu, 2013[150]	Yes	Yes	Yes	Unclear	No (for quantitative measures)	Yes (explant)	Unclear	Unclear	Yes	Yes	Moderate
Liu, 2012[151]	Yes	Yes	Yes	Unclear	Yes	Yes (explant)	Unclear	Unclear	Yes	Yes	Moderate
Liu, 2003[152]	Yes	No (all cases)	Yes	Unclear	Unclear	Yes (explant)	Unclear	Yes	Yes	Yes	Moderate
Lu CH, 2010[153]	Unclear	No (all cases)	Yes	Unclear	Unclear	Yes (explant)	Unclear	Yes	Yes	Yes	High
Luca, 2010[154]	Yes	Yes	Yes	Unclear	Yes	Yes (explant)	Yes (no radiological assistance)	Yes (mean 2 months)	Yes	Yes	Low
Luo, 2005[155]	Unclear	Yes	Yes	Yes	Unclear	Yes	Unclear	Unclear	Yes	Yes	Moderate
Luo W, 2009[156]	Yes	Yes	Yes	Yes	Yes	Yes	Unclear	Unclear	No	Yes	Moderate
Luo W, 2009 (2)[157]	Yes	Yes	Yes	Yes	Unclear	Yes	Unclear	Unclear	Yes	Yes	Moderate

Author, Year	Random or Consecutive Sample	Avoidance of Case-control Design	Avoidance of Inappropriate Exclusions	Index Test Results Interpreted Without Knowledge of Reference Standard	Use of Pre-specified Threshold or Definition for a Positive Test	Credible Reference Standard	Reference Standard Interpreted Independently From the Test Under Evaluation	Appropriate Interval Between Index Test and Reference Standard	Same Reference Standard Applied to All Patients	Were All Patients Included in the Analysis?	Overall Risk of Bias (Low, Moderate, High)
Luo W, 2009 (3)[158]	Unclear	Yes	Unclear (16 lesions excluded for unclear reasons)	Yes	Yes	Yes	Unclear	Unclear	No	Yes	Moderate
Lv, 2012[159]	Unclear	No (all cases)	Yes	Yes	Unclear	Yes	Unclear	Unclear	No	Yes	High
Lv, 2011[160]	Unclear	No (all cases)	Yes	Yes	Yes	Unclear	Unclear	Unclear	No	Yes	High
Maetani, 2008[161]	Yes	No (all cases)	Yes	Unclear	Yes	Yes (explant)	Unclear	Yes (mean 21 days)	Yes	Yes	High
Marin, 2009[162]	Yes	No (all cases)	Yes	Unclear	Yes	Yes	Unclear	Unclear	No	No (excluded 9 patients with inadequate CT)	Moderate
Marin, 2009 (2)[163]	Yes	No (all cases)	Yes	Yes	Yes	Yes	Unclear	Unclear	No	No	Moderate
Marrero, 2005[164]	Yes	Yes	Yes	Yes	No	Yes	Unclear	Unclear	No	Yes	Moderate
Matsuo, 2001[165]	Yes	Yes	Yes	Yes	Yes	Yes	Unclear	Yes	No	Yes	Moderate
Mita, 2010[166]	Unclear	No (all cases)	Yes	Yes	Yes	Yes	Unclear	Unclear	Yes	Yes	Moderate
Mok, 2004[167]	Unclear	Yes	Yes	Unclear	Unclear	Yes	Unclear	Unclear	Yes	Yes	Moderate
Monzawa, 2007[168]	Unclear	No (case-control)	Yes	Unclear	Yes	Yes	Unclear	Unclear	Yes	Yes	Moderate
Mori, 2005[169]	Yes	No (all cases)	Yes	Yes	Yes	Yes	Unclear	Yes	No	Yes	Moderate
Moriyasu, 2009[170]	Unclear	Yes	Unclear	Yes	Unclear	Unclear	Unclear	Unclear	Yes	Yes	High
Mortele, 2001[171]	Yes	Yes	Yes	Yes	Unclear	Yes (explant)	No (retrospective evaluation of pathology specimens for discordant results)	No (mean 103 days)	Yes	Yes	Moderate

Author, Year	Random or Consecutive Sample	Avoidance of Case-control Design	Avoidance of Inappropriate Exclusions	Index Test Results Interpreted Without Knowledge of Reference Standard	Use of Pre-specified Threshold or Definition for a Positive Test	Credible Reference Standard	Reference Standard Interpreted Independently From the Test Under Evaluation	Appropriate Interval Between Index Test and Reference Standard	Same Reference Standard Applied to All Patients	Were All Patients Included in the Analysis?	Overall Risk of Bias (Low, Moderate, High)
Motosugi, 2010[172]	Unclear	No (case-control)	Yes	Unclear	Yes	Unclear (CT only including lesions <2 cm)	Unclear	Unclear	No	Yes	High
Murakami, 2003[173]	Yes	No (48/49 cases)	Yes	Unclear	Yes	Yes	Unclear	Unclear	No	Yes	Moderate
Murakami, 2001[174]	Yes	Yes	Yes	Yes	Yes	Yes	Unclear	Unclear	No	Yes	Moderate
Nagaoka, 2006[175]	Unclear	Yes	Yes	Yes	Yes	Unclear	Unclear	Unclear	Unclear	Yes	High
Nakamura, 2013[176]	Unclear	No (all cases)	Yes	Unclear	Yes	Yes	Unclear	Unclear	Yes	Yes	High
Nakamura, 2000[177]	Unclear	No (all cases)	Yes	Unclear	Unclear	Unclear	Unclear	Unclear	Yes	No (denominator varied for different imaging tests)	High
Nakayama, 2001[178]	Unclear	No (all cases)	Yes	Unclear	Unclear	Yes	Unclear	Unclear	Yes	Yes	High
Noguchi, 2003[179]	Yes	No (all cases)	Yes	Unclear	Yes	Yes	Unclear	Unclear	No	Yes	Moderate
Noguchi, 2002[180]	Yes	No (all cases)	Yes	Yes	Yes	Yes	Unclear	Unclear	No	Yes	Moderate
Numata, 2014[181]	Yes	No (all cases)	Unclear	Yes	Yes	Yes	Unclear	Unclear	Yes	Yes	Moderate
Onishi, 2012[182]	Yes	No (>90% with HCC)	Yes	Yes	Yes	Unclear	Unclear	Unclear	No	Yes	Moderate
Ooi, 2010[183]	Unclear	Yes	Yes	Unclear	Yes	Yes	Unclear	Unclear	No	Yes	Moderate
Ooka, 2013[184]	Yes	No (all cases)	Yes	Unclear	Yes	Yes	Unclear	Unclear	Yes	Yes	Moderate
Park, 2013[185]	Yes	Yes	Yes	Yes	Yes	Yes	Unclear	Unclear	Yes	Yes	Moderate
Park, 2012[186]	Unclear	Yes	Yes	Unclear	Yes	Yes (explant)	Unclear	Yes	Yes	Unclear	Moderate
Park, 2011[187]	Unclear	Yes	Yes	Yes	Yes	Yes (explant)	Yes	Yes	Yes	Yes	Moderate

Author, Year	Random or Consecutive Sample	Avoidance of Case-control Design	Avoidance of Inappropriate Exclusions	Index Test Results Interpreted Without Knowledge of Reference Standard	Use of Pre-specified Threshold or Definition for a Positive Test	Credible Reference Standard	Reference Standard Interpreted Independently From the Test Under Evaluation	Appropriate Interval Between Index Test and Reference Standard	Same Reference Standard Applied to All Patients	Were All Patients Included in the Analysis?	Overall Risk of Bias (Low, Moderate, High)
Park, 2010[188]	Yes	No (all cases)	Yes	Yes	Yes	Yes	Unclear	Unclear	Yes	Yes	Moderate
Park G, 2010[189]	Yes	No (all cases)	Yes	Unclear	Yes	Unclear	Unclear	Unclear	Yes	Yes	Moderate
Park JW, 2008[190]	Unclear	No (all cases)	Yes	No	Yes	Unclear	Unclear	Yes	Yes	Yes	Moderate
Paul, 2007[191]	Unclear	Yes	Yes	Unclear	Unclear	Unclear	Unclear	Unclear	Yes	Yes	High
Pauleit, 2002[192]	Yes	Yes	Yes	Unclear	Yes	Yes	Unclear	Unclear	No	Yes	Moderate
Pei, 2013[193]	Unclear	No (case-control)	Unclear (only evaluated patients with optimum scanning nodules)	Yes	Yes	Yes	Unclear	Unclear	No	Yes	Moderate
Peterson, 2000[194]	Yes	No (all cases)	Yes	Yes	Unclear	Yes (explant)	Unclear	No (mean 107 days)	Yes	Yes	High
Petruzzi, 2013[195]	Unclear	Yes	Yes	Unclear	Yes	Yes (explant)	Unclear	Unclear	Yes	Yes	Moderate
Piana, 2011[196]	Unclear	No (all cases)	Yes	Unclear	Yes	Yes (histology or AASLD criteria)	Unclear	Yes	No	Yes	High
Pitton, 2009[197]	Unclear	No (all cases)	Yes	Yes	Yes	Yes (histology, except 3 patients)	Unclear	Unclear	Yes (3 patients did not have histology)	Yes	High
Pozzi Mucelli, 2006[198]	Yes	Yes	Yes	Unclear	Yes	Unclear (lab/imaging follow-up criteria not described)	Unclear	Unclear	No	Yes	Moderate
Pugacheva, 2011[199]	Yes	No (all cases)	Yes	Yes	Yes	Yes	Unclear	Unclear	No	Yes	Moderate
Quaia, 2009[200]	Unclear	Yes	No	Yes	Yes	Yes (histopathology)	Unclear	Yes	Yes	No (excluded 74 patients)	Moderate

Author, Year	Random or Consecutive Sample	Avoidance of Case-control Design	Avoidance of Inappropriate Exclusions	Index Test Results Interpreted Without Knowledge of Reference Standard	Use of Pre-specified Threshold or Definition for a Positive Test	Credible Reference Standard	Reference Standard Interpreted Independently From the Test Under Evaluation	Appropriate Interval Between Index Test and Reference Standard	Same Reference Standard Applied to All Patients	Were All Patients Included in the Analysis?	Overall Risk of Bias (Low, Moderate, High)
Quaia, 2003[201]	Unclear	Yes	Yes	Yes	Yes	Yes	Unclear	Unclear	Yes	Yes	Moderate
Rhee, 2012[202]	Yes	Yes	Unclear (excluded 49 lesions in which location on pathology did not match MRI)	Yes	No (for developing new criteria)	Yes	Unclear	Yes	No	Yes	Moderate
Rickes, 2003[203]	Unclear	Yes	Unclear (excluded 5 patients with obesity)	Yes	Yes	Unclear	Unclear	Unclear	No	No (excluded 10 patients due to loss to follow-up)	High
Rimola, 2012[204]	Unclear	Yes	Yes	Unclear	Yes	Yes (biopsy)	Unclear	Unclear	Yes	Yes	Moderate
Rizvi, 2006[205]	Unclear	Yes	Unclear	Yes	Unclear	Yes (explant)	Unclear	Unclear	Yes	No (excluded 2/21 for unclear reasons)	High
Rode, 2001[206]	Yes	Yes	Unclear	Unclear	Unclear	Yes (explant)	Yes	Yes (mean 50 days)	Yes	Yes	Moderate
Ronzoni, 2007[207]	Yes	Yes	Yes	Yes	Unclear	Yes (explant)	Unclear	Unclear	Yes	Unclear	Moderate
Sangiovanni, 2010[208]	Yes	Yes	Yes	No (for retrospective eval)	Yes	Yes (percutaneous biopsy)	Yes	Yes (<2 months)	Yes	Yes	Low
Sano, 2011[209]	Yes	No (all cases)	Yes	Yes	Yes	Yes (biopsy)	Yes	Yes	Yes	Yes	Moderate
Schima, 2006[210]	Yes	No (all cases)	Yes	Yes	Yes	Yes	Unclear	Unclear	Unclear	Yes	High
Secil, 2008[211]	Unclear	Yes	Yes	Unclear	Unclear	Yes	Unclear	Unclear	No (varied)	Yes	Moderate
Seitz, 2009[212]	Yes	Yes	Yes	Yes	Unclear (for CT)	Yes (biopsy, for cases included in analysis)	Unclear	Unclear	Yes (for cases included in analysis)	Yes	Moderate

Author, Year	Random or Consecutive Sample	Avoidance of Case-control Design	Avoidance of Inappropriate Exclusions	Index Test Results Interpreted Without Knowledge of Reference Standard	Use of Pre-specified Threshold or Definition for a Positive Test	Credible Reference Standard	Reference Standard Interpreted Independently From the Test Under Evaluation	Appropriate Interval Between Index Test and Reference Standard	Same Reference Standard Applied to All Patients	Were All Patients Included in the Analysis?	Overall Risk of Bias (Low, Moderate, High)
Seitz, 2010[213]	Yes	Yes	Yes	Unclear (for CT)	No (for MRI)	Yes (biopsy, for cases included in analysis)	Unclear	Unclear	Yes (for cases included in analysis)	Yes	Moderate
Serste, 2012[214]	Yes	Yes	Yes	Unclear (for MRI)	Yes	Yes	Yes	Yes	Yes	Yes	Low
Shah SA, 2006[215]	Yes	No	Yes	Yes; imaging done prior to transplant; its interpretation is part of qualifier for transplant	Yes	Yes	Unclear	Unclear	Yes	Yes; all that met inclusion criteria	Moderate
Simon, 2005[216]	Unclear	Yes	Yes	Yes	Unclear	Yes	Unclear	Unclear	No	Yes	Moderate
Singh, 2007[217]	Unclear	Yes	Yes	Yes	No	Yes	Unclear	Unclear	Yes	No	High
Sofue, 2011[218]	Yes	No (all cases)	Unclear (some exclusions of patients with equivocal CT/MRI findings)	Unclear	Yes	Unclear	Unclear	Unclear	No	No	High
Sorensen, 2011[219]	Unclear	Yes	Yes	Unclear	Yes	Yes (EASL criteria)	Unclear	Unclear	Unclear	Yes	High
Strobel, 2003[220]	Yes	Yes	Yes	Yes	Unclear	Unclear (imaging criteria not described)	Unclear	Unclear	No	Yes	High
Sugimoto, 2012[221]	Yes	No (case control)	Yes	Yes	Not applicable (only AUROC reported)	Yes	Unclear	Unclear	Yes	Yes	Moderate
Sugimoto, 2012 (2)[222]	Yes	No (all cases)	Yes	Yes	Yes	Yes	Unclear	Unclear	No	Yes	Moderate

Author, Year	Random or Consecutive Sample	Avoidance of Case-control Design	Avoidance of Inappropriate Exclusions	Index Test Results Interpreted Without Knowledge of Reference Standard	Use of Pre-specified Threshold or Definition for a Positive Test	Credible Reference Standard	Reference Standard Interpreted Independently From the Test Under Evaluation	Appropriate Interval Between Index Test and Reference Standard	Same Reference Standard Applied to All Patients	Were All Patients Included in the Analysis?	Overall Risk of Bias (Low, Moderate, High)
Sugiyama, 2004[223]	Unclear	No (case-control)	Yes	Unclear	Unclear	Unclear	Unclear	Unclear	No	Yes	High
Suh, 2011[224]	Unclear	Yes	Yes	Yes	No	Yes	Unclear	Unclear	No	Yes	Moderate
Sun, 2010[225]	Unclear	No (case-control)	Yes	Yes	Yes	Unclear	Unclear	Unclear	No	No	Moderate
Sun, 2009[226]	Unclear	Yes	Yes	Yes	Yes	Unclear	Unclear	Unclear	No	Yes	High
Suzuki, 2004 (2)[227]	Unclear	Yes	Yes	Unclear	Unclear	Yes	Unclear	Unclear	Yes	Yes	Moderate
Takahashi, 2013[228]	Unclear	Unclear	Unclear	Yes	Yes	Yes	Unclear	Unclear	Yes	Yes	Moderate
Talbot, 2010[229]	Unclear	Yes	Yes	Unclear	Yes	Yes	Unclear	Unclear	No	Yes	Moderate
Talbot, 2006[230]	Unclear	No (all cases)	Yes	Unclear	Yes	Yes	Unclear	Unclear	No	No	High
Tanaka, 2005[231]	Yes	Yes	Unclear	Unclear	Unclear	Unclear	Unclear	Unclear	No (varied)	Unclear	High
Tanaka, 2001[232]	Unclear	Yes	Yes	Unclear	Yes	No (some lesions based on single imaging test)	Unclear	Unclear	No	Yes	Moderate
Tang, 1999[233]	Unclear	No (all cases)	Unclear	Yes	Yes	Yes (based on biopsy or AFP, imaging findings, and response to treatment)	Unclear	Unclear (<1 month in patients with histological diagnosis)	No (varied)	Unclear	High
Tanimoto, 2002[234]	Yes	No (all cases)	Yes	Unclear	Yes	Unclear	Unclear	Unclear	No	Yes	High
Teefey, 2003[235]	Unclear	Yes	Unclear	Unclear	Yes	Yes (explant)	Unclear	No (mean 5.3 months)	Yes	No (10/37 excluded)	Moderate
Toyota, 2013[236]	Unclear	No (all cases)	Yes	Yes	Yes	Yes	Unclear	Unclear	Yes	Yes	Moderate

C-17

Author, Year	Random or Consecutive Sample	Avoidance of Case-control Design	Avoidance of Inappropriate Exclusions	Index Test Results Interpreted Without Knowledge of Reference Standard	Use of Pre-specified Threshold or Definition for a Positive Test	Credible Reference Standard	Reference Standard Interpreted Independently From the Test Under Evaluation	Appropriate Interval Between Index Test and Reference Standard	Same Reference Standard Applied to All Patients	Were All Patients Included in the Analysis?	Overall Risk of Bias (Low, Moderate, High)
Trojan, 1999[237]	Yes	No (all cases)	Yes	Yes	Unclear	Yes (histopathological)	Unclear	Unclear	Yes	Yes	Moderate
Tsurusaki, 2008[238]	Yes	No (all cases)	Yes	Unclear	Yes	Yes	Unclear	Unclear	No	Yes	Moderate
Valls, 2004[239]	Unclear	Yes	Yes	Unclear	Yes	Yes (explant)	Unclear	No (mean 6.6 months)	Yes	Yes	Moderate
Van Thiel, 2004[240]	Yes	Yes	Yes	Yes	Yes	Yes (explant)	Unclear	Unclear	Yes	Unclear	Moderate
Vandecaveye, 2009[241]	Yes	Yes	Yes	Unclear	Yes	Yes (surgical pathology, percutaneous biopsy, or follow-up MRI)	Unclear	No (median 4 months for explant)	No	Yes	Moderate
Verhoef, 2002[242]	Yes	Yes	Yes	Unclear	Yes	Yes (histopathological)	Unclear	Yes (<3 months)	Yes	Yes	Moderate
Wagnetz, 2011[243]	Yes	Yes	Yes	Unclear	Unclear	Yes (surgical biopsy)	Unclear	Yes	Yes	Yes	Moderate
Wang, 2008[244]	Yes	Yes	Yes	Unclear	Yes	Yes	Unclear	Unclear	Yes	Yes	Moderate
Wang, 2006[245]	Yes	Yes	Yes	Unclear	Unclear	Unclear	Unclear	Unclear	No	Yes	Moderate
Wolfort, 2010[246]	Yes	No (all cases)	Yes	Yes	Yes	Yes	Unclear	Unclear	Yes	No (denominator discrepancies in subgroup analyses)	High

Author, Year	Random or Consecutive Sample	Avoidance of Case-control Design	Avoidance of Inappropriate Exclusions	Index Test Results Interpreted Without Knowledge of Reference Standard	Use of Pre-specified Threshold or Definition for a Positive Test	Credible Reference Standard	Reference Standard Interpreted Independently From the Test Under Evaluation	Appropriate Interval Between Index Test and Reference Standard	Same Reference Standard Applied to All Patients	Were All Patients Included in the Analysis?	Overall Risk of Bias (Low, Moderate, High)
Wu, 2011[247]	Yes	No (all cases)	Yes	Unclear	Yes	Yes	Unclear	Unclear	No	Yes	Moderate
Wudel, 2003[248]	Yes	No (all cases)	Yes	Yes	Unclear	Unclear (not described for most patients)	Unclear	Unclear	No	Yes	High
Xiao, 2005[249]	Unclear	No (all cases)	Yes	Unclear	Unclear	Unclear	Unclear	Unclear	No	No	High
Xu, 2012[250]	Yes	Yes	Yes	Yes	Yes	Yes	Unclear	Unclear	No	Yes	Moderate
Xu, 2010[251]	Unclear	Yes	Yes	Yes	Yes	Yes	Unclear	Unclear	Yes	Yes	Moderate
Xu, 2009[252]	Unclear	No (all cases)	Yes	Yes	Yes	Yes	Unclear	Unclear	No	Yes	Moderate
Xu, 2008[253]	Yes	No (all cases)	Yes	Yes	Yes	Yes	Unclear	Unclear	No	Yes	Moderate
Yamamoto, 2008[254]	Yes	No (all cases)	Yes	Yes	Unclear	Unclear	Unclear	Yes (mean 22 days)	Unclear	Yes	High
Yamamoto, 2002[255]	Unclear	No (all cases)	Yes	Yes	Yes	Unclear	Unclear	Unclear	Unclear	Yes	High
Yan, 2002[256]	Unclear	No (all cases)	Yes	Unclear	Unclear	Unclear	Unclear	Unclear	No	Yes	High
Yoo, 2013[257]	Yes	No (all cases)	Yes	Unclear	Yes	Yes	Unclear	Unclear	Yes	Yes	Moderate
Yoo, 2009[258]	Yes	Yes	Yes	Unclear	Yes	Yes	Unclear	Yes	Yes	Yes	Moderate
Yoon, 2007[259]	Yes	Yes	Yes	Yes	Yes	Yes	Unclear	Unclear	Yes	Yes	Moderate
Yoshioka, 2002[260]	Yes	Yes	Yes	Unclear	Unclear	Yes	Unclear	Unclear	No	Yes	Moderate
Youk, 2004[261]	Unclear	No (all cases)	Yes	Yes	Yes	Yes	Unclear	Unclear	No	Yes	Moderate
Yu, 2013[262]	Unclear	Yes	Yes	Yes	Yes	Yes	Unclear	Unclear	Yes	Yes	Moderate
Yu, 2013 (2)[263]	Yes	No	Yes	Yes	No	Yes	Unclear	Unclear	Yes	Yes	Moderate
Yu, 2013 (3)[264]	Yes	No	Yes	Yes	No	Yes	Unclear	Unclear	Yes	Yes	Moderate
Yu, 2011[265]	Unclear	Yes	Yes	Yes	Unclear	Yes	Unclear (also not blinded to other imaging)	Unclear	Yes	Yes (<10% excluded)	Moderate

Author, Year	Random or Consecutive Sample	Avoidance of Case-control Design	Avoidance of Inappropriate Exclusions	Index Test Results Interpreted Without Knowledge of Reference Standard	Use of Pre-specified Threshold or Definition for a Positive Test	Credible Reference Standard	Reference Standard Interpreted Independently From the Test Under Evaluation	Appropriate Interval Between Index Test and Reference Standard	Same Reference Standard Applied to All Patients	Were All Patients Included in the Analysis?	Overall Risk of Bias (Low, Moderate, High)
Yu, 2009[266]	Yes	No (all cases)	Yes	Unclear	Yes	Yes	Unclear	Unclear	No	No (excluded 24 without reference standard diagnosis)	High
Yu, 2008[267]	Unclear	No (all cases)	Yes	Unclear	Yes	Yes	Unclear	Unclear	No	Yes	High
Yu, 2002[268]	Unclear	No (case-control)	Unclear (excluded patients with transvasal arterioportal shunt or gross portal vein thrombosis)	Unclear	Yes	Unclear	Unclear	Unclear	No	Yes	High
Yukisawa, 2007[269]	Yes	No (all cases)	Yes	Unclear	Yes	Yes	Unclear	Unclear	No	Yes	Moderate
Zacherl, 2002[270]	Yes	No (all cases)	Yes	Yes	Unclear	Yes (explant)	Unclear	Yes	Yes	Unclear	High
Zhao, 2007[271]	Unclear	No (all cases)	Unclear	Yes	Yes	Yes	Unclear	Unclear	No	Yes	High
Zhao, 2004[272]	Unclear	No (all cases)	Unclear	Yes	Yes	Yes	Unclear	Unclear	No	Yes	High
Zhao, 2003[273]	Unclear	No (all cases)	Yes	Unclear	Unclear	Unclear	Unclear	Unclear	No	Yes	High
Zheng, 2005[274]	Unclear	No (all cases)	Yes	Unclear	Unclear	Unclear	Unclear	Unclear	No	Yes	High
Zhou, 2002[275]	Unclear	No (all cases)	Yes	Unclear	Unclear	Unclear	Unclear	Unclear	Yes	Yes	High

Table C2. Risk of bias: Randomized controlled trials

Author, Year	Randomization Adequate?	Allocation Concealment Adequate?	Groups Similar at Baseline?	Eligibility Criteria Specified?	Outcome Assessors Masked?	Care Provider Masked?	Patient Masked?	Reporting of Attrition, Crossovers, Adherence, and Contamination
Pocha, 2013[276]	Yes	Unclear	Yes	Yes	Unclear	No	No	Attrition: yes Crossover: yes Adherence: yes Contamination: yes
Trinchet JC, 2011[277]	Yes	Yes	Yes	Yes	Unclear	Unclear	Unclear	Attrition: yes Crossover: no Adherence: yes Contamination: no
Wang JH, 2013[278]	Yes; computer-assisted randomization	Unclear	Yes; only age and bilirubin levels differ	Yes	Unclear	Unclear	Unclear	Attrition: no Crossover: no Adherence: yes Contamination: yes; 5 patients in 12-month surveillance group dx outside time schedule
Zhang BH, 2004[279]	Unclear	Unclear	Yes	Yes	Unclear	No	No	Attrition: no Crossover: no Adherence: yes Contamination: no

Author, Year	Loss to Followup: Differential/High	Analyze People in the Groups in Which They Were Randomized?	Post-Randomization Exclusions	Outcomes Prespecified	Funding Source	External Validity	Overall Risk of Bias (Low, Moderate, High)
Pocha, 2013[276]	No/no	Yes	Yes (2/165 had no imaging test and excluded from analysis)	Yes	Departement of Veterans Affairs	Moderate; American study, Veterans Affairs setting, all patients had cirrhosis	Moderate
Trinchet JC, 2011[277]	No/No	Yes	No (4% had lesion at inclusion and were excluded)	Yes	French Ministry of Health; French Ligue de Recherche contre le Cancer	Moderate; French study, all patients had cirrhosis	Moderate
Wang JH, 2013[278]	Not reported	Yes	No	Yes	National Scientific Council of Taiwan	Limited; study done in Taiwan; patients had low platelets and viral hepatitis	Moderate

| Zhang BH, 2004[279] | Not reported | Yes | No (4% of screening group refused to participate) | Yes | Not reported | Limited; study done in China | High |

Table C3. Risk of bias: Cohort study

Author, Year	Did the Study Attempt To Enroll All (Or a Random Sample of) Patients Meeting Inclusion Criteria, or a Random Sample (Inception Cohort)?	Were the Groups Comparable at Baseline on Key Prognostic Factors (E.G., by Restriction or Matching)?	Did the Study Use Accurate Methods for Ascertaining Exposures and Potential Confounders?	Were Outcome Assessors and/or Data Analysts Blinded to the Exposure Being Studied?	Did the Article Report Attrition?	Did the Study Perform Appropriate Statistical Analyses on Potential Confounders?	Is There Important Differential Loss to Followup or Overall High Loss to Followup?	Were Outcomes Pre-Specified and Defined, and Ascertained Using Accurate Methods?	Overall Risk of Bias (Low, Moderate, High)
Chen MH, 2007[280]	Unclear	Yes	Yes	Unclear	No	None performed	Unclear	Yes	High
Chen MH, 2007 (2)[281]	Unclear	Yes	No	Unclear	No	No	Unclear	Yes	High

Appendix D. Evidence Table: Diagnostic Accuracy Studies of Ultrasound Imaging

Table D1. Characteristics of diagnostic accuracy studies of ultrasound imaging

Author, Year	Reason for Ultrasound Imaging[a]	Contrast	Imaging Start Date	Reference Standard[b]	Country	Sample Size	Population Characteristics[c]		
Alaboudy, 2011[4]	2	Perflurobutane	2008	2	Japan	32	Age: 68	Male: 72%	HBV: 22%	Cirrhosis: NR
Bennett, 2002[11]	2	No contrast	1991	1	United States	200	Age: 50	Male: 67%	BV: 4.5%	Cirrhosis: 100%
Catala, 2007[14]	3	Sulfur hexafluoride	2002	2	Spain	77	NR			Cirrhosis: 100%
Chalasani, 1999[16]	1	No contrast	1994	4	United States	285	Age: 49	Male: 56%	HBV: NR	Cirrhosis: 100%
Dai, 2008[26]	3	Sulfur hexafluoride	2004	2	China	72	Age: 59	Male: 82%	HBV: NR	Cirrhosis: 100%
Di Martino, 2010[31]	2	No contrast	2007	4	Italy	140	Age: 59	Male: 74%	HBV: NR	Cirrhosis: 100%
D'Onofrio, 2005[32]	3	Sulfur hexafluoride	2002	4	Italy	NR	NR			
Egger, 2012[35]	3	Sulfur hexafluoride	2008	2	Germany	19	Age: median 63 Cirrhosis: 100%	Male: 84%	HBV: NR	
Forner, 2008[37]	3	Sulfur hexafluoride	2003	2	United States	89	Age: 65	Male: 60%	HBV: 6.7%	Cirrhosis: 100%
Fracanzani, 2001[39]	3	Galactose	1998	2	Italy	41	Age: 62	Male: 73%	HBV: NR	Cirrhosis: 100%
Freeman, 2006[40]	2, 5	NR	2003	1	United States	789	Age: 56	Male: 77%	HBV: NR	Cirrhosis: NR
Furuse, 2000[42]	1	No contrast	1996	2	Japan	37	Age: 64	Male: 86%	HBV: 3%	Cirrhosis: 89%
Gaiani, 2004[43]	3	Sulfur hexafluoride	2001	4	Italy	79	Age: 66	Male: 68%	HBV: 6%	Cirrhosis: NR
Gambarin-Gelwan, 2000[44]	2	No contrast	NR	1	United States	106	Age: 50	Male: 65%	HBV: 5.7%	Cirrhosis: 100%
Giorgio, 2004[47]	3	Sulfur hexafluoride	2002	2	Italy	74	Age: 67	Male: 81%	HBV: 7%	Cirrhosis: 100%
Giorgio, 2007[46]	3	Sulfur hexafluoride	2003	4	Italy	73	Age: 63	Male: 67%	HBV: 4.1%	Cirrhosis: 100%
Goto, 2012[50]	2	No contrast or perflurobutane	2007	3	Japan	100	Age: 68	Male: 60%	HBV: 9%	Cirrhosis: NR
Hatanaka, 2008 (2)[56]	3	Perfluorobutane	2007	4	Japan	214	Age: 68	Male: 63%	HBV: NR	Cirrhosis: NR
Iavarone, 2010[68]	2	Sulfur hexafluoride	2006	2	Italy	59	Age: 66	Male: 69%	HBV: 12%	Cirrhosis: 100%
Imamura, 1998[72]	2	No contrast	1995	2	Japan	114	Age: NR	Male: NR	HBV: 7.9%	Cirrhosis: 57%
Inoue, 2008[75]	2	Perflurobutane	NR	4	Japan	77	Age: 62	Male: 71%	HBV: 10%	Cirrhosis: 71%
Inoue, 2009[74]	3	No contrast	2002	2	Japan	50	Age: median 67	Male: 76%	HBV: 12%	Cirrhosis: 100%
Jang, 2009[80]	3	Perflurobutane	NR	4	Canada	59	Age: 56	Male: 73%	HBV: 47%	Cirrhosis: NR
Kawada, 2010[89]	2	Perflurobutane	2008	2	Japan	13	Age: median 67	Male: 77%	HBV: 7.7%	Cirrhosis: 100%
Khalili, 2011[92]	3	Perflutren lipid microsphere	2006	4	Canada	84	Age: 58	Male: 63%	HBV: 50%	Cirrhosis: 100%
Kim CK, 2001[95]	2	No contrast	1996	1	South Korea	52	Age: 45	Male: 77%	HBV: 94%	Cirrhosis: 100%
Kim PN, 2012[99]	2	No contrast	2008	3	South Korea	898	Age: 59	Male: 76%	HBV: 73%	Cirrhosis: 89%
Korenaga, 2009[122]	2	Perflurobutane	2007	2	Japan	43	Age: 67	Male: 70%	HBV: 9.3%	Cirrhosis: 81%
Kunishi, 2012[127]	2	No contrast or perflurobutane	2009	4	Japan	50	Age: 71	Male: 70%	HBV: 10%	Cirrhosis: 100%
Lee MW, 2010[139]	3	No contrast	2005	3	South Korea	93	Age: 59	Male: 70%	HBV: NR	Cirrhosis: NR
Li, 2007[140]	3	Sulfur hexafluoride	NR	2	China	109	Age: 46	Male: 66%	HBV: NR	Cirrhosis: NR
Libbrecht, 2002[144]	2, 5	No contrast	2000	1	Belgium	49	Age: 53	Male: 65%	HBV: 19%	Cirrhosis: 100%
Lim JH, 2006 (2)[145]	2	No contrast	1999	2	South Korea	103	Age: 53	Male: 83%	HBV: NR	Cirrhosis: 59%

Author, Year	Reason for Ultrasound Imaging[a]	Contrast	Imaging Start Date	Reference Standard[b]	Country	Sample Size	Population Characteristics[c]		
Liu, 2003[152]	2	No contrast	1996	1	South Korea	118	Age: 47	Male: 73%	HBV: 81%	Cirrhosis: 100%
Luo, 2005[155]	3	Galactose	2002	2	China	36	Age: 52	Male: 81%	HBV: 42%	Cirrhosis: NR
Luo W 2009 (3)[158]	3	Perfluorobutane	2007	4	Japan	84	Age: 70	Male: 66%	HBV: NR	Cirrhosis: 100%
Luo W, 2009[156]	3	Perfluorobutane	2007	4	Japan	152	Age: 71	Male: 55%	HBV: NR	Cirrhosis: NR
Luo W, 2009 (2)[157]	3	Perfluorobutane	2007	2	Japan	139	Age: 62	Male: 65%	HBV: NR	Cirrhosis: 53%
Mita, 2010[166]	3	Perfluorobutane	2008	2	Japan	29	Age: 70	Male: 45%	HBV: 3.4%	Cirrhosis: 100%
Mok, 2004[167]	1	No contrast	1997	2	China	103	Age: median 48	Male: 78%	HBV: 100%	Cirrhosis: NR
Moriyasu, 2009[170]	3	No contrast or perflurobutane	NR	4	Japan	190	Age: 63	Male: 67%	HBV: NR	Cirrhosis: NR
Numata, 2014[181]	2	Perflurobutane	2010	2	Japan	43	Age: 70	Male: 65%	HBV: 9.3%	Cirrhosis: 100%
Ooi, 2010[183]	3	Sulfur hexafluoride	2006	4	Singapore	73	Age: 64	Male: 75%	HBV: NR	Cirrhosis: NR
Paul, 2007[191]	1	No contrast	2001	4	India	301 (291 underwent US)	Age: NR	Male: NR	HBV: NR	Cirrhosis: 100%
Pei, 2012[193]	4	Sulfur hexafluoride	2005	2	China	100	Age: 51 Note: HCC group only	Male: 86%	HBV: NR	Cirrhosis: NR
Quaia, 2003[201]	3	Sulfur hexafluoride	NR	2	Italy	39	Age: 54	Male: 62%	HBV: NR	Cirrhosis: 100%
Quaia, 2009[200]	3	Sulfur hexafluoride	2009	2	Italy	106	Age: 70	Male: 64%	HBV: 80%	Cirrhosis: 100%
Rickes, 2003[203]	3	No contrast or galactose	1998	4	Germany	87	Age: 60	Male: 71%	HBV: 14%	Cirrhosis: 100%
Rode, 2001[206]	2	No contrast	1996	1	France	43	Age: 51	Male: 70%	HBV: 9.3%	Cirrhosis: 100%
Sangiovanni 2010[208]	3	Sulfur hexafluoride	2006	2	Italy	64	Age: NR	Male: NR	HBV: NR	Cirrhosis: 100%
Seitz, 2009[212]	3	Sulfur hexafluoride	2004	4	Germany	267	Age: 60	Male: 45%	HBV: NR	Cirrhosis: NR
Seitz, 2010[213]	3	Sulfur hexafluoride	2004	4	Germany	269	Age: 53	Male: 41%	HBV: NR	Cirrhosis: NR
Shah SA, 2006 (2)[215]	5	NR	NR	1	Canada	118	Age: NR	Male: 80%	HBV: 19%	Cirrhosis: NR
Singh, 2007[217]	1	No contrast	2005	2	United States	17	Age: 56	Male: NR	HBV: NR	Cirrhosis: 100%
Strobel, 2003[220]	3	Octafluoropropane	1998	4	Germany	90	NR			Cirrhosis: NR
Sugimoto, 2012[221]	4	Perflurobutane	2008	2	Japan	66	Age: 69	Male: 70%	HBV: 12%	Cirrhosis: NR
Sugimoto, 2012 (2)[222]	2	Perflurobutane	2008	2	Japan	54	Age: 70	Male: 54%	HBV: 5.6%	Cirrhosis: NR
Suzuki, 2004 (2)[227]	3	Galactose	2000	2	Japan	46	Age: 66	Male: 67%	HBV: NR	Cirrhosis: NR
Takahashi, 2013[228]	4	Perflurobutane	2008	2	Japan	56	Age: 66	Male: 71%	HBV: 14%	Cirrhosis: 79%
Tanaka, 2001[232]	3	Galactose	1999	2	Japan	107	Age: 62	Male: 75%	HBV: NR	Cirrhosis: NR
Teefey, 2003[235]	2	No contrast	1996	2	United States	25	Age: 47	Male: 65%	HBV: NR	Cirrhosis: 100%
Trojan, 1999[237]	2	No contrast	1996	2	Germany	14	Age: median 60	Male: 71%	HBV: 21%	Cirrhosis: NR
Van Thiel, 2004[240]	1	No contrast	1998	1	United States	100	Age: 52	Male: 68%	HBV: 2%	Cirrhosis: NR
Wang, 2006[245]	3	Galactose	2003	4	Taiwan	30	Age: 55	Male: 67%	HBV: 73%	Cirrhosis: 100%
Wang, 2008[244]	3	Sulfur hexafluoride	2005	4	China	52	Age: 45	Male: 65%	HBV: NR	Cirrhosis: 0%
Xu, 2008[253]	3	No contrast or sulfur hexafluoride (for HCC <2 cm)	2005	4	China	104	Age: 48	Male: 78%	HBV: NR	Cirrhosis: NR

Author, Year	Reason for Ultrasound Imaging[a]	Contrast	Imaging Start Date	Reference Standard[b]	Country	Sample Size	Population Characteristics[c]		
Xu, 2012[250]	3	No contrast or sulfur hexafluoride	2004	4	China	133	Age: 52	Male: 83%	HBV: 95%	Cirrhosis: 100%
Yamamoto, 2002[255]	3	Galactose	NR	4	Japan	41	Age: 65	Male: 54%	HBV: 2.4%	Cirrhosis: 95%
Yu, 2011[265]	2	No contrast	1999	1	United States	638	Age: 53	Male: 64%	HBV: 10%	Cirrhosis: NR
Zhou, 2002[275]	2	No contrast	1995	2	China	49	Age: NR	Male: 90%	HBV: NR	Cirrhosis: NR

HBV = hepatitis B virus; NR = not reported

[a] Reason for imaging key: 1=surveillance, 2=detection rate in patients undergoing surgery or with known HCC; 3=evaluation/characterization of liver mass; 4=differentiation between HCC and another type of lesion mass; 5=staging

[b] Reference standard key: 1=explanted livers only, 2=histological specimen (may include some explanted livers), 3=imaging and clinical criteria, 4=mixed histological and imaging/clinical criteria

[c] Age reported as mean (years), unless otherwise indicated

Appendix E. Evidence Table: Diagnostic Accuracy Studies of Computed Tomography Imaging

Table E1. Characteristics of diagnostic accuracy studies of computed tomography imaging

Author, Year	Reason for CT Imaging[a]	Scanner Type	Contrast Rate (ml/s)	Delayed Phase?	Delayed Phase Timing >120 s[b]	Section Thickness (mm)	Did Study Meet All Imaging Criteria?[c]	Imaging Start Date	Reference Standard[d]	Country	Number of Patients	Population Characteristics[e]	
Addley, 2011[1]	2	16- or 64-row multidetector CT	4	No	NA	1-2	No	2002	1	United Kingdom	39	Age: 56 HBV: 5.1%	Male: 72% Cirrhosis: NR
Akai, 2011[3]	2	64-row multidetector CT	3	Yes	No	5	No	2008	1	Japan	34	Age: 65 HBV: NR	Male: 79% Cirrhosis: NR
Alaboudy, 2011[4]	2	64-row multidetector CT	NR	No	NA	5	No	2008	2	Japan	32	Age: 68 HBV: 22%	Male: 72% Cirrhosis: NR
Baccarini U, 2006[7]	5	NR	NR	NR	NR	NR	No	NR	1	Italy	50	Age: median 57 HBV: NR	Male: 86% Cirrhosis: NR
Baek, 2012[8]	2	4-(n=6), 16-(n=9), or 64-row (n=36) multidetector CT	3-4	Yes	Yes	3-5	No	2008	4	South Korea	51	Age: NR, range 32-80 Male: 84% HBV: 80%	Cirrhosis: 100%
Bartolozzi, 2000[10]	2	Non-multidetector spiral CT	3	No	NA	7 (collimation)	No	1997	4	Italy	50	Age: 65 HBV: NR	Male: 64% Cirrhosis: 100%
Bhattacharjya, 2004[12]	2	Non-multidetector spiral CT	4	No	NA	7-10 (collimation)	No	1995	1	UK	30	Age: NR HBV: 23%	Male: NR Cirrhosis: 100%
Burrel, 2003[13]	2, 5	Non-multidetector spiral CT	4	Yes	Yes	5 (collimation)	No	2000	1	Spain	26	Age: 56 HBV: NR	Male: 66% Cirrhosis: 100%
Catala, 2007[14]	3	Non-multidetector spiral CT	4	Yes	Yes	5 (collimation)	No	2002	2	Spain	77	NR	
Chalasani, 1999[16]	1	Non-multidetector spiral CT	4	No	NA	5 (collimation)	No	1994	4	United States	285	Age: 49 HBV: None	Male: 56% Cirrhosis: 100%
Cheung, 2013[18]	2, 5	16-row multidetector CT	NR	Yes	NR	5	No	2004	2	China	43	Age: 60 HBV: 7.0%	Male: 79% Cirrhosis: NR
Colagrande, 2000[25]	3	Non-multidetector spiral CT	3-4	No	NA	8	No	1996	2	Italy	24	Age: 67 HBV: NR	Male: 92% Cirrhosis: 100%
Dai, 2008[26]	3	Non-multidetector spiral CT	3.5	Yes	120-240	5	No	2004	2	China	72	Age: 59 HBV: NR	Male: 82% Cirrhosis: 100%

Author, Year	Reason for CT Imaging[a]	Scanner Type	Contrast Rate (ml/s)	Delayed Phase?	Delayed Phase Timing >120 s[b]	Section Thickness (mm)	Did Study Meet All Imaging Criteria?[c]	Imaging Start Date	Reference Standard[d]	Country	Number of Patients	Population Characteristics[e]
de Ledinghen, 2002[27]	2	Non-multidetector spiral CT	3	No	NA	5 (collimation)	No	1997	1	France	34	Age: 54 Male: 71% HBV: 8.8% Cirrhosis: 100%
Denecke, 2009[29]	2	4-(n=9) or 16-row (n=23) multidetector CT	4	Yes	No	5 (4-row) or 1.25-5 (16-row)	No	2001	1	Germany	32	Age: 57 Male: 88% HBV: 16% Cirrhosis: NR
Di Martino, 2010[31]	2	64-row multidetector CT	4	Yes	Yes	3	Yes	2007	4	Italy	140	Age: 59 Male: 74% HBV: NR Cirrhosis: 100%
Di Martino, 2013[30]	2	64-row multidetector CT	4-5	Yes	Yes	3	Yes	2007	4	Italy	58	Age: 63 Male: 67% HBV: 14% Cirrhosis: 100%
Doyle, 2007[33]	2	8-row (n=8), 4-row (n=27), or non-multidetector CT (n=1)	5	No	NA	5 (collimation)	No	2001	2	Canada	36	Age: 55 Male: 67% HBV: 50% Cirrhosis: 100%
Egger, 2012[35]	3	16-row multidetector CT	NR	NR	NR	NR	No	2008	2	Germany	19	Age: Median 63 Male: 84% HBV: NR Cirrhosis: 100%
Fracanzani, 2001[39]	3	Non-multidetector spiral CT	NR	Yes	NR	NR	No	1998	2	Italy	41	Age: 62 Male: 73% HBV: NR Cirrhosis: 100%
Freeman, 2006[40]	2, 5	NR	NR	NR	NR	NR	No	2003	1	United States	789	Age: 56 Male: 77% HBV: NR Cirrhosis: NR
Freeny, 2003[41]	2	Non-multidetector spiral CT	5	Yes	Yes	3 (collimation)	No	1992	1	Switzerland	51	Age: 49 Male: 58% HBV: None Cirrhosis: 100% Note: only includes patients with hyperattenuating nodules on CT
Furuse, 2000[42]	1	Non-multidetector spiral CT	3	No	NA	NR	No	1996	2	Japan	37	Age: 64 Male: 86 HBV: 3% Cirrhosis: 89%
Giorgio, 2004[47]	3	Non-multidetector spiral CT	3	Yes	Yes	NR	No	2002	2	Italy	74	Age: 67 Male: 81% HBV: 7% Cirrhosis: 100%
Golfieri, 2009[48]	3	6-row multidetector CT	4	Yes	Yes	5	No	2003	2	Italy	63	Age: 64 Male: 84% HBV: 35% Cirrhosis: 100%
Haradome, 2011[52]	2	16-row multidetector CT	4	Yes	Yes	3	Yes	2008	2	Japan	75	Age: 55 Male: 80% HBV: 19% Cirrhosis: 72%
Hidaka, 2013[58]	2	64-row multidetector CT	4-5	Yes	NR	3	No	2008	1	Japan	11	Age: NR Male: NR HBV: 27% Cirrhosis: NR
Higashihara, 2012[59]	2	4- (n=5) or 64-row (n=25) multidetector CT	3-4	No	NA	5	No	2007	3	Japan	30	Age: 73 Male: 57% HBV: NR Cirrhosis: NR
Hirakawa, 2011[60]	2	4-row multidetector CT	2.5	Yes	Yes	5	No	1999	1	Japan	25	Age: 55 Male: 52% HBV: NR Cirrhosis: 100%

Author, Year	Reason for CT Imaging[a]	Scanner Type	Contrast Rate (ml/s)	Delayed Phase?	Delayed Phase Timing[b] >120 s	Section Thickness (mm)	Did Study Meet All Imaging Criteria?[c]	Imaging Start Date	Reference Standard[d]	Country	Number of Patients	Population Characteristics[e]
Hori, 1998[64]	2	Non-multidetector spiral CT	2	Yes	Yes	7-10	No	1995	3	Japan	50	Age: 65 HBV: 10% Male: 76% Cirrhosis: NR
Hori, 2002[63]	2	Non-multidetector spital CT	3-5	Yes	Yes	5,7	No	1995	4	Japan	41	Age: 64 HBV: 17% Male: 83% Cirrhosis:56%
Hwang, 2012[65]	2	64-row multidetector CT	3-4	Yes	Yes	5	Yes	2008	4	South Korea	54	Age: NR, range 33 to 81 years Male: 81% HBV: 70% Cirrhosis: NR
Iannaccone, 2005[67]	3	Multidetector CT, rows NR	5	Yes	Yes	3	No	2001	4	Italy	195	Age: 61 HBV: 19% Male: 66% Cirrhosis: 100%
Iavarone, 2010[68]	2	64-row multidetector CT	4	Yes	Yes	2.5	Yes	2006	2	Italy	59	Age: median 66 Male: 69% HBV: 12% Cirrhosis: 100%
Ichikawa, 2002[70]	2	16-row multidetector CT	3	No	NA	5	No	2001	2	Japan	59	Age: 58 HBV: NR Male: 59% Cirrhosis: 100%
Ichikawa, 2010[69]	2	Non-multidetector or multidetector CT, rows NR	2-4	Yes	Yes	NR	No	2001	4	Japan	151	Age: 66 HBV: NR Male: 72% Cirrhosis: 66%
Inoue, 2012[73]	2	64-row multidetector CT	NR	No	NA	5	No	2008	2	Japan	66	Age: 66 HBV: 30% Male: 64% Cirrhosis: 62%
Iwazawa, 2010[77]	2	16-row multidetector CT	3	No	NA	5	No	2007	4	Japan	69	Age: 68 HBV: NR Male: 58% Cirrhosis: NR
Jang, 2000[78]	2	Non-multidetector spiral CT	3	Yes	Yes	7 (collimation)	No	1996	2	South Korea	52	Age: 55 HBV: NR Male: 67% Cirrhosis: NR
Jang, 2013[79]	3	64-row multidetector CT	5	Yes	Yes	5	Yes	2006	4	Korea	96	Age: 58 HBV: 55% Male: 53% Cirrhosis: NR
Jeng, 2002[82]	2	Non-multidetector spiral CT	2	No	NA	10	No	1998	4	Taiwan	125	Age: 62 HBV: NR Male: 54% Cirrhosis: NR
Kakihara, 2013[86]	2	64-row multidetector CT	NR	Yes	Yes	1	No	2008	1	Japan	15	Age: Median 55 HBV: 27% Male: 73% Cirrhosis: 100%
Kang, 2003[88]	2	Non-multidetector spiral CT	3	Yes	Yes	7	No	1999	2	South Korea	70	Age: 52 HBV: NR Male: 84% Cirrhosis: 64%
Kawada, 2010[89]	2	64-row multidetector CT	3	No	NA	5	No	2008	2	Japan	13	Age: median 67 Male: 77% HBV: 7.7% Cirrhosis: NR

Author, Year	Reason for CT Imaging[a]	Scanner Type	Contrast Rate (ml/s)	Delayed Phase?	Delayed Phase Timing >120 s[b]	Section Thickness (mm)	Did Study Meet All Imaging Criteria?[c]	Imaging Start Date	Reference Standard[d]	Country	Number of Patients	Population Characteristics[e]	
Kawaoka, 2009[90]	5	16-row multidetector CT	3.5	Yes	Yes	NR	No	2005	4	Japan	34	Age: 59 HBV: 32%	Male: 82% Cirrhosis: NR
Kawata, 2002[91]	2	8-row multidetector CT	5	No	NA	5	No	1999	4	Japan	62 patients (analysis restricted to 43 patients with HCC)	Age: 64 HBV: NR	Male: 69% Cirrhosis: NR
Khalili, 2011[92]	3	64-row multidetector CT	5	Yes	Yes	5	Yes	2006	4	Canada	84	Age: 58 HBV: 50%	Male: 63% Cirrhosis: 100%
Khan, 2000[93]	2	Non-multidetector spiral CT	NR	No	NA	5-7 (collimation)	No	1995	2	United States	20	Age: 60 HBV: 18%	Male: 75% Cirrhosis: 75%
Kim KW, 2009[97]	2	16-row multidetector CT	NR	Yes	Yes	2-3	No	2005	4	South Korea	82	Age: 56 HBV: 92%	Male: 84% Cirrhosis: 100%
Kim SE, 2011[100]	4	Non-multidetector spiral CT	3.5	Yes	Yes	5	No	2006	2	South Korea	206	Age: 55 HBV: 67%	Male: 77% Cirrhosis: 52%
Kim SH, 2005[102]	2	4- (n=27) or 8-row (n=46) multidetector CT	4	Yes	Yes	5	No	2002	2	South Korea	73	Age: 53 HBV: NR	Male: 84% Cirrhosis: 48%
Kim SH, 2009[101]	2	16- (n=31), 40- (n=14), or 64-row (n=17) multidetector CT	3-4	Yes	Yes	5	Yes	2007	2	South Korea	62	Age: 55 HBV: 85%	Male: 87% Cirrhosis: 48%
Kim SJ, 2008[103]	2	4- (n=13), 8- (n=13), 16- (n=20), or 40-row (n=40) multidetector CT	4	Yes	Yes	5	No	2004	2	South Korea	86	Age: 52 Male: 81% HBV or HCV: 91% Cirrhosis: 48%	
Kim SK, 2002 (2)[104]	2	4-row multidetector CT	3	Yes	Yes	5	No	2000	4	South Korea	25	Age: 54 HBV: 84%	Male: 84% Cirrhosis: 64%
Kim T, 2002[105]	2	Non-multidetector spiral CT	3-5	Yes	Yes	5 (collimation)	No	1999	4	South Korea	106	NR	
Kim YK, 2006[116]	2	16-row multidetector CT	3	Yes	Yes	3	Yes	2003	4	South Korea	31	Age: 57 HBV: 97%	Male: 90% Cirrhosis: 100%
Kim YK, 2006 (2)[117]	2	16-row multidetector CT	3	Yes	Yes	3	Yes	2003	4	South Korea	44	Age: 56 HBV: 100%	Male: 82% Cirrhosis: 100%

Author, Year	Reason for CT Imaging[a]	Scanner Type	Con-trast Rate (ml/s)	Delayed Phase?	Delayed Phase Timing ≥120 s[b]	Section Thickness (mm)	Did Study Meet All Imaging Criteria?[c]	Imaging Start Date	Reference Standard[d]	Country	Number of Patients	Population Characteristics[e]
Kim YK, 2009 (2)[112]	2	16-row multidetector CT	3	Yes	Yes	3	Yes	2007	4	South Korea	62	Age: NR, range 40 to 74 Male: 81% HBV: 90% Cirrhosis: NR
Kitamura, 2008[120]	2	4-row multidetector CT	3	NR	NR	5	No	2000	4	Turkey	91	Age: 57 HBV: NR Male: 62% Cirrhosis: NR
Kumano, 2009[126]	2	8-row multidetector CT	4	No	NA	3	No	2002	4	Japan	28	Age: NR HBV: NR Male: 79% Cirrhosis: NR
Laghi, 2003[130]	2	Multidetector, rows NR	5	No	NA	3	No	2000	4	Italy	48	Age: 61 HBV: 36% Male: 73% Cirrhosis: NR
Lee CH, 2012[132]	2	16-row multidetector CT	3-4	Yes	Yes	5	Yes	2008	4	South Korea	46	Age: 57 HBV: 90% Male: 83% Cirrhosis: NR
Lee DH, 2009[133]	2	4-row (n=4), 8-row (n=23), 16-row (n=35), or 64-row (n=17) multidetector CT	2-5	No	NA	2.5-3	No	2005	1	South Korea	78	Age: 53 HBV: 89% Male: 74% Cirrhosis: 100%
Lee J, 2008[134]	2	Non-multidetector spiral CT (n=7), or 4- (n=3), 8- (n=2), or 16-row (n=4) multidetector CT	3	Yes	Yes	5-7	No	1997	2	South Korea	16	Age: 55 HBV: 81% Male: 81% Cirrhosis: 75%
Lee JE, 2012[135]	5	NR	NR	NR	NR	NR	No	2006	4	South Korea	138	Age: 69 HBV: 64% Male: 83% Cirrhosis: NR
Lee JM, 2003[136]	2	Non-multidetector spiral CT	3	No	NA	5	No	1998	4	South Korea	43	Age: NR HBV: NR Male: NR Cirrhosis: 100%
Li, 2007[140]	3	16-row multidetector CT	4	Yes	NR	NR	No	NR	2	China	109	Age: 46 HBV: NR Male: 66% Cirrhosis: NR
Li CS, 2006[142]	2	Non-multidetector spiral CT	2.5-3.5	Yes	No	7	No	2000	2	Taiwan	37	Age: 60 HBV: 60% Male: 68% Cirrhosis: 5%
Libbrecht, 2002[144]	2, 5	Non-multidetector spiral CT	2.5-4	No	NA	5	No	2000	1	Belgium	49	Age: 53 HBV: 19% Male: 65% Cirrhosis: 100%
Lim JH, 2000[147]	2	Non-multidetector spiral CT	3	Yes	Yes	7 (collimation)	No	1996	1	South Korea	41	Age: 49 HBV: 100% Male: 80% Cirrhosis: 100%
Lim JH, 2002[146]	2	Non-multidetector spiral CT	3	Yes	Yes	7	No	1996	2	South Korea	113	Age: 53 HBV: 68% Male: 82% Cirrhosis: 87%

Author, Year	Reason for CT Imaging[a]	Scanner Type	Contrast Rate (ml/s)	Delayed Phase?	Delayed Phase Timing >120 s[b]	Section Thickness (mm)	Did Study Meet All Imaging Criteria?[c]	Imaging Start Date	Reference Standard[d]	Country	Number of Patients	Population Characteristics[e]	
Lin MT, 2011[148]	2	Non-multidetector spiral CT	NR	NR	NR	5	No	2006	2	Taiwan	343	Age: 56 HBV: 57%	Male: 78% Cirrhosis: 47%
Liu, 2012[151]	2	8- or 16-row multidetector CT	4-5	Yes	Yes	3	Yes	2004	1	United States	24	Age: 53 HBV: 25%	Male: 83% Cirrhosis: 96%
Liu, 2013[150]	2	8-, 16-, or 64-row multidetector CT	4-5	Yes	Yes	3	Yes	2004	1	United States	24	Age: 53 HBV: 25%	Male: 83% Cirrhosis: NR
Lu CH, 2010[153]	2, 5	64-row multidetector CT	2.5-3	Yes	NR	NR	No	2006	1	Taiwan	57	Age: 51 HBV: NR	Male: 89% Cirrhosis: NR
Luca, 2010[154]	2, 5	16 or 64 row multidetector CT	5	Yes	Yes	2.5	Yes	2004	1	Italy	125	Age: 55 HBV: 20%	Male: 72% Cirrhosis: 100%
Luo W, 2009 (2)[157]	3	16-row multidetector CT	3	Yes	Yes	5	Yes	2007	2	Japan	152	Age: 71 HBV: NR	Male: 55% Cirrhosis: NR
Lv, 2011[160]	4	Spectral CT	3-4	No	NA	0.625 (collimation)	No	2010	4	China	49	Age: 53 HBV: NR	Male: 80% Cirrhosis: 18%
Lv, 2012[159]	2	Non-multidetector spiral CT with spectral mode	3-4	No	NA	1.25	No	2011	4	China	27	Age: 56 HBV: NR	Male: 81% Cirrhosis: 19%
Maetani, 2008[161]	2	8-row multidetector CT	2-3	Yes	No	2 (collimation)	No	2003	1	Japan	41	Age: 55 HBV: 32%	Male: 68% Cirrhosis: 100%
Marin, 2009[162]	2	64-row multidetector CT	5	Yes	Yes	3	Yes	2006	4	Italy	71	Age: 65 HBV: 25%	Male: 85% Cirrhosis: 100%
Marin, 2009 (2)[163]	2	64-row multidetector CT	5	Yes	Yes	3	Yes	2005	4	Italy	36	Age: 66 HBV: 29%	Male: 75% Cirrhosis: NR
Mita, 2010[166]	3	Non-multidetector spiral CT	3	Yes	No	5 (collimation)	No	2008	2	Japan	29	Age: 70 HBV: 3.4	Male: 45% Cirrhosis: 100%
Monzawa, 2007[168]	2	Non-multidetector spiral CT	4	Yes	Yes	5	No	1996	2	Japan	98	Age: 66 for cases, 61 for controls Male: 67% for cases, 59% for controls HBV: NR	Male: 66 for cases, 61 for controls Cirrhosis: 100%
Moriyasu, 2009[170]	3	Non-multidetector or multidetector CT, rows NR	NR	NR	NR	mean 6.9 (range 2-10 mm across centers)	No	2006	4	Japan	190	Age: 63 HBV: NR	Male: 67% Cirrhosis: NR
Mortele, 2001[171]	2	Non-multidetector spiral CT	2-4	No	NA	5 (collimation)	No	1991	1	Belgium	53	Age: 56 HBV: 11%	Male: 53% Cirrhosis: 100%
Murakami, 2001[174]	2	8-row multidetector CT	5	No	NA	5	No	1998	4	Japan	51	NR	
Murakami, 2003[173]	2	16-row multidetector CT	4	No	NA	5	No	2000	4	Japan	49	Age: 66 HBV: NR	Male: 63% Cirrhosis: NR

Author, Year	Reason for CT Imaging[a]	Scanner Type	Contrast Rate (ml/s)	Delayed Phase?	Delayed Phase Timing ≥120 s[b]	Section Thickness (mm)	Did Study Meet All Imaging Criteria?[c]	Imaging Start Date	Reference Standard[d]	Country	Number of Patients	Population Characteristics[e]	
Numata, 2014[181]	2	16- or 80-row multidetector CT	3	Yes	180	5	Yes	2010	2	Japan	43	Age: 70 HBV: 9.3%	Male: 65% Cirrhosis: 100%
Nagaoka, 2006[175]	5	NR	NR	NR	NR	NR	No	2004	3	Japan	21	Age (median): 64 Male: 76% HBV: 19%	Cirrhosis: NR
Nakamura, 2000[177]	2	Non-multidetector spiral CT	3	Yes	Yes	10	No	1997	3	Japan	30	Age: 63 HBV: NR	Male: 97% Cirrhosis: 83%
Nakamura, 2013[176]	2	16- or 64-row multidetector CT	NR	Yes	Yes	5	No	2008	1	Japan	11	Age: 69 HBV: 9.1%	Male: 73% Cirrhosis: 100%
Nakayama, 2001[178]	2	Non-multidetector spiral CT	3	No	NA	7-10 (collimation)	No	1993	4	Japan	69	Age: 64 HBV: NR Note: describes entire sample, not limited to those who underwent CT	Male: 74% Cirrhosis: NR
Noguchi, 2002[180]	2	4-row multidetector spiral CT	5	Yes	Yes	5	No	1999	4	Japan	29	Age: 64 HBV: NR	Male: 90% Cirrhosis: NR
Noguchi, 2003[179]	2	Non-multidetector spiral CT	5	Yes	Yes	5	No	2000	4	Japan	53	Age: 63 HBV: NR	Male: 68% Cirrhosis: 100%
Onishi, 2012[182]	2	8- or 64-row multidetector CT	3-5	Yes	Yes	5	Yes	2008	4	Japan	31	Age: 70 HBV: 13%	Male: 90% Cirrhosis: NR
Park, 2011[187]	2	Dual source 64-row multidetector CT	NR	No	NA	1.2 (collimation)	No	2008	1	South Korea	42	Age: 50 HBV: 64%	Male: 42% Cirrhosis: NR
Peterson, 2000[194]	2	Non-multidetector spiral CT	2.5-5	No	NA	7 (collimation)	No	1993	1	United States	59	Age: 57 HBV: 6.8%	Male: 69% Cirrhosis: 100%
Pitton, 2009[197]	2	64-row multidetector CT	5	No	NA	5	No	2006	4	Germany	28	Age: 67 years Male: 89% HBV: NR	Cirrhosis: NR
Pozzi Mucelli, 2006[198]	2	4-row multidetector CT	5	No	NA	5	No	2003	4	Italy	50	Age: 68 HBV: 24%	Male: 64% Cirrhosis: NR
Pugacheva, 2011[199]	2	64-row multidetector CT	3	Yes	Yes	2.5	Yes	2006	4	Japan	38 patients (only 30 underwent CT or MRI)	Age: 69 HBV: 7.9%	Male: 75% Cirrhosis: NR
Quaia, 2009[200]	3	64-row multidetector CT	5	Yes	Yes	0.3	Yes	2009	2	Italy	106	Age: 70 HBV: 80%	Male: 64% Cirrhosis: 100%
Rizvi, 2006[205]	2	NR	NR	NR	NR	NR	No	1995	1	United States	21	Age: 50 HBV: 4.8%	Male: 62% Cirrhosis: NR

Author, Year	Reason for CT Imaging[a]	Scanner Type	Contrast Rate (ml/s)	Delayed Phase?	Delayed Phase Timing >120 s[b]	Section Thickness (mm)	Did Study Meet All Imaging Criteria?[c]	Imaging Start Date	Reference Standard[d]	Country	Number of Patients	Population Characteristics[e]
Rode, 2001[206]	2	Non-multidetector spiral CT	4	No	NA	5	No	1996	1	France	43	Age: 51 HBV: 9.3%	Male: 70% Cirrhosis: 100%
Ronzoni, 2007[207]	2, 5	Multidetector, rows NR	3.4-4	Yes	Yes	3	No	2003	1	Italy	88	Age: 51 HBV: NR	Male: 80% Cirrhosis: NR
Sangiovanni, 2010[208]	3	64-row multidetector CT	4	Yes	Yes	2.5	Yes	2006	2	Italy	64	Age: NR HBV: NR	Male: NR Cirrhosis:100%
Sano, 2011[209]	2	16-row multidetector CT	2.6-5	Yes	Yes	5	No	2008	2	Japan	64	Age: 66 HBV: NR	Male: 73% Cirrhosis: NR
Schima, 2006[210]	2	4-, 8-, or 16-row multidetector CT	3	Yes	Yes	2.5-3	No	2003	4	6 European countries	97	Age: 64 HBV: 10%	Male: 81% Cirrhosis: 71%
Seitz, 2009[212]	3	Non-multidetector spiral CT (n=54) or ≥4-row multidetector CT (n=213)	≥3	No	NA	≤5	No	2004	4	Germany	267	Age: 60 HBV: NR	Male: 45 Cirrhosis: NR
Serste, 2012[214]	3	Multidetector CT, rows NR	NR	Yes	NR	NR	No	2005	2	France	74	Age: 60 HBV: 27%	Male: 78% Cirrhosis: 82%
Shah SA, 2006 (2)[215]	5	NR	NR	NR	NR	NR	No	NR	1	Canada	118	Age: NR HBV: 19%	Male: 80% Cirrhosis: NR
Singh, 2007[217]	1	Non-multidetector spiral CT	3	NR	NR	10 (collimation)	No	2005	2	United States	17	Age: 56 HBV: NR	Male: NR Cirrhosis: 100%
Sofue, 2011[218]	2	4-row multidetector CT	NR	Yes	Yes	10	No	2005	4	Japan	26	Age: 70 HBV: NR	Male: 81% Cirrhosis: 100%
Sun, 2010[225]	4	8-, 16-, or 64-row multidetector CT	3-5	Yes	Yes	2.5-3	Yes	2008	4	South Korea	69	Age: 56 HBV: 81%	Male: 82% Cirrhosis: 100%
Teefey, 2003[235]	2	Non-multidetector spiral CT	5	Yes	Yes	5	No	1996	2	United States	25	Age: 47 HBV: NR	Male: 65% Cirrhosis: 100%
Toyota, 2013[236]	2	64-row multidetector CT	NR	Yes	Yes	5	No	2008	2	Japan	50	Age: 69 HBV: 36%	Male: 64% Cirrhosis: NR
Trojan, 1999[237]	2	Non-multidetector spiral CT	NR	No	NA	NR	No	1996	2	Germany	14	Age: median 60 Male: 71% HBV: 21%	Cirrhosis: NR
Valls, 2004[239]	2, 5	Non-multidetector spiral CT	5	Yes	Yes	5 (collimation)	No	1995	1	Spain	85	Age: 55 HBV: 7.1%	Male: 65% Cirrhosis: 100%
Van Thiel, 2004[240]	1	Non-multidetector spiral CT	NR	NR	NR	NR	No	1998	1	United States	100	Age: 52 HBV: 2%	Male: 68% Cirrhosis: NR

Author, Year	Reason for CT Imaging[a]	Scanner Type	Contrast Rate (ml/s)	Delayed Phase?	Delayed Phase Timing ≥120 s[b]	Section Thickness (mm)	Did Study Meet All Imaging Criteria?[c]	Imaging Start Date	Reference Standard[d]	Country	Number of Patients	Population Characteristics[e]
Wagnetz, 2011[243]	2	64-row multidetector CT	5	No	NA	3	No	2005	2	Canada	292	Age: 60 HBV: NR Male: 38% Cirrhosis: NR
Xiao, 2005[249]	2	16-row multidetector CT	3	Yes	Yes	1.25	Yes	NR	4	China	56	Age: 56 HBV: NR Male: 66% Cirrhosis: NR
Yamamoto, 2002[255]	3	Non-multidetector spiral CT	3	No	NA	NR	No	NR	4	Japan	41	Age: 65 HBV: 2.4% Male: 54% Cirrhosis: 95%
Yan, 2002[256]	2	Non-multidetector spiral CT	3	Yes	Yes	NR	No	1996	4	China	53	Age: 61 HBV: NR Male: 79% Cirrhosis: NR
Yoo, 2013	2	64-row multidetector CT	3	Yes	Yes	5	Yes	2009	1	Korea	33	Age: 53 HBV: NR Male: 82% Cirrhosis: 100%
Yu, 2011[265]	2	Non-multidetector spiral CT or 4-, 16-, or 64-row multidetector CT	2-3	No	NA	7-7 (single, 4-row), 5 (16-, 64-row)	No	1999	1	United States	638	Age: 53 HBV: 10% Male: 64% Cirrhosis: NR
Yu, 2013[262]	4	64-row multidetector CT with spectral imaging mode	3-4	No	NA	0.625 (collimation)	No	2010	2	China	58	Age (median): 45 Male: 64% HBV: NR Cirrhosis: 24%
Yu, 2013 (2)[263]	4	64-row multidetector CT with spectral imaging mode	3-4	No	NA	0.625 (collimation)	No	2010	2	China	53	Age: 52 HBV: NR Male: 70% Cirrhosis: 29%
Yukisawa, 2007[269]	2	16-row multidetector CT	3	Yes	Yes	5	Yes	2004	4	Japan	25	Age: mean NR, range 53 to 76 Male: 76% HBV: NR Cirrhosis: 100%
Zacherl, 2002[270]	2, 5	Non-multidetector spiral CT	5	No	NA	5 (collimation)	No	1998	1	Austria	23	Age: 57 HBV: 17% Male: 87% Cirrhosis: 91%
Zhao, 2003[273]	2	4-row multidetector CT	3	No	NA	6.5	No	2001	4	China	75	Age: 49 HBV: NR Male: 89% Cirrhosis: NR
Zhao, 2004[272]	2	Multidetector CT, rows NR	3	No	NA	6.5	No	2001	4	China	40	Age: 49 HBV: NR Male: 85% Cirrhosis: NR
Zhao, 2007[271]	2	Multidetector CT, rows NR	3	No	NA	2.5	No	2002	4	China	24	Age: 56 HBV: NR Male: 78% Cirrhosis: 100% Note: describes entire sample, not limited to those in analysis
Zheng, 2005[274]	2	16-row multidetector CT	3	No	NA	NR	No	2003	4	China	28	Age: 49 HBV: NR Male: 86% Cirrhosis: NR
Zhou, 2002[275]	2	Non-multidetector spiral CT	3-4	No	NA	5-10 (collimation)	No	1995	2	China	49	Age: mean NR, range 21 to 75 Male: 90% HBV: NR Cirrhosis: NR

CT = computed tomography; HBV = hepatitis B virus; NA = not applicable; NR = not reported; s = second

[a] Reason for CT imaging key: 1=surveillance; 2=detection rate in patients undergoing surgery or with known HCC; 3=evaluation/characterization of liver mass; 4=differentiation between HCC and another type of lesion; 5=staging
[b] Delayed phase reported as time after contrast injection
[c] Imaging criteria = multidetector CT >8 rows; contrast rate >3 ml/s; delayed phase; timing of delayed phase >120 s after contrast injection; slice thickness <5 mm
[d] Reference standard key: 1=explanted livers only, 2=histological specimen (may include some explanted livers), 3=imaging and clinical criteria, 4=mixed histological and imaging/clinical criteria
[e] Age reported as mean (years), unless otherwise noted

Appendix F. Evidence Table: Diagnostic Accuracy Studies of Magnetic Resonance Imaging

Table F1. Characteristics of diagnostic accuracy studies of magnetic resonance imaging

Author, Year	Reason for MRI Imaging[a]	Scanner Type	Contrast, Rate	Delayed Phase?	Delayed Phase Timing >120 s[b]	Section Thickness (mm)	Did Study Meet All Imaging Criteria?[c]	Imaging Start Date	Reference Standard[d]	Country	Number of Patients	Population Characteristics[e]
Ahn, 2010[2]	2	1.5 T or 3 T	Gadoxetate disodium, rapid bolus	Yes	Yes	2	Yes	2007	4	South Korea	59	Age: 57, HBV: 76%, Male: 85%, Cirrhosis: 93%
Akai, 2011[3]	2	1.5 T	Gadoxetic acid disodium, rapid bolus	Yes	Yes	5	Yes	2008	1	Japan	34	Age: 65, HBV: NR, Male: 79%, Cirrhosis: NR
Alaboudy, 2011[4]	2	1.5 T or 3T	Gadoxetic acid disodium, 2 ml/s	Yes	Yes	NR	No	2008	2	Japan	32	Age: 68 years, HBV: 22%, Male: 72%, Cirrhosis: NR
An, 2012[6]	2	3.0 T	Gadoxetic acid disodium, 2 ml/s	Yes	Yes	2.5	Yes	2009	2	South Korea	175	Age: 57, HBV: 77%, Male: 79%, Cirrhosis: NR
An, 2013[5]	2	3.0 T	Gadoxetic acid disodium, 1-2 ml/s	No	NA	2.5	No	2008	2	South Korea	86	Age: 57, HBV: 87%, Male: 80%, Cirrhosis: 76%
Baek, 2012[8]	2	3 T	Gadoxetic acid disodium, 2 ml/s	Yes	Yes	2	Yes	2008	4	South Korea	51	Age: NR, range 32-80, Male: 84%, HBV: 80%, Cirrhosis: 100%
Baird, 2013[9]	2	1.5 T	Gadoxetic acid, 2 ml/s	Yes	Yes	3	Yes	2006	1	Australia	30	Age: 51, HBV: 6.7%, Male: 77%, Cirrhosis: 100%
Burrel, 2003[13]	2, 5	1.5 T	Gadodiamide, 2 ml/s	Yes	NR	4-5	No	2000	1	Spain	29	Age: 56, HBV: NR, Male: 66%, Cirrhosis: 100%
Cereser, 2010[15]	2	1.5 T	Gadobenate dimeglumine, 2 ml/s	Yes	Yes	4	Yes	2005	2	Italy	33	Age: 64, HBV: 6%, Male: 82%, Cirrhosis: 100%
Choi, 2001 (2)[21]	2	1.5 T	Gadopentetate disodium, rate NR	Yes	Yes	6-8	No	1998	2	South Korea	33	Age: 54, HBV: 70%, Male: 73%, Cirrhosis: 67%
Choi, 2008[20]	2	1.5 T	Gadobenate dimeglumine, rate NR	Yes	Yes	2.5	Yes	2003	1	South Korea	47	Age: 49, HBV: 79%, Male: 60%, Cirrhosis: 100%
Chou, 2011[22]	3	1.5 T	Gadopentetate dimeglumine, rapid bolus	Yes	Yes	8	No	2004	2	Taiwan	21	Age: 62, HBV: 43%, Male: 62%, Cirrhosis: 100%
Chung, 2010[24]	3	3.0 T	Gadoxetic acid, 1 or 2 ml/s	Yes	NR	2 or 3	No	2008	4	South Korea	62	Age: 59, HBV: 50%, Male: 68%, Cirrhosis: 48%

Author, Year	Reason for MRI Imaging[a]	Scanner Type	Contrast, Rate	Delayed Phase?	Delayed Phase Timing ≥120 s[b]	Section Thickness (mm)	Did Study Meet All Imaging Criteria?[c]	Imaging Start Date	Reference Standard[d]	Country	Number of Patients	Population Characteristics	Population Characteristics[e]
Chung, 2011[23]	3	1.5 T	Gadopentetate dimeglumine, 2 ml/s	Yes	Yes	6	No	2007	4	South Korea	46	Age: 60 HBV: 76%	Male: 78% Cirrhosis: 100%
de Ledinghen, 2002[27]	2	1.5 T	Gadopentetate dimeglumine, rate NR	No	NA	8-10	No	1997	1	France	34	Age: 54 HBV: 8.8%	Male: 71% Cirrhosis: 100%
Di Martino, 2010[31]	2	1.5 T	Gadobenate dimeglumine, 2 ml/s	Yes	Yes	3	Yes	2007	4	Italy	140	Age: 59 HBV: NR	Male: 74% Cirrhosis: 100%
Di Martino, 2013[30]	2	1.5 T	Gadoxetic acid disodium, 2 ml/s	Yes	Yes	3	Yes	2007	4	Italy	58	Age: 63 HBV: 14%	Male: 67% Cirrhosis: 100%
Filippone, 2010[36]	4	1.5 T	Gadoxetic acid, 2 ml/s	Yes	Yes	3	Yes	2007	4	Italy	34	Age: 59 HBV: NR	Male: 79% Cirrhosis: NR
Forner, 2008[37]	3	1.5 T	Gadodiamide, 2 ml/s	Yes	Yes	3	Yes	2003	2	United States	89	Age: Median 65 HBV: 6.7%	Male: 60% Cirrhosis: 100%
Freeman, 2006[40]	2, 5	NR	NR	NR	NR	NR	No	2003	1	United States	789	Age: 56 HBV: NR	Male: 77% Cirrhosis: NR
Gatto, 2012[45]	3	1.5 T	Gadobenate, 2.5 ml/s	Yes	Yes	3.8	Yes	NR	2	Italy	25	Age: 68 HBV: 24%	Male: 80% Cirrhosis: 100%
Giorgio, 2007[46]	3	1.5 T	Gadobenate dimeglumine, 3 ml/s	Yes	No	4	No	2003	4	Italy	73	Age: 63 HBV: 4.1%	Male: 67% Cirrhosis: 100%
Golfieri, 2009[48]	3	1.5 T	Ferucarbotran and gadopentetate dimeglumine, 2 ml/s	Yes	Yes	4-5	Yes	2003	2	Italy	63	Age: 64 HBV: 35%	Male: 84% Cirrhosis: 100%
Goshima S, 2004[49]	3	1.5 T	Gadopentetate dimeglumine, rapid bolus	Yes	Yes	8	No	1998	4	Japan	8	Age: 71 HBV: NR	Male: 63% Cirrhosis: NR
Guo, 2012[51]	2	3 T	Gadodiamide, 3 ml/s	Yes	No	4.8-5	No	2009	4	China	46	Age: 56 HBV: 89%	Male: 82% Cirrhosis: 100%
Haradome, 2011[52]	2	1.5 T	Gadoxetic acid disodium, 1 ml/s	Yes	Yes	4	Yes	2008	2	Japan	75	Age: 55 HBV: 19%	Male: 80% Cirrhosis: 72%
Hardie, 2011[53]	2	1.5 T	No contrast	No	NA	8	No	2008	1	United States	37	Age: 57 HBV: NR	Male: 68% Cirrhosis: 100%
Hardie, 2011 (2)[54]	2	1.5 T	Gadopentetate dimeglumine	Yes	Yes	NR	No	2008	1	United States	37	Age: 57 HBV: NR	Male: 73% Cirrhosis: NR
Hardie, 2011 (3)[55]	2	1.5 T	No contrast	No	NA	6, 10	No	2008	1	United States	25	NR	

Author, Year	Reason for MRI Imaging[a]	Scanner Type	Contrast, Rate	Delayed Phase?	Delayed Phase Timing ≥120 s[b]	Section Thickness (mm)	Did Study Meet All Imaging Criteria?[c]	Imaging Start Date	Reference Standard[d]	Country	Number of Patients	Population Characteristics[e]
Hecht, 2006[57]	2	1.5 T	Gadopentetate dimeglumine, 2 ml/s	Yes	Yes	2-3	Yes	1999	1	United States	38	Age: 54 Male: 74% HBV: 10% Cirrhosis: 100%
Hidaka, 2013[58]	2	1.5 T	Gadoxetic acid disodium, 1.5 ml/s	Yes	Yes	NR	No	2008	1	Japan	11	Age: NR Male: NR HBV: 27% Cirrhosis: NR
Hirakawa, 2011[60]	2	1.5 T	Gadopentetate dimeglumine, rate NR	Yes	Yes	NR	No	1999	1	Japan	25	Age: 55 Male: 52% HBV: NR Cirrhosis: 100%
Hori, 1998[64]	2	1.5 T	Gadopentetate dimeglumine, 1 ml/s	Yes	Yes	7-8	No	1995	3	Japan	50	Age: 65 Male: 76% HBV: 10% Cirrhosis: NR
Hwang, 2012[65]	2	3.0 T	Gadoxetic acid disodium, rate NR	Yes	Yes	2	Yes	2008	4	South Korea	54	Age: NR, range 33 to 81 Male: 81% HBV: 70% Cirrhosis: NR
Iavarone, 2010[68]	2	1.5 T	Gadobenate dimeglumine, 2 ml/s	Yes	Yes	3	Yes	2006	2	Italy	59	Age: median 66 Male: 69% HBV: 12% Cirrhosis: 100%
Ichikawa, 2010[69]	2	1.5 T	Gadoxetic acid disodium, rate NR	Yes	Yes	5-10	No	2001	4	Japan	151	Age: 66 years Male: 72% HBV: NR Cirrhosis: 66%
Inoue, 2012[73]	2	1.5 T or 3 T	Gadoxetic acid disodium, 2 ml/s	Yes	Yes	3-5	Yes	2008	2	Japan	66	Age: 66 Male: 64% HBV: 30% Cirrhosis: 62%
Ito, 2004[76]	4	1.5 T	Gadopentetate dimeglumine, 3 ml/s	No	NA	10	No	2002	4	Japan	40	Age: 62 Male: 58% HBV: NR Cirrhosis: NR
Jeong, 1999[84]	4	1.5 T	Gadopentetate dimeglumine, rapid bolus	Yes	Yes	8-10	No	1996	4	South Korea	51	Age: 54 Male: 67% HBV: NR Cirrhosis: NR
Jeong, 2011[83]	2	1.5 T	Gadobenate dimeglumine, 2 ml/s	Yes	Yes	3	Yes	2006	4	South Korea	19	Age: 54 Male: NR HBV: NR Cirrhosis: 100%
Jin, 2013[85]	5	NR	Gadoxetic acid disodium, 2 ml/s	Yes	NR	5-8	No	2009	4	South Korea	104	Age: 55 Male: 84% HBV: 73% Cirrhosis: NR
Kakihara, 2013[86]	2	1.5 T	Gadoxetic acid, variable rate	Yes	Yes	4	Yes	2008	1	Japan	15	Age: Median 55 Male: 73% HBV: 27% Cirrhosis: 100%
Kamura T, 2002[87]	4	1.5 T	Gadopentetate dimeglumine or gadodiamide, rate NR	Yes	Yes	4-5	Yes	1996	4	Japan	NR	NR

Author, Year	Reason for MRI Imaging[a]	Scanner Type	Contrast, Rate	Delayed Phase?	Delayed Phase Timing ≥120 s[b]	Section Thickness (mm)	Did Study Meet All Imaging Criteria?[c]	Imaging Start Date	Reference Standard[d]	Country	Number of Patients	Population Characteristics[e]
Kawada, 2010[89]	2	3.0 T	Gadoxetic acid disodium, 2 ml/s	Yes	Yes	5	Yes	2008	2	Japan	13	Age: median 67 Male: 77% HBV: 7.7% Cirrhosis: NR
Khalili, 2011[92]	3	1.5 T	Gadobenate dimeglumine, 2 ml/s	Yes	Yes	NR	No	2006	4	Canada	84	Age: 58 Male: 63% HBV: 50% Cirrhosis: 100%
Kim AY, 2012[94]	2	3.0 T	Gadoxetic acid disodium, 1 ml/s	Yes	Yes	2	Yes	2009	4	South Korea	189	Age: 63 Male: 77% HBV: 90% Cirrhosis: 100%
Kim DJ, 2012[96]	3	1.5 T	Gadopentetate dimeglumine, 3 ml/s	Yes	Yes	5	Yes	2008	4	South Korea	65	Age: NR, range 37-82 Male: 80% HBV: 69% Cirrhosis: 100%
Kim MJ, 2012[98]	2	3.0 T	Gadoxetic acid disodium, 2 ml/s	Yes	Yes	2	Yes	2008	2	South Korea	50	Age: 54 Male: 80% HBV: 84% Cirrhosis: 84%
Kim SH, 2009[101]	2	3.0 T	Gadoxetic acid disodium, 2 ml/s	Yes	Yes	2	Yes	2007	2	South Korea	62	Age: 55 Male: 87% HBV: 85% Cirrhosis: 48%
Kim TK, 2011[106]	3	1.5 T	Gadobenate dimeglumine, 2 ml/s	Yes	Yes	5	Yes	2006	4	South Korea	96	Age: 58 Male: 60% HBV: 53% Cirrosis: NR
Kim YK, 2004[118]	2	1.5 T	Gadopentetate dimeglumine and ferucarbotran	Yes	Yes	3.5-4	Yes	2002	4	South Korea	27	Age: 54 Male: 63% HBV: NR Cirrhosis: NR
Kim YK, 2004 (2)[119]	1	1.5 T	Gadobenate dimeglumine	Yes	Yes	2.3	Yes	2001	4	South Korea	29	Age: 58 Male: 66% HBV: NR Cirrhosis: 100%
Kim YK, 2006[116]	2	1.5 T	Gadopentetate dimeglumine, rate NR	Yes	Yes	3.5-4	Yes	2003	4	South Korea	31	Age: 57 Male: 90% HBV: 97% Cirrhosis: 100%
Kim YK, 2007[115]	2	1.5 T	Gadobenate dimeglumine, rate NR and ferucarbotran	Yes	Yes	3.5-4	Yes	2004	4	South Korea	29	Age: 56 Male: 72% HBV: 100% Cirrhosis: 100%
Kim YK, 2008[113]	2	1.5 T	Gadobenate dimeglumine, 2 mL/s	Yes	Yes	3.5-4	Yes	2004	4	South Korea	115	Age: NR, range 40 to 74 Male: 77% HBV: 96% Cirrhosis: 100%
Kim YK, 2008 (2)[114]	2	1.5 T	Gadobutrol, 2 ml/s	Yes	Yes	3.5-4	Yes	2005	4	South Korea	23	Age: NR, range 40 to 74 Male: 83% HBV: 100% Cirrhosis: 100%
Kim YK, 2009 (2)[112]	2	1.5 T	Gadoxetic acid disodium solution, 2 ml/s	Yes	Yes	2.5-3	Yes	2007	4	South Korea	62	Age: NR Male: 81% HBV: 90% Cirrhosis: NR

Author, Year	Reason for MRI Imaging[a]	Scanner Type	Contrast, Rate	Delayed Phase?	Delayed Phase Timing >120 s[b]	Section Thickness (mm)	Did Study Meet All Imaging Criteria?[c]	Imaging Start Date	Reference Standard[d]	Country	Number of Patients	Population Characteristics[e]
Kim YK, 2010[109]	2	1.5 T	Gadoxetic acid disodium, 1 ml/s or gadopentetate dimeglumine, 2 ml/s, and ferucarbotran	Yes	Yes	2.5-3	Yes	2009	4	South Korea	41 patients 41 (100%) with HCC 56 HCC lesions	Age (mean): not reported, range 40 to 74 years Male: 76% Cirrhosis: NR
Kim YK, 2010 (2)[110]	2	1.5 T	Gadoxetic acid disodium, 2 ml/s	Yes	Yes	2.5-3	Yes	2007	4	South Korea	89	Age: NR, range 40 to 74 Male: 70% HBV: 93% Cirrhosis: NR
Kim YK, 2011[107]	2	1.5 T or 3.0 T	Gadoxetic acid, 1 ml/s	Yes	Yes	3	Yes	2009	4	South Korea	40	Age: 63 HBV: 95% Male: 70% Cirrhosis: 95%
Kim YK, 2011 (2)[108]	2	1.5 T	Gadoxetic acid, 1 ml/s	Yes	Yes	2.5-3	Yes	2009	4	South Korea	14	Age: NR HBV: 100% Male: 71% Cirrhosis: 100%
Kondo, 2005[121]	2	1.5 T	Gadopentetate dimeglumine, 3 ml/s	Yes	Yes	8	No	1998	2	Japan	49	Age: 62 HBV: NR Male: 69% Cirrhosis: 100% Note: describes entire sample, including those not included in analysis
Koushima, 2002[123]	2	1.5 T	No contrast	No	NA	NA	No	1998	4	Japan	29	Age: 63 for cases, NR for controls Male: 76% of cases, 50% of controls HBV: 14% Cirrhosis: 100%
Krinsky, 2001[125]	2	1.5 T	Gadopentetate dimeglumine, 2 ml/s	Yes	No	5-8	No	1995	1	United States	71	Age: 50 HBV: 13% Male: 59% Cirrhosis: 100%
Krinsky, 2002[124]	2	1.5 T	Gadopentetate dimeglumine, 2 ml/s	Yes	NR	NR	No	1995	1	United States	24	Age: 52 HBV: NR Male: NR Cirrhosis: 100%
Kumano, 2009[126]	2	1.5 T	Gadopentetate dimeglumine, 2 ml/s	No	NA	7	No	2002	4	Japan	28	Age: NR HBV: NR Male: 79% Cirrhosis: NR
Kwak, 2004[129]	2	1.5 T	Gadopentetate dimeglumine, rapid bolus and ferumoxides	Yes	Yes	6	No	2000	4	South Korea	24	Age: 52 HBV: 100% Male: 75% Cirrhosis: NR
Kwak, 2005[128]	2	1.5 T	Gadopentetate dimeglumine, 3 ml/s and ferumoxides	Yes	Yes	2.3	Yes	2002	4	South Korea	49	Age: 57 HBV: 100% Male: 80% Cirrhosis: 100%
Lauenstein, 2007[131]	2	1.5 T	Gadopentetate dimeglumine, 2 ml/s	Yes	Yes	2-3	Yes	2004	1	United States	115	Age: 54 HBV: 9% Male: 67% Cirrhosis: NR

Author, Year	Reason for MRI Imaging[a]	Scanner Type	Contrast, Rate	Delayed Phase?	Delayed Phase Timing ≥120 s[b]	Section Thickness (mm)	Did Study Meet All Imaging Criteria?[c]	Imaging Start Date	Reference Standard[d]	Country	Number of Patients	Population Characteristics[e]	
Lee CH, 2012[132]	2	3.0 T	Gadoxetic acid disodium, 1 ml/s	Yes	Yes	5	Yes	2008	4	South Korea	46	Age: 57 HBV: 80%	Male: 83% Cirrhosis: NR
Lee JY, 2010[137]	2	3.0 T	Gadoxetic acid disodium, 2 ml/s and ferucarbotran	Yes	Yes	2	Yes	2007	2	South Korea	27	Age: 54 HBV: 93%	Male: 78% Cirrhosis: 52%
Lee MH, 2011[138]	4	3.0 T	Gadoxetic acid disodium, 2 ml/s	Yes	Yes	2	Yes	2008	2	South Korea	66	Age: 59 HBV: 68%	Male: 77% Cirrhosis: 100%
Libbrecht, 2002[144]	2, 5	1.5 T	Gadopentetate dimeglumine or gadoterate meglumine, 1.5 to 2 ml/s	No	NA	8	No	2000	1	Belgium	49	Age: 53 HBV: 19%	Male: 65% Cirrhosis: 100%
Lin MT, 2011[148]	2	NR	NR	NR	NR	NR	No	2006	2	Taiwan	343	Age: 56 HBV: 57%	Male: 78% Cirrhosis: 47%
Lu CH, 2010[153]	2, 5	1.5 T	Gadopentetate dimeglumine, 1.6-1.8 ml/s	Yes	No	5	No	2006	1	Taiwan	57	Age: 51 HBV: NR	Male: 89% Cirrhosis: NR
Marin, 2009 (2)[163]	2	1.5 T	Gadobenate dimeglumine, 2 ml/s	Yes	Yes	5	Yes	2005	4	Italy	36	Age: 66 HBV: 29% Note: described entire sample, including those excluded from analysis	Male: 75% Cirrhosis: NR
Marrero, 2005[164]	3	1.5 T	Gadopentetate dimeglumine, rate NR	Yes	Yes	NR	No	2002	2	United States	94	Age: 56 years HBV: 11%	Male: 69% Cirrhosis: NR
Matsuo, 2001[165]	2	1.5 T	Gadopentetate dimeglumine, rate NR	Yes	Yes	8-10	No	1998	4	Japan	53	Age: 64 HBV: NR	Male: 75% Cirrhosis: 90%
Mori, 2005[169]	2	1.5 T	Gadodiamide, 2.5 ml/s	Yes	Yes	8-9	No	2002	4	Japan	31	Age: 68 HBV: NR	Male: 84% Cirrhosis: NR
Motosugi, 2010[172]	4	1.5 T	Gadoxetic acid disodium, 1 ml/s	Yes	Yes	NR	No	2008	4	Japan	80	Age: 69 HBV: 19%	Male: 69% Cirrhosis: NR
Nakamura, 2000[177]	2	1.5 T	NR	NR	NR	8	No	1997	3	Japan	30	Age: 63 HBV: NR	Male: 97% Cirrhosis: 83%
Nakamura, 2013[176]	2	1.5 T	Gadoxetic acid disodium, 2 ml/s	Yes	Yes	5	Yes	2008	1	Japan	11	Age: 69 HBV: 9%	Male: 73% Cirrhosis: 100%
Noguchi, 2003[179]	2	1.5 T	Gadopentetate dimeglumine, 2 ml/s	Yes	Yes	NR	No	NR	4	Japan	53	Age: 63 HBV: NR	Male: 68% Cirrhosis: 100%

Author, Year	Reason for MRI Imaging[a]	Scanner Type	Contrast, Rate	Delayed Phase?	Delayed Phase Timing ≥120 s[b]	Section Thickness (mm)	Did Study Meet All Imaging Criteria?[c]	Imaging Start Date	Reference Standard[d]	Country	Number of Patients	Population Characteristics[e]
Onishi, 2012[182]	2	1.5 T or 3.0 T	Gadoxetic acid disodium, 1 ml/s	Yes	Yes	4	Yes	2008	4	Japan	31	Age: 70 HBV: 13% Male: 90% Cirrhosis: NR
Ooka, 2013[184]	2	1.5 T	Gadoxetic acid disodium, 2 ml/s	Yes	Yes	6	No	2008	2	Japan	54	Age: 69 HBV: 20% Male: 74% Cirrhosis: NR
Park G, 2010[189]	2	1.5 T	Gadopentetate dimeglumine, 3 ml/s or Gadoxetic acid disodium, 3 ml/s	Yes	Yes	2.5-3	Yes	2008	4	South Korea	43	Age: NR, range 44 to 70 Male: 65% HBV: 98% Cirrhosis: NR
Park, 2010[188]	2	3.0 T	Gadoxetic acid disodium and gadobenate dimeglumine, 2 ml/s	Yes	Yes	2	Yes	2007	2	South Korea	18	Age: 53 HBV: 89% Male: 94% Cirrhosis: 67%
Park, 2012[186]	2	1.5 T	No contrast or gadopentetate dimeglumine, rate NR	Yes	NR	2-3	No	2005	1	United States	52	Age: 57 HBV: NR Male: NR Cirrhosis: 100%
Park MJ, 2013[185]	4	3.0 T	Gadoxetic acid, 1 ml/s	Yes	Yes	2	Yes	2010	2	Korea	148	Age: 55 HBV: NR Male: 70% Cirrhosis: NR
Pauleit, 2002[192]	2	1.5 T	Gadopentetate dimeglumine, 5 ml/s and ferumoxides	Yes	Yes	8-9	No	NR	4	Germany	43	Age: 60 HBV: 23% Male: 79% Cirrhosis: 63%
Petruzzi, 2013[195]	2	1.5 T or 3.0 T	NR	Yes	NR	NR	No	2009	1	United States	45	NR
Piana, 2011[196]	2	1.5 T	No contrast or gadoterate meglumine, 2 ml/s	Yes	Yes	NR	No	2004	4	France	91	Age: 63 HBV: 20% Male: 74% Cirrhosis: NR
Pitton, 2009[197]	2	1.5 T	Gadopentetate dimeglumine, 2 ml/s	Yes	Yes	4	Yes	2006	4	Germany	28	Age: 67 HBV: NR Male: 89% Cirrhosis: NR
Pugacheva, 2011[199]	2	1.5 T	Gadopentetate dimeglumine, rate NR	Yes	Yes	NR	No	2006	4	Japan	38 (30 underwent CT or MRI)	Age: 69 HBV: 7.9% Male: 75% Cirrhosis: NR
Rhee, 2012[202]	4	3.0 T	Gadoxetic acid disodium, 2 ml/s	Yes	Yes	2	Yes	2008	2	South Korea	34	Age: 57 HBV: 82% Male: 88% Cirrhosis: 97%

Author, Year	Reason for MRI Imaging[a]	Scanner Type	Contrast, Rate	Delayed Phase?	Delayed Phase Timing >120 s[b]	Section Thickness (mm)	Did Study Meet All Imaging Criteria?[c]	Imaging Start Date	Reference Standard[d]	Country	Number of Patients	Population Characteristics[e]
Rimola, 2012[204]	3	1.5 T	Gadodiamide, 2 ml/s	Yes	NR	2.5	No	2003	2	Spain	159	Age: 63 HBV: 14% Male: 58% Cirrhosis: 100%
Rode, 2001[206]	2	1.5 T	Gadopentetate dimeglumine, rapid bolus	Yes	NR	6-8	No	1996	1	France	43	Age: 51 HBV: 9.3% Male: 70% Cirrhosis: 100%
Sangiovanni, 2010[208]	3	1.5 T	Gadobenate dimeglumine, 2 ml/s	Yes	Yes	3	Yes	2006	2	Italy	64	Age: NR HBV: NR Male: NR Cirrhosis:100%
Sano, 2011[209]	2	1.5 T	Gadoxetic acid, 1 ml/s	Yes	Yes	5	Yes	2008	2	Japan	64	Age: 66 HBV: NR Male: 73% Cirrhosis: NR
Secil, 2008[211]	2	1.5 T with and without dynamic subtraction	Gadopentetate dimeglumine, rapid bolus	Yes	NR	NR	No	NR	4	Turkey	32	Age: NR HBV: NR Male: NR Cirrhosis: 100%
Seitz, 2010[213]	3	1.5 T	Gadopentetate dimeglumine, rate NR	No	NA	5-8	No	2004	4	Germany	269	Age: 53 HBV: NR Male: 41 Cirrhosis: NR
Serste, 2012[214]	3	1.5 T	NR	Yes	NR	NR	No	2005	2	France	74	Age: 60 HBV: 27% Male: 78% Cirrhosis: 82%
Simon, 2005[216]	2	1.5 T	Gadopentetate dimeglumine, rate NR	Yes	No	4.4	No	1999	4	Germany	25	Age: 60 HBV: NR Male: 84% Cirrhosis: 84%
Singh, 2007[217]	1	1.5 T	Gadopentetate dimeglumine, 3 ml/s	NR	NR	NR	No	2005	2	United States	17	Age: 56 HBV: NR Male: NR Cirrhosis: 100%
Sugimoto, 2012[221]	4	1.5 T	Gadoxetic acid disodium, rate NR	Yes	Yes	3	Yes	2008	2	Japan	66	Age: 69 HBV: 12% Male: 70% Cirrhosis: NR
Sugimoto (2) 2012[222]	2	1.5 T	Gadoxetic acid, 2 ml/s	Yes	Yes	3	Yes	2008	2	Japan	54	Age: 70 HBV: 5.6% Male: 54% Cirrhosis: NR
Suh, 2011[224]	3	3.0 T	Gadoxetic acid disodium, rapid bolus	Yes	Yes	2	Yes	2007	4	South Korea	48	Age: 56 HBV: NR Male: 62% Cirrhosis: NR
Sun, 2010[225]	4	3.0 T	Gadoxetic acid disodium, 1.5 ml/s	Yes	Yes	4.8	Yes	2008	4	South Korea	69	Age: 56 HBV: 81% Male: 82% Cirrhosis: 100%
Takahashi, 2013[228]	4	1.5 T	Gadoxetic acid, 1.0 ml/s	Yes	Yes	4	No	2008	2	Japan	56	Age: 66 HBV: 14% Male: 71% Cirrhosis: 79%
Tanaka, 2005[231]	2	1.5 T	Gadopentetate dimeglumine, rate NR	Yes	Yes	6-9	No	NR	4	Japan	31	Age: 67 HBV: NR Male: 65% Cirrhosis: NR

Author, Year	Reason for MRI Imaging[a]	Scanner Type	Contrast, Rate	Delayed Phase?	Delayed Phase Timing >120 s[b]	Section Thickness (mm)	Did Study Meet All Imaging Criteria?[c]	Imaging Start Date	Reference Standard[d]	Country	Number of Patients	Population Characteristics[e]
Tang, 1999[233]	2	1.5 T	Gadopentetate dimeglumine, rapid bolus	Yes	Yes	8	No	1997	4	Japan	53	Age: 63 HBV: NR Male: 60% Cirrhosis: NR
Tanimoto, 2002[234]	2	1.5 T	Gadopentetate dimeglumine, 1 ml/s	Yes	Yes	NR	No	1998	4	Japan	50	Age: 63 HBV: NR Male: NR Cirrhosis: 60%
Teefey, 2003[235]	2	1.5 T	Gadodiamide, 2 ml/s	Yes	Yes	8	No	1996	2	United States	25	Age: 47 HBV: NR Male: 65% Cirrhosis: 100%
Toyota, 2013[236]	2	1.5 T	Gadoxetic acid, 2 ml/s	Yes	Yes	2	Yes	2008	2	Japan	50	Age: 69 HBV: 36% Male: 64% Cirrhosis: NR
Tsurusaki, 2008[238]	2	1.5 T with and without SENSE, high vs. low spatial resolution	Gadopentetate dimeglumine at 2 ml/s	No	NA	4	No	NR	4	Japan	35	Age: 65 HBV: NR Male: 69% Cirrhosis: NR
Vandecaveye, 2009[241]	4	1.5 T	Gadobenate dimeglumine, rate NR	Yes	NR	4	No	NR	4	Belgium	55	Age: NR HBV: 13% Male: NR Cirrhosis: 100%
Wagnetz, 2011[243]	2	1.5 T	Gadodiamide or gadobutrol, rate NR	Yes	No	5	No	2005	2	Canada	292	Age: 60 HBV: NR Male: 38% Cirrhosis: NR
Xu, 2009[252]	2	1.5 T	Gadopentetate dimeglumine, 2 ml/s	Yes	Yes	7	No	2005	4	China	37	Age: 46 HBV: NR Male: 95% Cirrhosis: NR
Xu, 2010[251]	4	1.5 T	Gadopentetate dimeglumine, 2 ml/s	Yes	Yes	7	No	2007	2	China	54	Age: 48 HBV: 100% Male: 85% Cirrhosis: NR
Yan, 2002[256]	2	1.5 T	Gadopentetate dimeglumine, rate NR	Yes	Yes	NR	No	1996	4	China	53	Age: 61 HBV: NR Male: 79% Cirrhosis: NR
Yoo, 2013[257]	2	3.0 T	Gadoxetic acid, 2 ml/s	Yes	Yes	2.8	Yes	2009	2	Korea	33	Age: 53 HBV: NR Male: 82% Cirrhosis: 100%
Yoshioka, 2002[260]	2	1.5 T with and without SENSE	Gadodiamide, 2.5 ml/s	Yes	Yes	8-10	No	2000	4	Japan	40	Age: 62 HBV: NR Male: 80% Cirrhosis: NR
Youk, 2004[261]	3	1.5 T	Gadopentetate, rate NR	Yes	Yes	7	No	2000	4	Korea	46	Age: 62 HBV: NR Male: 85% Cirrhosis: NR
Yu, 2002[268]	4	1.5 T	Gadopentetate dimeglumine, 3 ml/s	Yes	Yes	NR	No	NR	4	South Korea	120	Age: NR HBV: 77% Male: NR Cirrhosis: NR

Author, Year	Reason for MRI Imaging[a]	Scanner Type	Contrast, Rate	Delayed Phase?	Delayed Phase Timing ≥120 s[b]	Section Thickness (mm)	Did Study Meet All Imaging Criteria?[c]	Imaging Start Date	Reference Standard[d]	Country	Number of Patients	Population Characteristics[e]
Yu, 2008[267]	2	1.5 T	Gadopentetate dimeglumine, 3 ml/s	Yes	Yes	8-10	No	2000	1	United States	53	Age: 57 Male: 74% HBV: 85% Cirrhosis: NR
Yu, 2009[266]	2	1.5 T	Gadopentetate dimeglumine, 3 ml/s and ferucarbotran	Yes	Yes	8-10	No	2003	1	United States	42	Age: NR, range 44 to 73 Male: 70% HBV: 69% Cirrhosis: 86%
Yu, 2011[265]	2	1.5 T	Gadodiamide, rate NR	Yes	NR	NR	No	1999	1	United States	638	Age: 53 Male: 64% HBV: 10% Cirrhosis: NR
Yu, 2013 (3)[264]	2	1.5 T (n=39) or 3.0 T (n=33)	Gadoxetic acid, 1-1.5 ml/s	Yes	Yes	3.5-6.0	No	2009	4	Korea	68	Age: 62 Male: 81% HBV: NR Cirrhosis: NR
Zhao, 2007[271]	2	1.5 T	Gadopentetate dimeglumine, rapid bolus	Yes	Yes	7	No	2002	4	China	24	Age: 56 Male: 78% HBV: NR Cirrhosis: 100% Note: describes entire sample, including those excluded from analysis

HBV = hepatitis B virus; MRI = magnetic resonance imaging; NA = not applicable; NR = not reported; s = second; T = tesla

[a] Reason for MRI imaging key: 1=surveillance; 2=detection rate in patients undergoing surgery or with known HCC; 3=evaluation/characterization of liver mass; 4=differentiation between HCC and another type of lesion; 5=staging
[b] Delayed phase reported as time after gadolinium contrast injection
[c] Imaging criteria = 3.0 T MRI; delayed phase (or hepatobiliary for gadobenate or gadoxetic acid contrast); timing of delayed phase >120 s after contrast injection; slice thickness <5 mm
[d] Reference standard key: 1=explanted livers only; 2=histological specimen (may include some explanted livers); 3=imaging and clinical criteria; 4=mixed histological and imaging/clinical criteria
[e] Age reported as mean (years), unless otherwise noted

Appendix G. Evidence Table: Diagnostic Accuracy Studies of Positron Emission Tomography Imaging

Table G1. Characteristics of diagnostic accuracy studies of positron emission tomography imaging

Author, Year	Reason for PET Imaging[a]	Scan Tracer	Imaging Start Date	Reference Standard[b]	Country	Sample Size	Population Characteristics[c]		
Chen, 2005[17]	1	FDG	2000	4	Taiwan	26	Age: 61	Male: 81%	HBV: NR	Cirrhosis: NR
Cheung, 2011[19]	2	FDG or ^{11}C-acetate	2004	2	China	58	Age: NR	Male: 84%	HBV: 81%	Cirrhosis: NR
Cheung, 2013[18]	2, 4	FDG and ^{11}C-acetate or FDG or ^{11}C-acetate	2004	2	China	43	Age: 60	Male: 79%	HBV: 7%	Cirrhosis: NR
Delbeke, 1998[28]	3	FDG	NR	2	United States	110	Age: 59	Male: 55%	HBV: NR	Cirrhosis: NR
Eckel, 2009[34]	2	^{18}F-fluorothymidine	NR	4	Germany	18	Age: 67	Male: 94%	HBV: NR	Cirrhosis: NR
Ho, 2003[61]	2	FDG and or ^{11}C-acetate or FDG	NR	4	China	57	Age: 60	Male: 65%	HBV: 70%	Cirrhosis: NR
Ho, 2007[62]	4	FDG or ^{11}C-acetate or FDG and ^{11}C-acetate	2002	4	China	121	Age: 59	Male: 79%	HBV: NR	Cirrhosis: NR
Hwang, 2009[66]	2	FDG or ^{11}C-acetate	2006	4	South Korea	13	Age: 51	Male: 85%	HBV: 67%	Cirrhosis: NR
Ijichi, 2013[71]	2	FDG	2010	2	Japan	53	Age: 65	Male: 62%	HBV: NR	Cirrhosis: NR
Jeng, 2003[81]	3	FDG	NR	2	Taiwan	48	Age: NR, range 40 to 65	Male: 58%	HBV: 100%	Cirrhosis: NR
Kawaoka, 2009[90]	4	FDG	2005	4	Japan	34	Age: 59	Male: 82%	HBV: 32%	Cirrhosis: NR
Khan, 2000[93]	2	FDG	1995	2	United States	20	Age: 60	Male: 75%	HBV: 18%	Cirrhosis: 75%
Kim YK, 2010 (3)[111]	1	FDG	2005	4	South Korea	10	Age: median 48	Male: 100%	HBV: 100%	Cirrhosis: NR
Lee JE, 2012[135]	4	FDG	2006	4	South Korea	138	Age: 69	Male: 83%	HBV: 64%	Cirrhosis: NR
Li, 2006[141]	2	^{11}C-acetate	NR	2	Austria	21	Age: 64	Male: 90%	HBV: NR	Cirrhosis: NR
Liangpunsakul, 2003[143]	2	FDG	2000	4	United States	8	Age: 53	Male: 50%	HBV: NR	Cirrhosis: 100%
Lin WY, 2005[149]	2	FDG	NR	4	Taiwan	12	Age: 64	Male: 83%	HBV: 19%	Cirrhosis: NR
Nagaoka, 2006[175]	4	FDG	2004	3	Japan	21	Age: median 64	Male: 76%	HBV: 80%	Cirrhosis: NR
Park JW, 2008[190]	2, 4	FDG or ^{11}C-acetate	2006	2	South Korea	99	Age: 58	Male: 79%	HBV: 2.6%	Cirrhosis: 79%
Sorensen, 2011[219]	2, 4	FDG	NR	4	Denmark	39	Age: 61	Male: 59%	HBV: NR	Cirrhosis: NR
Sugiyama, 2004[223]	4	FDG	2000	4	Japan	19	Age: 69	Male: 79%	HBV: NR	Cirrhosis: NR
Sun, 2009[226]	1	FDG	2007	4	Cjoma	25	Age: 52	Male: 84%	HBV: NR	Cirrhosis: NR
Talbot, 2006[230]	2	FDG or ^{18}F-fluorocholine	2005	4	France	12	Age: NR	Male: 75%	HBV: 8.3%	Cirrhosis: 75%
Talbot, 2010[229]	2	FDG or ^{18}F-fluorocholine	2005	4	France	59	NR			

Author, Year	Reason for PET Imaging[a]	Scan Tracer	Imaging Start Date	Reference Standard[b]	Country	Sample Size	Population Characteristics[c]		
Teefey, 2003[235]	2	FDG	1996	2	United States	25	Age: 47	Male: 65%	HBV: NR	Cirrhosis: 100%
Trojan, 1999[237]	2	FDG	1996	2	Germany	14	Age: median 60	Male: 71%	HBV: 21%	Cirrhosis: NR
Verhoef, 2002[242]	2	FDG	2002	2	The Netherlands	13	Age: 54	Male: 85%	HBV: 46%	Cirrhosis: 92%
Wolfort, 2010[246]	4	FDG	2000	2	United States	20	NR			
Wu, 2011[247]	2, 4	FDG or FDG and ¹¹C-choline	2007	4	China	76	Age: 56	Male: 84%	HBV: NR	Cirrhosis: 60%
Wudel, 2003[248]	1, 2	FDG	1993	4	United States	91	Age: 60	Male: 79%	HBV: NR	Cirrhosis: NR
Yamamoto, 2008[254]	2	FDG or ¹¹C-choline	2007	2	Japan	12	Age: 71	Male: 42%	HBV: 17%	Cirrhosis: NR
Yoon, 2007[259]	4	FDG	2002	3	South Korea	87	Age: median 54	Male: 78%	HBV: 79%	Cirrhosis: NR

FDG = ¹⁸F-fluorodeoxyglucose; HBV = hepatitis B virus; NA = not applicable; NR = not reported; PET = positron emission tomography

[a] Reason for PET imaging key: 1=recurrence; 2=detection rate in patients undergoing surgery or with known HCC; 3=evaluation/characterization of liver mass; 4=staging/detection of metastatic disease

[b] Reference standard key: 1=explanted livers only; 2=histological specimen (may include some explanted livers); 3=imaging and clinical criteria; 4=mixed histological and imaging/clinical criteria

[c] Age reported as mean (years), unless otherwise noted

Appendix H. Evidence Table: Patient Outcomes for Staging (Randomized Controlled Trials)

Table H1. Characteristics of randomized controlled trials of patient outcomes for staging

Author, Year	Imaging Tests Used for Screening	Details of Imaging Tests	Definition of a Positive Test on Imaging and Followup	Population Characteristics	Eligibility Criteria	Country, Setting	Number Approached, Eligible, Enrolled, Analyzed
Trinchet JC, 2011[277]	Ultrasound Note: AFP was assesed but after analyses, high rates of AFP observed in 2 groups precluded interpretation based on AFP randomization and analysis was restricted to ultrasound randomization	Technical details of ultrasound not reported	In cases of focal liver lesions, diagnostic procedure using contrast-enhanced imaging, serum AFP, and/or guided biopsy was performed according to EASL guidelines; HCC diagnosis based on histology, if lesion >2 cm in diameter then early arterial hypervascularization on 2 contrast-enhanced methods, or when there was an association between serum AFP >400 ng/mL plus early arterial hypervascularization on one contrast-enhanced method; in case of increased AFP with no focal liver lesion on ultrasound, CT scan was performed	Age (mean): 55 years Male: 69% Race: NR Alcoholic cirrhosis: 39% HCV-related cirrhosis: 44% HBV-related cirrhosis: 13% Hemochromatosis-related cirrhosis: 1.6% Cirrhosis due to other etiology: 2.5% Note: other etiology = nonalcoholic steatohepatitis, primary biliary cirrhosis, autoimmune hepatitis, cryptogenic cirrhosis	Patients >18 years with histologically proven cirrhosis due to either excessive alcohol consumption, chronic HCV or HBV, or hereditary hemochromatosis, with no complications from cirrhosis, patients with Child-Pugh class A or B and no focal liver lesion. Excluded patients with Child-Pugh class C, severe uncontrolled extrahepatic disease resulting in estimated life expectancy <1 year, co-infection with HIV	France and Belgium; Selected from clinical centers in a cooperative group that included specialized liver disease centers	Overall (3-month surveillance vs. 6-month surveillance) Number approached: NR Number eligible: 1340 Number enrolled: 1340 (668 vs. 672) Number analyzed: 1278 (640 vs. 638)
Wang JH, 2013[278]	Ultrasound	Technical details of ultrasound not reported	Newly detected hepatic nodule on ultrasound >1cm in diameter suspicious for HCC; referred to medical centers for further diagositic procedures; followup by public health nurses; final diagnosis based on histology, EASL imaging criteria, or AASLD imaging criteria	Age (mean): 65.2 years Male: 50% Race: NR HBV: 28% HCV: 65% HBV and HCV: 7% Liver cirrhosis: 32%	Patients >40 years with either positive HBsAg or anti-HCV and a platelet count <150 (x109)/l. Excluded those with history of hepatic malignancy.	Taiwan; Selected from health data for 10 townships	Overall (4-month surveillance vs. 12-month surveillance) Number approached: 28,722 Number eligible: 1581 (785 vs. 796) Number enrolled: 744 (387 vs. 357) Number analyzed: 744 (387 vs. 357)
Zhang BH, 2004[279]	Ultrasound (in conjunction with AFP)	Technical details of ultrasound not reported	Solid liver lesion on ultrasound or AFP >20 mcg/l; individuals with an initial positive test underwent retesting; individuals with a positive retest underwent additional diagnostic evaluation (history, physical exam, serum AFP, ultrasound by senior doctor, CT or MRI as required); final diagnosis based on histology or long-term	Age (mean): 41.5[a] years Male: 63% Race: NR HBsAg positive: 64% Hepatitis: 27% HBsAg positive and hepatitis: 9%	People aged 35 to 59 years with serum evidence of HBV infection or a history of chronic hepatitis without HBV infection (abnormal biochemistry ≥6 months). Excluded those with history of HCC, or other malignant	China; Selected from medical records of primary care centers	Overall (screening vs. control) Number approached: NR Number eligible: 19,200 (9757 vs. 9373) Number enrolled: 18,816 (9373 vs. 9443) Number

H-1

Author, Year	Imaging Tests Used for Screening	Details of Imaging Tests	Definition of a Positive Test on Imaging and Followup	Population Characteristics	Eligibility Criteria	Country, Setting	Number Approached, Eligible, Enrolled, Analyzed
			followup		diseases, or serious illness.		analyzed:18,816 (9373 vs. 9443)

Author, Year	Duration of Followup	Attrition	Interventions	Outcomes	Adverse Events/Harms	Sponsor	Risk of Bias
Trinchet JC, 2011[277]	Mean followup 47.1 months in 3-month surveillance group vs. 46.8 months in 6-month surveillance group	0.9% (12/1340) patients lost to followup; 11.9% (143/1278) of patients not compliant with protocol; 14.6% (86/638) in 6-month surveillance group, 9.4% (57/640) in 3-month surveillance group Note: the raw numbers do not exactly equal the reported proportions for compliance	A: Ultrasound every 3 months B: Ultrasound every 6 months	A vs. B Cases of HCC/ new focal liver lesion 53/183 (30%) vs. 70/155 (45%) 2 and 5-year cumulative incidence of HCC 4.0%, 10.0% vs. 2.7%, 12.3% Prevalence and cumulative incidence of HCC <30 mm 79%, 7.8% vs. 70%, 9.1% Survival rates for all patients At 2 years: 95.8% vs. 93.5% At 5 years: 84.9% vs. 85.8% Cases of HCC-related mortality 17/72 (23.6%) vs. 12/82 (14.6%) Note: all associations were NS	NR	French Ministry of Health; French Ligue de Recherche contre le Cancer	Moderate
Wang JH, 2013[278]	4 years; individuals in 4-month surveillance scanned mean 7.13+/-2.0 times and individuals in 12-month surveillance scanned mean 2.53+/-0.5 times	NR: 27.4% of 4-month surveillance group and 45.7% of 12-month surveillance group attended all exams (67.6% in 4-month surveillance group attended >6 exams, 73.1% in 12-month surveillance group attended >2 exams)	A: Ultrasound every 4 months B: Ultrasound every 12 months	A vs. B Cases of HCC/ new hepatic nodule 24/46 (52%) vs. 15/28 (54%), including 5 patients diagnosed outside of surveillance schedule in B 3-year cumulative incidence of HCC 11.7% vs. 9.7% 1-,2-, and 4- year cumulative survival rates for patients with HCC 95.8%, 78.8%, 57.4% vs. 80%, 64%, 56%	NR	National Scientific Council of Taiwan	Moderate
Zhang BH, 2004[279]	5 years; all individuals offered screening 5 to 10 times	NR; Screened group completed 58% of offered screening (median: 5 screens)	A: Serum AFP test and ultrasound every 6 months B: No screening, usual care	A vs. B Cases (incidence per 100,000) of HCC 86 (223.7) vs. 67 (163.1); rate ratio, 1.37 (95% CI 0.41 to 0.98); Cases (incidence per 100,000) of HCC-associated death 32 (83.2) vs. 54 (131.5); rate ratio, 0.63 (95% CI 0.41 to 0.98)	NR	NR	High

AASLD = American Association for the Study of Liver Disease; AFP = alphafetoprotein; CT = computed tomography; EASL = European Association for the Study of the Liver; HBV = hepatitis B virus; HBsAg = hepatitis B surface antigen; HBsAb = antibody to hepatitis B surface antigen; HBcAb = antibody to hepatitis B core antigen; HBeAg = hepatitis B e antigen; HBeAb = antibody to hepatitis B e antigen; HCC = hepatocellular cancer; NR = not reported; NS = not significant
a Calculated

Appendix I. Evidence Table: Comparative Effectiveness of Imaging Strategies on Clinical Decisionmaking and Patient Outcomes (Cohort Studies)

Table I1. Characteristics of cohort studies of effectiveness of imaging strategies on clinical decisionmaking and patient outcomes

Author, Year	Imaging Tests Evaluated	Details of Imaging Tests	Definition of a Positive Test on Imaging and Followup	Population Characteristics	Eligibility Criteria	Country, Setting	Number Approached, Eligible, Enrolled, Analyzed
Chen MH, 2007[280]	A: CEUS B: Conventional US in control group plus contrast-enhanced CT or MRI within one week of RFA	Contrast-enhanced US Operator: Performed by 3 experienced sonographers Contrast: sulfur hexafluoride (Sonovue) administered as 2.4 ml bolus over 2 to 3 s Transducer frequency: 2.5 to 5.0 MHz (3 systems used) Contrast-enhanced CT 64-slice spiral CT scanner used, other details NR; Images read by 3 experienced radiologists MRI 1.5 T MRI scanner, other details NR; Images read by 3 experienced radiologists	On CEUS, quick enhancement in arterial phase with fast washout in portal or parenchymal phase; repeat CEUS was done if first CEUS suspicious for new tumor; patients selected for RFA on basis of tumor size, number, position, and anatomic relationship with surrounding structures	Age (mean): 67.2[a] years Male: 62% Race: NR	Patients with HCC diagnosed on imaging or histology	China; enrolled patients, source not reported	18 to 50 months
Chen MH, 2007 (2)[281]	A: CEUS plus contrast (n=81) B: Ultrasound without contrast plus CT (n=86)	Contrast-enhanced US Operator: 2 radiologists with experience in interventional US and CEUS Contrast: sulfur hexaflouride (Sonovue) suspension (2.4 ml) administered through by bolus injection in 1-3 s Transducer frequency: approximately 2.5-5 MHz. MI used in CEUS imaging: 0.04 to 0.1. Contrast-enhanced CT Technical information not reported	RFA was considered successful if no arterial and portal enhancement was seen in and around the tumor; ultrasound guided biopsy was performed to confirm the pathology of recurrent or new lesions; complete necrosis was defined by CECT examination as the absence of viable tissue in the treated tumor upon 1 year follow-up	Age (mean): 60.2[a] years Male: 82% Race: NR	Patients with HCC meeting 5 criteria: no more than four lesions; tumor diameter less than 8 cm; nothrombosis in the main branch of the portal vein and no extrahepatic metastases; prothrombin time ratio greater than 50% of normal and platelet count greater than	China Setting: Not reported Duration of follow-up: 1 year	Number approached and eligible: Not reported Number enrolled and analyzed: 167 (81 vs. 86)

I-1

Author, Year	Comparison Groups	Adjusted Variables for Statistical Analysis	Outcomes		Adverse Events	Funding Source	Risk of Bias
				50,000/ml; biopsy proof of malignancy for at least one hepatic lesion			
Chen MH, 2007[280]	Screening: CEUS plus contrast-enhanced CT (n=81) or MRI (n=11) Control: conventional ultrasound plus contrast-enhanced CT (n=74) or MRI (n=13)	No adjustments	Screening vs. control Local tumor progression rate, % (n) 7.2 (6/83) vs. 18.3 (15/82); p=0.033; RR[a], 0.40 (95% CI 0.16 to 0.87) New HCC rate, % (n) 15.7 (13/83) vs. 35.4 (29/82); p=0.004; RR[a], 0.44 (95% CI 0.25 to 0.79) Mean local progression-free survival (months) 40.5 (SD 1.9) vs. 33.3 (2.2); p=0.015 New tumor-free survival (months) 38.1 (SD 2.0) vs. 26.4 (SD 2.0); p<0.001		Not reported for screening	NR	High
Chen MH, 2007 (2)[281]	A: CEUS plus contrast (n=81) B: Ultrasound without contrast plus CT (n=86)	NR	CEUS vs. US without contrast Detection rates for small (≤2 cm) HCC lesions , % (n) 94.7 vs. 81.6: p=0.001 (36 vs. 31) Complete tumor necrosis rate 1 year after RFA: 92%(106/115) vs. 83% (93/112 lesions), p=0.036		None reported	NR	High

CT = computed tomography; HCC = hepatocellular cancer; MRI = magnetic resonance imaging; NR = not reported; RFA = radiofrequency ablation; US = ultrasound
[a] Calculated

Appendix J. Strength of Evidence

Key Question 1. Surveillance

Table J1. Key Question 1a: Test performance

	Imaging Modality or Comparison	Number of Studies	Risk of Bias (Low, Moderate, High)	Consistency (Consistent or Inconsistent)	Directness (Direct or Indirect)	Precision (Precise or Imprecise)	Number of Subjects/Lesions	Strength of Evidence (High, Moderate, Low, Insufficient)
Surveillance settings *Unit of analysis: patients with HCC*	US without contrast	Sens: 4 Spec: 3	Moderate	Inconsistent	Indirect	Imprecise	Sens: 540 Spec: 488	Sens: Low Spec: Low
Surveillance settings *Unit of analysis: patients with HCC*	CT	Sens: 2 Spec: 2	Moderate	Consistent	Indirect	Imprecise	Sens: 385 Spec: 385	Sens: Low Spec: Low
Surveillance settings *Unit of analysis: patients with HCC*	MRI or PET	No evidence	--	--	--	--	--	Insufficient
Surveillance settings *Unit of analysis: HCC lesions*	US without contrast	Sens: 1 Spec: 0	Moderate	Sens: Inconsistent Spec: No studies	Indirect	Sens: Imprecise Spec: No studies	Sens: 42 Spec: --	Sens: Low Spec: Insufficient
Surveillance settings *Unit of analysis: HCC lesions*	CT	Sens: 1 Spec: 0	Moderate	Sens: Single study Spec: No studies	Indirect	Sens: Imprecise Spec: No studies	Sens: 42 Spec: --	Sens: Low Spec: Insufficient
Surveillance settings *Unit of analysis: HCC lesions*	MRI or PET	No evidence	--	--	--	--	--	Insufficient
Nonsurveillance settings *Unit of analysis: patients with HCC*	US without contrast	Sens: 8 Spec: 6	Moderate	Inconsistent	Indirect	Imprecise	Sens: 975 Spec: 858	Sens: Low Spec: Low

	Imaging Modality or Comparison	Number of Studies	Risk of Bias (Low, Moderate, High)	Consistency (Consistent or Inconsistent)	Directness (Direct or Indirect)	Precision (Precise or Imprecise)	Number of Subjects/Lesions	Strength of Evidence (High, Moderate, Low, Insufficient)
Nonsurveillance settings *Unit of analysis: patients with HCC*	CT	Sens: 16 Spec: 11	Moderate	Inconsistent	Indirect	Precise	Sens: 1277 Spec: 1095	Sens: Moderate Spec: Moderate
Nonsurveillance settings *Unit of analysis: patients with HCC*	MRI	Sens: 10 Spec: 8	Moderate	Inconsistent	Indirect	Precise	Sens: 1066 Spec: 974	Sens: Moderate Spec: Moderate
Nonsurveillance settings *Unit of analysis: patients with HCC*	PET	Sens: 15 Spec: 5	Moderate	Inconsistent	Indirect	Sens: Precise Spec: Imprecise	Sens: 559 Spec: 144	Sens: Moderate Spec: Low
Nonsurveillance settings *Unit of analysis: HCC lesions*	US without contrast	Sens: 11 Spec: 2	Moderate	Inconsistent	Indirect	Sens: Precise Spec: Imprecise	Sens: 1996 Spec: 323	Sens: Moderate Spec: Low
Nonsurveillance settings *Unit of analysis: HCC lesions*	US with contrast	Sens: 8 Spec: 0	Moderate	Sens: Inconsistent Spec: No studies	Indirect	Sens: Imprecise Spec: No studies	Sens: 374 Spec: ---	Sens: Low Spec: Insufficient
Nonsurveillance settings *Unit of analysis: HCC lesions*	CT	Sens: 79 Spec: 21	Moderate	Inconsistent	Indirect	Precise	Sens: 8090 Spec: 2893	Sens: Moderate Spec: Moderate
Nonsurveillance settings *Unit of analysis: HCC lesions*	MRI	Sens: 75 Spec: 16	Moderate	Inconsistent	Indirect	Precise	Sens: 6664 Spec: 1984	Sens: Moderate Spec: Moderate
Nonsurveillance settings *Unit of analysis: HCC lesions*	PET	Sens: 9 Spec: 1	Moderate	Sens: Inconsistent Spec: Single study	Indirect	Sens: Precise Spec: Imprecise	Sens: 674 Spec: 104	Sens: Moderate Spec: Low

	Imaging Modality or Comparison	Number of Studies	Risk of Bias (Low, Moderate, High)	Consistency (Consistent or Inconsistent)	Directness (Direct or Indirect)	Precision (Precise or Imprecise)	Number of Subjects/Lesions	Strength of Evidence (High, Moderate, Low, Insufficient)
Direct (within-study) comparisons of imaging modalities *Unit of analysis: patients with HCC*	US without contrast vs. CT	Sens: 6 Spec: 5	Moderate	Inconsistent	Direct	Precise	Sens: 899 (US) Sens: 838 (CT) Spec: 885 (US) Spec: 824 (CT)	Sens: Moderate Spec: Moderate For the 2 studies in surveillance settings, the strength of evidence is low for sensitivity and specificity.
Direct (within-study) comparisons of imaging modalities *Unit of analysis: patients with HCC*	US without contrast vs. MRI	Sens: 3 Spec: 3	Moderate	Consistent	Direct	Precise	Sens: 712 (US) Sens: 712 (MRI) Spec: 712 (US) Spec: 712 (MRI)	Sens: Moderate Spec: Moderate
Direct (within-study) comparisons of imaging modalities *Unit of analysis: patients with HCC*	MRI vs. CT	Sens: 4 Spec: 4	Moderate	Inconsistent	Direct	Precise	Sens: 318 (MRI) Sens: 484 (CT) Spec: 318 (MRI) Spec: 484 (CT)	Sens: Moderate Spec: Moderate
Direct (within-study) comparisons of imaging modalities *Unit of analysis: HCC lesions*	US without contrast vs. CT	Sens: 3 Spec: 2	Moderate	Inconsistent	Direct	Precise	Sens: 535 (US) Sens: 539 (CT) Spec: 323 (US) Spec: 323 (CT)	Sens: Moderate Spec: Moderate
Direct (within-study) comparisons of imaging modalities *Unit of analysis: HCC lesions*	US without contrast vs. MRI	Sens: 3 Spec: 2	Moderate	Consistent	Direct	Precise	Sens: 660 (US) Sens: 660 (MRI) Spec: 323 (US) Spec: 323 (MRI)	Sens: Moderate Spec: Moderate

	Imaging Modality or Comparison	Number of Studies	Risk of Bias (Low, Moderate, High)	Consistency (Consistent or Inconsistent)	Directness (Direct or Indirect)	Precision (Precise or Imprecise)	Number of Subjects/Lesions	Strength of Evidence (High, Moderate, Low, Insufficient)
Direct (within-study) comparisons of imaging modalities *Unit of analysis: HCC lesions*	US with contrast vs. CT	Sens: 4 Spec: 0	Moderate	Sens: Inconsistent Spec: No studies	Direct	Sens: Precise Spec: No studies	Sens: 217 (US) Sens: 217 (CT) Spec: --	Sens: Moderate Spec: Insufficient
Direct (within-study) comparisons of imaging modalities *Unit of analysis: HCC lesions*	US with contrast vs. MRI	Sens: 3 Spec: 0	Moderate	Sens: Consistent Spec: No studies	Direct	Sens: Imprecise Spec: No studies	Sens: 172 (US) Sens: 170 (MRI) Spec: --	Sens: Moderate Spec: Insufficient
Direct (within-study) comparisons of imaging modalities *Unit of analysis: HCC lesions*	MRI vs. CT	Sens: 31 Spec: 7	Moderate	Inconsistent	Direct	Precise	Sens: 2947 (MRI) Sens: 3233 (CT) Spec: 819 (MRI) Spec: 787 (CT)	Sens: Moderate Spec: Moderate
Multiple imaging modalities	Various combinations	Sens: 2 Spec: --	Moderate	Sens: Inconsistent Spec: No studies	Indirect	Sens: Imprecise Spec: No studies	Sens: 112 Spec: --	Sens: Insufficient Spec: Insufficient

Table J2. Key Question 1a.i: Effects of reference standard on test performance (based on HCC lesions as the unit of analysis)

Imaging Modality or Comparison	Number of Studies	Risk of Bias (Low, Moderate, High)	Consistency (Consistent or Inconsistent)	Directness (Direct or Indirect)	Precision (Precise or Imprecise)	Number of Subjects/Lesions	Strength of Evidence (High, Moderate, Low, Insufficient)
US without contrast	Sens: 9 Spec: --	Moderate	Sens: Inconsistent Spec: No studies	Indirect	Sens: Precise Spec: No studies	Sens: 982 Spec: --	Sens: Moderate Spec: Insufficient
US with contrast	Sens: 5 Spec: --	Moderate	Sens: Inconsistent Spec: No studies	Indirect	Sens: Imprecise Spec: No studies	Sens: 315 Spec: --	Sens: Low Spec: Insufficient
CT	Sens: 72 Spec: 19	Moderate	Inconsistent	Indirect	Precise	Sens: 7094 Spec: 2528	Sens: Moderate Spec: Moderate
MRI	Sens: 63 Spec: 15	Moderate	Inconsistent	Indirect	Precise	Sens: 5688 Spec: 1732	Sens: Moderate Spec: Moderate
PET	Sens: 5 Spec: 0	Moderate	Sens: Inconsistent Spec: No studies	Indirect	Sens: Imprecise Spec: No studies	Sens: 169 Spec: --	Sens: Low Spec: Insufficient

Table J3. Key Question 1a.ii: Effects of patient, tumor, technical, and other factors on test performance

	Imaging Modality or Comparison	Number of Studies	Risk of Bias (Low, Moderate, High)	Consistency (Consistent or Inconsistent)	Directness (Direct or Indirect)	Precision (Precise or Imprecise)	Number of Subjects/Lesions	Strength of Evidence (High, Moderate, Low, Insufficient)
Lesion Size	US without contrast	Sens: 9 Spec: 2	Moderate	Inconsistent	Direct	Sens: Precise Spec: Imprecise	Sens: 1013 Spec: 323	Sens: Moderate Spec: Low
Lesion Size	US with contrast	Sens: 5 Spec: 1	Moderate	Sens: Inconsistent Spec: Single study	Direct	Imprecise	Sens: 553 Spec: 70	Sens: Low Spec: Low
Lesion Size	CT	Sens: 34 Spec: 4	Moderate	Inconsistent	Direct	Sens: Precise Spec: Imprecise	Sens: 3550 Spec: 596	Sens: Moderate Spec: Low
Lesion Size	MRI	Sens: 29 Spec: 8	Moderate	Inconsistent	Direct	Precise	Sens: 2723 Spec: 790	Sens: Moderate Spec: Moderate

	Imaging Modality or Comparison	Number of Studies	Risk of Bias (Low, Moderate, High)	Consistency (Consistent or Inconsistent)	Directness (Direct or Indirect)	Precision (Precise or Imprecise)	Number of Subjects/Lesions	Strength of Evidence (High, Moderate, Low, Insufficient)
Lesion Size	PET	Sens: 5 Spec: 0	Moderate	Sens: Inconsistent Spec: No studies	Direct	Sens: Imprecise Spec: No studies	Sens: 182 Spec: --	Sens: Low Spec: Insufficient
Degree of tumor differentiation	US with contrast	Sens: 3 Spec: 0	Moderate	Sens: Inconsistent Spec: No studies	Direct	Sens: Imprecise Spec: No studies	Sens: 165 Spec: --	Sens: Low Spec: Insufficient
Degree of tumor differentiation	CT	Sens: 5 Spec: 0	Moderate	Sens: Inconsistent Spec: No studies	Direct	Sens: Imprecise Spec: No studies	Sens: 320 Spec: --	Sens: Low Spec: Insufficient
Degree of tumor differentiation	MRI	Sens: 3 Spec: 0	Moderate	Sens: Consistent Spec: No studies	Direct	Sens: Imprecise Spec: No studies	Sens: 160 Spec: --	Sens: Low Spec: Insufficient
Degree of tumor differentiation	PET	Sens: 6 Spec: 0	Moderate	Sens: Inconsistent Spec: No studies	Direct	Sens: Imprecise Spec: No studies	Sens: 309 Spec: --	Sens: Low Spec: Insufficient
Other factors	US	1 to 3, depending on factor	Moderate	Inconsistent	Direct	Imprecise	N/A	Low
Other factors	CT	4-8, depending on factor	Moderate	Inconsistent	Direct	Imprecise	N/A	Low
Other factors	MRI	2-8, depending on factor	Moderate	Inconsistent	Direct	Imprecise	N/A	Low
Other factors	PET	1-8, depending on factor	Moderate	Inconsistent	Direct	Imprecise	N/A	Low

Table J4. Key Question 1b: Clinical decisionmaking

Imaging Modality or Comparison	Number of Studies	Risk of Bias (Low, Moderate, High)	Consistency (Consistent or Inconsistent)	Directness (Direct or Indirect)	Precision (Precise or Imprecise)	Number of Subjects/Lesions	Strength of Evidence (High, Moderate, Low, Insufficient)
All	1 RCT	Moderate	Single study	Direct	Imprecise	163	Low

Table J5. Key Question 1c: Clinical and patient-centered outcomes

Imaging Modality or Comparison	Number of Studies	Risk of Bias (Low, Moderate, High)	Consistency (Consistent or Inconsistent)	Directness (Direct or Indirect)	Precision (Precise or Imprecise)	Number of Subjects/Lesions	Strength of Evidence (High, Moderate, Low, Insufficient)
US plus serum AFP	1 RCT	High	Single study of surveillance vs. no surveillance	Direct	Precise	18816	Low
US screening at different intervals, mortality	3 RCTs	Moderate	Consistent	Direct	Precise	2185	Moderate

Table J6. Key Question 1d: Harms

Imaging Modality or Comparison	Number of Studies	Risk of Bias (Low, Moderate, High)	Consistency (Consistent or Inconsistent)	Directness (Direct or Indirect)	Precision (Precise or Imprecise)	Number of Subjects/Lesions	Strength of Evidence (High, Moderate, Low, Insufficient)
MRI, CT, US	2	Moderate	Inconsistent	Direct	Imprecise	248	Insufficient

Key Question 2. Diagnosis

Table J7. Key Question 2a: Test performance

	Imaging Modality or Comparison	Number of Studies	Risk of Bias (Low, Moderate, High)	Consistency (Consistent or Inconsistent)	Directness (Direct or Indirect)	Precision (Precise or Imprecise)	Number of Subjects/Lesions	Strength of Evidence (High, Moderate, Low, Insufficient)
Evaluation of focal liver lesion *Unit of analysis: patients with HCC*	US with contrast	Sens: 12 Spec: 8	Moderate	Inconsistent	Indirect	Precise	Sens: 836 Spec: 678	Sens: Moderate Spec: Moderate
Evaluation of focal liver lesion *Unit of analysis: patients with HCC*	US without contrast	Sens: 1 Spec: 0	Moderate	Sens: Consistent Spec: No studies	Indirect	Sens: Imprecise Spec: No studies	Sens: 93 Spec: --	Sens: Low Spec: Insufficient
Evaluation of focal liver lesion *Unit of analysis: patients with HCC*	CT	Sens: 8 Spec: 5	Moderate	Inconsistent	Indirect	Sens: Precise Spec: Imprecise	Sens: 656 Spec: 471	Sens: Moderate Spec: Low
Evaluation of focal liver lesion *Unit of analysis: patients with HCC*	MRI	Sens: 4 Spec: 4	Moderate	Consistent	Indirect	Imprecise	Sens: 308 Spec: 308	Sens: Low Spec: Low
Evaluation focal liver lesion *Unit of analysis: HCC lesions*	US with contrast	Sens: 21 Spec: 10	Moderate	Inconsistent	Indirect	Precise	Sens: 1652 Spec: 1175	Sens: Moderate Spec: Moderate
Evaluation focal liver lesion *Unit of analysis: HCC lesions*	CT	Sens: 13 Spec: 6	Moderate	Inconsistent	Indirect	Precise	Sens: 1196 Spec: 591	Sens: Moderate Spec: Moderate
Evaluation focal liver lesion *Unit of analysis: HCC lesions*	MRI	Sens: 14 Spec: 11	Moderate	Inconsistent	Indirect	Precise	Sens: 1185 Spec: 1014	Sens: Moderate Spec: Moderate
Evaluation focal liver lesion *Unit of analysis: HCC lesions*	PET	Sens: 2 Spec: 2	Moderate	Consistent	Indirect	Imprecise	Sens: 168 Spec: 168	Sens: Low Spec: Low

	Imaging Modality or Comparison	Number of Studies	Risk of Bias (Low, Moderate, High)	Consistency (Consistent or Inconsistent)	Directness (Direct or Indirect)	Precision (Precise or Imprecise)	Number of Subjects/Lesions	Strength of Evidence (High, Moderate, Low, Insufficient)
For distinguishing HCC lesions from non-HCC hepatic lesions	US with contrast	Sens: 2 Spec: 2	Moderate	Inconsistent	Indirect	Imprecise	Sens: 167 Spec: 167	Sens: Low Spec: Low
For distinguishing HCC lesions from non-HCC hepatic lesions	CT	Sens: 5 Spec: 5	Moderate	Inconsistent	Indirect	Imprecise	Sens: 467 Spec: 467	Sens: Low Spec: Low
For distinguishing HCC lesions from non-HCC hepatic lesions	MRI	Sens: 12 Spec: 10	Moderate	Inconsistent	Indirect	Precise	Sens: 1025 Spec: 908	Sens: Moderate Spec: Moderate
Direct (within-study) comparisons of imaging modalities *Unit of analysis: Patients with HCC*	US without contrast vs. CT	Sens: 1 Spec: 0	Moderate	Sens: Single study Spec: No studies	Direct	Sens: Imprecise Spec: No studies	Sens: 121 Spec: 0	Sens: Low Spec: Insufficient
Direct (within-study) comparisons of imaging modalities *Unit of analysis: Patients with HCC*	US with contrast vs. CT	Sens: 5 Spec: 2	Moderate	Consistent	Direct	Sens: Precise Spec: Imprecise	Sens: 956 Spec: 586	Sens: Moderate Spec: Low
Direct (within-study) comparisons of imaging modalities *Unit of analysis: Patients with HCC*	MRI vs. CT	Sens: 1 Spec: 1	Moderate	Single study	Direct	Imprecise	Sens: 74 Spec: 74	Sens: Low Spec: Low

	Imaging Modality or Comparison	Number of Studies	Risk of Bias (Low, Moderate, High)	Consistency (Consistent or Inconsistent)	Directness (Direct or Indirect)	Precision (Precise or Imprecise)	Number of Subjects/Lesions	Strength of Evidence (High, Moderate, Low, Insufficient)
Direct (within-study) comparisons of imaging modalities *Unit of analysis: HCC lesions*	US with contrast vs. CT	Sens: 4 Spec: 0	Moderate	Sens: Inconsistent Spec: No studies	Direct	Sens: Imprecise Spec: No studies	Sens: 446 Spec: 0	Sens: Moderate Spec: Insufficient
Direct (within-study) comparisons of imaging modalities *Unit of analysis: HCC lesions*	US with contrast vs. MRI	Sens: 1 Spec: 1	Moderate	Single study	Direct	Imprecise	Sens: 162 Spec: 162	Sens: Low Spec: Low
Direct (within-study) comparisons of imaging modalities *Unit of analysis: HCC lesions*	MRI vs. CT	Sens: 1 Spec: 1	Moderate	Single study	Direct	Imprecise	Sens: 123 Spec: 123	Sens: Low Spec: Low
Multiple imaging modalities	Various combinations	7	Moderate	Consistent	Direct	Imprecise	552	Moderate

Table J8. Key Question 2a.i: Effects of reference standard on test performance (based on HCC lesions as the unit of analysis)

Imaging Modality or Comparison	Number of Studies	Risk of Bias (Low, Moderate, High)	Consistency (Consistent or Inconsistent)	Directness (Direct or Indirect)	Precision (Precise or Imprecise)	Number of Subjects/Lesions	Strength of Evidence (High, Moderate, Low, Insufficient)
All	Sens: 23 (US) Spec: 11 (US) Sens: 13 (CT) Spec: 6 (CT) Sens: 14 (MRI) Spec: 11 (MRI)	Moderate	Inconsistent	Indirect	Precise	Sens: 1871 (US) Spec: 1322 (US) Sens: 1218 (CT) Spec: 294 (CT) Sens: 1064 (MRI) Spec: 908 (MRI)	Sens: Moderate Spec: Moderate

Table J9. Key Question 2a.ii: Effects of patient, tumor, technical, and other factors on test performance

Imaging Modality or Comparison		Number of Studies	Risk of Bias (Low, Moderate, High)	Consistency (Consistent or Inconsistent)	Directness (Direct or Indirect)	Precision (Precise or Imprecise)	Number of Subjects/Lesions	Strength of Evidence (High, Moderate, Low, Insufficient)
Other factors	US	1-2, depending on factor	Moderate	Inconsistent	Direct	Imprecise	N/A	Low
Other factors	CT	1-3, depending on factor	Moderate	Inconsistent	Direct	Imprecise	N/A	Low
Other factors	MRI	5-8, depending on factor	Moderate	Inconsistent	Direct	Imprecise	N/A	Low

Table J10. Key Question 2b: Clinical decisionmaking

Imaging Modality or Comparison	Number of Studies	Risk of Bias (Low, Moderate, High)	Consistency (Consistent or Inconsistent)	Directness (Direct or Indirect)	Precision (Precise or Imprecise)	Number of Subjects	Strength of Evidence (High, Moderate, Low, Insufficient)
All	No evidence	--	--	--	--	--	Insufficient

Table J11. Key Question 2c: Clinical and patient-centered outcomes

Imaging Modality or Comparison	Number of Studies	Risk of Bias (Low, Moderate, High)	Consistency (Consistent or Inconsistent)	Directness (Direct or Indirect)	Precision (Precise or Imprecise)	Number of Subjects	Strength of Evidence (High, Moderate, Low, Insufficient)
All	No evidence	--	--	--	--	--	Insufficient

Table J12. Key Question 2d: Harms

Imaging Modality or Comparison	Number of Studies	Risk of Bias (Low, Moderate, High)	Consistency (Consistent or Inconsistent)	Directness (Direct or Indirect)	Precision (Precise or Imprecise)	Number of Subjects	Strength of Evidence (High, Moderate, Low, Insufficient)
US and CT	1	High	Single study	Direct	Imprecise	190	Insufficient

Key Question 3. Staging

Table J13. Key Question 3a: Test performance

	Imaging Modality or Comparison	Number of Studies	Risk of Bias (Low, Moderate, High)	Consistency (Consistent or Inconsistent)	Directness (Direct or Indirect)	Precision (Precise or Imprecise)	Number of Subjects	Strength of Evidence (High, Moderate, Low, Insufficient)
Staging accuracy, using TNM criteria	CT	6	Moderate	Inconsistent	Indirect	Precise	985	Moderate
Staging accuracy, using TNM criteria	MRI	3	Moderate	Inconsistent	Indirect	Imprecise	960	Low
Staging accuracy, using TNM criteria	PET	1	Moderate	Single study	Indirect	Imprecise	43	Low
Staging accuracy, using TNM criteria	MRI vs. CT	2	Moderate	Inconsistent	Direct	Imprecise	831	Low
Identification of metastatic disease *Unit of analysis: Patients with metastatic HCC*	PET	Sens: 6 Spec: 5	Moderate	Inconsistent	Indirect	Imprecise	Sens: 375 Spec: 356	Sens: Low Spec: Low
Identification of metastatic	PET/CT vs. CT	3	Moderate	Inconsistent	Direct	Imprecise	183	Low

	Imaging Modality or Comparison	Number of Studies	Risk of Bias (Low, Moderate, High)	Consistency (Consistent or Inconsistent)	Directness (Direct or Indirect)	Precision (Precise or Imprecise)	Number of Subjects	Strength of Evidence (High, Moderate, Low, Insufficient)
disease *Unit of analysis: Patients with Metastatic HCC lesions*								
Identification of metastatic disease *Unit of analysis: Metastatic HCC lesions*	PET	Sens: 5 Spec: 0	Sens: Moderate Spec: No studies	Consistent	Indirect	Sens: Imprecise Spec: No studies	Sens: 237 Spec: --	Sens: Low Spec: Insufficient

Table J14. Key Question 3.a.i: Effects of reference standard on test performance

Imaging Modality or Comparison	Number of Studies	Risk of Bias (Low, Moderate, High)	Consistency (Consistent or Inconsistent)	Directness (Direct or Indirect)	Precision (Precise or Imprecise)	Number of Subjects	Strength of Evidence (High, Moderate, Low, Insufficient)
CT, MRI, PET	6	Moderate	Consistent	Indirect	Imprecise	Sens: 375 Spec: 356	Sens: Insufficient Spec: Insufficient

J-13

Table J15. Key Question 3.a.ii: Effects of patient, tumor, and technical factors on test performance

Imaging Modality or Comparison	Number of Studies	Risk of Bias (Low, Moderate, High)	Consistency (Consistent or Inconsistent)	Directness (Direct or Indirect)	Precision (Precise or Imprecise)	Number of Subjects	Strength of Evidence (High, Moderate, Low, Insufficient)
CT, MRI, PET	No evidence	--	--	--	--	--	Insufficient
PET	1-8, depending on factor	Moderate	Inconsistent	Indirect	Imprecise	N/A	Low

Table J16. Key Question 3b: Clinical decisionmaking

	Imaging Modality or Comparison	Number of Studies	Risk of Bias (Low, Moderate, High)	Consistency (Consistent or Inconsistent)	Directness (Direct or Indirect)	Precision (Precise or Imprecise)	Number of Subjects	Strength of Evidence (High, Moderate, Low, Insufficient)
Transplant eligibility, using Milan criteria	CT	7	Moderate	Consistent	Indirect	Imprecise	442	Moderate
Transplant eligibility, using Milan criteria	CT vs. MRI	1	Moderate	Single study	Direct	Imprecise	57	Low
Transplant eligibility, using Milan criteria	PET vs. CT	1	Moderate	Single study	Direct	Imprecise	43	Low
Use of resection and ablative therapies	MRI vs. CT	1	High	Single study	Direct	Imprecise	50	Low

Table J17. Key Question 3c: Clinical and patient-centered outcomes

Imaging Modality or Comparison	Number of Studies	Risk of Bias (Low, Moderate, High)	Consistency (Consistent or Inconsistent)	Directness (Direct or Indirect)	Precision (Precise or Imprecise)	Number of Subjects	Strength of Evidence (High, Moderate, Low, Insufficient)
US with contrast vs. US without contrast plus CT	1	High	Single study	Direct	Imprecise	167	Low

Table J18. Key Question 3d: Harms

Imaging Modality or Comparison	Number of Studies	Risk of Bias (Low, Moderate, High)	Consistency (Consistent or Inconsistent)	Directness (Direct or Indirect)	Precision (Precise or Imprecise)	Number of Subjects	Strength of Evidence (High, Moderate, Low, Insufficient)
All	No evidence	--	--	--	--	--	Insufficient

AFP = alpha-fetoprotein; CT = computed axial tomography; HCC = hepatocellular carcinoma; MRI = magnetic resonance imaging; PET = positron emission tomography; RCT = randomized control trial; Sens = sensitivity; Spec = specificity; TNM = tumor, node, metastasis staging sytem; US = ultrasound; vs. = versus

Appendix K. Appendix References

1. Addley HC, Griffin N, Shaw AS, et al. Accuracy of hepatocellular carcinoma detection on multidetector CT in a transplant liver population with explant liver correlation. Clin Radiol. 2011 Apr;66(4):349-56. PMID: 21295772.

2. Ahn SS, Kim M-J, Lim JS, et al. Added value of gadoxetic acid-enhanced hepatobiliary phase MR imaging in the diagnosis of hepatocellular carcinoma. Radiology. 2010 May;255(2):459-66. PMID: 20413759.

3. Akai H, Kiryu S, Matsuda I, et al. Detection of hepatocellular carcinoma by Gd-EOB-DTPA-enhanced liver MRI: comparison with triple phase 64 detector row helical CT. Eur J Radiol. 2011 Nov;80(2):310-5. PMID: 20732773.

4. Alaboudy A, Inoue T, Hatanaka K, et al. Usefulness of combination of imaging modalities in the diagnosis of hepatocellular carcinoma using Sonazoid(R)-enhanced ultrasound, gadolinium diethylene-triamine-pentaacetic acid-enhanced magnetic resonance imaging, and contrast-enhanced computed tomography. Oncology. 2011;81 Suppl 1:66-72. PMID: 22212939.

5. An C, Park MS, Kim D, et al. Added value of subtraction imaging in detecting arterial enhancement in small (<3 cm) hepatic nodules on dynamic contrast-enhanced MRI in patients at high risk of hepatocellular carcinoma. Eur Radiol. 2013;23:924-30. PMID: 23138382.

6. An C, Park M-S, Jeon H-M, et al. Prediction of the histopathological grade of hepatocellular carcinoma using qualitative diffusion-weighted, dynamic, and hepatobiliary phase MRI. Eur Radiol. 2012 Aug;22(8):1701-8. PMID: 22434421.

7. Baccarani U, Adani GL, Avellini C, et al. Comparison of clinical and pathological staging and long-term results of liver transplantation for hepatocellular carcinoma in a single transplant center. Transplant Proc. 2006 May;38(4):1111-3. PMID: 16757280.

8. Baek CK, Choi JY, Kim KA, et al. Hepatocellular carcinoma in patients with chronic liver disease: a comparison of gadoxetic acid-enhanced MRI and multiphasic MDCT. Clin Radiol. 2012 Feb;67(2):148-56. PMID: 21920517.

9. Baird AJ, Amos GJ, Saad NF, et al. Retrospective audit to determine the diagnostic accuracy of Primovist-enhanced MRI in the detection of hepatocellular carcinoma in cirrhosis with explant histopathology correlation. J Med Imaging Radiat Oncol. 2013;57(3):314-20. PMID: 23721140.

10. Bartolozzi C, Donati F, Cioni D, et al. MnDPDP-enhanced MRI vs dual-phase spiral CT in the detection of hepatocellular carcinoma in cirrhosis. Eur Radiol. 2000;10(11):1697-702. PMID: 11097390.

11. Bennett GL, Krinsky GA, Abitbol RJ, et al. Sonographic detection of hepatocellular carcinoma and dysplastic nodules in cirrhosis: correlation of pretransplantation sonography and liver explant pathology in 200 patients. AJR Am J Roentgenol. 2002 Jul;179(1):75-80. PMID: 12076908.

12. Bhattacharjya S, Bhattacharjya T, Quaglia A, et al. Liver transplantation in cirrhotic patients with small hepatocellular carcinoma: an analysis of pre-operative imaging, explant histology and prognostic histologic indicators. Dig Surg. 2004;21(2):152-9; discussion 9-60. PMID: 15166485.

13. Burrel M, Llovet JM, Ayuso C, et al. MRI angiography is superior to helical CT for detection of HCC prior to liver transplantation: an explant correlation. Hepatology. 2003 Oct;38(4):1034-42. PMID: 14512891.

14. Catala V, Nicolau C, Vilana R, et al. Characterization of focal liver lesions: comparative study of contrast-enhanced ultrasound versus spiral computed tomography. Eur Radiol. 2007 Apr;17(4):1066-73. PMID: 17072617.

15. Cereser L, Furlan A, Bagatto D, et al. Comparison of portal venous and delayed phases of gadolinium-enhanced magnetic resonance imaging study of cirrhotic liver for the detection of contrast washout of hypervascular hepatocellular carcinoma. J

16. Chalasani N, Horlander JC, Sr., Said A, et al. Screening for hepatocellular carcinoma in patients with advanced cirrhosis. Am J Gastroenterol. 1999 Oct;94(10):2988-93. PMID: 10520857.

17. Chen Y-K, Hsieh D-S, Liao C-S, et al. Utility of FDG-PET for investigating unexplained serum AFP elevation in patients with suspected hepatocellular carcinoma recurrence. Anticancer Res. 2005 Nov-Dec;25(6C):4719-25. PMID: 16334166.

18. Cheung TT, Ho CL, Lo CM, et al. 11C-acetate and 18F-FDG PET/CT for clinical staging and selection of patients with hepatocellular carcinoma for liver transplantation on the basis of milan criteria: Surgeon's perspective. J Nucl Med. 2013;54(2):192-200. PMID: 23321459.

19. Cheung TT, Chan SC, Ho CL, et al. Can positron emission tomography with the dual tracers [11 C]acetate and [18 F]fludeoxyglucose predict microvascular invasion in hepatocellular carcinoma? Liver Transpl. 2011 Oct;17(10):1218-25. PMID: 21688383.

20. Choi SH, Lee JM, Yu NC, et al. Hepatocellular carcinoma in liver transplantation candidates: detection with gadobenate dimeglumine-enhanced MRI. AJR Am J Roentgenol. 2008 Aug;191(2):529-36. PMID: 18647927.

21. Choi D, Kim SH, Lim JH, et al. Detection of hepatocellular carcinoma: combined T2-weighted and dynamic gadolinium-enhanced MRI versus combined CT during arterial portography and CT hepatic arteriography. J Comput Assist Tomogr. 2001 Sep-Oct;25(5):777-85. PMID: 11584240.

22. Chou C-T, Chen R-C, Chen W-T, et al. Characterization of hyperintense nodules on T1-weighted liver magnetic resonance imaging: comparison of Ferucarbotran-enhanced MRI with accumulation-phase FS-T1WI and gadolinium-enhanced MRI. J Chin Med Assoc. 2011 Feb;74(2):62-8. PMID: 21354082.

23. Chung J, Yu J-S, Kim DJ, et al. Hypervascular hepatocellular carcinoma in the cirrhotic liver: diffusion-weighted imaging versus superparamagnetic iron oxide-enhanced MRI. Magn Reson Imaging. 2011 Nov;29(9):1235-43. PMID: 21907517.

24. Chung S-H, Kim M-J, Choi J-Y, et al. Comparison of two different injection rates of gadoxetic acid for arterial phase MRI of the liver. J Magn Reson Imaging. 2010 Feb;31(2):365-72. PMID: 20099350.

25. Colagrande S, Fargnoli R, Dal Pozzo F, et al. Value of hepatic arterial phase CT versus lipiodol ultrafluid CT in the detection of hepatocellular carcinoma. J Comput Assist Tomogr. 2000 Nov-Dec;24(6):878-83. PMID: 11105704.

26. Dai Y, Chen MH, Fan ZH, et al. Diagnosis of small hepatic nodules detected by surveillance ultrasound in patients with cirrhosis: Comparison between contrast-enhanced ultrasound and contrast-enhanced helical computed tomography. Hepatol Res. 2008 Mar;38(3):281-90. PMID: 17908168.

27. de Ledinghen V, Laharie D, Lecesne R, et al. Detection of nodules in liver cirrhosis: spiral computed tomography or magnetic resonance imaging? A prospective study of 88 nodules in 34 patients. Eur J Gastroenterol Hepatol. 2002 Feb;14(2):159-65. PMID: 11981340.

28. Delbeke D, Martin WH, Sandler MP, et al. Evaluation of benign vs malignant hepatic lesions with positron emission tomography. Arch Surg. 1998 May;133(5):510-5; discussion 5-6. PMID: 9605913.

29. Denecke T, Grieser C, Froling V, et al. Multislice computed tomography using a triple-phase contrast protocol for preoperative assessment of hepatic tumor load in patients with hepatocellular carcinoma before liver transplantation. Transpl Int. 2009 Apr;22(4):395-402. PMID: 19000231.

30. Di Martino M, De Filippis G, De Santis A, et al. Hepatocellular carcinoma in cirrhotic patients: prospective comparison of US, CT and MR imaging. Eur Radiol. 2013;23:887-96. PMID: 23179521.

31. Di Martino M, Marin D, Guerrisi A, et al. Intraindividual comparison of gadoxetate disodium-enhanced MR imaging and 64-section multidetector CT in the Detection of hepatocellular carcinoma in patients with cirrhosis. Radiology. 2010 Sep;256(3):806-16. PMID: 20720069.

32. D'Onofrio M, Rozzanigo U, Masinielli BM, et al. Hypoechoic focal liver lesions: characterization with contrast enhanced ultrasonography. J Clin Ultrasound. 2005 May;33(4):164-72. PMID: 15856516.

33. Doyle DJ, O'Malley ME, Jang H-J, et al. Value of the unenhanced phase for detection of hepatocellular carcinomas 3 cm or less when performing multiphase computed tomography in patients with cirrhosis. J Comput Assist Tomogr. 2007 Jan-Feb;31(1):86-92. PMID: 17259838.

34. Eckel F, Herrmann K, Schmidt S, et al. Imaging of proliferation in hepatocellular carcinoma with the in vivo marker 18F-fluorothymidine. J Nucl Med. 2009 Sep;50(9):1441-7. PMID: 19690030.

35. Egger C, Goertz RS, Strobel D, et al. Dynamic contrast-enhanced ultrasound (DCE-US) for easy and rapid evaluation of hepatocellular carcinoma compared to dynamic contrast-enhanced computed tomography (DCE-CT)--a pilot study. Ultraschall Med. 2012;33(6):587-92. PMID: 23154871.

36. Filippone A, Cianci R, Patriarca G, et al. The Value of Gadoxetic Acid-Enhanced Hepatospecific Phase MR Imaging for Characterization of Hepatocellular Nodules in the Cirrhotic Liver. European Journal of Clinical & Medical Oncology. 2010;2(4):1-8. PMID: 69823585.

37. Forner A, Vilana R, Ayuso C, et al. Diagnosis of hepatic nodules 20 mm or smaller in cirrhosis: Prospective validation of the noninvasive diagnostic criteria for hepatocellular carcinoma.[Erratum appears in Hepatology. 2008 Feb;47(2):769]. Hepatology. 2008 Jan;47(1):97-104. PMID: 18069697.

38. Fowler KJ, Karimova EJ, Arauz AR, et al. Validation of organ procurement and transplant network (OPTN)/united network for organ sharing (UNOS) criteria for imaging diagnosis of hepatocellular carcinoma. Transplantation. 2013;95(12):1506-11. PMID: 23778569.

39. Fracanzani AL, Burdick L, Borzio M, et al. Contrast-enhanced Doppler ultrasonography in the diagnosis of hepatocellular carcinoma and premalignant lesions in patients with cirrhosis. Hepatology. 2001 Dec;34(6):1109-12. PMID: 11731999.

40. Freeman RB, Mithoefer A, Ruthazer R, et al. Optimizing staging for hepatocellular carcinoma before liver transplantation: A retrospective analysis of the UNOS/OPTN database. Liver Transpl. 2006 Oct;12(10):1504-11. PMID: 16952174.

41. Freeny PC, Grossholz M, Kaakaji K, et al. Significance of hyperattenuating and contrast-enhancing hepatic nodules detected in the cirrhotic liver during arterial phase helical CT in pre-liver transplant patients: radiologic-histopathologic correlation of explanted livers. Abdom Imaging. 2003 May-Jun;28(3):333-46. PMID: 12719903.

42. Furuse J, Maru Y, Yoshino M, et al. Assessment of arterial tumor vascularity in small hepatocellular carcinoma. Comparison between color doppler ultrasonography and radiographic imagings with contrast medium: dynamic CT, angiography, and CT hepatic arteriography. Eur J Radiol. 2000 Oct;36(1):20-7. PMID: 10996754.

43. Gaiani S, Celli N, Piscaglia F, et al. Usefulness of contrast-enhanced perfusional sonography in the assessment of hepatocellular carcinoma hypervascular at spiral computed tomography. J Hepatol. 2004 Sep;41(3):421-6. PMID: 15336445.

44. Gambarin-Gelwan M, Wolf DC, Shapiro R, et al. Sensitivity of commonly available screening tests in detecting hepatocellular carcinoma in cirrhotic patients undergoing liver transplantation. Am J Gastroenterol. 2000 Jun;95(6):1535-8. PMID: 10894592.

45. Gatto A, De Gaetano AM, Giuga M, et al. Differentiating hepatocellular carcinoma from dysplastic nodules at gadobenate dimeglumine-enhanced hepatobiliary-phase magnetic resonance imaging. Abdom Imaging. 2013;38(4):736-44. PMID: 22986351.

46. Giorgio A, De Stefano G, Coppola C, et al. Contrast-enhanced sonography in the characterization of small hepatocellular carcinomas in cirrhotic patients: comparison with contrast-enhanced ultrafast magnetic resonance imaging. Anticancer Res. 2007 Nov-Dec;27(6C):4263-9. PMID: 18214030.

47. Giorgio A, Ferraioli G, Tarantino L, et al. Contrast-enhanced sonographic appearance

of hepatocellular carcinoma in patients with cirrhosis: Comparison with contrast-enhanced helical CT appearance. AJR Am J Roentgenol. 2004;183(5):1319-26. PMID: 15505297.

48. Golfieri R, Marini E, Bazzocchi A, et al. Small (≤ 3 cm) hepatocellular carcinoma in cirrhosis: the role of double contrast agents in MR imaging vs. multidetector-row CT. Radiol Med (Torino). 2009 Dec;114(8):1239-66. PMID: 19697104.

49. Goshima S, Kanematsu M, Matsuo M, et al. Nodule-in-nodule appearance of hepatocellular carcinomas: comparison of gadolinium-enhanced and ferumoxides-enhanced magnetic resonance imaging. J Magn Reson Imaging. 2004 Aug;20(2):250-5. PMID: 15269950.

50. Goto E, Masuzaki R, Tateishi R, et al. Value of post-vascular phase (Kupffer imaging) by contrast-enhanced ultrasonography using Sonazoid in the detection of hepatocellular carcinoma. J Gastroenterol. 2012;47(4):477-85. PMID: 22200940.

51. Guo L, Liang C, Yu T, et al. 3 T MRI of hepatocellular carcinomas in patients with cirrhosis: does T2-weighted imaging provide added value? Clin Radiol. 2012 Apr;67(4):319-28. PMID: 22099524.

52. Haradome H, Grazioli L, Tinti R, et al. Additional value of gadoxetic acid-DTPA-enhanced hepatobiliary phase MR imaging in the diagnosis of early-stage hepatocellular carcinoma: comparison with dynamic triple-phase multidetector CT imaging. J Magn Reson Imaging. 2011 Jul;34(1):69-78. PMID: 21598343.

53. Hardie AD, Kizziah MK, Boulter DJ. Diagnostic accuracy of diffusion-weighted MRI for identifying hepatocellular carcinoma with liver explant correlation. J Med Imaging Radiat Oncol. 2011 Aug;55(4):362-7. PMID: 21843170.

54. Hardie AD, Kizziah MK, Rissing MS. Can the patient with cirrhosis be imaged for hepatocellular carcinoma without gadolinium?: Comparison of combined T2-weighted, T2*-weighted, and diffusion-weighted MRI with gadolinium-enhanced MRI using liver explantation standard. J Comput Assist Tomogr. 2011 Nov-Dec;35(6):711-5. PMID: 22082541.

55. Hardie AD, Nance JW, Boulter DJ, et al. Assessment of the diagnostic accuracy of T2*-weighted MR imaging for identifying hepatocellular carcinoma with liver explant correlation. Eur J Radiol. 2011 Dec;80(3):e249-52. PMID: 21112710.

56. Hatanaka K, Kudo M, Minami Y, et al. Differential diagnosis of hepatic tumors: value of contrast-enhanced harmonic sonography using the newly developed contrast agent, Sonazoid. Intervirology. 2008;51 Suppl 1:61-9. PMID: 18544950.

57. Hecht EM, Holland AE, Israel GM, et al. Hepatocellular carcinoma in the cirrhotic liver: gadolinium-enhanced 3D T1-weighted MR imaging as a stand-alone sequence for diagnosis. Radiology. 2006 May;239(2):438-47. PMID: 16641353.

58. Hidaka M, Takatsuki M, Okudaira S, et al. The expression of transporter OATP2/OATP8 decreases in undetectable hepatocellular carcinoma by Gd-EOB-MRI in the explanted cirrhotic liver. Hepatology International. 2012:1-7.

59. Higashihara H, Osuga K, Onishi H, et al. Diagnostic accuracy of C-arm CT during selective transcatheter angiography for hepatocellular carcinoma: comparison with intravenous contrast-enhanced, biphasic, dynamic MDCT. Eur Radiol. 2012 Apr;22(4):872-9. PMID: 22120061.

60. Hirakawa M, Yoshimitsu K, Irie H, et al. Performance of radiological methods in diagnosing hepatocellular carcinoma preoperatively in a recipient of living related liver transplantation: comparison with step section histopathology. Jpn J Radiol. 2011 Feb;29(2):129-37. PMID: 21359938.

61. Ho C-L, Yu SCH, Yeung DWC. 11C-acetate PET imaging in hepatocellular carcinoma and other liver masses. J Nucl Med. 2003 Feb;44(2):213-21. PMID: 12571212.

62. Ho C-l, Chen S, Yeung DWC, et al. Dual-tracer PET/CT imaging in evaluation of metastatic hepatocellular carcinoma. J Nucl Med. 2007 Jun;48(6):902-9. PMID: 17504862.

63. Hori M, Murakami T, Kim T, et al. Detection of hypervascular hepatocellular carcinoma: comparison of SPIO-enhanced MRI with dynamic helical CT. J Comput

Assist Tomogr. 2002 Sep-Oct;26(5):701-10. PMID: 12439302.

64. Hori M, Murakami T, Oi H, et al. Sensitivity in detection of hypervascular hepatocellular carcinoma by helical CT with intra-arterial injection of contrast medium, and by helical CT and MR imaging with intravenous injection of contrast medium. Acta Radiol. 1998 Mar;39(2):144-51. PMID: 9529444.

65. Hwang J, Kim SH, Lee MW, et al. Small (≤ 2 cm) hepatocellular carcinoma in patients with chronic liver disease: comparison of gadoxetic acid-enhanced 3.0 T MRI and multiphasic 64-multirow detector CT. Br J Radiol. 2012 Jul;85(1015):e314-22. PMID: 22167508.

66. Hwang KH, Choi D-J, Lee S-Y, et al. Evaluation of patients with hepatocellular carcinomas using [(11)C]acetate and [(18)F]FDG PET/CT: A preliminary study. Appl Radiat Isot. 2009 Jul-Aug;67(7-8):1195-8. PMID: 19342249.

67. Iannaccone R, Laghi A, Catalano C, et al. Hepatocellular carcinoma: role of unenhanced and delayed phase multi-detector row helical CT in patients with cirrhosis. Radiology. 2005 Feb;234(2):460-7. PMID: 15671002.

68. Iavarone M, Sangiovanni A, Forzenigo LV, et al. Diagnosis of hepatocellular carcinoma in cirrhosis by dynamic contrast imaging: the importance of tumor cell differentiation. Hepatology. 2010 Nov;52(5):1723-30. PMID: 20842697.

69. Ichikawa T, Saito K, Yoshioka N, et al. Detection and characterization of focal liver lesions: a Japanese phase III, multicenter comparison between gadoxetic acid disodium-enhanced magnetic resonance imaging and contrast-enhanced computed tomography predominantly in patients with hepatocellular carcinoma and chronic liver disease. Invest Radiol. 2010 Mar;45(3):133-41. PMID: 20098330.

70. Ichikawa T, Kitamura T, Nakajima H, et al. Hypervascular hepatocellular carcinoma: can double arterial phase imaging with multidetector CT improve tumor depiction in the cirrhotic liver? AJR Am J Roentgenol. 2002 Sep;179(3):751-8. PMID: 12185057.

71. Ijichi H, Shirabe K, Taketomi A, et al. Clinical usefulness of 18F-fluorodeoxyglucose positron emission tomography/computed tomography for patients with primary liver cancer with special reference to rare histological types, hepatocellular carcinoma with sarcomatous change and combined hepatocellular and cholangiocarcinoma. Hepatol Res. 2013;43(5):481-7. PMID: 23145869.

72. Imamura M, Shiratori Y, Shiina S, et al. Power Doppler sonography for hepatocellular carcinoma: factors affecting the power Doppler signals of the tumors. Liver. 1998 Dec;18(6):427-33. PMID: 9869398.

73. Inoue T, Kudo M, Komuta M, et al. Assessment of Gd-EOB-DTPA-enhanced MRI for HCC and dysplastic nodules and comparison of detection sensitivity versus MDCT. J Gastroenterol. 2012 Sep;47(9):1036-47. PMID: 22526270.

74. Inoue T, Kudo M, Maenishi O, et al. Value of liver parenchymal phase contrast-enhanced sonography to diagnose premalignant and borderline lesions and overt hepatocellular carcinoma. AJR Am J Roentgenol. 2009 Mar;192(3):698-705. PMID: 19234266.

75. Inoue T, Kudo M, Hatanaka K, et al. Imaging of hepatocellular carcinoma: Qualitative and quantitative analysis of postvascular phase contrast-enhanced ultrasonography with sonazoid. Oncology. 2008;75(SUPPL. 1):48-54. PMID: 19092272.

76. Ito K, Fujita T, Shimizu A, et al. Multiarterial phase dynamic MRI of small early enhancing hepatic lesions in cirrhosis or chronic hepatitis: Differentiating between hypervascular hepatocellular carcinomas and pseudolesions. AJR Am J Roentgenol. 2004;183(3):699-705. PMID: 15333358.

77. Iwazawa J, Ohue S, Hashimoto N, et al. Detection of hepatocellular carcinoma: comparison of angiographic C-arm CT and MDCT. AJR Am J Roentgenol. 2010 Oct;195(4):882-7. PMID: 20858813.

78. Jang HJ, Lim JH, Lee SJ, et al. Hepatocellular carcinoma: are combined CT during arterial portography and CT hepatic arteriography in addition to triple-phase helical CT all necessary for preoperative

evaluation? Radiology. 2000 May;215(2):373-80. PMID: 10796910.

79. Jang HJ, Kim TK, Khalili K, et al. Characterization of 1- to 2-cm liver nodules detected on hcc surveillance ultrasound according to the criteria of the american association for the study of liver disease: Is quadriphasic CT necessary? AJR Am J Roentgenol. 2013;201(2):314-21. PMID: 23883211.

80. Jang HJ, Kim TK, Wilson SR. Small nodules (1-2 cm) in liver cirrhosis: characterization with contrast-enhanced ultrasound. Eur J Radiol. 2009 Dec;72(3):418-24. PMID: 18834687.

81. Jeng L-B, Changlai S-P, Shen Y-Y, et al. Limited value of 18F-2-deoxyglucose positron emission tomography to detect hepatocellular carcinoma in hepatitis B virus carriers. Hepatogastroenterology. 2003 Nov-Dec;50(54):2154-6. PMID: 14696485.

82. Jeng C-M, Kung C-H, Wang Y-C, et al. Spiral biphasic contrast-enhanced computerized tomography in the diagnosis of hepatocellular carcinoma. J Formos Med Assoc. 2002 Aug;101(8):588-92. PMID: 12440092.

83. Jeong WK, Byun JH, Lee SS, et al. Gadobenate dimeglumine-enhanced liver MR imaging in cirrhotic patients: quantitative and qualitative comparison of 1-hour and 3-hour delayed images. J Magn Reson Imaging. 2011 Apr;33(4):889-97. PMID: 21448954.

84. Jeong MG, Yu JS, Kim KW, et al. Early homogeneously enhancing hemangioma versus hepatocellular carcinoma: differentiation using quantitative analysis of multiphasic dynamic magnetic resonance imaging. Yonsei Med J. 1999 Jun;40(3):248-55. PMID: 10412337.

85. Jin Y, Nah S, Lee J, et al. Utility of Adding Primovist Magnetic Resonance Imaging to Analysis of Hepatocellular Carcinoma by Liver Dynamic Computed Tomography. Clin Gastroenterol Hepatol. 2013;11(2):187-92. PMID: 23142203.

86. Kakihara D, Nishie A, Harada N, et al. Performance of gadoxetic acid-enhanced MRI for detecting hepatocellular carcinoma in recipients of living-related-liver-transplantation: Comparison with dynamic multidetector row computed tomography and angiography-assisted computed tomography. J Magn Reson Imaging. 2013 Nov [Epub ahead of print]. PMID: 24259437.

87. Kamura T, Kimura M, Sakai K, et al. Small hypervascular hepatocellular carcinoma versus hypervascular pseudolesions: Differential diagnosis on MRI. Abdom Imaging. 2002;27(3):315-24. PMID: 12173363.

88. Kang BK, Lim JH, Kim SH, et al. Preoperative depiction of hepatocellular carcinoma: ferumoxides-enhanced MR imaging versus triple-phase helical CT. Radiology. 2003 Jan;226(1):79-85. PMID: 12511672.

89. Kawada N, Ohkawa K, Tanaka S, et al. Improved diagnosis of well-differentiated hepatocellular carcinoma with gadolinium ethoxybenzyl diethylene triamine pentaacetic acid-enhanced magnetic resonance imaging and Sonazoid contrast-enhanced ultrasonography. Hepatol Res. 2010;40(9):930-6. PMID: 20887598.

90. Kawaoka T, Aikata H, Takaki S, et al. FDG positron emission tomography/computed tomography for the detection of extrahepatic metastases from hepatocellular carcinoma. Hepatol Res. 2009;39(2):134-42. PMID: 19208034.

91. Kawata S, Murakami T, Kim T, et al. Multidetector CT: diagnostic impact of slice thickness on detection of hypervascular hepatocellular carcinoma. AJR Am J Roentgenol. 2002 Jul;179(1):61-6. PMID: 12076906.

92. Khalili K, Kim TK, Jang H-J, et al. Optimization of imaging diagnosis of 1-2 cm hepatocellular carcinoma: an analysis of diagnostic performance and resource utilization. J Hepatol. 2011 Apr;54(4):723-8. PMID: 21156219.

93. Khan MA, Combs CS, Brunt EM, et al. Positron emission tomography scanning in the evaluation of hepatocellular carcinoma. J Hepatol. 2000 May;32(5):792-7. PMID: 10845666.

94. Kim AY, Kim YK, Lee MW, et al. Detection of hepatocellular carcinoma in gadoxetic acid-enhanced MRI and diffusion-weighted MRI with respect to the severity of

95. Kim CK, Lim JH, Lee WJ. Detection of hepatocellular carcinomas and dysplastic nodules in cirrhotic liver: accuracy of ultrasonography in transplant patients. J Ultrasound Med. 2001 Feb;20(2):99-104. PMID: 11211142.

96. Kim DJ, Yu JS, Kim JH, et al. Small hypervascular hepatocellular carcinomas: value of diffusion-weighted imaging compared with "washout" appearance on dynamic MRI. Br J Radiol. 2012 Oct;85(1018):e879-86. PMID: 22573299.

97. Kim KW, Lee JM, Klotz E, et al. Quantitative CT color mapping of the arterial enhancement fraction of the liver to detect hepatocellular carcinoma. Radiology. 2009 Feb;250(2):425-34. PMID: 19188314.

98. Kim M-J, Lee M, Choi J-Y, et al. Imaging features of small hepatocellular carcinomas with microvascular invasion on gadoxetic acid-enhanced MR imaging. Eur J Radiol. 2012 Oct;81(10):2507-12. PMID: 22137613.

99. Kim PN, Choi D, Rhim H, et al. Planning ultrasound for percutaneous radiofrequency ablation to treat small (≤ 3 cm) hepatocellular carcinomas detected on computed tomography or magnetic resonance imaging: a multicenter prospective study to assess factors affecting ultrasound visibility. J Vasc Interv Radiol. 2012 May;23(5):627-34. PMID: 22387030.

100. Kim SE, Lee HC, Shim JH, et al. Noninvasive diagnostic criteria for hepatocellular carcinoma in hepatic masses >2 cm in a hepatitis B virus-endemic area. Liver Int. 2011 Nov;31(10):1468-76. PMID: 21745284.

101. Kim SH, Kim SH, Lee J, et al. Gadoxetic acid-enhanced MRI versus triple-phase MDCT for the preoperative detection of hepatocellular carcinoma. AJR Am J Roentgenol. 2009 Jun;192(6):1675-81. PMID: 19457834.

102. Kim SH, Choi D, Kim SH, et al. Ferucarbotran-enhanced MRI versus triple-phase MDCT for the preoperative detection of hepatocellular carcinoma. AJR Am J Roentgenol. 2005 Apr;184(4):1069-76. PMID: 15788575.

103. Kim SJ, Kim SH, Lee J, et al. Ferucarbotran-enhanced 3.0-T magnetic resonance imaging using parallel imaging technique compared with triple-phase multidetector row computed tomography for the preoperative detection of hepatocellular carcinoma.[Erratum appears in J Comput Assist Tomogr. 2008 Jul-Aug;32(4):615]. J Comput Assist Tomogr. 2008 May-Jun;32(3):379-85. PMID: 18520541.

104. Kim SK, Lim JH, Lee WJ, et al. Detection of hepatocellular carcinoma: comparison of dynamic three-phase computed tomography images and four-phase computed tomography images using multidetector row helical computed tomography. J Comput Assist Tomogr. 2002 Sep-Oct;26(5):691-8. PMID: 12439300.

105. Kim T, Murakami T, Hori M, et al. Small hypervascular hepatocellular carcinoma revealed by double arterial phase CT performed with single breath-hold scanning and automatic bolus tracking. AJR Am J Roentgenol. 2002 Apr;178(4):899-904. PMID: 11906869.

106. Kim TK, Lee KH, Jang H-J, et al. Analysis of gadobenate dimeglumine-enhanced MR findings for characterizing small (1-2-cm) hepatic nodules in patients at high risk for hepatocellular carcinoma. Radiology. 2011 Jun;259(3):730-8. PMID: 21364083.

107. Kim YK, Kim CS, Han YM, et al. Detection of small hepatocellular carcinoma: intraindividual comparison of gadoxetic acid-enhanced MRI at 3.0 and 1.5 T.[Erratum appears in Invest Radiol. 2011 Sep;46(9):600]. Invest Radiol. 2011 Jun;46(6):383-9. PMID: 21467946.

108. Kim YK, Kim CS, Han YM, et al. Detection of liver malignancy with gadoxetic acid-enhanced MRI: is addition of diffusion-weighted MRI beneficial?.[Erratum appears in Clin Radiol. 2011 Oct;66(10):1006]. Clin Radiol. 2011 Jun;66(6):489-96. PMID: 21367403.

109. Kim YK, Kim CS, Han YM, et al. Detection of small hepatocellular carcinoma: can gadoxetic acid-enhanced magnetic resonance imaging replace combining gadopentetate dimeglumine-enhanced and superparamagnetic iron oxide-enhanced magnetic resonance imaging? Invest Radiol. 2010 Nov;45(11):740-6. PMID: 20644488.

110. Kim YK, Kim CS, Han YM, et al. Comparison of gadoxetic acid-enhanced MRI and superparamagnetic iron oxide-enhanced MRI for the detection of hepatocellular carcinoma. Clin Radiol. 2010 May;65(5):358-65. PMID: 20380933.

111. Kim Y-K, Lee K-W, Cho SY, et al. Usefulness 18F-FDG positron emission tomography/computed tomography for detecting recurrence of hepatocellular carcinoma in posttransplant patients. Liver Transpl. 2010 Jun;16(6):767-72. PMID: 20517911.

112. Kim YK, Kim CS, Han YM, et al. Detection of hepatocellular carcinoma: gadoxetic acid-enhanced 3-dimensional magnetic resonance imaging versus multi-detector row computed tomography. J Comput Assist Tomogr. 2009 Nov-Dec;33(6):844-50. PMID: 19940648.

113. Kim YK, Lee YH, Kim CS, et al. Added diagnostic value of T2-weighted MR imaging to gadolinium-enhanced three-dimensional dynamic MR imaging for the detection of small hepatocellular carcinomas. Eur J Radiol. 2008 Aug;67(2):304-10. PMID: 17714904.

114. Kim YK, Lee YH, Kim CS, et al. Double-dose 1.0-M gadobutrol versus standard-dose 0.5-M gadopentetate dimeglumine in revealing small hypervascular hepatocellular carcinomas. Eur Radiol. 2008 Jan;18(1):70-7. PMID: 17404740.

115. Kim YK, Kwak HS, Han YM, et al. Usefulness of combining sequentially acquired gadobenate dimeglumine-enhanced magnetic resonance imaging and resovist-enhanced magnetic resonance imaging for the detection of hepatocellular carcinoma: comparison with computed tomography hepatic arteriography and computed tomography arterioportography using 16-slice multidetector computed tomography. J Comput Assist Tomogr. 2007 Sep-Oct;31(5):702-11. PMID: 17895780.

116. Kim YK, Kim CS, Chung GH, et al. Comparison of gadobenate dimeglumine-enhanced dynamic MRI and 16-MDCT for the detection of hepatocellular carcinoma. AJR Am J Roentgenol. 2006 Jan;186(1):149-57. PMID: 16357395.

117. Kim YK, Kwak HS, Kim CS, et al. Hepatocellular carcinoma in patients with chronic liver disease: comparison of SPIO-enhanced MR imaging and 16-detector row CT. Radiology. 2006 Feb;238(2):531-41. PMID: 16371577.

118. Kim YK, Kim CS, Kwak HS, et al. Three-dimensional dynamic liver MR imaging using sensitivity encoding for detection of hepatocellular carcinomas: comparison with superparamagnetic iron oxide-enhanced mr imaging. J Magn Reson Imaging. 2004 Nov;20(5):826-37. PMID: 15503325.

119. Kim YK, Kim CS, Lee YH, et al. Comparison of superparamagnetic iron oxide-enhanced and gadobenate dimeglumine-enhanced dynamic MRI for detection of small hepatocellular carcinomas. AJR Am J Roentgenol. 2004 May;182(5):1217-23. PMID: 15100122.

120. Kitamura T, Ichikawa T, Erturk SM, et al. Detection of hypervascular hepatocellular carcinoma with multidetector-row CT: single arterial-phase imaging with computer-assisted automatic bolus-tracking technique compared with double arterial-phase imaging. J Comput Assist Tomogr. 2008 Sep-Oct;32(5):724-9. PMID: 18830101.

121. Kondo H, Kanematsu M, Itoh K, et al. Does T2-weighted MR imaging improve preoperative detection of malignant hepatic tumors? Observer performance study in 49 surgically proven cases. Magn Reson Imaging. 2005 Jan;23(1):89-95. PMID: 15733793.

122. Korenaga K, Korenaga M, Furukawa M, et al. Usefulness of Sonazoid contrast-enhanced ultrasonography for hepatocellular carcinoma: Comparison with pathological diagnosis and superparamagnetic iron oxide magnetic resonance images. J Gastroenterol. 2009;44(7):733-41. PMID: 19387532.

123. Koushima Y, Ebara M, Fukuda H, et al. Small hepatocellular carcinoma: assessment with T1-weighted spin-echo magnetic resonance imaging with and without fat suppression. Eur J Radiol. 2002 Jan;41(1):34-41. PMID: 11750150.

124. Krinsky GA, Lee VS, Theise ND, et al. Transplantation for hepatocellular carcinoma and cirrhosis: Sensitivity of magnetic resonance imaging. Liver Transpl. 2002;8(12):1156-64. PMID: 12474156.

125. Krinsky GA, Lee VS, Theise ND, et al. Hepatocellular carcinoma and dysplastic nodules in patients with cirrhosis: prospective diagnosis with MR imaging and explantation correlation. Radiology. 2001 May;219(2):445-54. PMID: 11323471.

126. Kumano S, Uemura M, Haraikawa T, et al. Efficacy of double arterial phase dynamic magnetic resonance imaging with the sensitivity encoding technique versus dynamic multidetector-row helical computed tomography for detecting hypervascular hepatocellular carcinoma. Jpn J Radiol. 2009 Jul;27(6):229-36. PMID: 19626408.

127. Kunishi Y, Numata K, Morimoto M, et al. Efficacy of fusion imaging combining sonography and hepatobiliary phase MRI with Gd-EOB-DTPA to detect small hepatocellular carcinoma. AJR Am J Roentgenol. 2012 Jan;198(1):106-14. PMID: 22194485.

128. Kwak H-S, Lee J-M, Kim Y-K, et al. Detection of hepatocellular carcinoma: comparison of ferumoxides-enhanced and gadolinium-enhanced dynamic three-dimensional volume interpolated breath-hold MR imaging. Eur Radiol. 2005 Jan;15(1):140-7. PMID: 15449000.

129. Kwak H-S, Lee J-M, Kim C-S. Preoperative detection of hepatocellular carcinoma: comparison of combined contrast-enhanced MR imaging and combined CT during arterial portography and CT hepatic arteriography. Eur Radiol. 2004 Mar;14(3):447-57. PMID: 14531005.

130. Laghi A, Iannaccone R, Rossi P, et al. Hepatocellular carcinoma: detection with triple-phase multi-detector row helical CT in patients with chronic hepatitis. Radiology. 2003 Feb;226(2):543-9. PMID: 12563152.

131. Lauenstein TC, Salman K, Morreira R, et al. Gadolinium-enhanced MRI for tumor surveillance before liver transplantation: center-based experience. AJR Am J Roentgenol. 2007 Sep;189(3):663-70. PMID: 17715115.

132. Lee CH, Kim KA, Lee J, et al. Using low tube voltage (80kVp) quadruple phase liver CT for the detection of hepatocellular carcinoma: two-year experience and comparison with Gd-EOB-DTPA enhanced liver MRI. Eur J Radiol. 2012 Apr;81(4):e605-11. PMID: 22297180.

133. Lee DH, Kim SH, Lee JM, et al. Diagnostic performance of multidetector row computed tomography, superparamagnetic iron oxide-enhanced magnetic resonance imaging, and dual-contrast magnetic resonance imaging in predicting the appropriateness of a transplant recipient based on milan criteria: correlation with histopathological findings. Invest Radiol. 2009 Jun;44(6):311-21. PMID: 19462486.

134. Lee J, Won JL, Hyo KL, et al. Early hepatocellular carcinoma: Three-phase helical CT features of 16 patients. Korean J Radiol. 2008;9(4):325-32. PMID: 18682670.

135. Lee JE, Jang JY, Jeong SW, et al. Diagnostic value for extrahepatic metastases of hepatocellular carcinoma in positron emission tomography/computed tomography scan. World J Gastroenterol. 2012 Jun 21;18(23):2979-87. PMID: 22736922.

136. Lee J-M, Kim I-H, Kwak H-S, et al. Detection of small hypervascular hepatocellular carcinomas in cirrhotic patients: comparison of superparamagnetic iron oxide-enhanced MR imaging with dual-phase spiral CT. Korean J Radiol. 2003 Jan-Mar;4(1):1-8. PMID: 12679628.

137. Lee JY, Kim SH, Jeon YH, et al. Ferucarbotran-enhanced magnetic resonance imaging versus gadoxetic acid-enhanced magnetic resonance imaging for the preoperative detection of hepatocellular carcinoma: initial experience. J Comput Assist Tomogr. 2010 Jan;34(1):127-34. PMID: 20118735.

138. Lee MH, Kim SH, Park MJ, et al. Gadoxetic acid-enhanced hepatobiliary phase MRI and high-b-value diffusion-weighted imaging to distinguish well-differentiated hepatocellular carcinomas from benign nodules in patients with chronic liver disease. AJR Am J Roentgenol. 2011 Nov;197(5):W868-75. PMID: 22021534.

139. Lee MW, Kim YJ, Park HS, et al. Targeted sonography for small hepatocellular carcinoma discovered by CT or MRI: factors affecting sonographic detection. AJR Am J Roentgenol. 2010 May;194(5):W396-400. PMID: 20410384.

140. Li R, Guo Y, Hua X, et al. Characterization of focal liver lesions: comparison of pulse-inversion harmonic contrast-enhanced sonography with contrast-enhanced CT. J Clin Ultrasound. 2007 Mar-Apr;35(3):109-17. PMID: 17295272.

141. Li S, Beheshti M, Peck-Radosavljevic M, et al. Comparison of (11)C-acetate positron emission tomography and (67)Gallium citrate scintigraphy in patients with hepatocellular carcinoma. Liver Int. 2006 Oct;26(8):920-7. PMID: 16953831.

142. Li CS, Chen RC, Tu HY, et al. Imaging well-differentiated hepatocellular carcinoma with dynamic triple-phase helical computed tomography. Br J Radiol. 2006 Aug;79(944):659-65. PMID: 16641423.

143. Liangpunsakul S, Agarwal D, Horlander JC, et al. Positron emission tomography for detecting occult hepatocellular carcinoma in hepatitis C cirrhotics awaiting for liver transplantation. Transplant Proc. 2003 Dec;35(8):2995-7. PMID: 14697959.

144. Libbrecht L, Bielen D, Verslype C, et al. Focal lesions in cirrhotic explant livers: pathological evaluation and accuracy of pretransplantation imaging examinations. Liver Transpl. 2002 Sep;8(9):749-61. PMID: 12200773.

145. Lim JH, Kim SH, Lee WJ, et al. Ultrasonographic detection of hepatocellular carcinoma: Correlation of preoperative ultrasonography and resected liver pathology. Clin Radiol. 2006;61(2):191-7. PMID: 16439225.

146. Lim JH, Choi D, Kim SH, et al. Detection of hepatocellular carcinoma: value of adding delayed phase imaging to dual-phase helical CT. AJR Am J Roentgenol. 2002 Jul;179(1):67-73. PMID: 12076907.

147. Lim JH, Kim CK, Lee WJ, et al. Detection of hepatocellular carcinomas and dysplastic nodules in cirrhotic livers: accuracy of helical CT in transplant patients. AJR Am J Roentgenol. 2000 Sep;175(3):693-8. PMID: 10954452.

148. Lin M-T, Chen C-L, Wang C-C, et al. Diagnostic sensitivity of hepatocellular carcinoma imaging and its application to non-cirrhotic patients. J Gastroenterol Hepatol. 2011 Apr;26(4):745-50. PMID: 21418303.

149. Lin W-Y, Tsai S-C, Hung G-U. Value of delayed 18F-FDG-PET imaging in the detection of hepatocellular carcinoma. Nucl Med Commun. 2005 Apr;26(4):315-21. PMID: 15753790.

150. Liu YI, Shin LK, Jeffrey RB, et al. Quantitatively defining washout in hepatocellular carcinoma. AJR Am J Roentgenol. 2013 Jan;200(1):84-9. PMID: 23255745.

151. Liu YI, Kamaya A, Jeffrey RB, et al. Multidetector computed tomography triphasic evaluation of the liver before transplantation: importance of equilibrium phase washout and morphology for characterizing hypervascular lesions. J Comput Assist Tomogr. 2012 Mar-Apr;36(2):213-9. PMID: 22446362.

152. Liu WC, Lim JH, Park CK, et al. Poor sensitivity of sonography in detection of hepatocellular carcinoma in advanced liver cirrhosis: accuracy of pretransplantation sonography in 118 patients. Eur Radiol. 2003 Jul;13(7):1693-8. PMID: 12835987.

153. Lu CH, Chen CL, Cheng YF, et al. Correlation between imaging and pathologic findings in explanted livers of hepatocellular carcinoma cases. Transplant Proc. 2010 Apr;42(3):830-3. PMID: 20430183.

154. Luca A, Caruso S, Milazzo M, et al. Multidetector-row computed tomography (MDCT) for the diagnosis of hepatocellular carcinoma in cirrhotic candidates for liver transplantation: prevalence of radiological vascular patterns and histological correlation with liver explants.[Erratum appears in Eur Radiol. 2011 Jul;21(7):1574 Note: Grutttadauria, Salvatore [corrected to Gruttadauria, Salvatore]]. Eur Radiol. 2010 Apr;20(4):898-907. PMID: 19802612.

155. Luo BM, Wen YL, Yang HY, et al. Differentiation between malignant and benign nodules in the liver: use of contrast C3-MODE technology. World J Gastroenterol. 2005 Apr 28;11(16):2402-7. PMID: 15832408.

156. Luo W, Numata K, Kondo M, et al. Sonazoid-enhanced ultrasonography for evaluation of the enhancement patterns of focal liver tumors in the late phase by intermittent imaging with a high mechanical

index. J Ultrasound Med. 2009 Apr;28(4):439-48. PMID: 19321671.

157. Luo W, Numata K, Morimoto M, et al. Focal liver tumors: characterization with 3D perflubutane microbubble contrast agent-enhanced US versus 3D contrast-enhanced multidetector CT. Radiology. 2009 Apr;251(1):287-95. PMID: 19221060.

158. Luo W, Numata K, Morimoto M, et al. Three-dimensional contrast-enhanced sonography of vascular patterns of focal liver tumors: pilot study of visualization methods. AJR Am J Roentgenol. 2009 Jan;192(1):165-73. PMID: 19098197.

159. Lv P, Lin XZ, Chen K, et al. Spectral CT in patients with small HCC: investigation of image quality and diagnostic accuracy. Eur Radiol. 2012 Oct;22(10):2117-24. PMID: 22618521.

160. Lv P, Lin XZ, Li J, et al. Differentiation of small hepatic hemangioma from small hepatocellular carcinoma: recently introduced spectral CT method. Radiology. 2011 Jun;259(3):720-9. PMID: 21357524.

161. Maetani YS, Ueda M, Haga H, et al. Hepatocellular carcinoma in patients undergoing living-donor liver transplantation. Accuracy of multidetector computed tomography by viewing images on digital monitors. Intervirology. 2008;51 Suppl 1:46-51. PMID: 18544948.

162. Marin D, Catalano C, De Filippis G, et al. Detection of hepatocellular carcinoma in patients with cirrhosis: added value of coronal reformations from isotropic voxels with 64-MDCT. AJR Am J Roentgenol. 2009 Jan;192(1):180-7. PMID: 19098199.

163. Marin D, Di Martino M, Guerrisi A, et al. Hepatocellular carcinoma in patients with cirrhosis: qualitative comparison of gadobenate dimeglumine-enhanced MR imaging and multiphasic 64-section CT. Radiology. 2009 Apr;251(1):85-95. PMID: 19332848.

164. Marrero JA, Hussain HK, Nghiem HV, et al. Improving the prediction of hepatocellular carcinoma in cirrhotic patients with an arterially-enhancing liver mass. Liver Transpl. 2005 Mar;11(3):281-9. PMID: 15719410.

165. Matsuo M, Kanematsu M, Itoh K, et al. Detection of malignant hepatic tumors: comparison of gadolinium-and ferumoxide-enhanced MR imaging. AJR Am J Roentgenol. 2001 Sep;177(3):637-43. PMID: 11517061.

166. Mita K, Kim SR, Kudo M, et al. Diagnostic sensitivity of imaging modalities for hepatocellular carcinoma smaller than 2 cm. World J Gastroenterol. 2010 Sep 7;16(33):4187-92. PMID: 20806437.

167. Mok TSK, Yu SCH, Lee C, et al. False-negative rate of abdominal sonography for detecting hepatocellular carcinoma in patients with hepatitis B and elevated serum alpha-fetoprotein levels. AJR Am J Roentgenol. 2004 Aug;183(2):453-8. PMID: 15269040.

168. Monzawa S, Ichikawa T, Nakajima H, et al. Dynamic CT for detecting small hepatocellular carcinoma: usefulness of delayed phase imaging. AJR Am J Roentgenol. 2007 Jan;188(1):147-53. PMID: 17179357.

169. Mori K, Yoshioka H, Takahashi N, et al. Triple arterial phase dynamic MRI with sensitivity encoding for hypervascular hepatocellular carcinoma: comparison of the diagnostic accuracy among the early, middle, late, and whole triple arterial phase imaging. AJR Am J Roentgenol. 2005 Jan;184(1):63-9. PMID: 15615952.

170. Moriyasu F, Itoh K. Efficacy of perflubutane microbubble-enhanced ultrasound in the characterization and detection of focal liver lesions: phase 3 multicenter clinical trial. AJR Am J Roentgenol. 2009 Jul;193(1):86-95. PMID: 19542399.

171. Mortele KJ, De Keukeleire K, Praet M, et al. Malignant focal hepatic lesions complicating underlying liver disease: dual-phase contrast-enhanced spiral CT sensitivity and specificity in orthotopic liver transplant patients. Eur Radiol. 2001;11(9):1631-8. PMID: 11511882.

172. Motosugi U, Ichikawa T, Sou H, et al. Distinguishing hypervascular pseudolesions of the liver from hypervascular hepatocellular carcinomas with gadoxetic acid-enhanced MR imaging. Radiology. 2010 Jul;256(1):151-8. PMID: 20574092.

173. Murakami T, Kim T, Kawata S, et al. Evaluation of optimal timing of arterial phase imaging for the detection of hypervascular hepatocellular carcinoma by using triple arterial phase imaging with multidetector-row helical computed tomography. Invest Radiol. 2003 Aug;38(8):497-503. PMID: 12874516.

174. Murakami T, Kim T, Takamura M, et al. Hypervascular hepatocellular carcinoma: detection with double arterial phase multi-detector row helical CT. Radiology. 2001 Mar;218(3):763-7. PMID: 11230652.

175. Nagaoka S, Itano S, Ishibashi M, et al. Value of fusing PET plus CT images in hepatocellular carcinoma and combined hepatocellular and cholangiocarcinoma patients with extrahepatic metastases: preliminary findings. Liver Int. 2006 Sep;26(7):781-8. PMID: 16911459.

176. Nakamura Y, Tashiro H, Nambu J, et al. Detectability of hepatocellular carcinoma by gadoxetate disodium-enhanced hepatic MRI: Tumor-by-tumor analysis in explant livers. J Magn Reson Imaging. 2013;37(3):684-91. PMID: 23055436.

177. Nakamura H, Ito N, Kotake F, et al. Tumor-detecting capacity and clinical usefulness of SPIO-MRI in patients with hepatocellular carcinoma. J Gastroenterol. 2000;35(11):849-55. PMID: 11085494.

178. Nakayama A, Imamura H, Matsuyama Y, et al. Value of lipiodol computed tomography and digital subtraction angiography in the era of helical biphasic computed tomography as preoperative assessment of hepatocellular carcinoma. Ann Surg. 2001 Jul;234(1):56-62. PMID: 11420483.

179. Noguchi Y, Murakami T, Kim T, et al. Detection of hepatocellular carcinoma: comparison of dynamic MR imaging with dynamic double arterial phase helical CT. AJR Am J Roentgenol. 2003 Feb;180(2):455-60. PMID: 12540451.

180. Noguchi Y, Murakami T, Kim T, et al. Detection of hypervascular hepatocellular carcinoma by dynamic magnetic resonance imaging with double-echo chemical shift in-phase and opposed-phase gradient echo technique: comparison with dynamic helical computed tomography imaging with double arterial phase. J Comput Assist Tomogr. 2002 Nov-Dec;26(6):981-7. PMID: 12488747.

181. Numata K, Fukuda H, Miwa H, et al. Contrast-enhanced ultrasonography findings using a perflubutane-based contrast agent in patients with early hepatocellular carcinoma. Eur J Radiol. 2014PMID: 24176532.

182. Onishi H, Kim T, Imai Y, et al. Hypervascular hepatocellular carcinomas: detection with gadoxetate disodium-enhanced MR imaging and multiphasic multidetector CT. Eur Radiol. 2012 Apr;22(4):845-54. PMID: 22057248.

183. Ooi C-C, Low S-C, Schneider-Kolsky M, et al. Diagnostic accuracy of contrast-enhanced ultrasound in differentiating benign and malignant focal liver lesions: a retrospective study. J Med Imaging Radiat Oncol. 2010 Oct;54(5):421-30. PMID: 20958940.

184. Ooka Y, Kanai F, Okabe S, et al. Gadoxetic acid-enhanced MRI compared with CT during angiography in the diagnosis of hepatocellular carcinoma. Magn Reson Imaging. 2013;31(5):748-54 Epub 2012 Dec 5. PMID: 23218794.

185. Park MJ, Kim YK, Lee MH, et al. Validation of diagnostic criteria using gadoxetic acid-enhanced and diffusion-weighted MR imaging for small hepatocellular carcinoma (≤ 2.0 cm) in patients with hepatitis-induced liver cirrhosis. Acta Radiol. 2013;54(2):127-36. PMID: 23148300.

186. Park M-S, Kim S, Patel J, et al. Hepatocellular carcinoma: detection with diffusion-weighted versus contrast-enhanced magnetic resonance imaging in pretransplant patients. Hepatology. 2012 Jul;56(1):140-8. PMID: 22370974.

187. Park JH, Kim SH, Park HS, et al. Added value of 80 kVp images to averaged 120 kVp images in the detection of hepatocellular carcinomas in liver transplantation candidates using dual-source dual-energy MDCT: results of JAFROC analysis. Eur J Radiol. 2011 Nov;80(2):e76-85. PMID: 20875937.

188. Park Y, Kim SH, Kim SH, et al. Gadoxetic acid (Gd-EOB-DTPA)-enhanced MRI versus gadobenate dimeglumine (Gd-BOPTA)-enhanced MRI for preoperatively detecting hepatocellular carcinoma: an

initial experience. Korean J Radiol. 2010 Jul-Aug;11(4):433-40. PMID: 20592927.

189. Park G, Kim YK, Kim CS, et al. Diagnostic efficacy of gadoxetic acid-enhanced MRI in the detection of hepatocellular carcinomas: comparison with gadopentetate dimeglumine. Br J Radiol. 2010 Dec;83(996):1010-6. PMID: 20682591.

190. Park J-W, Kim JH, Kim SK, et al. A prospective evaluation of 18F-FDG and 11C-acetate PET/CT for detection of primary and metastatic hepatocellular carcinoma. J Nucl Med. 2008 Dec;49(12):1912-21. PMID: 18997056.

191. Paul SB, Gulati MS, Sreenivas V, et al. Evaluating patients with cirrhosis for hepatocellular carcinoma: value of clinical symptomatology, imaging and alpha-fetoprotein. Oncology. 2007;72 Suppl 1:117-23. PMID: 18087192.

192. Pauleit D, Textor J, Bachmann R, et al. Hepatocellular carcinoma: detection with gadolinium- and ferumoxides-enhanced MR imaging of the liver. Radiology. 2002 Jan;222(1):73-80. PMID: 11756708.

193. Pei XQ, Liu LZ, Xiong YH, et al. Quantitative analysis of contrast-enhanced ultrasonography: Differentiating focal nodular hyperplasia from hepatocellular carcinoma. Br J Radiol. 2013 Mar;86(1023):20120536 Epub 2013 Feb 7. PMID: 23392189.

194. Peterson MS, Baron RL, Marsh JW, Jr., et al. Pretransplantation surveillance for possible hepatocellular carcinoma in patients with cirrhosis: epidemiology and CT-based tumor detection rate in 430 cases with surgical pathologic correlation. Radiology. 2000 Dec;217(3):743-9. PMID: 11110938.

195. Petruzzi N, Mitchell D, Guglielmo F, et al. Hepatocellular carcinoma likelihood on MRI exams. Evaluation of a standardized categorization System. Acad Radiol. 2013 Jun;20(6):694-8 Epub 2013 Mar 28. PMID: 23541479.

196. Piana G, Trinquart L, Meskine N, et al. New MR imaging criteria with a diffusion-weighted sequence for the diagnosis of hepatocellular carcinoma in chronic liver diseases. J Hepatol. 2011 Jul;55(1):126-32. PMID: 21145857.

197. Pitton MB, Kloeckner R, Herber S, et al. MRI versus 64-row MDCT for diagnosis of hepatocellular carcinoma. World J Gastroenterol. 2009 Dec 28;15(48):6044-51. PMID: 20027676.

198. Pozzi Mucelli RM, Como G, Del Frate C, et al. Multidetector CT with double arterial phase and high-iodine-concentration contrast agent in the detection of hepatocellular carcinoma. Radiol Med (Torino). 2006 Mar;111(2):181-91. PMID: 16671376.

199. Pugacheva O, Matsui O, Kozaka K, et al. Detection of small hypervascular hepatocellular carcinomas by EASL criteria: comparison with double-phase CT during hepatic arteriography. Eur J Radiol. 2011 Dec;80(3):e201-6. PMID: 20855175.

200. Quaia E, Alaimo V, Baratella E, et al. The added diagnostic value of 64-row multidetector CT combined with contrast-enhanced US in the evaluation of hepatocellular nodule vascularity: implications in the diagnosis of malignancy in patients with liver cirrhosis. Eur Radiol. 2009 Mar;19(3):651-63. PMID: 18815790.

201. Quaia E, Bertolotto M, Calderan L, et al. US characterization of focal hepatic lesions with intermittent high-acoustic-power mode and contrast material. Acad Radiol. 2003 Jul;10(7):739-50. PMID: 12862283.

202. Rhee H, Kim MJ, Park MS, et al. Differentiation of early hepatocellular carcinoma from benign hepatocellular nodules on gadoxetic acid-enhanced MRI. Br J Radiol. 2012 Oct;85(1018):e837-44. PMID: 22553295.

203. Rickes S, Schulze S, Neye H, et al. Improved diagnosing of small hepatocellular carcinomas by echo-enhanced power Doppler sonography in patients with cirrhosis. Eur J Gastroenterol Hepatol. 2003 Aug;15(8):893-900. PMID: 12867800.

204. Rimola J, Forner A, Tremosini S, et al. Non-invasive diagnosis of hepatocellular carcinoma ≤ 2 cm in cirrhosis. Diagnostic accuracy assessing fat, capsule and signal intensity at dynamic MRI. J Hepatol. 2012 Jun;56(6):1317-23. PMID: 22314420.

205. Rizvi S, Camci C, Yong Y, et al. Is post-Lipiodol CT better than i.v. contrast CT scan for early detection of HCC? A single liver

206. Rode A, Bancel B, Douek P, et al. Small nodule detection in cirrhotic livers: evaluation with US, spiral CT, and MRI and correlation with pathologic examination of explanted liver. J Comput Assist Tomogr. 2001 May-Jun;25(3):327-36. PMID: 11351179.

207. Ronzoni A, Artioli D, Scardina R, et al. Role of MDCT in the diagnosis of hepatocellular carcinoma in patients with cirrhosis undergoing orthotopic liver transplantation. AJR Am J Roentgenol. 2007 Oct;189(4):792-8. PMID: 17885047.

208. Sangiovanni A, Manini MA, Iavarone M, et al. The diagnostic and economic impact of contrast imaging techniques in the diagnosis of small hepatocellular carcinoma in cirrhosis. Gut. 2010 May;59(5):638-44. PMID: 19951909.

209. Sano K, Ichikawa T, Motosugi U, et al. Imaging study of early hepatocellular carcinoma: usefulness of gadoxetic acid-enhanced MR imaging. Radiology. 2011 Dec;261(3):834-44. PMID: 21998047.

210. Schima W, Hammerstingl R, Catalano C, et al. Quadruple-phase MDCT of the liver in patients with suspected hepatocellular carcinoma: Effect of contrast material flow rate. AJR Am J Roentgenol. 2006;186(6):1571-9. PMID: 16714645.

211. Secil M, Obuz F, Altay C, et al. The role of dynamic subtraction MRI in detection of hepatocellular carcinoma. Diagn Interv Radiol. 2008 Dec;14(4):200-4. PMID: 19061165.

212. Seitz K, Strobel D, Bernatik T, et al. Contrast-Enhanced Ultrasound (CEUS) for the characterization of focal liver lesions - prospective comparison in clinical practice: CEUS vs. CT (DEGUM multicenter trial). Parts of this manuscript were presented at the Ultrasound Dreilandertreffen 2008, Davos. Ultraschall Med. 2009 Aug;30(4):383-9. PMID: 19688670.

213. Seitz K, Bernatik T, Strobel D, et al. Contrast-enhanced ultrasound (CEUS) for the characterization of focal liver lesions in clinical practice (DEGUM Multicenter Trial): CEUS vs. MRI--a prospective comparison in 269 patients. Ultraschall Med. 2010 Oct;31(5):492-9. PMID: 20652854.

214. Serste T, Barrau V, Ozenne V, et al. Accuracy and disagreement of computed tomography and magnetic resonance imaging for the diagnosis of small hepatocellular carcinoma and dysplastic nodules: role of biopsy. Hepatology. 2012 Mar;55(3):800-6. PMID: 22006503.

215. Shah SA, Tan JC, McGilvray ID, et al. Accuracy of staging as a predictor for recurrence after liver transplantation for hepatocellular carcinoma. Transplantation. 2006 Jun 27;81(12):1633-9. PMID: 16794527.

216. Simon G, Link TM, Wortler K, et al. Detection of hepatocellular carcinoma: comparison of Gd-DTPA- and ferumoxides-enhanced MR imaging. Eur Radiol. 2005 May;15(5):895-903. PMID: 15800773.

217. Singh P, Erickson RA, Mukhopadhyay P, et al. EUS for detection of the hepatocellular carcinoma: results of a prospective study. Gastrointest Endosc. 2007 Aug;66(2):265-73. PMID: 17543307.

218. Sofue K, Tsurusaki M, Kawasaki R, et al. Evaluation of hypervascular hepatocellular carcinoma in cirrhotic liver: comparison of different concentrations of contrast material with multi-detector row helical CT--a prospective randomized study. Eur J Radiol. 2011 Dec;80(3):e237-42. PMID: 21067880.

219. Sørensen M, Frisch K, Bender D, et al. The potential use of 2-[18F]fluoro-2-deoxy-D-galactose as a PET/CT tracer for detection of hepatocellular carcinoma. Eur J Nucl Med Mol Imaging. 2011;38(9):1723-31. PMID: 21553087.

220. Strobel D, Raeker S, Martus P, et al. Phase inversion harmonic imaging versus contrast-enhanced power Doppler sonography for the characterization of focal liver lesions. Int J Colorectal Dis. 2003 Jan;18(1):63-72. PMID: 12458384.

221. Sugimoto K, Moriyasu F, Saito K, et al. Comparison of Kupffer-phase Sonazoid-enhanced sonography and hepatobiliary-phase gadoxetic acid-enhanced magnetic resonance imaging of hepatocellular carcinoma and correlation with histologic

grading. J Ultrasound Med. 2012 Apr;31(4):529-38. PMID: 22441909.

222. Sugimoto K, Moriyasu F, Shiraishi J, et al. Assessment of arterial hypervascularity of hepatocellular carcinoma: comparison of contrast-enhanced US and gadoxetate disodium-enhanced MR imaging. Eur Radiol. 2012 Jun;22(6):1205-13. PMID: 22270142.

223. Sugiyama M, Sakahara H, Torizuka T, et al. 18F-FDG PET in the detection of extrahepatic metastases from hepatocellular carcinoma. J Gastroenterol. 2004;39(10):961-8. PMID: 15549449.

224. Suh YJ, Kim M-J, Choi J-Y, et al. Differentiation of hepatic hyperintense lesions seen on gadoxetic acid-enhanced hepatobiliary phase MRI. AJR Am J Roentgenol. 2011 Jul;197(1):W44-52. PMID: 21700994.

225. Sun HY, Lee JM, Shin CI, et al. Gadoxetic acid-enhanced magnetic resonance imaging for differentiating small hepatocellular carcinomas (≤ 2 cm in diameter) from arterial enhancing pseudolesions: special emphasis on hepatobiliary phase imaging. Invest Radiol. 2010 Feb;45(2):96-103. PMID: 20057319.

226. Sun L, Guan YS, Pan WM, et al. Metabolic restaging of hepatocellular carcinoma using whole-body F-FDG PET/CT. World J Hepatol. 2009 Oct 31;1(1):90-7. PMID: 21160970.

227. Suzuki S, Iijima H, Moriyasu F, et al. Differential diagnosis of hepatic nodules using delayed parenchymal phase imaging of levovist contrast ultrasound: comparative study with SPIO-MRI. Hepatol Res. 2004 Jun;29(2):122-6. PMID: 15163434.

228. Takahashi M, Maruyama H, Shimada T, et al. Characterization of hepatic lesions (≤ 30 mm) with liver-specific contrast agents: a comparison between ultrasound and magnetic resonance imaging. Eur J Radiol. 2013;82(1):75-84. PMID: 23116806.

229. Talbot J, Fartoux L, Balogova S, et al. Detection of hepatocellular carcinoma with PET/CT: a prospective comparison of 18F-fluorocholine and 18F-FDG in patients with cirrhosis or chronic liver disease. J Nucl Med. 2010 Nov;51(11):1699-706. PMID: 20956466.

230. Talbot J, Gutman F, Fartoux L, et al. PET/CT in patients with hepatocellular carcinoma using [(18)F]fluorocholine: preliminary comparison with [(18)F]FDG PET/CT. Eur J Nucl Med Mol Imaging. 2006 Nov;33(11):1285-9. PMID: 16802155.

231. Tanaka O, Ito H, Yamada K, et al. Higher lesion conspicuity for SENSE dynamic MRI in detecting hypervascular hepatocellular carcinoma: analysis through the measurements of liver SNR and lesion-liver CNR comparison with conventional dynamic MRI. Eur Radiol. 2005 Dec;15(12):2427-34. PMID: 16041592.

232. Tanaka S, Ioka T, Oshikawa O, et al. Dynamic sonography of hepatic tumors. AJR Am J Roentgenol. 2001 Oct;177(4):799-805. PMID: 11566675.

233. Tang Y, Yamashita Y, Arakawa A, et al. Detection of hepatocellular carcinoma arising in cirrhotic livers: comparison of gadolinium- and ferumoxides-enhanced MR imaging. AJR Am J Roentgenol. 1999 Jun;172(6):1547-54. PMID: 10350287.

234. Tanimoto A, Yuasa Y, Jinzaki M, et al. Routine MR imaging protocol with breath-hold fast scans: diagnostic efficacy for focal liver lesions. Radiat Med. 2002 Jul-Aug;20(4):169-79. PMID: 12296432.

235. Teefey SA, Hildeboldt CC, Dehdashti F, et al. Detection of primary hepatic malignancy in liver transplant candidates: prospective comparison of CT, MR imaging, US, and PET. Radiology. 2003 Feb;226(2):533-42. PMID: 12563151.

236. Toyota N, Nakamura Y, Hieda M, et al. Diagnostic capability of gadoxetate disodium-enhanced liver MRI for diagnosis of hepatocellular carcinoma: Comparison with multi-detector CT. Hiroshima J Med Sci. 2013;62(3):55-61. PMID: 24279123.

237. Trojan J, Schroeder O, Raedle J, et al. Fluorine-18 FDG positron emission tomography for imaging of hepatocellular carcinoma. Am J Gastroenterol. 1999 Nov;94(11):3314-9. PMID: 10566736.

238. Tsurusaki M, Semelka RC, Uotani K, et al. Prospective comparison of high- and low-spatial-resolution dynamic MR imaging with sensitivity encoding (SENSE) for hypervascular hepatocellular carcinoma. Eur

Radiol. 2008 Oct;18(10):2206-12. PMID: 18446347.

239. Valls C, Cos M, Figueras J, et al. Pretransplantation diagnosis and staging of hepatocellular carcinoma in patients with cirrhosis: value of dual-phase helical CT. AJR Am J Roentgenol. 2004 Apr;182(4):1011-7. PMID: 15039179.

240. Van Thiel DH, Yong S, Li SD, et al. The development of de novo hepatocellular carcinoma in patients on a liver transplant list: frequency, size, and assessment of current screening methods. Liver Transpl. 2004 May;10(5):631-7. PMID: 15108254.

241. Vandecaveye V, De Keyzer F, Verslype C, et al. Diffusion-weighted MRI provides additional value to conventional dynamic contrast-enhanced MRI for detection of hepatocellular carcinoma. Eur Radiol. 2009 Oct;19(10):2456-66. PMID: 19440718.

242. Verhoef C, Valkema R, de Man RA, et al. Fluorine-18 FDG imaging in hepatocellular carcinoma using positron coincidence detection and single photon emission computed tomography. Liver. 2002 Feb;22(1):51-6. PMID: 11906619.

243. Wagnetz U, Atri M, Massey C, et al. Intraoperative ultrasound of the liver in primary and secondary hepatic malignancies: comparison with preoperative 1.5-T MRI and 64-MDCT. AJR Am J Roentgenol. 2011 Mar;196(3):562-8. PMID: 21343497.

244. Wang ZL, Tang J, Weskott HP, et al. Undetermined focal liver lesions on gray-scale ultrasound in patients with fatty liver: characterization with contrast-enhanced ultrasound. J Gastroenterol Hepatol. 2008 Oct;23(10):1511-9. PMID: 18713302.

245. Wang J-H, Lu S-N, Hung C-H, et al. Small hepatic nodules (≤ 2 cm) in cirrhosis patients: characterization with contrast-enhanced ultrasonography. Liver Int. 2006 Oct;26(8):928-34. PMID: 16953832.

246. Wolfort RM, Papillion PW, Turnage RH, et al. Role of FDG-PET in the evaluation and staging of hepatocellular carcinoma with comparison of tumor size, AFP level, and histologic grade. Int Surg. 2010 Jan-Mar;95(1):67-75. PMID: 20480845.

247. Wu H-b, Wang Q-s, Li B-y, et al. F-18 FDG in conjunction with 11C-choline PET/CT in the diagnosis of hepatocellular carcinoma. Clin Nucl Med. 2011 Dec;36(12):1092-7. PMID: 22064078.

248. Wudel LJ, Jr., Delbeke D, Morris D, et al. The role of [18F]fluorodeoxyglucose positron emission tomography imaging in the evaluation of hepatocellular carcinoma. Am Surg. 2003 Feb;69(2):117-24; discussion 24-6. PMID: 12641351.

249. Xiao X-g, Han X, Shan W-d, et al. Multi-slice CT angiography by triple-phase enhancement in preoperative evaluation of hepatocellular carcinoma. Chin Med J (Engl). 2005 May 20;118(10):844-9. PMID: 15989766.

250. Xu HX, Lu MD, Liu LN, et al. Discrimination between neoplastic and non-neoplastic lesions in cirrhotic liver using contrast-enhanced ultrasound. Br J Radiol. 2012 Oct;85(1018):1376-84. PMID: 22553290.

251. Xu P-J, Yan F-H, Wang J-H, et al. Contribution of diffusion-weighted magnetic resonance imaging in the characterization of hepatocellular carcinomas and dysplastic nodules in cirrhotic liver. J Comput Assist Tomogr. 2010 Jul;34(4):506-12. PMID: 20657216.

252. Xu P-J, Yan F-H, Wang J-H, et al. Added value of breathhold diffusion-weighted MRI in detection of small hepatocellular carcinoma lesions compared with dynamic contrast-enhanced MRI alone using receiver operating characteristic curve analysis. J Magn Reson Imaging. 2009 Feb;29(2):341-9. PMID: 19161186.

253. Xu H-X, Xie X-Y, Lu M-D, et al. Contrast-enhanced sonography in the diagnosis of small hepatocellular carcinoma ≤ 2 cm. J Clin Ultrasound. 2008 Jun;36(5):257-66. PMID: 18088056.

254. Yamamoto Y, Nishiyama Y, Kameyama R, et al. Detection of hepatocellular carcinoma using 11C-choline PET: Comparison with 18F-FDG PET. J Nucl Med. 2008 Aug;49(8):1245-8. PMID: 18632827.

255. Yamamoto K, Shiraki K, Deguchi M, et al. Diagnosis of hepatocellular carcinoma using digital subtraction imaging with the contrast agent, Levovist: comparison with helical

CT, digital subtraction angiography, and US angiography. Oncol Rep. 2002 Jul-Aug;9(4):789-92. PMID: 12066210.

256. Yan FH, Shen JZ, Li RC, et al. Enhancement patterns of small hepatocellular carcinoma shown by dynamic MRI and CT. Hepatobiliary Pancreat Dis Int. 2002 Aug;1(3):420-4. PMID: 14607719.

257. Yoo SH, Choi JY, Jang JW, et al. Gd-EOB-DTPA-enhanced MRI is better than MDCT in decision making of curative treatment for hepatocellular carcinoma. Ann Surg Oncol. 2013;20(9):2893-900. PMID: 23649931.

258. Yoo HJ, Lee JM, Lee JY, et al. Additional value of SPIO-enhanced MR imaging for the noninvasive imaging diagnosis of hepatocellular carcinoma in cirrhotic liver. Invest Radiol. 2009 Dec;44(12):800-7. PMID: 19838119.

259. Yoon KT, Kim JK, Kim DY, et al. Role of 18F-fluorodeoxyglucose positron emission tomography in detecting extrahepatic metastasis in pretreatment staging of hepatocellular carcinoma. Oncology. 2007;72 Suppl 1:104-10. PMID: 18087190.

260. Yoshioka H, Takahashi N, Yamaguchi M, et al. Double arterial phase dynamic MRI with sensitivity encoding (SENSE) for hypervascular hepatocellular carcinomas. J Magn Reson Imaging. 2002 Sep;16(3):259-66. PMID: 12205581.

261. Youk JH, Lee JM, Kim CS. MRI for detection of hepatocellular carcinoma: comparison of mangafodipir trisodium and gadopentetate dimeglumine contrast agents. AJR Am J Roentgenol. 2004 Oct;183(4):1049-54. PMID: 15385303.

262. Yu Y, Lin X, Chen K, et al. Hepatocellular carcinoma and focal nodular hyperplasia of the liver: differentiation with CT spectral imaging. Eur Radiol. 2013 Jun;23(6):1660-8 Epub 2013 Jan 10. PMID: 23306709.

263. Yu Y, He N, Sun K, et al. Differentiating hepatocellular carcinoma from angiomyolipoma of the liver with CT spectral imaging: A preliminary study. Clin Radiol. 2013;68(9):e491-e7. PMID: 23702491.

264. Yu MH, Kim JH, Yoon JH, et al. Role of C-arm CT for transcatheter arterial chemoembolization of hepatocellular carcinoma: Diagnostic performance and predictive value for therapeutic response compared with gadoxetic acid-enhanced MRI. AJR Am J Roentgenol. 2013;201(3):675-83. PMID: 23971463.

265. Yu NC, Chaudhari V, Raman SS, et al. CT and MRI improve detection of hepatocellular carcinoma, compared with ultrasound alone, in patients with cirrhosis. Clin Gastroenterol Hepatol. 2011 Feb;9(2):161-7. PMID: 20920597.

266. Yu JS, Chung JJ, Kim JH, et al. Small hypervascular hepatocellular carcinomas: value of "washout" on gadolinium-enhanced dynamic MR imaging compared to superparamagnetic iron oxide-enhanced imaging. Eur Radiol. 2009 Nov;19(11):2614-22. PMID: 19513719.

267. Yu JS, Lee JH, Chung JJ, et al. Small hypervascular hepatocellular carcinoma: limited value of portal and delayed phases on dynamic magnetic resonance imaging. Acta Radiol. 2008 Sep;49(7):735-43. PMID: 18608015.

268. Yu JS, Kim KW, Park MS, et al. Transient peritumoral enhancement during dynamic MRI of the liver: Cavernous hemangioma versus hepatocellular carcinoma. J Comput Assist Tomogr. 2002 May-Jun;26(3):411-7. PMID: 12016371.

269. Yukisawa S, Okugawa H, Masuya Y, et al. Multidetector helical CT plus superparamagnetic iron oxide-enhanced MR imaging for focal hepatic lesions in cirrhotic liver: a comparison with multi-phase CT during hepatic arteriography. Eur J Radiol. 2007 Feb;61(2):279-89. PMID: 17070663.

270. Zacherl J, Pokieser P, Wrba F, et al. Accuracy of multiphasic helical computed tomography and intraoperative sonography in patients undergoing orthotopic liver transplantation for hepatoma: what is the truth? Ann Surg. 2002 Apr;235(4):528-32. PMID: 11923609.

271. Zhao H, Yao J-L, Wang Y, et al. Detection of small hepatocellular carcinoma: comparison of dynamic enhancement magnetic resonance imaging and multiphase multirow-detector helical CT scanning. World J Gastroenterol. 2007 Feb 28;13(8):1252-6. PMID: 17451209.

272. Zhao H, Yao JL, Han MJ, et al. Multiphase hepatic scans with multirow-detector helical CT in detection of hypervascular hepatocellular carcinoma. Hepatobiliary Pancreat Dis Int. 2004 May;3(2):204-8. PMID: 15138110.

273. Zhao H, Zhou K-R, Yan F-H. Role of multiphase scans by multirow-detector helical CT in detecting small hepatocellular carcinoma. World J Gastroenterol. 2003 Oct;9(10):2198-201. PMID: 14562377.

274. Zheng X-H, Guan Y-S, Zhou X-P, et al. Detection of hypervascular hepatocellular carcinoma: Comparison of multi-detector CT with digital subtraction angiography and Lipiodol CT. World J Gastroenterol. 2005 Jan 14;11(2):200-3. PMID: 15633215.

275. Zhou K-R, Yan F-H, Tu B-W. Arterial phase of biphase enhancement spiral CT in diagnosis of small hepatocellular carcinoma. Hepatobiliary Pancreat Dis Int. 2002 Feb;1(1):68-71. PMID: 14607626.

276. Pocha C, Dieperink E, McMaken KA, et al. Surveillance for hepatocellular cancer with ultrasonography vs. computed tomography - A randomised study. Aliment Pharmacol Ther. 2013;38(3):303-12. PMID: 23750991.

277. Trinchet JC, Chaffaut C, Bourcier V, et al. Ultrasonographic surveillance of hepatocellular carcinoma in cirrhosis: a randomized trial comparing 3- and 6-month periodicities. Hepatology. 2011 Dec;54(6):1987-97. PMID: 22144108.

278. Wang JH, Chang KC, Kee KM, et al. Hepatocellular carcinoma surveillance at 4- vs. 12-month intervals for patients with chronic viral hepatitis: a randomized study in community. Am J Gastroenterol. 2013 Mar;108(3):416-24. PMID: 23318478.

279. Zhang BH, Yang BH, Tang ZY. Randomized controlled trial of screening for hepatocellular carcinoma. J Cancer Res Clin Oncol. 2004 Jul;130(7):417-22. PMID: 15042359.

280. Chen MH, Wu W, Yang W, et al. The use of contrast-enhanced ultrasonography in the selection of patients with hepatocellular carcinoma for radio frequency ablation therapy. J Ultrasound Med. 2007;26(8):1055-63. PMID: 17646367.

281. Chen MH, Yang W, Yan K, et al. The role of contrast-enhanced ultrasound in planning treatment protocols for hepatocellular carcinoma before radiofrequency ablation. Clin Radiol. 2007 Aug;62(8):752-60. PMID: 17604763.

www.ingramcontent.com/pod-product-compliance
Lightning Source LLC
Chambersburg PA
CBHW081718170526
45167CB00009B/3615